Mothering Occupations

Challenge, Agency, and Participation

Mothering Occupations

Challenge, Agency, and Participation

Susan A. Esdaile, PhD, MAPS, AccOT, OTR, SROT

Professor, Department of Occupational Therapy
Eugene Applebaum College of Pharmacy and Health Sciences
Wayne State University
Detroit, Michigan
Honorary Professor
School of Occupation and Leisure Sciences
University of Sydney
Lidcombe, New South Wales, Australia

Judith A. Olson, PhD, OTR

Associate Professor, Occupational Therapy Program
College of Health and Human Services
Eastern Michigan University
Ypsilanti, Michigan

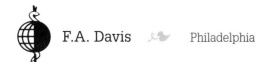 F.A. Davis Philadelphia

F. A. Davis Company
1915 Arch Street
Philadelphia, PA 19103
www.fadavis.com

Printed in the United States of America

Last digit indicates print number: 10 9 8 7 6 5 4 3 2 1

Acquisitions Editor: Margaret Biblis
Developmental Editor: Peg Waltner
Production Editor: Jessica Howie Martin
Cover Designer: MW Design

As new scientific information becomes available through basic and clinical research, recommended treatments and drug therapies undergo changes. The authors and publisher have done everything possible to make this book accurate, up to date, and in accord with accepted standards at the time of publication. The authors, editors, and publisher are not responsible for errors or omissions or for consequences from application of the book, and make no warranty, expressed or implied, in regard to the contents of the book. Any practice described in this book should be applied by the reader in accordance with professional standards of care used in regard to the unique circumstances that may apply in each situation. The reader is advised always to check product information (package inserts) for changes and new information regarding dose and contraindications before administering any drug. Caution is especially urged when using new or infrequently ordered drugs.

Library of Congress Cataloging-in-Publication Data

Esdaile, Susan A.
   Mothering occupations : challenge, agency, and participation / Susan A. Esdaile, Judith A. Olson.
      p. ; cm.
   Includes bibliographical references and index.
   ISBN 0-8036-1105-6 (hard cover : alk. paper)
      1. Occupational therapy. 2. Motherhood. 3. Mothers. 4. Mother and child. 5. Parents with disabilities. 6. Mothers of exceptional children. 7. Children with disabilities—Care. 8. Children with social disabilities—Care 9. Child development. 10. Child rearing. 11. Feminism. 12. Family social work. I. Olson, Judith A. II. Title.
   [DNLM: 1. Child Rearing. 2. Maternal Behavior. 3. Mother-Child Relations. 4. Mothers—psychology. 5. Occupational Therapy—psychology. 6. Professional-Family Relations. WS 105.5.F2 E75d 2004]
   RM735.4E77 2004
   615.8′515—dc22

                                                         2003055530

We dedicate this book to Kathleen, the first,
and all the other mothers with whom we have worked.

Foreword

Elizabeth J. Yerxa, EdD, LHD, ScD, MDHC, OTR, FAOTA
Distinguished Professor Emerita
Department of Occupational Science and Occupational Therapy
University of Southern California

This book contains an international mosaic of knowledge of what it is to be a mother and engage in the occupation of mothering in a rapidly changing, globalized society. It fills an important need for understanding the incomprehensible complexity of actually being a mother under differing demands and levels of challenge, requiring "craft and grit" (Llewellyn & McConnell, p.175). Thus, this work is on the cutting edge, contributing new knowledge and wisdom to the practice of occupational therapy and the occupational science that supports it.

The content, written by a group of world-class scientist-practitioners, is appropriately broad in scope, giving voice to mothers whose experience and insight are sought and valued. The authors reflect an optimistic view of human capability and respect for mothers' ability to meet both everyday challenges of daily living and the more demanding challenges of special needs through agency and participation. Although mothering occupations are carried out in myriad ways under diverse environmental conditions, commonalities are also revealed; for example, mothers' needs for support, the lifelong nature of mothering, the issue of social expectations of maternal control and responsibility, along with self comparisons to an "ideal" of maternal perfection, and the profound impact of becoming a mother on a woman's entire lifestyle and trajectory ("My old life died," Griffin, p. 53).

As is typical of other occupations, mothering is often viewed as commonplace, self-evident, and therefore unworthy of serious study since everyone already knows all about it. This work stands as evidence to the contrary. Changing gender, familial, and occupational roles negate much folk knowledge and require new creativity in developing mothering strategies to orchestrate occupations for successful performance. This is where occupational scientists and therapists might employ their understanding in support of and serving mothers. A revealing aspect of the content of this book is its implications for occupational therapy practice with and for mothers. The authors are of one voice in recognizing the changing role of the professional from that of "expert possessor of knowledge" to that of a partner who sensitively facilitates and empowers mothers or serves as their advocates when the going gets rough. Many of these authors reflected on the responsibility of occupational therapists to engage in "mother-focused work" (Esdaile & Olson, p. 393) that seeks to understand the mothers' perspectives on both the meaning of professional intervention and their need for agency.

The *process* of scholarship and research displayed in this book seems to me to represent occupational science at its fullest. The chapters are well documented and thoughtful without reducing the occupation of mothering either to some internal psychological dimension or externally observed behavior. Rather, they present an integral portrait of real human beings acting in interaction with their environments in order to flourish. The science presented here is congruent with the sort of integral science required to support a complex, dynamic practice of occupational therapy focused on occupation. Wilber (1998), a philosopher, envisioned such a science: "We are looking for a deep science that includes not just the exteriors of ITs but the interiors of I and We. We are looking for a deep science of self and self-expression and aesthetics; of morals and values and meaning; as well as of objects and ITs and processes and systems" (p. 176). The science revealed in this book is not non-rigorous but, as Esdaile observed, "differently rigorous" (p. 101). It is appropriately rigorous for a complex, newly developing, integral occupational science. Whoever reads it will gain a fuller understanding of what it is to be a mother in today's world and how mothers continue to engage in meeting the challenges of mothering occupations through their agency and participation. I did. I congratulate this international group of authors on their rich research and insightful writing about a deeply significant but little understood aspect of occupation.

Reference

Wilber, K. (1998). *The marriage of sense and soul.* New York: Broadway Books.

Preface

Working with mothers and concerns about issues related to the health and welfare of mothers and their children have been major occupations in our professional lives. For me (Susan), it started early in my career, several years before I became a mother. I was working in the cardiopulmonary unit of a major university teaching hospital in Australia when I became aware of the fact that many women with chronic heart disease had huge difficulties managing their childcare and household occupations. I learned a lot about mothering under challenging circumstances from one of these women, Kathleen, who had three children and was repeatedly readmitted to the unit. When she died at age 29, I was devastated and felt compelled to try to do something. That was how I first got involved in doing research.

For me (Judith), my interest in mothering began when I was a novice caseworker in a residential facility for children who were described as severely and profoundly retarded. I saw with sadness the loss of mothering occupations as women were unable to feed, clothe, bathe, and sometimes even cuddle their children as a result of their child's medical fragility, their own fears of incompetence, and sometimes even as a defense against the pain of the loss of their imagined child. I, too, felt compelled to try to do something to restore a sense of occupational competence.

Mothering Occupations: Challenge, Agency, and Participation is our response to Arendell's invitation to study "the experiences and activities of mothering" (2000, p. 1202). This text is the result of many years of work with moth-

ers and their children, some of it clinical and some research; a lot of reading; teaching about the topic to our students; and much reflection. Mothering is one of the most important occupations of women, and yet helping professions, such as occupational therapy, had all but neglected it as a topic for research and scholarship until recently. Other disciplines, such as sociology and psychology, have for the past 25 years examined mothering and its multiple facets (e.g., Chodorow, 1978; Chodorow & Contratto, 1982; Hochschild, 1989; Oakley, 1974; Phoenix et al., 1991; Polakow, 1993; Rich, 1976; Ruddick, 1980, 1995; Thurer, 1994).

Given the huge potential scope of this subject, we are conscious of the fact that what we have included in this text is a very thin slice taken from a particular perspective. However, we believe that this could be said about any important, complex area of human concern, and that an honest exploration of a topic from a limited perspective is a valid contribution to the subject matter. In fact, we have deliberately narrowed our scope to maintain a limited, but clear, focus.

Our book examines mothering through the lens of the helping professions from a feminist, phenomenological perspective. That is not to say that all the contributors are feminists, but that we, as the editors, embraced this perspective. We encouraged our invited authors to speak about themselves and their ideas and to work from a first-person perspective, thereby claiming their own agency with respect to their writing. We are not certain that all of the authors of the chapters of this book would consider themselves feminist in perspective. But we are sure that they would agree with the use of the Australian scholar Dale Spender's identification of the core feminist idea "... that there is no one truth, no one authority, no one objective method which leads to the production of pure knowledge" (1985, pp. 5–6).

The authors in this text do not speak for mothers, but they speak out for mothers, just as Reinharz has written that feminist researchers do (1992, p. 16). Many of the chapters in this book, therefore, reflect what Arendell (2000) has called the "...interpretive, critical, hermeneutic, qualitative and feminist" perspective (p. 1193). We wanted to honor the stories of mothering occupations that these authors share in their writing as important sources of knowledge about mothering. We hope that, hearing the voices of mothers who speak in the chapters of our book, readers will recognize their own voices and those of their mothers, sisters, clients, and friends. We believe that these voices are raising broad human concerns, not just the concerns of women who are mothers. The fact that 10 out of the 22 of us who wrote chapters in this book (45 percent) are not mothers, or in the case of the one male contributor, a father, speaks to the fact that mothering also encompasses a more universal metaphor of concern and caring, one that speaks to all of us.

Mothering is often considered a ubiquitous concept. However, we believe that it is different from the concept of parenting. We are following in the ideological path of Sara Ruddick as she sees the essence of mothering as an individual commitment to meet three universal demands of children for preservation, nurturance, and training to take their place in society (Ruddick, 1995), irrespective of gender, biology, or social role. We also agree with Ruddick that: "Anyone who commits her or himself to children's demands, and makes the work of response a considerable part of her or his life, is a mother" (xxii). Thus we accept Primeau's quote of a statement by Oprah Winfrey in Chapter 6 of this text that: "Biology is the least of what makes someone a mother". In this book you will find various examples and definitions of mothering. You may delib-

erate, as we have, for example, over Llewellyn and McConnell's use of the term "mothering" in Chapter 9 in regard to a random act of kindness by a stranger who engages an upset child at a bus stop. You may or may not agree with this idea, but the intellectual pearl rests in the thinking that this idea stimulated. You will have the opportunity to consider other differing perspectives, for example, in regard to concepts of mothering co-occupations.

Although we freely accept the concept that mothering is done by women and men who are not mothers, in congruence with Ruddick (1995), we "recognize and honor the fact that even now, and certainly through most of history, women have been the mothers. To speak of 'parenting' obscures that historical fact, while to speak evenhandedly of mothers and fathers suggests that women's history has no importance" (p. 44). It also denies the unique historical contribution of fathers, whose primary roles have been to procreate, provide, and protect. They represent the moral, legal world of the child, and thus fathering "is more a role determined by cultural demands than a kind of work determined by children's needs "(p.42). The terms parenting, mothering, and fathering, are often used collectively and interchangeably by professionals who work with mothering women and men and with men and women who are fulfilling a fathering role. In this text, we have tried to avoid these generalizations.

We invited contributors to focus on mothers in occupational engagement because we have been strongly influenced by the recent development of the discipline of occupational science, which has centralized occupation as its major concept (Yerxa et al., 1989). There is growing interest in mothering research among occupational scientists, and we discuss this in Chapter 1.

In this text we aim to make a unique contribution to the identification, explication, and application of knowledge about mothering occupations. Within this focus, we have a range of issues that we hope will speak to mothering more broadly and highlight concerns to which many women and men can relate. The topics we have collected within this umbrella of occupation touch on what mothers do within the context of their mothering, the everyday and special challenges that this occupation brings, and mothers' ability to claim agency in order to participate fully with their children in the communities in which they live. We have used the term "agency" because it "implies the conduct of action under the sway of intentional states"(Bruner, 1990, p.9). The term "participation" as used in this text is congruent with its use in the World Health Organization's International Classification for Functioning, Disability and Health, known as ICF (2001), because it acknowledges that participation is improved when societal hindrances are removed and social supports and facilitators are provided.

Mothering is embedded in a particular historical time and is shaped by culture, ethnicity, class, and gender, as well as economic, geographical, and political factors. The cultural perspective of this text is essentially that from western industrialized countries. Although we have not included mothers from developing countries, many chapters speak for women who are living in poverty or are incarcerated, disadvantaged, or subject to discrimination. Some have been homeless and others could become homeless.

Although many of the authors are from the United States, others are from other countries, such as Australia, Mexico, and the United Kingdom, and they have brought some clear and subtle cultural differences to this text. Within these different perspectives, there are the ever-present threads of whimsy, poignancy, heartache, and ambivalence, as well as a darker side, which, in this text, is expressed particularly in chapters that relate to mothers living in extreme poverty, as described by LeRoy in Chapter 18, or who are in jail, as described by Jose-Kampfner in Chapter 13. Mothering is like a rich tapestry: the warp and weft of the weave are strong and constant, but the patterns change as you hold it to light, shade, or dark. It's all there, but looks different.

There are many topics that we would like to have included in this book but didn't, mainly because there was a limit to the size of the text and the time to write and edit it. For example, we say nothing directly about mothering and

sexuality. Although the topic is outside our own professional expertise, we acknowledge its importance and know that it is being addressed by other mothering researchers (e.g., a special issue on "Mothering, sex, and sexuality" of the *Journal of the Association for Research on Mothering*, volume 4, number 1, 2002). We had planned to include a chapter on lesbian mothers and co-mothers, but unfortunately, people knowledgeable about this topic could not make themselves available to this project. Therefore we refer readers to another special issue of the *Journal of the Association for Research on Mothering*, volume 1, number 2, 1999: Lesbian Mothering. Many of the topics we have included, as well as the ones we have not, including those described above and others such as adopting mothers and surrogate mothers, are complex topics that could fill many books.

Most of the contributors are qualitative researchers, and therefore they present their own perspective in a more or less agentic manner, in the genre of this type of scholarship. People were invited to present their own work and their own perspective within the context of mothering occupations. Not all chapters reflect the use of qualitative methodology. We welcome this diversity of research approaches and trust that you will use this diversity to broaden your understanding of mothering occupations. Whatever their research methodology, all the authors in this text have written respectfully of context, theory, and history and have legitimized women and people of color as participants in the construction of knowledge.

Many of our authors framed their theoretical perspective as social constructionist (Primeau, Chapter 6; Francis-Connolly, Chapter 8; Llewellyn and McConnell, Chapter 9), and we acknowledge that our thinking about mothering parallels social constructivism. Yet there are several chapters, or parts thereof, that are written in the classic positivistic methodology of social science. That is, they involve statistical methodologies (Esdaile, Chapter 5; LeRoy, Chapter 18). But you will find that even these authors do not take the stance of objectivity that is characteristic of positivistic inquiry.

☙ How This Book Is Organized

Mothering occupations are not a static bundle of neatly organized activities. They vary with the mothering individuals and those who are mothered. They change with age and time. We discuss a range of those mothering activities in this book, from the general activities of all mothers to the specific activities of mothers who have particular challenges of their own or whose children have particular challenges and needs.

This book is organized into three sections. Section A includes Chapters 1 through 8 and highlights the everyday challenges of mothering. In this section you will find a discussion of the anticipating occupations of mothering (Chapter 1), the co-occupations of mothers and their young children (Chapter 2), the physical care occupations related to young children (Chapter 3), maternal management of play spaces (Chapter 4), the co-occupation of play (Chapter 5), mothering occupations in the context of unpaid work and play (Chapter 6), the conflicting occupations of teenage mothers (Chapter 7), and a discussion of mothering through the lifecourse (Chapter 8).

Section B includes Chapters 9 through 13. In this section, the special challenges of mothers as they engage in their mothering occupations are described. These include mothers with intellectual disabilities and how they affect and are affected by the social milieu (Chapter 9), mothers with disabilities (Chapter 10), mothers with chronic illness (Chapter 11), and mothers with mental illness (Chapter 12). This section of the book ends with the environmental challenge to women of mothering from prison (Chapter 13).

Section C is the concluding section that includes Chapters 14 through 18. This section describes the special challenges that mothers experience when their children have special needs. These needs include disabilities that create the mothering occupation of activism (Chapter 14), disabilities that require sensitive navigation through the American health care system (Chapter 15), children with attention deficit hyperactivity disorder and the construction of mother time (Chapter 16), and

the creation of family-centered therapy programs (Chapter 17). This section ends with another environmental challenge to mothering, a discussion of the impact of welfare on mothers of children with disabilities (Chapter 18).

Thus, mothering and the mothering occupations are a series of challenges that last a lifetime but that also lead to agency. From the mothering occupations that provide the daily physical care and play of very young children through struggles with poverty and disability, either the mother's disability or the child's, mothers develop agency, the self-knowledge that they should and can act for their own and their children's best interests. In this way, they develop the ability and the intent to claim their agency. Then they act to participate in their children's lives and in their communities. This is why we have called this book *Mothering Occupations: Challenge, Agency, and Participation.*

You will notice that either a picture or a drawing and a poem distinctly separate the sections. We feel that visual and poetic representations also speak eloquently about mothering. These provide you with an interlude—a clear statement of the change—between the sections.

In the concluding pages of this book you will find the epilogue. We have reserved this place for our final words, which contain our wish list for action on behalf of mothers.

References

Arendell, T. (2000). Conceiving and investigating motherhood: The decade's scholarship. *Journal of Marriage and the Family, 62,* 1192–1207.

Bruner, J. (1990). *Acts of meaning.* Cambridge, MA: Harvard University Press.

Chodorow, N. (1978). *The reproduction of mothering.* Berkeley, CA: University of California Press.

Chodorow, N., & Contratto, S. (1982). The fantasy of the perfect mother. In B. Thorne & M. Yalom (Eds.). *Rethinking the family* (p 54–75). New York: Longman.

Hochschild, A. (1989). *The second shift.* New York: Avon.

Oakley, A. (1974). *The sociology of housework.* New York: Pantheon.

Phoenix, A., Woollett, A., & Lloyd, E. (1991). *Motherhood: Meanings, practices and Ideologies.* Thousand Oaks, CA: Sage.

Polakow, V. (1993). *Lives on the edge: Single mothers and their children in the other America.* Chicago: The University of Chicago Press.

Reinharz, S. (1992). *Feminist methods in social research.* Oxford: Oxford University Press.

Rich, A. (1976). *Of women born: Motherhood as experience and institution.* New York: W. W. Norton & Co., Inc.

Ruddick, S. (1980). Maternal thinking. *Feminist Studies, 6,* 342–367.

Ruddick, S. (1995). *Maternal thinking: Toward a politics of peace.* Boston: Beacon Press.

Spender, D. (1985). *For the record: The meaning and making of feminist knowledge.* London (UK): Women's Press.

Thurer, S. L. (1994). *The myths of motherhood.* Boston: Houghton Mifflin Co.

World Health Organization (2001). Fifty-fourth World Health Assembly for international use on 22 May 2001. (Resolution WHA54.21). Author: Geneva, Switzerland.

Yerxa, E. , Clark, F., Frank, G., Jackson, J., Parham, D., Pierce, D., Stein, C. , & Zemke, R. (1989). An introduction to occupational science, a foundation for occupational therapy in the 21st century. *Occupational Therapy in Health Care, 6* (4), 14–30.

Susan A. Esdaile
Judith A. Olson

Acknowledgments

The idea of writing a book about mothers grew out of our work with mothering women, so we first want to thank all the mothers and mothering individuals with whom we have worked, as well as the students with whom we have shared our experiences and learning. Next we gratefully acknowledge the contributions of our children: Anna, Lucy, Eric, Megan, Jeanette, and Kathryn, for grounding our professional knowledge about mothering. Because writing and editing are time-consuming tasks that spill into all areas of a person's life, we want to thank our families and friends for their support, interest, and encouragement. We are also grateful to our employers and colleagues for their support and interest. We cannot name everyone, but would like to acknowledge colleagues with whom we have discussed this text, who were not able to contribute to it, but whose research and practice has also focused on mothering occupations: Ellen Cohn, Elizabeth Larson, Terry Crowe, and Diane Kellegrew. We extend our very special thanks to Mary Wilcox for helping us hone our thinking, and to the knowledgeable, friendly, and supportive team of publishing experts at F. A Davis. We extend our grateful thanks to Dr. Elizabeth J. Yerxa, the founding scholar of the discipline of occupational science, for writing the foreword to this text. Our colleagues, listed in the next section, generously gave their time to review chapters and provide constructive feedback to the contributing authors. We would also like to thank Janice Fialka for her closing poem to Section C entitled "Advice to Professionals Who Must Conference Cases." This poem can be found in the booklet *It Matters: Lessons from My Son.* Janice Fialka also co-authored the book *Do You Hear What I Hear? Parents and Professional Working Together for Children with Special Needs.*

Reviewers

Caroline Robinson Brayley, PhD, FAOTA
Associate Professor Emeritus, Department of
 Occupational Therapy
University of Pittsburgh
Pittsburgh, Pennsylvania

Gerry E. Conti, MS, OTR
Assistant Professor, Department of
 Occupational Therapy
Eugene Applebaum College of Pharmacy and
 Health Sciences
Wayne State University
Detroit, Michigan

Virginia A. Dickie, PhD, OTR/L, FAOTA
Associate Professor, Division of Occupational
 Science
Department of Allied Health Sciences
University of North Carolina at Chapel Hill
Chapel Hill, North Carolina

Louise Farnworth, PhD, AccOT
Senior Lecturer, School of Occupational
 Therapy
Faculty of Health Sciences
La Trobe University
Bundoora, Victoria, Australia

Ruth Hansen, PhD, FAOTA
Professor, Occupational Therapy Program
College of Health and Human Services
Eastern Michigan University
Ypsilanti, Michigan

Maralynne D. Mitcham, PhD, OTR/L, FAOTA
Professor and Director, Occupational
 Therapy Program
Department of Rehabilitation Sciences
College of Health Professions
Charleston, South Carolina

Heather Neff, PhD
Professor, Department of English
College of Arts & Sciences
Eastern Michigan University
Ypsilanti, Michigan

Gretchen Dahl Reeves, PhD, OT, FAOTA
Associate Professor, Occupational Therapy
 Program
College of Health & Human Services
Eastern Michigan University
Ypsilanti, Michigan

Linda M. Roth, PhD
Associate Professor, Department of Family
 Medicine
School of Medicine
Wayne State University
Detroit, Michigan

Susan E. Ryan, MS, OTR, SROT, AccOT
Professor of Occupational Therapy
Faculty of Medicine and Health
University College of Cork
Cork, Ireland

Karen E. Stagnitti, PhD, AccOT
Senior Lecturer, Education and Training
Greater Green Triangle University
 Department of Rural Health
Warrnambool, Victoria, Australia

Contributors

Gillian Brown, MSc, DipCOT, SROT
Head Occupational Therapist, Barking
  Havering and Redbridge NHS Trust
Community Paedatrics, Redbridge
  Children's Centre
Associate Lecturer, University of East
  London, UK

Ruth S. Farber, PhD, MSW, OTR
Associate Professor, Department of
  Occupational Therapy
Temple University
Philadelphia, Pennsylvania

Elizabeth Farrell, MBMS, FRANZCOG,
  FRCOG
Head, Menopause Unit, Monash Medical
  Centre and the Jean Hailes Foundation
Monash University
Clayton, Victoria, Australia

Elizabeth B. Francis-Connolly, PhD, OTR
Associate Professor & Director, Occupational
  Therapy Program
College of Health and Human Services
Eastern Michigan University
Ypsilanti, Michigan

Susan D. Griffin, PhD, MA(Hons),
    BAppSc(OT),GradDipAppBehSc
Senior Lecturer, School of Occupation and
  Leisure Sciences
University of Sydney
Lidcombe, New South Wales, Australia

Doreen Y. Head, MS, OTR
Assistant Professor, Department of
  Occupational Therapy
Eugene Applebaum College of Pharmacy
  and Health Sciences
Wayne State University
Detroit, Michigan

Cristina Jose-Kampfner, PhD
Professor, Department of Teacher Education
College of Education
Eastern Michigan University
Ypsilanti, Michigan

Mary C. Lawlor, ScD, OTR, FAOTA
Professor, Department of Occupational
  Science and Occupational Therapy
University of Southern California
Los Angeles, California

Barbara W. LeRoy, PhD
Director, Developmental Disabilities Institute
Wayne State University
Detroit, Michigan

Gwynnyth Llewellyn, PhD
Sesquicentenary Professor of Occupation
  and Leisure Sciences
School of Occupation and Leisure Sciences
University of Sydney
Lidcombe, New South Wales, Australia

Amy Marshall, BS, OTR/L
Graduate Assistant, Department of
  Occupational Therapy
Eastern Kentucky University
Richmond, Kentucky

David McConnell, PhD, BAppSc (OT)
  Hons, ARC Postdoctoral Research
  Fellow
Research Manager, Family Support & Services
  Project
School of Occupation and Leisure Sciences
University of Sydney
Lidcombe, New South Wales, Australia

Elizabeth Anne McKay, PhD, MSc,
  DipCOT, SROT
Head, Department of Occupational Therapy
Faculty of Science
University of Limerick
Limerick, Ireland

Karin J. Opacich, PhD, MHPE, OTR/L,
  FAOTA
Opacich Consultative Services
Chicago, Illinois, USA

Doris Pierce, PhD, OTR/L, FAOTA
Endowed Chair in Occupational Therapy
Department of Occupational Therapy
Eastern Kentucky University,
Richmond, Kentucky

Loree A. Primeau, PhD, OTR, OT(C)
Associate Professor and Chair, Department of
  Occupational Therapy
University of Texas Medical Branch
Galveston, Texas

Teresa A. Savage, PhD, RN
Associate Director, Center for the Study of
  Disability Ethics
Rehabilitation Institute of Chicago
Assistant Professor—Research
Maternal-Child Nursing
University of Illinois at Chicago, College of
  Nursing
Chicago, Illinois

Ruth Segal, PhD, OTR
Assistant Professor, Department of
  Occupational Therapy
The Steinhardt School of Education
New York University
New York, New York

Kirsty Thompson, BAppSc (OT) Hons.
Lecturer, School of Occupation and Leisure
  Sciences
University of Sydney
Lidcombe, New South Wales, Australia

Samantha Whybrow, BAppSc (OT) Hons.
Research Officer, School of Occupation and
  Leisure Sciences
University of Sydney
Lidcombe, New South Wales, Australia

Contents

The Everyday Challenges of Mothering Occupations

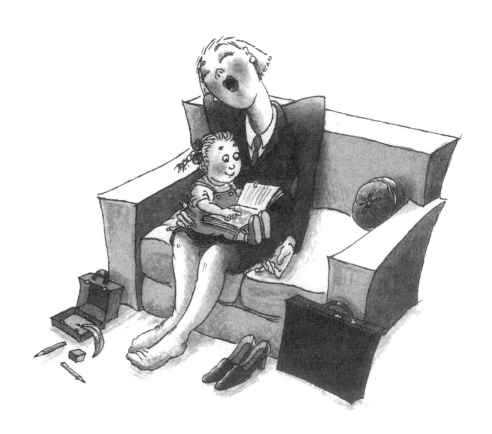

Drawing by Mary Leunig, reprinted with permission.

CHAPTER *1*

Anticipating Occupations of Mothering and the Development of Agency

Susan A. Esdaile, PhD, MAPS, AccOT, OTR, SROT

Elizabeth A. Farrell, MBMS, FRANZCOG, FRCOG

Judith A. Olson, PhD, OTR

 Anticipated Outcomes

We anticipate that, after reading this chapter, readers will:

- Have an increased understanding of the implication of decision making as it affects women who choose to become mothers in current western societies

- Have an increased understanding of the concept of lifestyle redesign from a number of perspectives

- Have increased their ability to understand the implication of pregnancy and birthing stories in their own lives, within their circle of family and friends, and the clients with whom they work

- Have an increased understanding of the historical contexts and ideologies that have shaped mothering in the 21st century

ᕲ Introduction

In this chapter we explore the anticipating occupations of mothering, how women plan for motherhood, and the societal and familial influences that impinge on women during these stages of becoming pregnant and anticipating the birth of their child. We highlight themes of choice, preferences of occupational engagement, and lifestyle redesign, as current mothers-to-be negotiated paradoxical options in order to make decisions with lifelong implications. Sifting information to make life-altering choices is a central, anticipating occupation for mothers-to-be living in industrialized western societies in the 21st century: first, deciding when is the right time to have a baby; second, selecting from the options for managing a career and a baby or choosing to be a full-time mother; and third, making health-related choices before and during pregnancy. For many women, the anticipating occupations of mothering include decisions about genetic testing, in vitro fertilization (IVF), and possibly termination of the pregnancy. To provide illustrations and points for discussion, we tell stories from our professional perspective or experience. Susan reflects on a colleague's experience of lifestyle redesign as she planned for her first pregnancy and the birth of her child. Elizabeth describes her reasons for becoming an obstetrician, presents three vignettes of former patients, with changes to protect their identity, and discusses why she has given up this side of her medical practice. Judith discusses the outcomes of an interview with a mother who had triplets as a result of IVF. In the third section of the chapter, we explore theoretical issues related to our themes of challenge, agency, and participation. We conclude with a summary, propose implications for research and practice, and pose questions for further discussion.

Figure 1–1 presents an overview of our concept. Birth giving and its anticipating occupations occur within the social, biological, cultural, and historical experiences of a mother's milieu. These are the contextual influences of mothering that she shares with

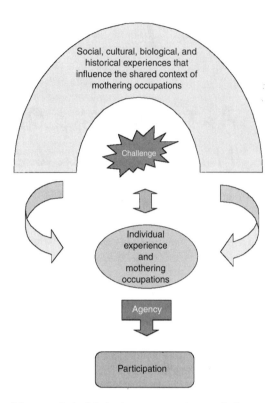

Figure 1–1. *Mothering occupations: challenge, agency, and participation.*

her peers, and that shape her mothering occupations. Thus, for example, in the 1950s middle-class white mothers in the United States and other similar industrialized western countries assumed or supported the idea of mothering as a full-time occupation. However, they may not have included breast-feeding among these occupations. Experiences within a woman's family of origin also shape her own mothering. So the individual experience of mothering is a reflection of shared experience.

Mothering always negotiates challenge. Biology is an inescapable challenge. It is unpredictable, and often violent in comparison with a protected, structured western lifestyle. Whatever the situation of birth giving, there is always challenge associated with pain, whether it is physical, or mental, or both. Society also challenges mothers-to-be, setting out the latest empirical data and prescribed conditions for healthy pregnancy, healthy infants and children, and optimal childcare and child-rearing practices. The challenge of making the right choices is daunting. For some mothers the challenge includes making ethically difficult, life-altering choices, enduring lengthy periods of discomfort, and technical intrusion. For some it is a matter of surviving against the odds of criticism, ostracism, and even violence.

Faced with a myriad of challenges, mothers draw close to the supporting, nurturing elements within their milieu: their families, friends, physicians, healthcare professionals, and other supports, and try to ensure the success of their pregnancy. During pregnancy the relational self and the importance of connectedness with significant others become emphasized (Smith, 1999). They attempt to create a context in which the individual experience of anticipating birth will be successful, with both mother and baby in good health. The just-right balance in mothering occupations needs planning, and is not often achieved with ease. The assumptions of it happening naturally, by tacit design of nature, often causes the harshest of reality checks for new mothers in western countries in the 21st century. Faced with the occupations of childcare that are most readily learned through role modeling, they are often flipped from feeling like a competent adult to a state of vulnerable confusion.

However, most mothers do persevere, seek out their support systems, and learn to be assertive about their needs and the needs of their children. They do what they have to do and find their voice, their agency. Bruner (1990), in common with other cognitive scientists, has stated his belief in the goal-directed nature of behavior and "'agency' [that] implies the conduct of action under the sway of intentional states" (p. 9). The paths mothers take to achieve agency and move forward to participate in life, on their own terms, are echoed in the voices of many mothers in the chapters of this text. In telling their stories we have attempted to follow Bruner's four injunctions in regard to narrative: first, in emphasizing human agency; second, in attempting to create a conceptually sequential order; third, in being sensitive and not violating the "canonicality" in human interaction (p. 77); and finally, in acknowledging our own perspective, our voice and bias.

For many women this acquisition of agency, leading to participation, has been a power struggle against oppression, marginalization, and trivialization. Even historically, when women had few, if any legal rights, this has applied, although less so to educated, financially secure women. Today it still applies to many women "on the edge" because of poverty, racial diversity, or lifestyle. It certainly applies to millions of women outside western industrialized societies. In this text we take a phenomenological perspective, explicating meaning from individual experience. We give voice to women facing the everyday challenges of mothering occupations, as well as those challenged by their own illness or disability or that of their child or children. In our attempt to give voice to these women, we bring our own perspectives. As suggested by Ruddick (1983), we identify ourselves as middle-aged, middle-class women with postgraduate qualifications: one is a physician specialized in surgery, obstetrics, and gynecology; two are occupational therapists with graduate qualifications in behavioral sciences, infant mental health and education; and all of us have been educated within western societies. Two of us live and work in the United States (Susan and Judith); and one (Elizabeth) lives and works in Australia. Two of us (Elizabeth and Susan) were educated in Australia.

What Factors Influence the Timing of Pregnancy and "Beginning" of Motherhood?

In this chapter we share information on the timing and beginning of motherhood from two perspectives: the United States and Australia. According to the National Center for Health Statistics in the United States, as reported by the March of Dimes, the birth rate for women between the ages of 35 and 39 during the period between 1978 and 1997 rose 90 percent. Even more significant is that during the period between 1981 and 1997, the birth rate increased 87 percent for women in their 40s (March of Dimes, 1999). Why are we seeing what seems almost to be a pattern of delayed pregnancy?

Susan Coady (cited in Recker, 1998), faculty member at the Ohio State University, has studied this phenomenon and suggests a number of reasons. She has found that women who wait to have a child do so to: secure their financial futures, develop emotional maturity sufficient to the task of parenting, and to have the time needed to focus on both their marriage and career before their attention can be shifted to children. Deferring marriage also contributes to delayed pregnancy. A large chunk of a woman's reproductive life is gone if she has delayed marriage. Additionally, there is a dauntingly high divorce rate in America that cautions thoughtful individuals to have a stable marriage before childbearing. Other factors that have contributed to delayed pregnancy include national economic insecurity, abortion as a choice, and effective contraception (Recker, 1998).

From my clinical experience in Australia, I (Elizabeth) have found that the average age of first pregnancy is older than a generation ago and pregnancy is more likely to be deferred until the early 30s, with an increasing number of women choosing pregnancy in their 40s. Women are often well established in a career and a relationship, having experienced a period of adulthood and independence before maternity. They appear to want to have more time to study and achieve some qualification, establish a career outside the home, travel and experience different cultures, "have a good time" without the responsibility of children, or develop a relationship with more equality of roles and commitment. The women and their partners may wish to have bought a home and achieved some financial security. One woman told me (Elizabeth), "We just haven't discussed it, and maybe when we do it might be too late; I'll be 40 next year," as she shrugged her shoulders.

In Australia, the birth rate is falling and there is negative population growth, which may reflect an attitude that it is not necessary to have children in adulthood as the woman above suggests (Evans, 2002). Australia's fertility rate is 1.7 babies per woman, with 1 in 4 women never giving birth. Also, a majority of couples are choosing to have only one or two children. There are many safe forms of contraception available now, and pregnancy can be delayed safely with the risk of unwanted pregnancy reduced. Termination of pregnancy (although illegal under statute law but available under common law) is also freely and safely available in Australia. In some states in the United States, termination of pregnancy is unavailable and illegal.

Formal Education for Birth Giving and Early Baby Care: Australia and the United States Compared

In Australia, most obstetric hospitals provide antenatal (prenatal) education preparing women for their labor and delivery, as well as instruction on the care of the baby in the early neonatal period, so as to give women knowledge and understanding to feel more in control of their own experience in becoming a mother. Some of the programs aimed at special groups such as adolescents may also include parenting skills training. These programs may also continue postnatally. The classes usually focus on a healthy pregnancy; being fit; learning about normal labor; reducing anxiety and fear about labor and delivery; analgesia in labor; and relaxation and breathing techniques for labor aided by the partner, family member, or other support person. Classes also discuss baby care and breastfeeding.

In the United States, prenatal classes, or preparation for labor and delivery classes as they are sometimes called, are accessible to mothers-to-be and their partners in various ways. Hospitals and various specialty groups, such as midwifery programs, offer prenatal classes on a regular basis to women who are between 1 and 2 months predelivery. The issues that are addressed in these classes are varied and range from preparation for labor and delivery and related information about medications and breathing techniques to breastfeeding, infant massage, and bathing and caring for the newborn infant. Also, in the United States there are some managed care organizations that have recognized the nation's new emphasis on health promotion. Conceptualizing prenatal care as healthcare promotion has led to the reimbursement of hospitals for prenatal education as in the case of Priority Health (Priority Health 2002). In addition, some high schools provide prenatal classes to adolescents. Often these classes include the traditional topics identified previously and, in addition, offer education on contraception; the consequences of unsafe sex such as sexually transmitted diseases and AIDS; the affective components of values; and methods of enhancing self-esteem, assertion, and the development of one's own sexuality.

When Biology Challenges Participation

Many women want a biological child and the experience of birth giving. Additionally, although society is not as rigid as in the past, there is still societal pressure to have children. This pressure affects women individually and differently. Most women still expect to have children of their own and to be their primary caregivers. When a woman decides to have children and discovers that she is infertile, it has a profound impact on her emotionally, psychologically, and even socially. Although it is beyond the scope of this chapter to do anything more than acknowledge that infertility can affect one's self-image and purpose in life and can engender feelings of helplessness, depression, and emptiness, the depth of the impact these factors can have on a woman cannot be overstated.

Today there is an array of treatments, ranging from pharmacology to surgery and new reproductive technologies such as IVF, to reduce the physical obstacles interfering with the satisfaction of the human desire to have a child (Sher, Davis, & Stoess, 1995). The various other reproductive technologies, like donor insemination, which is not truly new, provide alternative pathways to motherhood (Cooper & Glazer, 1994). For an increasing number of other individuals who once may have been considered sterile, there are even third-party parenting options such as ovum or sperm donation, surrogacy, or gestational care (Cooper & Glazer, 1994).

Sandelowski and associates have termed this process of deciding on a route to motherhood as "mazing" and define it as "the torturous process of negotiating the paths to parenthood" (1989, p. 220). This maze includes, but is not limited to, fertility drugs and assistive reproductive technologies, including the consideration of adoption.

The opportunity to achieve pregnancy through human decision and intervention by the use of these new technologies rather than biological destiny must affect the occupations of the birth giver. There is a paucity of literature about this experience and the anticipating occupations, which must, of necessity, include medical procedures, medication regimens, and some degree of anxiety about whether they will work. In Sharon's story we will get a glimpse into the experience of one woman's route to achieving biological motherhood.

✎ Stories from the Chapter Authors

Susan's Story: Lifestyle Redesign and Occupational Balance

My interest in this topic was stimulated by my experience as a mother and a health professional working with mothers. Becoming a mother is full of pain and full of joy, and women will tell and retell their birth-giving stories. For mothers who have less-than-perfect children, the birthing and pregnancy stories often involve repeated reliving of the pregnancy and birth experience, examining the details of what may have been and what could have been changed if only they had known or the doctor had known. I heard many of these stories, and hoped that what I said was a positive validation of the experience and somehow, by my role as a witness, would validate the reality of the stories, acknowledging the mothers' agency and enabling them to participate in their chosen roles. The belief that most of us do our best but are often seriously limited by knowledge and circumstances is poignantly true in respect to pregnancy and birth giving for many women. Given the rate at which new advances in medicine have changed the whole experience of having a baby, even when the event and outcome are without undue trauma, mothers compare their experiences with those of other mothers, weighing the gains and losses of past and present. For example, the benefits of the more leisurely experience of a week in hospital, getting to know the baby without distractions, as was the practice a generation ago, also carried medical risks associated with the less advanced technology existing at that time.

Early in my career, I worked with a friend and colleague, Jane, who became pregnant a few months after we started working together. Although our careers have taken different trajectories, we have kept in touch over the years, and she has given me permission to tell her story, because I think that it illustrates agency in making a conscious decision to undertake lifestyle redesign as an anticipating occupation of mothering. (Clark et al., 2001; 1997; Clark, Ennevor, & Richardson, 1996; Jackson et al., 1998). As with the other mothers whose stories we tell, her name and some details have been changed to protect her anonymity.

⌘ Vignette: **Jane**

Jane took a part-time position as an occupational therapist in a large children's hospital that also served as a university teaching hospital, where I then worked. Her working hours were Monday through Friday from 8:15 AM to 12 noon. Because the hospital offered regular lunchtime seminars, and had an extensive library, Jane often stayed until 2 PM to take advantage of these learning opportunities. It was an intellectually stimulating environment, with a high degree of collaboration and social interaction between departments, especially between occupational and physical therapy. We all enjoyed the work and the companionship of our colleagues. We were young, energetic, and enthusiastic. In addition to working together, we took turns to arrange social events such as barbecues, and as a group participated in other fund-raising social functions. So Jane and I had lots of opportunities to talk, and because I was planning to have children myself, I was interested in the way she had consciously redesigned her lifestyle. Jane had moved to our department from a demanding job as the head occupational therapist in a community hospital, where she had found both the politics and the extended travel draining. She told me that she had moved because she was hoping to become pregnant, and had decided to change her

lifestyle and create occupational balance for herself, with more free time to renovate their 80-year-old house; rest when tired; and play tennis, a game she enjoyed. She later mentioned that she had needed to have surgery (a myomectomy to remove uterine fibroids) so that she could become pregnant. Therefore she decided to make achieving and maintaining her pregnancy a priority.

Not working full-time meant that Jane could engage in non–work-related occupations in which she was interested. She played tennis regularly, three afternoons during the week. She had time for house renovating, her favorite occupation being the restoration of the cedar-wood balustrade and a glass-fronted, built-in cabinet in their old house. She also made curtains and many of her clothes, seemed to read extensively, and often walked to and from work. When she became pregnant about 4 to 5 months into this redesigned life, she still appeared to have plenty of time to prepare a nursery and to rest when she was tired. She certainly never appeared hassled. Because Jane was the only pregnant woman in our department, we were very interested in her condition. I was possibly the most interested. A generation ago, it was the custom for pregnant women to leave work at the end of the second trimester of their pregnancy. However, as Jane felt well, and worked part-time, she decided to continue working until 3 weeks before her baby was due. This extended my opportunity to observe the latter stages of her pregnancy more closely and to realize that the problem that had necessitated her to have surgery did cause her to worry about her capacity to carry her infant to term and have a safe delivery.

When compared with the anticipating occupations of mothering now, a generation later, Jane's were minimally medical and nontechnical, very similar to Speier's (2001) description of her experience in 1974. Then "the process seemed to be a much simpler one, and the decisions reflected that relative simplicity (p. 7)". Jane did not have a birth plan, something mothers-to-be now develop as a matter of course, as illustrated in Elizabeth's story later in this chapter. Jane described her obstetrician as competent, well known, and respected in the local medical community, but she found him remote, and she certainly didn't have a close relationship with him. She was pragmatic about this and made the best of what was available without too much fuss. She had a few relatively noninvasive tests, was prescribed folic acid tablets, and attended childbirth preparation classes conducted by a physical therapist. These were focused entirely on the experience of giving birth. Jane enjoyed them and found that she was really good at performing all the exercises, especially the more complex, cross-lateral relaxation patterns that she got to demonstrate to the rest of the prenatal class (and her colleagues in the occupational and physical therapy departments at the hospital where we worked). Jane appeared very well physically, and read the relatively few childbirth preparation books that were then available. She seemed to enjoy what she described as "my life of occupational balance."

However, later she said that, apart from being able to competently breathe and relax her way through a physiologically normal delivery, even on her back, "feeling like a large beetle," as was then the custom, she was not prepared for the next phase of motherhood. Her baby was born 4 weeks early, but the hospital had the wrong due date, so like many mothers before and since (Brown, Lumley, Small, & Astbury, 1994), she was not able to convince anyone that she was in labor too early. As she later said, "my baby had to turn blue to demonstrate that he had indeed arrived too early." At this point, Jane became a disruptive patient and was sedated. She wasn't allowed visitors for the first 2 days after her son was born, and I had a sense that this was a most difficult time for her, a direct challenge to her agency, a time of disempowerment. Years later, she said that, in hindsight, she believed that both her obstetrician and pediatrician did their best, and that they, she and these two men, were limited by their lack of knowledge. In this Jane was referring to her son's respiratory problems, associated with his premature birth, and the severe bouts of asthma during his childhood that made Jane constantly watchful for his health.

When social change accelerates, and technical knowledge increases rapidly, the 20/20 vision of hindsight approaches rapidly to highlight past omissions. So it becomes easy to view our past actions and those of others without compassion, forgetting that we do our best with the knowledge and values that are available to us at a given time. One of the tragedies of life is that the knowledge and skills we have may not be adequate, and the future can make this abundantly and painfully clear. In past generations, when knowledge advanced less rapidly, we were more secure in the correctness of medical opinion. Educated people are now much more critical, sometimes unfairly, as illustrated later in Elizabeth's story.

For Jane, the most challenging part of mothering came next. Like many young women in "advanced" western societies, she was separated from her mother and family of origin by 800 miles, which then meant a 12-hour drive, an equally long train trip, or expensive airfare that she could not easily afford often. Her new friends and colleagues, like me, were either working or lived too far away for her to meet them easily. I only realized how lonely she had been years later, when I became more aware of the importance of social support for new mothers (Smith, 1999), and the potential for a loss of a sense of competence following a birth-giving experience associated with loss of control (Mackey, 1999). She had also felt rather intimidated by her neighbors, many of whom had been at university with the then newly famous Germaine Greer, author of *The Female Eunuch*. They seemed to be able to do everything with ease, enfolding childcare with busy professional lives. They kept their support networks well hidden, giving the impression that they did it all alone. The first wave of feminists was still influential; their focus was directed towards political and sexual liberation. Motherhood was viewed as something that women managed along the way, not as the focus of their life (Speier, 2001). But mothering occupations had become the focus of Jane's life, and the sense of competence and well-being that she had enjoyed during pregnancy vanished very quickly. She felt very inadequate and lonely, and had to work hard to master all the day-to-day occupations of mothering, from breast-feeding a preterm infant to the best routine for diaper washing. It took her effort and time to regain a sense of competence.

Reflection

When I discussed this chapter with Jane recently, she said that she still looks back on her first pregnancy as a period when her occupational engagements were in complete balance. She said that this occupationally balanced lifestyle was associated with a great sense of physical and emotional well-being and of competence. As an occupational therapist, Jane has remained very interested in the concept of lifestyle. In thinking about Jane's comments, I wonder whether the disruption of this occupational balance experienced by many mothers with whom I've spoken is caused by the unsupportive cultural context in which we live rather than by the birth of a baby per se.

Jane's experience of the anticipating occupations of mothering seems to have been quite leisurely and technologically unsophisticated. However, she was lonely and isolated as a new mother. Her story, and the professional experience I've had since working with mothers, left me convinced that mothers of infants and young children need extensive community support as a matter of course, not just in the case of illness and special needs. When I worked in Australia, we were fortunate to have an excellent maternal and child health service, with clinics within walking distance for most people. Thus, vaccinations, dental care for children, and advice about infant and child-feeding care were free and easily available. When Jane's son was born, the service was more medically focused, with an emphasis on regular weighing of infants to ensure that they gained weight. These services became more holistic and expanded to include educational programs offered by nutritionists, occupational and physical therapists, speech and language pathologists, social workers, and psychologists. I was fortunate to work part-time for 12 years as a member of such a community-based child and family service. This work with mothers and infants was a pivotal time of my professional life. The nonthreatening nature of these programs made them both available and accessible to new mothers, who could participate without feeling intimidated by experts. Although the papers that I published about this work were mainly about mothers of preschoolers (Esdaile & Greenwood, 1995a & b), I also worked extensively with new and expectant mothers. I think that creating occupational balance through the anticipating occupations of mothering and the care of infants and young children remains a challenge within our western culture. We have adopted a male model of emotional separateness, replacing the connectedness that is an integral part of women's social and biological development (Gilligan, 1982; Mayo Clinic Women's Health Source, 2002; Shrewsbury, 1987; Smith, 1999).

Transition

Jane's story of her anticipating occupations of mothering involved little medical technology; for her it was a time of occupational balance and well-being. Fortunately, she was in good health. However, in hindsight, she agreed that the availability of ultrasound and more rigorous monitoring could have avoided the complications for her infant that followed. At least, with more empirical evidence, it would have been harder to miscalculate the dates by a month. Elizabeth's story highlights the fact that advances in medical knowledge and technology have had many positive outcomes, but they have also created additional burdens of high expectations placed on physicians. The challenge is not always equal to the agency because many factors associated with the anticipating occupations of mothering remain outside our control.

Elizabeth's Story: An Obstetrician's Perspective

As an obstetrician and gynecologist, I have seen many women progress through pregnancy, deliver their babies, and then return for their postnatal review with their young infants. It is the most joyous of medical specialties, watching and facilitating a woman's successful transition through the "inside baby" stage to the "outside baby" lifelong phase. But it is the most heartbreaking when a woman's biology lets her down and there are pregnancy or birthing complications, at worst the death of a baby or (thankfully, these days occurring extremely rarely in western cultures) the death of a mother.

I chose to train as an obstetrician and gynecologist because of the immense fulfillment experienced in working with women at all ages of their lives. In many ways, obstetrics is really a nurturing, mothering specialty in which the doctor has an intimate and very personal relationship with each woman, looking after both her and her unborn child. The obstetrician has to have skills not only in obstetrics, but also in medicine, surgery, psychology, and psychiatry. So many times after a baby is born, a woman will thank her doctor "for her baby" when it is the woman and her partner who have conceived the baby, nurtured and nourished it in utero, and experienced the labor and delivery. The doctor is merely the facilitator, but with a very special place in a woman's life.

However, I chose to stop practicing obstetrics for a number of reasons:

- I developed "burnout," becoming terrified of complications occurring because I might miss something, or that a baby or mother might die.
- The expectations of many couples were for a perfect pregnancy, labor, and delivery, and that it would all fit into their anticipated timetables and "birth plans," and if it all "didn't happen," then the obstetrician was to blame.
- Increasing insurance costs, resulting from increased litigation and the large payments ordered by the courts, have created an environment of defensive medicine.
- The unpredictability of obstetrics had become more frustrating because I could never plan my life or expect to be able to attend the entirety of my children's school activities or any social outings without being called away.
- As a single parent working full-time, I was dependent on nannies to be responsible and available. This came to a head at a very stressful time in my life and precipitated me into ceasing obstetrics in 1994.
- Last, I believe that the role of the obstetrician is undervalued in Australia by the general community and by government, shown both in their lack of acknowledg-

ment of the training, skill, and commitment required and in the fees set down by the government compared to those for other medical specialties such as heart bypass surgery. It seems that the facilitation of a new member into our community is much less valued.

Vignette: *Leanne*

This story relates the evolution of a young mother's adjustment to motherhood with each successive pregnancy, feeling more and more comfortable in her intimate relationship with her unborn child and her mothering of each child after birth. Leanne's first pregnancy was unplanned and took place when she was 30 years old and still in a training position as a physician at a city hospital. The pregnancy was unexpected. She had mixed feelings about the timing and lack of planning, and even more anxiety when the diagnosis of a twin pregnancy was made at 12 weeks. Each time she worked a night shift, she had some bleeding and felt that the pregnancy was very fragile. At 17 weeks of gestation she was admitted to hospital because of major bleeding and uterine contractions. At this time Leanne's husband was away at a conference and her mother found it hard to help appropriately, so Leanne felt very alone and frightened. She submitted her resignation and took leave from professional training. She expressed feelings of insecurity about her pregnancy, her job, and her incomplete training, but all the time felt an exhilaration that she had achieved a pregnancy and that her biology actually worked. Leanne told me that throughout her adult life she had wondered whether she was capable of becoming pregnant, so even though the pregnancy was extremely complicated and its chances of survival limited, she nevertheless felt successful.

Sadly, at 23 weeks another hemorrhage occurred, and a blood transfusion and intravenous medications to suppress uterine contractions were given. Labor subsequently began because the membranes had ruptured at the time of the hemorrhage, and twin boys were delivered. Both died some hours after delivery because of their prematurity. The sadness and grief following the loss of the pregnancy compelled Leanne to want another child immediately. She continued to feel alone within her family because her mother's way of coping was to dismiss the loss and "get on with life," and her husband refused to discuss the loss of the babies and was uncomfortable when she openly talked about their loss. After her discharge from hospital, she was unemployed, but her husband encouraged her to complete her training.

Some 5 years later, when Leanne was in practice as a primary care physician, she and her husband decided it was an appropriate time for them to have a child. Initially she had a miscarriage at 5 weeks' gestation, which seemed to confirm to her that she was unable to achieve maternity. Two cycles later, she was pregnant again. She expressed great anxiety and fear that she would not be able to maintain the pregnancy despite ultrasound evidence of a normal fetus. Throughout pregnancy she felt insecure, which was also manifested by uncomfortable Braxton-Hicks contractions requiring regular medications to control them. At times, Leanne told me, she had feelings of invasion, distress caused by discomfort as her body shape changed, and painful fetal movements. She also felt a sense of disequilibrium with the *inside baby*. There was a state of an *uneasy truce*. The labor progressed uneventfully, but the delivery was complicated by a rotational forceps delivery under a local anesthetic. It was a very painful experience, but the baby, a little girl, was fit and healthy. Leanne felt elated to have achieved the delivery of such a healthy baby. All the family were thrilled, and her mother was so happy to have her first grandchild.

In the postpartum period, she experienced mothering as relatively comfortable, but as is common with the first child, there was a lack of the experience and confidence that one obtains with subsequent children. Leanne felt that there was such a pressure to do the right thing, be organized, and have the perfect baby. As time went by, there were problems in delineating clear boundaries between herself and the baby—when the baby cried, she cried. Putting the baby to sleep became a battle of separation, so much so that Leanne would stay and stay until the baby settled, feeling unable to leave her unless she was calm and sleepy. This created conflict within the household, particularly with her husband, because he felt that the baby was taking up *couple time* in the evenings. When the baby was 2 months old, Leanne went back to work, having arranged for the baby to be cared for by a nanny at home.

At about 5 months postpartum, Leanne found it increasingly difficult to manage and had to take leave in order to have some rest. However, the marriage relationship was unhappy; there were frequent arguments about time spent with the child, and Leanne questioned her ability to function as a mother, wife, and medical practitioner. Her friendship with other mothers was limited, and her life outside of work seemed to evolve almost totally around the household, leading to feelings of isolation and lack of support.

Three years later, during a time of marital stability, another pregnancy occurred. As the pregnancy progressed, it became a very tumultuous time in the marriage, leading to separation in the week before delivery. Despite the trauma of the collapse of the marriage, Leanne's experience of the pregnancy was quite different. From the beginning of the pregnancy, she felt in complete oneness, with an immediate acceptance of her inside baby. At 13 weeks she had an amniocentesis and found out she was having a son. She had no sense of vulnerability and felt invincible, with great strength that the pregnancy would continue successfully to term. Throughout the pregnancy there were many stresses and traumas that imposed enormous strain on her physical and emotional well-being; however, at no time did she feel insecure about the pregnancy. In the last trimester, it was agreed that the marriage should end, and arrangements were made to separate. This took place 2 days before delivery. During this time, Leanne had pregnancy euphoria and was *untouched* by the drama and stress—she had great strength and energy. By then, she also had a live-in nanny who was a great support and help, particularly with her daughter. After a normal delivery, Leanne came home to a half-empty house but had complete confidence in her ability to manage. Her son was a calm baby, quite placid, but he gave clear communication as to his wants and was easy to settle in to a routine.

There was an evolution of acceptance in

Leanne's experience of motherhood from the first unsuccessful pregnancy to some acceptance of the internal child with the second pregnancy and an immediate bond with the internal child and a great sense of partnership with the third. This second case study illustrates the desire of a professional woman to program her maternity, her pregnancy, and the progress of her antenatal time, labor, and delivery to fit in with her lifestyle, career, and desire for motherhood.

⌘ *Vignette:* **Amanda**

Amanda, an attorney in commercial law, decided at age 38 that a pregnancy would fit in with her lifestyle at this time. Her marriage was stable; she had been married for 10 years to her accountant husband, who was keen to have children. She discussed with me, her obstetrician, the optimal time for conception and, after three cycles off the contraceptive pill, she became pregnant. The pregnancy progressed well until she had a threatened miscarriage at 14 weeks while in the midst of a protracted court case, which was expected to run for 4 months. Amanda refused to have an ultrasound as she felt the pregnancy would be *all right* and deemed the test unnecessary. Unfortunately, she had to take time off work and rest at home until the bleeding settled. She became irritable and frustrated with having to rest because she saw it as a waste of time. Another lawyer had to take her place, and she lost the case. Once she returned to work, she was advised not to work long hours; she ignored this advice because she had always worked long hours to develop her reputation as a very competent lawyer.

All the subsequent antenatal investigations were normal, including an ultrasound at 19 weeks, when she found out she was having a boy. By 20 weeks the pregnancy seemed stable; the baby moved well and she went back to her routine activities. At this time, Amanda started reading about exercises, attending prenatal classes with her husband, and planning the labor and delivery. In the prenatal classes she was encouraged to develop a *birth plan* outlining the type of labor and delivery she would prefer. The *birth plan* would contain her choice of analge-

sia, if any; her preferred birthing position; whether she wished to have an oxytocic for the placental delivery; if the baby was to be given Vitamin K; and which pediatrician should perform the neonatal examination.

When Amanda was 30 weeks pregnant, she accepted a case that was to last about 4 to 6 weeks but instead went on until after the expected date of her delivery. Because there was to be a court vacation break when she was at 38 to 39 weeks' gestation, she requested induction of labor on a particular date to fit in with the court closing. An adjournment was sought for the 2 weeks after the break so that she could return to the case when the baby was 3 weeks old. It seemed imperative to her to finish the case. A week before her induction date, her membranes ruptured just before she was to cross-examine a senior businessman who was a key witness. She was confused, vulnerable, and angry, and got no support from her male colleagues, who thought it was a great joke. Luckily, she was quick-witted and turned it to her advantage. The contractions had only begun by the time the case finished for the day.

The labor progressed slowly, Amanda was tired and irritable after her day in court, and her husband had flown interstate on business. He was not able to return until the next morning. The staff found her difficult, and she complained about everything. After refusing analgesia for some hours, she was quite exhausted and eventually agreed to an epidural anesthetic, but only by a specific anesthesiologist whom she had *checked out*. While Amanda slept, the labor progressed more rapidly, and in the morning she was ready for delivery but had no energy to push the baby out. Her husband arrived just as I applied the forceps to deliver the baby.

The baby was quite big, and Amanda's episiotomy tore, with some heavy bleeding. Her husband was overjoyed at the sight of the baby, and Amanda immediately gave the baby to him. She was so tired, overwhelmed, and sore. The next day her episiotomy was very painful and she couldn't walk comfortably. The baby fed well but wanted to suck constantly. After 24 hours, Amanda had cracked nipples and was exhausted. All her time during her hospital stay was spent feeding, bathing, or changing diapers, and the large bag of files she had brought with her remained unopened. She was feeling very tired and frustrated. She disliked all the menial tasks associated with caregiving and got her husband to do them when he visited. One of the first tasks she did learn was to express her breast milk so that her husband could feed the baby.

The staff were very worried about Amanda's behavior and her management of her baby because she always seemed impatient, hurrying and wanting everything, including care of the baby, to go smoothly and fit in with her routine. She never relaxed with the baby, and he was often irritable, so she felt that she was a failure because she believed that a *perfect mother* would be able to organize and control her child. Every day she talked about getting back to her court case and that she and the baby must be organized by then. The pressure she imposed on herself was immense. When she went home, her husband took over much of the role of caregiving for the baby, except for the breast-feeding. He remained at home for the first month, even after Amanda returned to court. Despite her very supportive husband and a nanny in the daytime, after the court case finished she became quite depressed, requiring psychiatric intervention. During her admission to hospital, she tried to accept that she could not do everything or expect her body, her mind, and her baby to fit rigidly into her perceived structure. She chose to have only one child.

Amanda's story illustrates some of the issues that women need to consider before pregnancy. The choice of having a baby should be made responsibly, including questioning one's ability to nurture and nourish a new person who will be dependent for many years. It seems that Amanda had been motivated to become pregnant because she felt obliged to fulfill her biological function and *complete the family unit.* The feeling conveyed by her was that the baby was like an object that would acquiesce to her work and rigid life structure so that she remained totally in control. She had not developed any contingency plans for complications that could occur. The conflict between her work and pregnancy and then the baby interfered with her ability to function effectively in both of her current major life occupations, mothering and professional work. She seemed to have no capacity

for flexibility or for putting the baby's needs above her own. However, she was able to continue work because of her nurturing husband, who looked after the baby with great love and care.

Reflection

In reflecting over the years of my practice as an obstetrician, I believe that there are a number of issues that a woman needs to consider before deciding whether to become pregnant. These are:

- The appropriate age for her first pregnancy in the context of her life
- Whether she is ready to limit her personal freedom
- Whether she likes children
- Whether the timing is right if she has an established career or owns a business
- Whether she has the support of her partner and family
- The level of her flexibility to cope if there are complications
- Whether she plans to stay at home for a long period after the birth
- Her childcare needs if returning to work

Motherhood is a very special role, but it may be best expressed as a nurturing responsibility. Looking after the physical, psychological, and social development of children while helping them to become functioning, independent adults requires long-term, dedicated effort and the ability to place the needs of dependent children first.

Transition

Elizabeth's story has highlighted a number of issues that are common to the experience of many mothers. These include the unpredictability of biology, causing a limit to the degree to which anyone can plan for a pregnancy or foresee what will be involved in order to live through it successfully. The desire to control pregnancy and birthing is not new, and emerges in different forms throughout history. We know that when agency is thwarted and women lose their sense of control during labor, their experience of giving birth becomes unfavorable (Mackey, 1999). Some cultures, and some individuals, are better able to flexibly approach the rhythms of human biology than others. Feminists have written extensively about the medical control of women and the process of reproduction. Historical perspectives are provided by Ulrich (1990), and further accounts describe mothers' current situations (e.g., Oakley, 1993; Brown, et al., 1994). In questioning the control exerted over women by the medical profession, many women have now moved from being the oppressed to being the oppressor, and expect, even demand, that their obstetrician control nature to their specification. Thus, we seem to have moved from one extreme to another, often losing sight of the fact that although childbirth is natural, without the benefits of current medical expertise it is risky and can even be fatal. Lack of support is a theme that occurs in Elizabeth's story of Leanne and was evident in Susan's story of Jane. This is common to the mothering narratives of women living in industrialized western cultures, and reflects the loneliness and emotional pain of becoming a mother in a society that does not provide adequate support to mothers (e.g. Crittenden, 2001; Esdaile & Greenwood, 1995a).

In the next story, told by Judith, the entire focus is on the occupation of achieving pregnancy and enfolding the demands of medical technology into a busy life and a lifestyle redesign to achieve pregnancy, rather than anticipate mothering, that can be highly stressful, and is seldom tranquil.

Judith's Story: Achieving Pregnancy and Medical Technology

I had four opportunities to experience the anticipating occupations of pregnancy, and had been remarkably well for each pregnancy. I recall the pleasure and the exhilaration these times of anticipation brought. However, working with mothers made me very aware that not every pregnancy is easy or filled with the pleasurable anticipating occupations. The uniqueness of the individual experience of pregnancy, with its concomitant potential for change, has always held a fascination for me. The story I have chosen to tell is very different from mine. Instead, I will share Sharon's story.

Sharon was a participant in a small qualitative research study that investigated the anticipatory occupations of women who used assistive reproductive technologies to become pregnant. So this story is actually about the anticipatory occupations of pregnancy rather than mothering per se. In the following vignette about Sharon and George, we hear about one couple's experience of participation in an IVF Program and the anticipatory occupations that resulted from Sharon's wish to have a baby of her own.

✄ Vignette: *Sharon*

Sharon and George hadn't really planned to have children. They were a career-oriented couple who thought that they would never want children. But then, as Sharon realized that she was getting older and that if she did want children, the decision would need to be made now, she changed her mind. She decided that she did want a child.

Sharon had always known that having a child in her marriage to George would require artificial insemination. A previous condition had resulted in his sterility. So Sharon knew that conceiving would require some additional planning. Furthermore, she knew that this planning included timing, and she had decided that she would like to conceive in the fall of the coming year. Sharon had no difficulty finding medical help because she was living in a large metropolitan area and working at a university hospital doing veterinary research. She was sure that, give or take 3 months, she could plan on a baby. This was going to be easy, almost natural even. All she needed was a sperm donor. Of course, that would take careful consideration because she wanted a child who would have visible physical characteristics connecting him or her to George and herself.

Financial considerations were minimal for this couple. Fortunately, they had insurance and lived in a state where insurance had to cover the medical expenses. Without much ado, Sharon made an appointment with an obstetrics and gynecology group. Early in her medical evaluation, Sharon was shocked to learn that she had cervical cancer in situ and her plans for conceiving would have to be on hold until she had surgery and recovered.

It was 6 months before insemination could be attempted. But Sharon did not become pregnant after the initial procedure, or indeed after several more. As her biological clock continued to tick away, and with no mechanical problems found to explain the lack of conception, Sharon began to realize how great her investment was in having a biological child of her own. This was when she and George agreed to in vitro fertilization (IVF). A full year and a half after her decision to have a child, Sharon became part of an IVF program. She began charting temperatures and managing the IVF program appointments during her 1-hour break at work. She was fortunate that her job allowed her the flexibility to come and go without questions being asked.

Sharon began a series of subcutaneous daily injections. The need for these injections resulted in several difficult situations for her. For example, on the first day of the first series, although George had been taught to give the injection, and he was competent at this task, he just could not do it. So Sharon had to contact a friend who was a nurse, tell her about the IVF Program, and ask her assistance. Another complication of the daily injections was that they needed to be given at a specific time of the day. On one particular occasion, Sharon had a business trip that occurred unscheduled. She had two choices: either cancel the trip or ask someone else to give her the injection, which meant sharing her situation with yet another person. She opted for the second and asked a medical practitioner who was on the trip to give her the injections. Sharon then had to return from her trip promptly so that the eggs could be harvested within 48 hours. The next step of the IVF procedure was placing the harvested eggs in a Petri dish with donor sperm for 48 hours. Sharon then had to return to the hospital for the replacement of the embryos in her uterus. During the replacement procedure, Sharon recalled being asked how many embryos to replace. In our interview, she described to me her confusion as she tried to make a judgment about this question.

After the replacement, Sharon had to remain in the hospital with her feet elevated. The position was difficult enough, but the environment made it worse for Sharon. In this facility, she was surrounded by women who were in various stages of labor and delivery because in this hospital the IVF facilities were merely rooms that adjoined the labor and delivery suite. Within a few days of the embryo replacement, Sharon was experiencing pain that resulted in a trip to the emergency room of her local hospital. The doctors there were reluctant to treat her because she had just had an embryo transfer. Eventually she was given morphine, but she needed to go to the university hospital. There the doctors did a laparoscopy and found that she had an ovarian cyst that had ruptured.

This first attempt at conception was unsuccessful. Nevertheless, Sharon was not dissuaded from continuing. In the meantime, concerns about finances were mounting because her insurance coverage did have limits. In addition, Sharon and George were just about to close on the purchase of a house that they needed for their family. Now, yet another sperm donor had to be chosen. When the arrangements were completed, a second cycle was instituted. But this time the process was successful. Sharon was pregnant at last.

After the news of this success, Sharon was plagued with concerns about her risk factors. After all, she was overweight, older, and had a potential for a multiple pregnancy: twins, triplets, or even quadruplets were possible. Then, at 6 weeks, Sharon and George learned that they were expecting twins. They had been aware of the increased likelihood of a multiple pregnancy, and now the likelihood had been confirmed. It was now time to tell their friends and family that they were expecting twins. Sharon began to consider what having twins would mean to their lives. What about their annual canoe trip? Would they need to change the house that they just purchased? What about Sharon's desire to have a vaginal delivery?

Sharon began to buy clothes that were bigger but that were not traditional maternity clothes. She began to take pregnancy preparation classes for delivery and breast-feeding. Reactions to her desire to breast-feed were mainly negative. People wondered whether she would be able to manage breast-feeding twins.

Fortunately, one lactation counselor was reassuring, noting that historically wet nurses could provide for up to six infants. The reality of twins had just been accepted when, at her next prenatal visit, a third heartbeat was discovered. They were going to have triplets. Although Sharon's science background had helped her to understand the possibility of multiple births, she was numbed by the notion of three babies. As she shared this news with friends and family, she found herself deluged with bags of clothing, along with offers of cribs and other items of equipment. Sharon and George felt that they would have no need to shop for anything for their babies.

During this entire time, Sharon had continued to work and even changed jobs. She had planned to work until the delivery date. But with the realization of the implications of having triplets, she knew that a cesarean delivery would now be required. In addition, she was told that her plan to continue working was not an acceptable option. At around 7 months, she would be required to go on bed rest. Sharon balked at this and considered that maybe she would reduce her work time to half-time, but monetary realities had to be considered. She could receive disability payment for loss of salary if she remained on bed rest, but she would receive nothing if she chose to work part-time. Sharon acknowledged later that she was living in a state of denial. She could not imagine stopping work, and was unable to prepare for it. Despite a strong science education and an intellectual understanding of her situation, Sharon was emotionally and psychologically incapable of considering the implications of triplets or the mothering occupations of caregiving that would be required after their birth.

Reflections

Sharon's is a story of a woman having different needs at different times in her life (Rothman, 1989). As her story began, Sharon had not wanted children. In her early 30s, she had pursued her career and the establishment of a stable relationship, seeming to have settled the question of whether or not to have children. Life reassessment comes at different times, but this came particularly at a time when society views a woman's biological clock as winding down for certain decisions. So, in her reassessment, in her late 30s, Sharon considered the tremendous number of factors—psychological, economic, and physical—that have an impact on having children and the various alternative ways that women who had previously chosen to be childless can mother. Then she asked herself the all-important question—what do I really want? Knowing that she still did have choices, Sharon chose to have a child. Her story then becomes one of self-determination, of allowing a woman to have control over her entry into the experience of being pregnant through the use of technology.

In technologically advanced countries such as the United States, where Sharon lived, giving birth could be a chosen occupation even when there was a lack or diminishment of the biological abilities of ovulating, conceiving, and gestating. Sharon did not have the biological conditions that resulted in an easy conception. She did, however, have social, environmental, and personal strengths. Her story is an example of how a woman with financial means, excellent health care, a high level of education, and know-how had the agency that was needed to navigate the maze of assistive reproductive technologies. She was able to overcome many challenges in order to participate in the process of pregnancy and birth giving, her chosen occupation.

Sharon's story has little mention of preparation for the mothering identity. Caught of necessity in the medicalized world of assistive reproductive technology, her focus was on conceiving and gestating. When that was successful, Sharon faced the cost of her choice; she was expecting three children instead of just the one that she had wanted. Sharon described herself as numbed by this discovery. Unable to consider the implications of multiple births, Sharon turned her energy to her career, even planning to work up to the moment of delivery. Reflecting on her situation during our interview, Sharon recognized that she had been in denial. This denial negated the possibility of lifestyle redesign before birth giving. This was something she had to face later.

﹋ The Theoretical Context

In the following section we discuss the major theoretical influences on our thinking about mothering occupations within the social, cultural, biological, and historical experience that mothers share with their peers. These theoretical influences have led us to view mothering occupations from a phenomenological, feminist perspective of power and agency.

A Phenomenological, Feminist Perspective of Power and Agency

Feminist research and literature have led to the development of a number of theoretical perspectives in relation to women generally and mothers in particular. Dowling (1982) explored issues of dependency in *The Cinderella Complex,* suggesting that, in wishing to be saved and protected from challenge and stress and assuming a supportive rather than an active role, women risked becoming helpless to the point of being dysfunctional. In contrast, this myth of women's wish for protection and dependency has been questioned by those writing from a feminist psychotherapy perspective (Eichenbaum & Orbach, 1985), as well as others (Oakley, 1993) who have suggested that women are actually caught in a double bind situation between conflicting role demands of home and workplace. The wish for protection and the seeming negation of agency to achieve it have deep-rooted historical antecedents. Given the state of almost continuous pregnancy and high infant and maternal mortality with which all married women once lived (Fraser, 1984), the need for protection was a harsh reality. However, educated women with financial means, like the mid-18th century woman of letters, Lady Mary Wortley Montagu (Halsband, 1986), were still able to ensure that their voices were heard. Other women, who worked for a living, for example the late 18th and early 19th century New England midwife Martha Ballard (Ulrich, 1990), had some degree of independence and

kept their own earnings. However, Mistress Ballard still deferred to the mothers in her care in relation to their husbands, whom she acknowledged as the head of the family. Before the 20th century, women had little legal power, but we should not forget that this situation also applied to men without property.

The negation of agency by women appears to have become stronger during the latter part of the 19th century than it had been during the more robust, less sentimental time 100 or so years earlier. The way in which Jane Addams wrote about her carefully planned and executed welfare work as something that happened to her serendipitously, by chance, has been strongly criticized by current feminists, who believe that women still have not recovered from this role modeling and learned to fully claim their agency (e.g., Heilbrun, 1988; Ker Conway, 1998). Our work has led us to believe that when the cause is urgent, the motivation strong, and the action on behalf of dependent others, especially a woman's own children or other children, women's agency is readily visible (e.g., Olson & Esdaile, 2000). The aim of activism within a feminist context is power: "...as the ability to take one's place in whatever discourse is essential to action and the right to have one's part matter." (Heilbrun, 1988, p. 18). In Chapter 14 of this book, Llewellyn, Thompson, and Whybrow describe an example of mothers' occupation of activism.

Women's power struggle against the tyranny of experts is historically long and well recorded. These experts appear in every generation, telling mothers how to behave during their pregnancy and how to bring up their children. Frequently the experts undermine women's confidence and contradict each other, creating confusion (Hardyment, 1983). Feminists have argued that presenting women as incompetent, in need of expert guidance, has enabled the professions of obstetrics and pediatrics to flourish. However, by the first quarter of the 20th century, it also became possible for women to practice in these branches of the medical profession (Deacon, 1985; Reiger, 1986). We believe that finding a balance in this argument is essential; otherwise it can become oversimplified. Scientific development in the medical profession has made pregnancy and birth giving safer, and has also contributed to the reduction of infant mortality, a critical indicator of the health of a population. Reality is always multifaceted because, despite advanced medical technology, poverty is still associated with health risk, especially high infant mortality. Thus, in some parts of the United States, infant mortality, especially for African-Americans, remains as high as in a Third-World country (Shirilla, 2002). Additionally, mothers who live in poverty, on the edge of a wealthy society, are infantilized and trivialized as well as marginalized (Coll, Surrey, & Weingarten, 1998; Polakow, 1993).

It also seems that the valuing of fecundity still exerts power over women. During previous times, there was a strong connection between childbearing and Divine grace because it was believed that, through childbearing, women could atone for the sins they inherited from Eve. So childless women bewailed their fate and resorted to many remedies that today we would consider bizarre (Fraser, 1984). Poor women in some cultures still suffer greatly from the consequences of infertility (Inhorn, 2000). In our industrial culture, we believe in the inherent goodness of research and the technological advances that it can generate. The fact that we also have the resources to support research has lead to sophisticated technological advances in enabling fertility (Sher, Davis, & Stoess, 1995). Because of our tacit message that research and its outcomes are good, we now overtly, or covertly, encourage childless women to endure extraordinary intrusion to their lives in order to achieve pregnancy. Therefore it can still be said that women endure the *tyranny* of experts, often male and—in historical sequence— from the disciplines of theology, medicine, and technology. Claiming their agency in order to participate fully in society, on their own terms remains a challenge for many women.

Given the conflicting challenges that women experience, especially in regard to mothering, it isn't surprising that motherhood is associated with ambivalence. The heartache of this ambivalence and the powerlessness of mothers in a patriarchal society have been most eloquently described by Rich

(1995). Others have suggested that the ambivalence is not about mothering itself, but mothering under the conditions of isolation, in a nuclear family, with a particular set of beliefs about mothering that are self-negating and lead to feelings of incompetence and stress (Davis & Welch, 1986). This enforced isolation that separates women from support is heard in the voices of many women in this and other chapters of this text. Isolation is a contradiction of female development for which connectedness is so important (Gilligan, 1982; Smith, 1999). This connectedness is so important because, without it, motherhood cannot be supported adequately and so becomes a misery of loneliness. The male paradigm of seeking separateness, connected by rules (Shrewsbury, 1987) is not readily applicable to the occupations of mothering.

Mothering Viewed Through an Occupational Lens

In this perspective we focus on mothers' occupational engagement within the context of their mothering, adopting an occupational science definition of *occupation*, as units of meaningful activity that can be named in the lexicon of the culture (Clark et al., 1991; Yerxa et al., 1989; Zemke & Clark, 1996). Occupational science has its roots in occupational therapy, and has drawn theoretically and methodologically on biological and social sciences. Occupation is rich in symbolic meaning, and for this reason, Yerxa, who is credited with founding the emerging discipline of occupational science, believes that qualitative methods of inquiry are more suited to this discipline than experimental methods (1991). Currently emerging shifts in the conceptualization of social and behavioral sciences that acknowledge the importance of rich, reflexive analysis as the appropriate form of inquiry support her views. Attempting to emulate the methodology of physical and biological sciences to study human behavior, values, and power can lead to a diminished perspective of them (Flyvbjerg, 2001).

Because occupation is such an ubiquitous concept, it can be rendered meaningless if viewed outside its sociocultural, historical and individual context. For example, many western women wear *make-up* on their face. A hundred years ago, *respectable* women did not wear make-up, and in some cultures this still applies, or the wearing of facial decoration is expressed differently. How women in our culture practice this occupation of facial enhancement varies with individuals; some do it daily, others for special social occasions. Among some groups of affluent North American women, facial enhancement involving surgery is an acceptable, meaningful occupation. A number of distinct constructs and views about occupation have emerged under the umbrella of occupational science during the past decade. Some of these are discussed below.

Health through occupation is not a new notion. Wilcock (1999, 2001) has provided an informed account of the way the lifestyle of individuals was believed to influence their health, and how a set of rules for health, the *Regimen Sanitatis*, was developed in the Middle Ages. The moral philosophies of the 18th and 19th centuries, and reformers such as Thomas Carlyle and Octavia Hill, recognized the relationship between health and meaningful occupation. They provided the philosophical and theoretical as well as the practical impetus to the development of the profession of occupational therapy. Wilcock believes that the consideration of humans as occupational beings needs to be an essential concern of societies and must be addressed at the policy-making level to ensure the health of communities (Wilcock, 1998).

Occupational engagement by itself may not promote well-being; it is also important to achieve occupational balance. The notion of an optimal level of occupational engagement had been emphasized by the founders of the profession of occupational therapy, and was incorporated into treatment plans for patients with mental illness (Christiansen, 1996). The concept of occupational balance has been described in relation to adaptation and time use and as the balance in the relationship of life tasks. A common perspective on occupational balance that Christiansen has questioned is the time budget approach, in which activities have intrinsic meaning for the individual, so longer time engagement in the valued occupations is thought to promote well-being.

Another view of balance that he describes is based on chronobiology, suggesting that balance is achieved when internal clocks and external behaviors are synchronized. The mother-child co-occupation of feeding and eating, discussed by Olson in Chapter 2 of this book, supports this perspective of balance. A third perspective, offered by Christiansen, is based on the work of Little et al. (1983) and presents a view of occupational balance as the degree of congruence between an individual's goal-oriented *personal projects* and investment, plus success in the achievement of these projects.

The concept of lifestyle redesign has been central to occupational therapy practice since the inception of the profession and relates directly to earlier concepts of health through occupation (Clark, 1993; Meyer, 1977; Wilcock, 1998; 1999; 2001). In her 1993 Eleanor Clark Slagle lecture, Clark quoted Penny Richardson, stroke survivor, who said that occupational therapy involved "recycling the old me into the new one" (Clark, Ennevor & Richardson, 1996, p. 374). This concept was further elaborated by Clark and her associates (Clark et al., 1997; Jackson et al., 1998) in their study of well elderly people in the Los Angles area, in which they demonstrated empirically that lifestyle redesign, assisted through individually prescribed occupational therapy, can maintain and enhance health and well-being. In this chapter, we have extended this concept to include health and well-being in the anticipating occupations of mothering.

A recognition of the relationships between health and occupational engagement has led to the consideration of occupational deprivation and occupational justice. Townsend has explored the differences and similarities between social justice and occupational justice, and the feasibility of a utopian world in which everyone has opportunities for meaningful occupation (1992). Whiteford (2000) has further described the effect of global and national economic forces that have led to social changes, resulting in marginalization of some groups in society. These groups are being excluded from paid employment and participation in leisure activities as a consequence of unemployment. Thus, people on the edge of both rural and urban societies are rendered occupationally deprived. Discourse about occupational justice is often community focused, exploring ways to expand occupational opportunities. The exclusion of the poor and educationally disadvantaged from occupational opportunities is reminiscent of feminist discourse about the marginalization and exclusion of women in general, and mothering women more particularly (e.g. Coll, et al., 1998; Polakow, 1993).

Feminism and mothering are both dynamic concepts that continue to be reconceptualized and reinvented. Holloway (1999), predicating her argument on a body of late 20th century feminist literature, postulates that motherhood is an invented construct that has been differently defined with different rules, expectations and limits. Even the most cursory exploration of motherhood in a historical context (e.g., Fischer, 1989; Fraser, 1984) will support the concept that: "far from being a simple, natural experience, motherhood is a complex social phenomenon: it varies over time and space, and is intimately bound up with normative ideas of femininity" (Holloway, 1999, p. 91) that are culturally determined. As an ideology, feminism has evolved from a focus on the equality of women that considered the role of women as wives and mothers "oppressive" (Speier, 2001). A more current view of feminism is as "an inclusive model of liberation for all people, with particular attention given to the status of women and the elimination of sexism" (Hamlin, Loukas, Froehlich, & McRae, 1992, p. 967). Women of color have made a major contribution to feminist debate through their traditional valuing of mothering, and in presenting the perspective of working class and minority women (Hill Collins, 1991).

Anthropologists have described mothering occupations extensively. A more recent example is the concept of enfolded occupations (Bateson, 1990) to describe the way women, and particularly mothers, enfold household work and childcare, simultaneously attending to and executing both. Recent research in neuroscience supports the fact that gender differences in women's behavior are biologically, as well as socially, determined. Medical

scientists have monitored brain activity using advanced imaging devices such as positron emission tomography (PET) and functional magnetic resonance imaging (MRI) to demonstrate that women are able to listen to several things at once more readily than men (Mayo Clinic Women's Health Source, 2002). Others discuss the application of this construct in research about mothers in chapters of this text, for example Griffin in Chapter 3, and Pierce and Marshall in Chapter 4. Occupational scientists and occupational therapists have written about mothering occupations from a variety of perspectives, using mainly qualitative methodology "to generate knowledge by unpacking the storied nature of occupation that would have lost its richness if quantified." (Zemke & Clark, 1996, p. viii). Their philosophical framework shared similarities with Ruddick's (1995) ideas about the nature of maternal thinking, in believing that "unity of thought, judgment, and emotion emanates from everyday practices." (Zemke & Clark, 1996, p. viii).

Several of these authors have written chapters in this book. Pierce (2000) has used techniques derived from primatology research to examine the way in which mothers create play space for their children. Mothering children with special needs has been described by several occupational scientists/therapists. Pierce and Frank (1992) used feminist analysis to describe the family-centered care given by a mother to her child with severe, multiple disabilities. Larson (2000) has described mothers' orchestration of daily occupations in terms of the specialized maternal work of caring for a child with a disability, and implications for mothers' sense of well-being. She has also explored the paradox of meaning associated with family concepts of disability (1998). Kellegrew (2000) used ecocultural theory to examine the influence of ecological constraints and cultural values in mothers' construction of daily routines for their children with disabilities. Segal (2000) has described the adaptive strategies of mothers who have children with attention deficit hyperactivity disorder in terms of enfolding and unfolding occupations. Cohn (2001) used the experience of mothers waiting for treatment for their child to explore the transition from waiting to meaningful relating with others and the benefits of peer support. We (Olson & Esdaile, 2000) have looked at the influence of a challenging urban environment on mothering occupations for women who have children with disability. These are examples, not a comprehensive literature review. Many of these themes will be discussed further by some of the above-mentioned authors, who are also contributors to this text.

Giving Birth and Mothering

Ruddick's (1994) distinction between giving birth and mothering provides a starting point for understanding some of the anticipating occupations of mothering and their antecedent factors. Women who give birth are birth givers, and it is true that most birth givers do become mothers. Yet the occupations of preparing for giving birth and mothering are not necessarily the same. Both require commitment and responsibility, but neither is a necessary condition, nor is one the necessary consequence of the other. This distinction allows us to consider these two occupations as separate although connected. Ruddick (1994) offers us three thoughts about birth giving. First, she considers the occupation of giving birth as a choice. In technologically sophisticated countries like the United States, giving birth has the possibility of being a chosen occupation. There will always be exceptions, as in the case of women who would choose to terminate a pregnancy, but because of financial, religious, or other circumstances, do not. In general, though, giving birth can be an occupation that a woman can choose, even if it requires technological support. Second, there are "demands" that pregnancy and giving birth make on women. We would suggest that Ruddick's demands could be recast as anticipatory occupations. These include waiting as an occupation, preparing for the birthing experience, and preparing for the homecoming and establishment of a new person within an already existing family. And, finally, Ruddick speculates that giving birth gives rise to the acquisition of certain cognitive and emotional capacities. Here we use Ruddick's three thoughts about birth giving to structure the discussion of the anticipatory occupations of mothering and its antecedent factors.

Pregnant women are typically referred to as *expecting*. This seems to be an appropriate term because the 9 months (more or less) of pregnancy are a time of anticipation of the new life that is to come. "Pregnancy is an active, receptive waiting..." (Ruddick, 1994, p. 39). Furthermore, this "active waiting has an intrinsic relational character" (Ruddick, p. 39). The waiting is not a solitary experience but an occupation of caring for the developing fetus as the mother simultaneously cares for herself. During this waiting time, many health-related choices must be made. This may include weighing medical evidence about moderate social drinking during pregnancy and the effects of smoking on the fetus.

Stern and Bruschweiler-Stern have developed the concept of the "motherhood mindset" (1998, p. 6). This is comparable to Ruddick's thought about the acquisition of new cognitive and emotional capacities (1994). The Sterns have written that the development of the motherhood mindset is not an automatic process, but requires active participation and acknowledgment that lifestyle and self are truly being irrevocably transformed, thus supporting the notion of lifestyle redesign. They further believe that this mindset becomes a permanent part of a woman and is used extensively at first when children are young. Although this mindset may recede, it lasts a lifetime, always ready to come forward when needed, such as when a child is sick (Stern, 1999; Stern & Bruschweiler-Stern, 1998). As an example, in Chapter 8 of this text, Francis-Connolly discusses the ongoing nature of mothering across the lifecourse.

✍ Challenges from Current Reading

The limited literature available on mothering that was described in Susan's story and supported by Speier (2001) is in sharp contrast with the current situation. Women who consider becoming mothers have a large volume of publications to consider. Additionally, there are Web sites and a range of media sources.

Much of the information presented by those who write for the general public is contradictory. An editorial in the New York Times stated that: "Not since the Victorians gave us the Angel in the House has motherhood been so fashionable. Every female celebrity worth her Psion is dropping or preparing to drop." (the *New York Times,* June 29, 2002, p.25). The article names several well known women in their late 30s, late 40s, and early 50s who have had or are having their first child, suggesting that babies have become a status symbol for mature women with established careers. However, Hewlett (2002) has been causing controversy by stating that postponing motherhood until a woman is over 30 is risky because it can lead to childlessness, despite the advances in reproductive technology. The fact that Hewlett herself had her last child when over 40 has added fuel to the debate. The tone of her book and the debate it has generated are far removed from Frydman's (1987) celebration of the fact that she and her fellow mature-age mothers were able to become mothers in midlife without criticism or medical risk.

Other popular authors, such as Wolf (2001) and Cusk (2001), present motherhood with considerable ambivalence. They highlight the emotional burdens, the physical violence of birth itself, and the difficulty of finding a cooperative as well as competent obstetrician. Wolf is additionally very critical of other writers like Eisenberg, Murkoff and Hathaway (1996), who have written an extensive book on preparing for motherhood that Wolf believes presents an unrealistic picture, glossing over the realities. Wolf's account of her search for the right obstetrician adds weight to Elizabeth's reasons for giving up the practice of obstetrics. Wolf also describes the life-altering choices that women are able to make, and do make, with the aid of genetic testing, amniocentesis tests and the availability and the possibility of terminating the pregnancy if the child has a genetic defect. She tells the story of a woman who wanted to ensure that her child did not inherit a gene for progressive deafness from her husband. As this gene affects only males, and there is no specific test for it, she had three pregnancies of male embryos terminated. Cusk even questions whether motherhood is of real interest to anyone. Her view is echoed by Crittenden (2001), an economics journalist, who argues that women have been liberated but mothers have not. Possibly the most ethically challenging aspect of the paradoxical choices created through advanced technology is that the anticipating occupation of mothering, for some people, includes a quest for a child with no potential health problems. There are many ethical questions that remain unanswered in regard to how the diversity of disability is accepted or rejected.

Women who want to be mothers are left with a paradox of choices and possibilities. They are urged to have children earlier than most professional women now do, but assailed by powerful and glamorous role models who are having children at a life stage when they could biologically be grandmothers. Having made the decision to have a child, or children, they then need to negotiate an emotional and technological minefield of choices in health care. For many, such as Sharon, the mother of IFV triplets whose story was told by Judith, this includes the maze of reproductive technology. Making ethically complex, emotionally charged, life-altering choices is a major anticipating occupation of mothering for women in industrialized, western cultures in the 21st century.

✎ Conclusion

Women engage in a variety of occupations to overcome challenges to become mothers, claim their agency during pregnancy and birth giving, and participate in society as mothering caregivers. We have used the stories of four women, Jane, Leanne, Amanda, and Sharon, to create threads that weave through this chapter and illustrate our theoretical assumptions. The importance of acknowledging and respecting individual experience is an important factor that we acknowledge. Occupational balance is essential for health, a sense of well-being, and a sense of competence, but individuals achieve it differently. For Jane, it involved choosing to work part-time. But this was not an option that the other mothers whose stories we told had chosen. However, in their different ways, they all identified problems associated with a lack of support, and added emphasis to the relational nature of mothering. Influenced by an ideology that encourages autonomy, the four mothers whose stories we told anticipated autonomy but experienced lack of support as a challenge in their role as mothering caregivers. Jane was separated from her family and close friends; Leanne had to deal with the breakup of her marriage; Amanda's mothering was contingent on her more nurturing partner; and Sharon, who had been totally focused on achieving pregnancy, also faced these issues, although later than the other three mothers.

In countries such as the United States, there are no universal maternal and child health services available to all mothers on a drop-in, self-referral basis. There are excellent services available, but they are not centrally located and, being differently organized in different locations, are less easy to access. They also tend to be more problem based, predicated on the assumption that mothers can cope alone, with visits to a pediatrician and support from their own families, or from fee-based childcare services. In many neighborhoods mothers get together and form support groups. However, the mothers who form these support groups tend to be the better educated, more financially secure mothers who have the time and initiative to organize. The Internet has made it easier for all mothers to locate their local group. However, often those experiencing the most urgent problems are the ones least likely to seek out a support group of women they do not know. The fact that many mothers with "normal" infants still have problems was a major factor in the development of Infant Mental Health Services. The work of infant mental health specialists and mothers' experience of this service is discussed in Chapter 2.

Pregnancy and birth giving continue to be areas in which much research is needed. Any discussion about this in respect to the physical and biological sciences is beyond the scope of this chapter. Given my interest in the lived, everyday experiences of mothers and the challenges inherent in these experiences, I (Susan) have often been asked why these seemingly common-sense concerns need to be researched. Why do we need research to support the "obvious," basic human needs that intrinsically (at "gut level") most of us acknowledge, and in our hearts know to be true? My answer is: because every generation has to understand and distill basic, fundamental truths within its own cultural and historical context in order to suit its needs and focus. There has to be a scholarly, disciplined, objective and rigorous way to do this. In order to make it available, and meaningful to others, we have to distill "the truth" through a scholarly process. Without this discipline, it remains amorphous, and unintelligible. Research is one such scholarly process that is held in high regard and accepted by our age. Literature and the arts also provide options for this disciplinary process, as do the disciplines of philosophy and theology; we just happen to value them less at the turn of the 21st century.

Discussion Questions

■ Do you think that lifestyle redesign should be a part of the anticipating occupations of mothering?

■ Describe an experience related to anticipating mothering from your own life or work and compare this with the experience of one of the mothers described in this chapter.

■ Do you agree that mothers generally lack support? What could you do to compensate for this within your sphere of work?

■ Why are mothers ambivalent about mothering? Do you believe that this is an acceptable fact, or would you want to change this perception? Support your response with empirical and theoretical evidence.

References

Bateson, M.C. (1990). *Composing a life*. New York, NY: A Plume Book.

Brown, S., Lumley, J., Small, R., & Astbury, J. (1994). *Missing voices. The experience of motherhood*. Oxford, UK: Oxford University Press.

Bruner, J. (1990). *Acts of meaning*. New York: Routledge.

Christiansen, C. (1996). Three perspectives on balance in occupation. In R. Zemke & F. Clark (1996) (Eds.). *Occupational science. The evolving discipline.* Philadelphia: F. A. Davis, pp. 431–451.

Clark, F.A. (1993). Occupation embedded in a real life: Interweaving occupational science and occupational therapy. 1993 Eleanor Clark Slagle lecture. *American Journal of Occupational Therapy, 47,* 1067–1078.

Clark, F., Azen, S., Carlson, M., Mandel, D., LaBree, L., Zemke, R., Hay, J., Jackson, J., & Lipson, L. (2001). Embedding health-promoting changes into the daily lives of independent-living older adults: Long-term follow-up of occupational therapy intervention. *Journal of Gerontology, 56B,* 60–63.

Clark, F., Azen, S., Zemke, R., Jackson, J., Carlson, M., Mandel, D., Hay, J., Josephson, K., Cherry, B., Hessel, C., Palmer, J., & Lipson, L. (1997). Occupational therapy for independent-living older adults: A randomized controlled trial. *Journal of the American Medical Association, 278,* 1321–1326.

Clark, F., Ennevor, B. L., & Richardson, P.L. A grounded theory of techniques for occupational storytelling and occupational story making. In R. Zemke & F. Clark (1996) (Eds.). *Occupational science. The evolving discipline.* Philadelphia: F. A. Davis, pp 373–392.

Clark, F. A., Parham, D., Carlson, M. E., Frank, G., Jackson, J., Pierce, D., Wolfe, R., & Zemke, R. (1991). Occupational science: An academic innovation in the service of occupational therapy's future. *American Journal of Occupational Therapy, 45,* 300–310.

Cohn, E. S. (2001). From waiting to relating: Parents' experiences in the waiting room of an occupational therapy clinic. *American Journal of Occupational Therapy, 55,* 167–174.

Coll, C. G., Surrey, J. L., & Weingarten, K. (Eds.) (1998). *Mothering against the odds. Diverse voices of contemporary mothers.* New York: The Guilford Press.

Cooper, S., & Glazer, E. (1994). *Beyond infertility: The new pathways to parenthood.* NY: Lexington Books.

Crittenden, A. (2001). *The price of motherhood. Why the most important job in the world is least valued.* New York: Metropolitan Books.

Cusk, R. (2001). *A life's work. Becoming a mother.* New York: Picador, USA.

Davis, B., & Welch, D. (1986). Motherhood and feminism: Are they compatible? The ambivalence of mothering. *Australian and New Zealand Journal of Sociology, 22*(3), 411–426.

Deacon, D. (1985). "Taylorism" in the home: The medical profession, the infant welfare movement and the deskilling of women. *Australian and New Zealand Journal of Sociology, 21,* 161–173.

Dowling, C. (1982). *The Cinderella complex.* Blackburn Victoria, Australia: Fontana.

Eichenbaum, L., & Orbach, S. (1985). *Understanding women.* Harmondsworth, UK: Penguin.

Eisenberg, A., Murkoff, H. F., & Hathaway, S. E. (1996). *What to expect when you are expecting.* New York: Workman Publishing.

Esdaile, S. A., & Greenwood, K. M. (1995a) Issues of parenting stress: A study involving mothers of toddlers. *Journal of Family Studies, 1*(2), 153–165.

Esdaile, S. A, & Greenwood, K. (1995b). A survey of mothers' relationship with their preschoolers. *Occupational Therapy International, 2*(3), 204–219.

Evans, K. The mother of all myths. Melbourne, Victoria, Australia: *The Sunday Age Magazine.* 2002, Jan 27, 17–19.

Fischer, D.H. (1989). *Albion's seed. Four British folkways in America.* New York: Oxford University Press.

Flyvbjerg, B. (2001). *Making social science matter. Why social inquiry fails and how it can succeed again.* Cambridge, UK: Cambridge University Press.

Fraser, A. (1984). *The weaker vessel. Woman's lot in seventeenth-century England.* London, UK: Methuen.

Frydman, G. (1987). *Mature-age mothers.* Ringwood Victoria: Penguin Australia.

Gilligan, C. (1982). *In a different voice: Psychological theory and women's development.* Cambridge, MA: Harvard University Press.

Halsband, R. (Ed.) (1986). *The selected letters of Lady Mary Wortley Montagu.* Harmondsworth, UK: Penguin.

Hamlin, R. B., Loukas, K. M., Froehlich, J., & MacRae, N. (1992). Feminism: An inclusive perspective. *American Journal of Occupational Therapy, 46*(11), 967–970.

Hardyment, C. (1983). *Dream babies. Childcare from Locke to Spock.* London, UK: Jonathan Cape.

Heilbrun, C. (1988). *Writing a woman's life.* New York: Ballantine Books.

Hewlett, S.A. (2002). *Creating a life. Professional women and the quest for children.* New York: Talk Miramax Books.

Hill Collins, P. (1991). *Black feminist thought. Knowledge, consciousness, and the politics of empowerment.* New York: Routledge.

Holloway, S. L. (1999). Reproducing motherhood. In N. Laurie, C. Dwyer, S. L. Holloway, & F. M. Smith (Eds). *Geographies of new femininities.* New York: Pearson Education Ltd.

Inhorn, M.C. (2000). Missing motherhood: Infertility, technology, and poverty in Egyptian women's lives. In H. Ragoné & F. Winddance Twine (2000). *Ideologies and technologies of motherhood. Race, class, sexuality, nationalism.* New York: Routledge, pp 139–168.

Jackson, J., Carlson, M., Mandel, D., Zemke, R., & Clark, F. (1998). Occupation in lifestyle redesign: The well-elderly study occupational therapy program. *American Journal of Occupational Therapy, 52,* 326–336.

Kellegrew, D. H. (2000). Constructing daily routines: A qualitative examination of mothers with young children with disability. *American Journal of Occupational Therapy, 54,* 252–259.

Ker Conway, J. (1998) *When memory speaks. Exploring the art of autobiography.* New York: Vintage Books.

Larson, E.A. (2000). The orchestration of occupation: The dance of mothers. *American Journal of Occupational Therapy, 54,* 269–280.

Larson, E.A. (1998). Reframing the meaning of disability to families: The embrace of paradox. *Social Science and Medicine, 47,* 865–875.

Little, B. R. (1983). Personal projects: A rationale and method for investigation. *Environment and Behavior, 15,* 273–309.

Mackey, M. (1999). Women's evaluation of the labor and delivery experience. *Nursing Connections, 11,* 19–32.

March of Dimes (1999). Pregnancy after age 35. Retrieved August 26, 2002 from *noah-health.org/english/pregnancy/march_of_dimes/pre_preg.plan/after30.html*

Mayo Clinic Women's Health Source (2002). Women are different from men. It's a matter of biology. *Mayo Clinic Women's Health Source, 6.* (9), 1–2.

Meyer, A. (1977). The philosophy of occupation therapy. *American Journal of Occupational Therapy, 31,* 639–642.

New York Times (June 29, 2002). Dad's mags. Lads have much to learn from dads. New York: the *New York Times,* p. 25.

Oakley, A. (1993). *Essays on women, medicine and health.* Edinburgh, UK: University of Edinburgh Press.

Olson, J. A., & Esdaile, S. A. (2000). Mothering young children with disabilities in a challenging urban environment. *American Journal of Occupational Therapy, 54,* 307–314.

Pierce, D. (2000). Maternal management of the home as a developmental play space for infants and toddlers. *American Journal of Occupational Therapy, 54,* 290–299.

Pierce D., & Frank, G. (1992). A mother's work: Two levels of feminist analysis of family centered care. *American Journal of Occupational Therapy, 46,* 972–980.

Polakow, V. (1993). *Lives on the edge. Single mothers and their children in the other America.* Chicago: The University of Chicago Press.

Priority Health. (2002). Expanded prenatal education services. Insights. Retrieved October 27, 2002 from *priority-health.com/providers/newsletters/insights/current//05.htm*

Recker, N. (1998). Delayed parenting. The Ohio State University Fact Sheet FLM-FS-9-98. Retrieved August 26, 2002 from *ohioline.osu.edu/flm98/fs09.html*

Reiger, K. (1986). Mothering deskilled? Australian child rearing and the "experts." *Community Health Studies, X,* (1), 39–46.

Rich, A. (1995). *Of woman born. Motherhood as experience and institution.* New York: W. W. Norton & Company.

Rothman, B. (1989). *Recreating motherhood.* New Brunswick: Rutgers University Press.

Ruddick, S. (1995). *Maternal thinking. Toward a politics of peace.* Boston, MA: Beacon Press.

Ruddick, S. (1994). *Thinking mothers/conceiving birth .*In D. Bassin, M. Honey, & M. Kaplan (Eds.). *Representations of motherhood* (pp. 29–45). New Haven: Yale University Press.

Ruddick, S. (1983). Maternal thinking. In J. Treblicot (Ed.), *Mothering: Essays in feminist theory.* (pp. 213–230). Savage, MD: Rowan & Littlefield.

Sandelowski , M., Harris, B. G., Holditch-Davis, D. (1989). Mazing: Infertile couples and the quest for a child. *Image: Journal of Nursing Scholarship, 21,* 220–226.

Segal, R. (2000). Adaptive strategies of mothers with children with attentions deficit hyperactivity disorder: Enfolding and unfolding occupations. *American Journal of Occupational Therapy, 54,* 300–306.

Sher, G., Davis, V., & Stoess, J. (1995). *In vitro fertilization: The A. R. T. of making babies.* NY: Facts on File.

Shirilla, J. (2002). Infant mortality. *The Infant Voice.* Metropolitan Detroit Association for Infant Mental Health. Winter, 2002, 2.

Shrewsbury, C. M. (1987). What is feminist pedagogy? *Women's Studies Quarterly, XV,* 3 & 4 (Fall/Winter), 6–13.

Smith, J. A. (1999). Towards a relational self: Social engagement during pregnancy and psychological preparation for motherhood. *British Journal of Social Psychology, 38,* 409–426.

Speier, D. (2001). Becoming a mother. *Journal of the Association for Research on Mothering, 3*(1), 7–18.

Stern, D.L. (1999). *The motherhood constellation.* New York: Basic Books.

Stern, D., & Burnschweiler-Stern, N. (1998). *The birth of a mother.* New York: Basic Books.

Townsend, E. (1992). Institutional ethnography: Explicating the social organization of professional health practices intending client empowerment. *Canadian Journal of Occupational Therapy, 55,* 65–70.

Ulrich, L.T. (1990). *A midwife's tale. The life of Martha Ballard based on her diary 1785–1812.* New York: Vintage Books.

Whiteford, G. (2000). Occupational deprivation: Global challenge in the new millennium. *British Journal of Occupational Therapy, 63,* 200–204.

Wilcock, A. (1998). *An occupational perspective on health.* Thorofare, NJ: Slack Inc.

Wilcock, A. (1999). *Occupation for health, Volume 1. A journey from self health to prescription.* London, UK: College of Occupational Therapists.

Wilcock, A. (2001). *Occupation for health, Volume 2. A journey from to prescription to self health.* London, UK: College of Occupational Therapists.

Wolf, N. (2001). *Misconceptions. Truth, lies and the unexpected journey to motherhood.* New York: Doubleday.

Yerxa, E.J. (1991). Nationally speaking: Seeking a relevant, ethical and realistic way of knowing for occupational therapy. *American Journal of Occupational Therapy, 45,* 199–204

Yerxa, E. J., Clark, F., Frank, G., Jackson, J., Praham, D., Pierce, D., Stein, C., & Zemke, R. (1989). An introduction to occupational science, a foundation for occupational therapy in the 21st century. *Occupational Therapy in Health Care, 6,* 1.

Zemke, R., & Clark, F. (1996) (Eds.). *Occupational science. The evolving discipline.* Philadelphia: F.A. Davis.

Additional Readings

GENERAL

Barnard, K. E., & Martell, L. K. (1995). *Mothering.* In M. H. Bornstein (Ed.). *Handbook of parenting volume 3. Status and social conditions of parenting.* New Jersey: Lawrence Erlbaum Associates, Inc., pp. 3–26.

Boulton, M. G. (1983). *On being a mother. A study of women with preschool children.* London: Tavistock Publications.

Chodorow, N. J. (1999). *The reproduction of mothering.* Berkeley and Los Angeles, CA: University of California Press.

Daly, B., & Reddy, M. T. (Eds.). (1991). *Narrating mothers. Theorizing maternal subjectivities.* Knoxville, TE: University of Tennessee Press.

Glenn, E. N., Chang, G., & Forcey, L. R. (1994). *Mothering, ideology, experience, and agency.* New York: Routledge.

Hattery, A. (2001). *Women, work and family. Balancing and weaving.* Thousand Oaks, CA: Sage Publications.

Hrdy, S. B. (1999). *Mother nature. A history of mothers, infants, and natural selection.* New York: Random House Inc.

Nicholson, J. (1983). *The heartache of motherhood.* Ringwood: Penguin Australia.

Placksin, S. (1998). *Mothering the new mother.* 2nd edition. New York: New Market Press.

Ragoné, H., & Winddance Twine, F. (2000). *Ideologies and technologies of motherhood. Race, class, sexuality, nationalism.* New York: Routledge.

Teicher, M.H. (2002). Scars that won't heal: The neurobiology of child abuse. *Scientific American, 286*(3), 68–75.

Watson, P. (2001). *The modern mind. An intellectual history of the 20th century.* New York: Harper Collins.

Articles from the *Journal of the Association of Research on Mothering.* Volume 1(1) (1999): Mothering and motherhood; Volume 3, (1)(2001): Becoming a mother, and other issues. Also, visit the web site for the *Association for Research on Mothering.* http://www.yorku.ca/crm

TRANSITION TO PARENTHOOD

Ball, R. E. (1993). Children and marital happiness of Black Americans. *Journal of Marriage and and the Family, 55*, 203–218.

Belsky, J., Lang, M., & Rovine, M. (1985). Stability and change in marriage across the transition to parenthood: A second study. *Journal of Marriage and the Family, 47*, 855–865.

Belsky, J., Lang, M., & Huston, T. L. (1986). Sex typing and division of labor as determinants of Marital change across the transition to parenthood. *Journal of Personality and Social Psychology, 50*, 517–522.

Belsky, J., & Rovine, M. (1990). Patterns of marital change across the transition to parenthood: Pregnancy to three years postpartum. *Journal of Marriage and the Family, 52*, 5–19.

Broman, C. L. (1988) Satisfaction among Blacks: The significance of marriage and parenthood. *Journal of Marriage and the Family, 50*, 63–72.

Cowan, C. P., & Cowan, P. A. (1992). *When partners become parents: The big life change for Couples.* New York: Basic Books, Inc.

Dyer, E. D. (1963). Parenthood as crisis: A re-study. *Marriage and Family Living, 25*, 196–201.

Glenn, N. D. & McLanahan, S. (1982). Children and marital happiness: A further specification of the relationship. *Journal of Marriage and the Family, 42*, 63–72.

Heaton, T. B. (1990). Marital stability throughout the childrearing years. *Demography, 2*, 55–63.

Hobbs, D. F., & Cole, S. P. (1976). Transition to parenthood: A decade replication. *Journal of Marriage and the Family, 38*, 723–731.

LeMasters, E. E. (1957). Parenthood as crisis. *Marriage and Family Living, 19*, 353–355.

MacDermid, S. M., Huston, T. L., & McHale, S. M. (1990). Changes in marriage associated with the transition to parenthood: Individual differences as a function of sex-role attitudes and changes in the division of household labor. *Journal of Marriage and the Family, 5* 475–486.

Rossi, A. S. (1968). Transition to parenthood. *Journal of Marriage and the Family, 30*, 26–39.

Schwartz, A. (1994). Taking the nature out of mother. In D. Bassin, M. Honey, & M. M. Kaplan (Eds.). *Representations of Motherhood* (pp. 240–255). New Haven: Yale University Press.

White, L. K., Booth, A., & Edwards, J. N. (1986). Children and marital happiness: Why the negative correlation? *Journal of Family Issues, 7*, 131–147.

CHAPTER **2**

Mothering Co-occupations in Caring for Infants and Young Children

Judith A. Olson, PhD, OTR

 Anticipated Outcomes

I anticipate that, after reading this chapter, readers will:

- Have deepened their understanding of the co-occupations of mothers and their young children

- Have increased their understanding of those factors that affect the co-occupations of mothers and their young children

- Have considered the implications of recent research from the neurosciences that will affect their understanding of the development of co-occupations

Introduction

I have been mothering now for 26 years. My oldest child was 25 this year. Yet I remember when he was first born and those early mothering occupations of feeding, dressing, and bathing. I remember the thrill of having my first baby. I also remember vividly our early struggles with breast-feeding, its attendant feelings of incompetence, and my worries about being a good mother. This probably led to my interest in the area of early mothering. This is part of the personal history that I bring to this chapter.

Additionally, I am a white, married, upper-middle class, university faculty member teaching in an occupational therapy program. As an occupational therapist, I have looked to our profession to address mothering because it is one of the most significant occupations and one that profoundly affects all of us—men, women, and children alike.

During my career, I have worked with mothers of young children. As an occupational therapy educator, I have worked with students to understand the co-occupations of mothers and their young children. Therefore, in this chapter, I will explore some early co-occupations of mothering infants and young children. I will use the stories that mothers told me during my dissertation work to illustrate important concepts and issues. And, finally, I will explore the literature related to early brain development and early emotional development for their contributions to the discussion of co-occupations. The major objective of this chapter is to describe the co-occupations of mothers and their young children as the crucibles within which a young child's neuropsychobiological systems develop his or her ability to self-regulate.

Background

Within the past 20 years in the United States, there has been a societal sentiment that getting children off to a good start contributes to their healthy development. By extension, our culture is ensuring its survival. Yet we seem to be grappling with what a good start means and, conversely, what happens when a good start is not always possible.

The way we think about early childhood development has become more complex. At one time it seemed that child development was almost synonymous with the acquisition of developmental milestones. If children rolled over on time, said their first words on time, and walked on time (or thereabouts), they were considered well on their way to healthy development. This way of conceiving of devel-

opment was taught in our classrooms and supported by well-baby visits to the pediatrician. It formed a common belief within society. Our current understanding of child development, however, is much more complex.

According to a maturational perspective, on an individual level, development unfolds consistent with timetables that are dependent on an individual child's innate capacities and environmental tasks and challenges. It would seem, then, that development does proceed in a series of linear ages and stages or developmental milestones. And yet, within this perspective, development results from the growth of brain/body systems that allow the individual new abilities and greater capacity for dealing with the environment (Davies, 1999).

Sameroff's transactional model of development brings further insight into the complexity of development. His model suggests that development occurs because of "the interplay between child and context across time, in which the state of one affects the next state of the other in a continuous dynamic process" (Sameroff, 1993, p.6). In this model, development results from biological givens in dynamic interplay with other factors such as quality of caregiving interactions, social and economic circumstances, and the wider culture that includes the historical context of the time (Sameroff & Chandler, 1975). Both the young child and the parents are active participants in the process of development. This implies that the parents' relationship, their relational histories, and their individual characteristics and circumstances also affect child development.

Bronfenbrenner's ecological model has conceptualized development in much the same way (Bronfenbrenner, 1979; Bronfenbrenner & Morris, 1988). He has further elaborated on the contribution of the environment to development as he has demonstrated the widening circle of transactions that any individual has with his or her immediate environment of the home, and then the child-care center, school, and eventually even sports teams, social organizations, and perhaps blended families. Bronfenbrenner's model includes those broader social forces that result from national and state government policies or laws, cultural practices, and economic conditions. This model helps us to understand the complexity of a child's transactions with his or her environment and to appreciate that the mother's and father's transactions within their environment affect child development as well.

Finally, since the 1990s, which was dubbed the decade of the brain, our understanding of the way brain function unfolds has increased. This too has increased our understanding of child development. What was once thought to be a biological given—that is, how the brain develops—is now being conceptualized as a transactional process. Some of the latest research is demonstrating that the transactional processes of physical touching, social interaction, and sensory stimulation actually promote physical brain growth and can increase brain function (Diamond, 1991; Greenspan, 1997).

Occupational therapy has contributed the essential concept of occupation to our consideration of development. A plethora of definitions of occupation exist. For this chapter, I will use a definition of occupation that includes all ". . . groups of activities and tasks of everyday life, named, organized, and given value and meaning by individuals and a culture" (Law, Polatajko, Baptiste, & Townsend, 1997, p. 34). Vergara has suggested a definition of infant occupations as "…any tasks and activities that are valued within the family (or Neonatal Intensive Care Unit—NICU) culture in which the infant is expected to engage" (2002, p.9). We can use this understanding of infant occupations to identify those tasks and activities that an infant can engage in and, further, we can identify those factors that encourage or interfere with the infant's participation.

ᴧᴠ About the Occupations of Young Children

When we think of the occupations of young children, it is most obvious that they are carried out with another person. This other person is typically the primary caregiver. And in western society, the primary caregiver is most often the mother (Coltrane & Adams, 2001). So in this chapter I will use "mother" to mean the primary caregiver. Caregiving occupa-

tions, in particular, seem to take up much of mother-infant time. Typically, these occupations have been viewed as involving activity on the part of the caregiver and passive receiving on the part of the child (Zemke & Clarke, 1996).

However, Zemke and Clarke have urged us to reconsider the true nature of these interactions. In fact, in every occupation of caregiving, there are two actors. For example, consider feeding, an activity that occupies much time for the mother of a young child. The mother feeds, but the baby eats. Both play active parts. Therefore, feeding and eating can be considered co-occupations (Zemke & Clarke, 1996).

Dunlea (1996) helps us to further understand this notion of co-occupation; she has written that "the principal occupations of mothers and infants center on the repertoire of social interactive routines that evolve within the mother-infant dyad" (p. 228). Basic interactive routines that form the daily lives of mothers and their infants are these co-occupations. It is important to distinguish passive activities from co-occupations. For example, sleeping is obviously a passive activity and, though purposeful, should not be considered an occupation. Nevertheless, the falling-asleep process, or the transition that occurs between arousal states, can be considered an occupation (Vergara, 2002).

Last, an important assumption of this chapter is that the nature of development is relational. Therefore co-occupations and development can be discussed only within a relationship. For this chapter, the mother-infant relationship is the space in which co-occupations will be discussed.

In this chapter, three co-occupations of mothers and their young children will be presented: feeding/eating, getting to sleep and maintaining sleep, and crying and consoling. Each of these co-occupations will be introduced by stories based on my research with mothers and then discussed (Olson, 1998). Pseudonyms have been provided for the individuals described in these stories, and identifying information has been changed to protect confidentiality. These stories were developed from my doctoral dissertation work. All the mothers and young children were already receiving services in infant mental health programs in a large metropolitan area for problems often observed in these early co-occupations.

The mothers and their children were receiving home-visiting services provided as prevention-intervention services. Therefore, there were no formal diagnoses for either the mothers or the children. In fact, even though these mothers sought infant mental health services, the problems that they described were comparable to the challenges experienced by all mothers as part of the everyday challenges of their mothering occupations.

Infant mental health programs provide services to young children and their families in order to support stable child-family relationships and to promote secure attachments (Weatherston & Tableman, 1989). The services that are provided include emotional support for the caregivers; concrete assistance (food and clothing, for example); guidance to parents about individual baby's behaviors and needs; advocacy on behalf of the health, development, and well-being of the mothers and their young children; and relationship-focused psychotherapy. The families in my study received these services in their own homes, but infant mental health services can be provided in hospitals, schools, foster care, and daycare by professionals with postprofessional training in the area of infant mental health. The patterns of service delivery are individualized and vary with need from once weekly to as many as three times weekly. Some of the interventions are of brief duration (six visits), but some may be long in duration and complex, requiring 1 to 2 years of intensive support.

❧ Feeding/Eating

Vignette: *Margharita and José*

Margharita married when she was 35 years old. She considered this late because most of her Mexican relatives had married much earlier. Margharita and her husband, Edward, had wanted to be professionally qualified as well as financially secure before marrying. Edward had several post-baccalaureate degrees and was very highly regarded by his company, so he was certain of advancement and financial rewards. Margharita and Edward lived in an upper–middle-class suburban neighborhood in a large house—another sign of their success.

Margharita had always wanted a child. She wanted to be a mother. This was her dream. Margharita waited 7 years to become pregnant, and she and Edward were delighted when it happened. Margharita enjoyed her pregnancy. She was healthy and happy throughout. She loved Edward, felt financially secure, and went about her pregnancy eagerly, planning and outfitting a nursery.

Her son José was born after an uncomplicated labor and delivery. Margharita had looked forward to breast-feeding her child. She was supported in this decision by her husband, the rest of her family, and her cultural upbringing. Within a few hours after delivery, José had his first feeding. Margharita felt that he was eager to nurse but seemed to be having some trouble. She could not figure out what was really happening: either he was having difficulty latching onto her nipple or he just wasn't breathing right. She quickly called a nurse, who observed the feeding for a few minutes and recommended that they discontinue. She explained that José was looking "dusky" and had an increased respiratory rate. Margharita was not sure what "dusky" meant, but she trusted the nurse's knowledge and authority and immediately discontinued the feeding. Meanwhile, the nurse took José away from Margharita and to the neonatologist.

The next day, Margharita and Edward were told that José had a hole in his heart. They heard the words "congenital heart disease." They were told that at some point José would need to have cardiac surgery to repair his heart, but that, for now, Margharita was to bottle-feed him with a superformula that was guaranteed to build him up for the surgery. In the meantime, she was to take José home, feed him, love him, and bring him back for his newborn check-ups. Margharita was told that bottle-feeding would be easier for him than breast-feeding; he wouldn't have to work so hard and use up so many critically needed growth calories.

Bottle-feeding did not prove that easy. José did not seem to like the nipples. There was something wrong with either the shapes of the nipples or the materials that they were made of. Through trial and error, Margharita eventually found an acceptable nipple.

During this early period, Margharita fed José on a demand schedule. She felt that all she did was feed José. He took only small amounts of formula at any one feeding, and he was clearly losing weight. At his first post-hospitalization visit to the doctor, he was weighed officially, and she was told that he was losing weight. Margharita was told that she must bring José back daily so that they could track his weight. And so she did.

Daily weigh-ins were the rule. On those days when José registered even a small amount of weight gain, Margharita would be exultant and breathed a sigh of relief. But those days were indeed few. On most days, she would hear that his weight had either decreased or stayed the same. All this effort for such minimal return! She was trying so hard to be a good mother, and José wasn't gaining weight. She worried that the doctors and nurses did not believe that she was actually feeding José when, in fact, that was all she seemed to do.

Margharita received a lot of advice and solicitude from her family. Everyone seemed to feel that they knew how to feed her baby except her. The daily weigh-ins were excruciatingly painful emotionally because José would gain minimally one day but might lose a bit by the next day. Eventually, he began to gain very small amounts regularly, and the daily weigh-ins ended.

After 6 months, Margharita was exhausted. José was still gaining minimally. She and Edward had remained firm in their decision not to start solid foods until then, but it had been painful. Everyone had suggestions: put corn syrup in his formula; add cereal to all feedings; make your own mashed potatoes; applesauce is the answer. She graciously accepted these suggestions outwardly; inwardly, she felt incompetent but determined to feed José her way. So, at 6 months, under her pediatrician's direction, she began offering solid foods, conscientiously offering only one new food substance at a time, and re-offering it for several days. José seemed to accept each new food, but without interest or ea-

gerness. In fact, Margharita felt that he didn't want any of it. He fussed, cried, and eventually thrashed around from side to side in his highchair as she tried to get him to eat more than one bite. Margharita did not understand this behavior. How could she have an infant who didn't want to eat? Margharita felt that she was living an oxymoron: how could she, an excellent cook, from a culture that enjoyed food and focused daily activities as well as celebrations around food and eating, have a child who didn't like to eat? This was not the fun she had envisioned; this was not what she had wanted all of her life.

Margharita sought help in her local school district and was provided with an early intervention program that included occupational therapy and speech therapy in a playgroup setting. However, José's feeding issues were never directly addressed. Margharita then sought additional help in an infant mental health program. With support from her infant mental health specialist, Margharita arranged for private occupational therapy for José because she knew from her previous work experience that occupational therapy was helpful to families when their children had feeding problems. Today José is slight in build, but is a vigorous child who is steadily increasing the variety of foods that he will accept.   ⌘

⌘ Vignette: *Maeghan and Mary*

Maeghan and John married after meeting in an exchange program while both were in graduate school and in their late 20s. Maeghan was from Ireland and John from the United States. After they were married, Maeghan left her friends and family and moved to the United States, where her daughter Mary was born.

Mary was born after a healthy, happy pregnancy and full-term labor with uncomplicated delivery. Having researched the issue of infant feeding, that is, breast versus bottle, John and Maeghan decided on breast feeding for Mary. As a strong, full-term infant, Mary was able to suck well. So she should have been able to breast-feed successfully. Yet she was fussy in the hospital and slept poorly. She was discharged with her mother a few days after delivery.

The first days at home were difficult. Although Mary seemed to be feeding, she was not happy, crying often and inconsolably and sleeping poorly. At her first check-up within days of discharge, Mary was found to have lost more than a pound, and this brought concern from the pediatrician and worry for Meaghan and John. They were both already exhausted from lack of sleep, and they described their life as disorganized. They had been jointly focusing all of their efforts on feeding Mary, but she was fretful and losing weight.

John and Meaghan had agreed before Mary's birth that they wanted to be equal partners in her care. John did not want to be a "Sunday dad." So both Meaghan and John had been getting up for all of Mary's feedings, and they were at least every 2 hours, maybe even more often than that, and now they were both as exhausted as their infant.

John was worried about Mary's weight loss. He had an older sister who was married with young children and knew that Mary should be gaining weight. John's mother and father lived close by and visited often. After all, this was the first grandchild in their only son's family, so Mary held a special place in their hearts. They saw Mary's fretfulness and difficulty with feeding and were eager to help. John's family prided themselves on their educational achievements—everyone had done some graduate work. John's mother took an academic approach to Mary's feeding problems and looked into issues related to breast-feeding. She was particularly struck by what she read about the diet of nursing mothers, and she took it upon herself to scrutinize Meaghan's diet. John and his sister were united in supporting Meaghan, who was beginning to feel like a culprit. Everyone was aware of Mary's pitiful wailing, difficulty sleeping, and lack of weight gain. It was the topic of all family conversations. It seemed to Meaghan that she was the cause of Mary's unhappiness. At least, Meaghan's mother-in-law implied that what she was eating was causing Mary's intestinal distress.

So Meaghan began eliminating foods from her diet. First she dropped meats, then certain vegetables, and finally she was eating nothing but rice cereal with milk and a few other milk-based products. Mary and Meaghan were both miserable. Meaghan was distressed by the thought that it was her breast milk that was bad for her child.

In the meantime, John was eager to have Meaghan accept the suggestion of their pediatrician to see a lactation specialist. John was relieved when Meaghan agreed and delighted when the lactation specialist suggested a breast pump. This would solve the problem, he was certain. Now Meaghan was eating a very limited diet and pumping regularly. And still Mary was unhappy. Meaghan found Mary's wailing totally disorganizing. She felt as if she just couldn't do anything right. Here she was, far from her home and her mother, a stay-at-home mother, without benefit of her personal network of friends, and she was failing at being a mother. She felt that it was all her fault.

Meaghan became so desperate that she even called John at work one day and told him that she just couldn't do anything with Mary. She cried all the time and was inconsolable. John believed that Meaghan was at her wit's end. What should he do? It was at this point that Meaghan and John found help through an infant mental health program. After a few visits, Mary was growing adequately. Meaghan was able to reinterpret Mary's crying as a plea for rest from stimulation and to provide her with an environment that allowed more rest and sleep. She was taught to do infant massage and was successful in using this technique to facilitate relaxation, which, in turn, fostered more time spent in mutually satisfying co-occupations.

The Infant and Eating as a Co-occupation

I have chosen to illustrate the co-occupations of feeding/eating with the stories of Margharita and José and Meaghan and Mary. In these stories, both actors, the mothers and their young children, were engaged in the co-creation of their feeding/eating occupation. Imms defines occupational performance as the ". . . ability of a person to perform an activity in a satisfactory way [as being] influenced by factors in three domains: the person, his or her environment, and the occupation itself" (Imms, 2001, p. 278). In infant feeding, two actors coordinate the occupations of feeding and eating. Therefore, both bring their personal, cognitive, physical, and affective skills to this endeavor. I will use Imms' definition of occupational performance as a lens through which to consider the co-occupations of feeding/eating in the stories presented.

In the stories of Margharita and José and Maeghan and Mary, the physical factors contributing to occupational performance were obvious. In the example of Margharita and José, the most relevant physical component of their co-occupation was José's inability to develop a good suck-swallow-breathe sequence, as evidenced on that first occasion of breast-feeding (Kimball, 1999). He responded by turning dusky—a clear physical sign. Another physical sign was that José was easily fatigued by the work of sucking and had a general decrease in activity tolerance. These were signs of the physical condition of his heart. He had a small hole in his heart, a congenital defect. He must grow physically before the surgical intervention needed to repair the defect could be performed.

It is necessary that infants begin to physically sense hunger and to initiate those actions that signify a need for food, including crying. We can only speculate that José's ability to sense hunger and to initiate actions that would result in satiation might have been diminished.

Imms considers the actual communication of hunger-satiation and pleasure-displeasure as cognitive skills (Imms, 2001). The repetition of transactions initiated by an infant crying and a mother responding with actions that lead to the infant's satisfaction are early experiences with cause and effect. These are cognitive experiences that provide the groundwork for early affective experiences. Successful experiences with feeding/eating reinforce the infant's growing image of himself or herself as a successful actor who can affect his or her environment.

Simultaneously, successful feeding experiences support the mother's developing image of herself as a good mother who is effective in one of the most basic occupations of mothering, feeding her infant. Feeding is a highly emotionally charged occupation, as we saw in the stories of Margharita and José and of Maeghan and Mary. Feeding is the foundation of the infant's survival and, furthermore, the elemental occupation that leads to maternal confidence and competence. Feeding is one of the most important visible occupations signifying a mother's public role.

Feeding is one of the earliest co-occupations between a mother and her infant. It directly contributes to feelings of pleasure and satisfaction. For it is within the context of the earliest co-occupations, which also include bathing and dressing—the daily routines of care—that the infant and his or her mother build emotional routines that form their relationship. It is within this relationship that an infant elicits responses from his or her mother that are contingent on and responsive to a particular need.

The Mother and Feeding as a Co-occupation

Margharita had made a deliberate choice to breast-feed José. For Margharita's part, she was physically capable of breast-feeding and stated that this was what she had looked forward to doing all her life. She was supported in this decision by her culture, her family's cultural values, and her husband. Additionally, Margharita's cultural background promoted the affective pleasures of feeding/eating. She was surrounded by cultural reminders that feeding and eating were occupations that were to be enjoyed, celebrated, and shared in various social ways, such as family get-togethers and so forth.

However, these cultural notions about feeding/eating only heightened Margharita's stress around feeding José. Within this context of support for her choice of an infant feeding method, Margharita had invested a lifetime of meaning into the idea of breast-feeding her child. To her, that was the way infants fed, and now she was told to discontinue breast-feeding.

In the feeding/eating story of Maeghan and Mary, we find another feeding partner, the father. John was eager to look to a feeding expert outside of his own family for help with feeding Mary. He personally felt helpless to contribute to the resolution of the difficulty.

He was relieved by the consultation with the lactation specialist and the technological solution of a breast pump. In the medical–model-based system of health care that pervades North American society, John eagerly embraced a suggestion by their pediatrician, a culturally recognized expert in pediatric feeding problems. John was even more relieved when a technological solution to the problem could be made concrete in the form of a breast pump.

In our technically advanced western society, many find relief in technological solutions instead of such interventions as additional support for the mother to continue breast-feeding by, for example, a referral to the La Leche League. This is an extension of the medicalization of infant feeding that began in the mid-19th century, along with the greater availability of breast milk substitutes, the introduction of scientific approaches to children's needs, and the emergence of the expert role of the medical doctor in areas that included infant feeding (Obermeyer & Castle, 1997). Yet it is known that the conditions that are especially important for the successful initiation and maintenance of breast-feeding include additional supports for the mother. This may be in the form of a helper who would provide instruction, advice, or even assistance with other responsibilities like housework (Dettwyler, 1987).

Our society tells new mothers that their primary responsibility to their baby is to ensure survival (Hrdy, 1999). This realization develops during pregnancy. For many women, it becomes their ultimate responsibility. Stern and Bruschweiler-Stern (1998) have written that a mother's first and unavoidable task is to keep the baby alive. Ruddick has written further about this as the child's demand for preservation and growth (Ruddick, 1980). Survival is so basic that it is a responsibility shared by all animals. The survival of a baby is necessary for the survival of the larger family unit that passes its genes down through the generations in each new life. This is part of the socially constructed understanding of what mothers do.

A mother's primary occupation, then, is to care for her child. This is an awesome responsibility, one that is meant to be shared. The woman's partner shares a portion of this responsibility. Other support systems can include extended family members, friends, and even medical professionals (consider the doctor and lactation specialist in the story of Meaghan and Mary). Nevertheless, the feeling exists in our society that the mother is ultimately responsible.

A secondary set of concerns centers on the question of whether or not the baby will grow physically—that is, gain weight and stay healthy (Stern & Bruschweiler-Stern, 1998). This concern is intimately connected with feeding and raises issues that include, but are not limited to, choice of feeding method, outward signs of growth, timing of adding solid foods, and selection and use of utensils. These issues will be considered separately in the next section, but we must realize that in the everyday experiences of living with a baby, these issues do not operate in isolation from each other.

New mothers, especially first-timers, must consider how they will feed their infant—bottle or breast. If breast-feeding is their choice, they will struggle with the societal myth that breast-feeding is natural and easy (Obermeyer & Castle, 1997). If a woman has been raised in a culture that supports breast-feeding and has witnessed examples of women and babies in this co-occupation, it might be an easier choice for her. The choice of a feeding method is a deliberate act, often made jointly with a partner. This choice begins a chain of events that starts with nipple care for the breast-feeding mother, or bottle selection and care for the mother choosing bottle-feeding. Physical positioning for either method needs to be experimented with and sometimes even problem-solved around. For example, mothers who had cesarean sections might find certain holds difficult and/or painful.

When babies do not gain weight, serious concern is raised about their current and future well-being. If appropriate weight gain does not occur, there is a potential for failure to thrive and hospitalization (Dawson, 1992). These are concerns specifically related to the health of the young child's physical body. For the mother, the baby's lack of weight gain provides a serious challenge to her image as a competent mother. She can perceive that she has failed as a mother because she has not met her primary responsibility to feed her baby (Humphrey, 1991).

Feeding/Eating and the Impact of the Environment

Since the 1980s and the publication of the pivotal writings of Vygotsky (1978) and Bronfenbrenner (1979), we have been more conscious of the extent to which occupations are affected by their cultural contexts that are part of the larger concept of environment. Culture includes, but is not limited to, ideas, beliefs, and values held by parents, as well as the rituals and practices that result from them (Shonkoff & Phillips, 2000). These rituals and practices are embodied in the routines of everyday life.

Cultural considerations related to infant feeding affect how a baby is fed (breast versus bottle), what food substances are introduced and when, the nature of the response to infant signals about need (demand versus schedule feeding), the physical location of feeding, and the equipment used for feeding. In addition, geographical location affects feeding. In the !Kung San culture, a hunter-gatherer Kalahari Desert society, an infant is fed breast milk in small quantities every 15 minutes. He or she is in constant contact with the mother, and any fussing is responded to immediately so that the crying stage is never reached (Shonkoff & Phillips, 2000). In the United States, a greater variety of patterns for responding to fussing and feeding exists.

When occupations like feeding and responding to fussy behavior are repeated over time, they become routines. According to Fiese (2002), routines typically involve what needs to be done; that is, they are instrumental in nature. She has further written that when they are repeated over time, routines lead to the development of habits. Kubicek supports this concept of routines by defining them as "…patterned interactions that occur with predictable regularity in the course of everyday living" (Kubicek, 2002, p. 4). I suggest that, when these routinized occupations become habitual behavior, they are more than

just predictable patterns of action. They are also predictable patterns of emotional responses. Later in this chapter I will address the emotional environment of occupations and its implications for mothers and infants.

Imms' conceptualization of feeding as "… an interactive process between a caregiver and an infant that ensures nutritional intake and provides social and emotional experiences to support the development of the infant's physical, cognitive, and affective performance components" (2001, p. 280) supports the notion of a co-occupation. As the infant is eating, the mother is feeding. If these actions are surrounded by a positive emotional climate, the beginnings of a new and highly desired affective relationship are strengthened.

⁂ Getting to and Settling for Sleep

⌘ Vignette: *Barbara and David*

Barbara was an unmarried 22-year-old when her first son, David, was born. David's father, Dwayne, was not at the delivery, nor did he live with Barbara after the birth. In fact, Barbara and Dwayne were no longer seeing each other. Barbara's experiences of pregnancy and delivery were unremarkable, although she felt incredibly alone during the delivery. David came home to live with Barbara in a small apartment. Barbara continued to feel the loneliness that had so marked her delivery experience, and she was uncertain of her new role as a mother. But she had wanted David, and she wanted to have him close to her. She easily fell into a pattern of having David in bed with her. After all, co-sleeping facilitated breast-feeding, and she needed to arrange their lives to make it easier for her to care for him alone. Besides, co-sleeping provided them both with contact comfort, and it diminished her loneliness.

Barbara admitted that there was no type of schedule in their house early in David's life. Sometimes David went to bed very late because that was when she put him to bed. Sometimes he just fell asleep during an evening's activities. There was no such thing as a bedtime routine. This pattern worked well for Barbara and David until Dwayne wanted to resume his previous relationship with Barbara during David's second year of life. Dwayne had remained peripherally in touch with mother and son during the previous year. Now, Barbara and Dwayne both wanted to get back together, and so they married. This called for a reorganization of the co-sleeping arrangement. Barbara tried to begin a bedtime routine. She began by putting David into his own crib at night—a new sleeping environment for David. He responded by waking, crying, and appearing to need feeding. Barbara fed him and then returned to her own bed, but David soon awakened again. Often she fed him again after changing him, for he would be soaked and cold. And then she tried to resettle him, and stayed in his room with him until he fell asleep. Then, "like a thief in the night," she tried to steal away. If that did not work, which it most often did not, she brought David to their bed, placing him between her and Dwayne. After David fell asleep, she lifted him carefully and carried him back to his room and ever so gently deposited him back into his crib, trying not to awaken him. Barbara had to become expert at the gentle movements, quiet steps, and calm, controlled breathing that would not unsettle her sleeping infant.

Despite these efforts, David slept for only a few hours, and then the sequence of changing, feeding, and moving from bed to bed was repeated. Sometimes these actions were repeated as often as seven times a night. Barbara referred to this behavior as bed-hopping. She was exhausted; Dwayne was losing patience; and David was establishing a routine of short periods of sleep, frequent nighttime feedings, and frequent irritability. Barbara felt that the only answer to this problem was to stop breast-feeding, and that is exactly what she did. One evening, she just gave David a bottle and continued to bottle-feed him at every feeding after that. Barbara described this as the "cold turkey" method of discontinuing nursing. However, this did not resolve the sleeping pattern. Barbara sought infant mental health services and, with supportive counseling and much trial and error, she developed a bedtime routine that facilitated David's sleeping in his own crib for gradually lengthening periods.　⌘

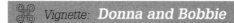

⌘ *Vignette:* **Donna and Bobbie**

Donna, another mother, brought her new son, Bobbie, home to the lovely apartment that she and her husband had tenderly prepared together. She, too, had chosen to breast-feed and had been provided at the hospital with instructions about feeding and the proper positioning of the baby for feeding. Positioning was particularly important to Donna because she had had a cesarean delivery. Bobbie's bassinet had been arranged in their bedroom. Bobbie seemed to sleep fitfully, needing to nurse regularly. To Donna, it seemed as if it was every 15 minutes. She did not even consider this as sleeping and felt that, at best, they were napping. No one was getting any sleep—everyone in the family was exhausted. Conscious of the deleterious effects of lack of sleep on her husband, who had to go to work every day, Donna moved the bassinet and herself out of the bedroom and into the living room, where she made a bed for herself on the couch and placed Bobbie's bassinet next to her.

Donna awakened to every cry, actually to every sound. She was afraid to miss Bobbie's waking, and soon she was not sleeping at all. Why bother when Bobbie would awaken within 15 minutes? Donna vividly remembered living at home with her mother and father, who were now divorced, but who had been together when she was a teenager. It had seemed to her that her father's every wish was more like a command that had to be attended to immediately. Now it felt like that again with Bobbie. As the days went on, Donna felt like a zombie, going unconsciously through the motions of everyday life. She felt as if she were going crazy. There was no rhythm to their lives. She could not see a pattern of daily activities. Donna felt disorganized. She felt as though she had no control. Bobbie cried often, fed often, but slept little. She wondered: was she a prisoner—held captive by her infant son?

Donna sought help from an infant mental health program, and during her first phone call to initiate service, she was assisted to develop a plan that provided her with outside help with Bobbie so that she could get some sleep.　⌘

Getting the Infant to Sleep: The Mothering Co-occupation

Both of the infants in the stories presented were experiencing sleep problems. Getting the infant ready for sleep is often seen as the mother's co-occupation; getting to sleep and remaining asleep in a location that fits the family's plan for appropriate sleeping arrangements are the infant's co-occupations (Sadeh & Anders, 1993). Mothers often raise issues about sleep and crying during the early period from birth through age 3 months, and these issues raise the question of infant pathology versus the style of caregiving in our North American culture. In fact, 20 to 30 percent of all babies and their parents experience some type of sleep disturbances (Sadeh, 2001).

Barbara and Donna had normal and uncomplicated pregnancies, labors, and deliveries. Both had looked forward to bringing their sons home. And, within a few days of coming home, both mothers were exhausted, disorganized, and feeling that their lives and those of the other members of their families were out of control. Both mothers even questioned their mental health. Barbara and Donna had chosen an infant feeding method that brought with it the expectation of night-time wakings for feeding. But neither mother had anticipated how this would affect their sleeping and the sleep of their spouses. It is well known that early sleep and crying issues raise serious challenges within a family. These early sleeping concerns create strain and tension among family members, potentially allow negative perceptions of the infant to develop, and erode the parenting confidence of both mothers and fathers (Shonkoff & Phillips, 2000).

Young babies do not know the difference between day and night. We do not really understand why this is so. What we do know is that it is the mother and the family that help the infant differentiate between night and day. We do have information about the structure and temporal organization of sleep during the first 4 months of life. Typically, newborns sleep between 16 and 17 hours per day, and the structure of sleep-wakefulness resembles a 90-minute rest-activity cycle more than a diurnal rhythm (Sadeh, 2001). However, by age 3 months, total sleeping time has decreased to 14 to 15 hours with lengthened and consolidated periods of sleeping and waking. The longest sleep period shortly after birth is about 4 hours, but by age 3 months, for normal full-term infants at least, a sleep period of 8 to 10 hours can occur, often during night hours (Anders et al., 1992).

In addition, there is initial evidence that babies who fall asleep in their own cribs establish their own pattern of self-settling, whereas babies who fall asleep in contact with their mothers awake to circumstances that are different from those when they fell asleep (Sadeh, 2001). This may present a novel situation to an infant that interests and wakens him or her. It has also been found that mothers and their infants do not sleep as soundly when they sleep together (McKenna et al., 1993, 1994). The development of a self-settling pattern is also influenced by feeding patterns (Wright et al., 1983). Breast-fed babies are a bit slower to lengthen their sleep cycle (Sadeh, 2001). However, it is doubtful whether all new mothers have this knowledge and understanding of their infant's sleep-wakefulness organization. Lacking this knowledge and its implications for the establishment of a daily routine may have contributed to some of the problems experienced by Donna and Barbara. Neither mother had instituted a bedtime routine with their infant, nor were they able to establish a structure on their own round of daily activities. The establishment of a bedtime ritual is important because getting settled for sleep is truly a social learning process in which the mother sends signals to her infant that night is for sleeping. The mother then reinforces this by certain signals that could include darkening and quieting the room, terminating dialogue, and a variety of other individually selected signals (Sadeh, 2001).

Donna had speculated on the possibility that she had the "baby blues," that is, some degree of postpartum depression that leads to depressed activity level, a propensity for crying, a generally more negative affect, and a lack of sleep. Maternal depression is common and potentially serious in respect to the development of the mother-infant relationship and ultimately to child development. We know that approximately 1 in 10 women with young children experiences depression (Dickstein et al., 1998; Gelfand et al., 1996). Depression is certainly not a static condition; it varies in severity, with periods when symptoms are decreased. It is also known that depression in adults changes the neural activity in the frontal area of the brain, which controls emotion regulation (Davidson, 1994) as well as altering sleeping, eating, and cortisol production. In the light of the knowledge of neurobiology and neuroendocrinology associated with maternal depression, both Donna's speculation about baby blues and Barbara's behavior in trying to settle David need to be taken seriously. We know that babies are sensitive to their mothers' emotional situations (Sadeh, 2001) and vulnerable to the negative effects of maternal depression (Dawson & Ashman, 1997; Dawson et al., 1992).

The emotional availability of a mother and the emotional tenor of her interactions with her baby are affected by depression. Mothers who are depressed demonstrate disrupted interaction patterns. In addition, their perceptions of their ability to parent competently are affected, which increases the likelihood that they will perceive their infants as difficult (Teti et al., 1996). Additionally, mothers who are depressed demonstrate a greater tendency to withdraw from their children, to respond to them with little energy, or to become intrusive and hostile (Frankel & Harmon, 1996; Tronick & Weinberg, 1997; Zeanah et al., 1997). What we also know, though, is that these adverse effects of maternal depression are not uniform. That is, some mothers who are depressed can be caring and competent.

Getting to Sleep and Remaining Asleep: The Infant's Co-occupations

Sleep consolidation, the settling and sustaining of "...sleep in a continuous fashion for an age-appropriate period," and sleep regulation, "...the ability of the infant to transition smoothly from wakefulness to sleep" (Sadeh & Anders, 1993, p. 17), were difficult for two-thirds of the infants in my study (Olson, 1998). This is not surprising because the programs in which these families were enrolled were for mothers and infants with problems related to

feeding, sleeping, and consoling. I would suggest, though, that all mothers must negotiate feeding, sleeping, and consoling with their young children during everyday living. However, for some mothers, these challenges just become too much. They are no longer in the realm of the "just-right" challenge range.

A very young infant must contend with the multiple factors involved in sleep arrangements. These include: sleeping alone or with others, feeding pattern, type of nutrition, lighting, and sound conditions (Sadeh, 2001). This is certainly nowhere near an exhaustive list of the environmental factors related to sleeping. In addition, the child has his or her own traits, sometimes referred to as temperament, that play a role in the ability to adjust to change. Going to sleep is a change. It is also a separation from the primary caregiver with whom the infant has had much contact throughout the day. Therefore, getting to sleep is merely one more occupation that can be challenging for very young children, who have difficulty with change in general.

Getting an infant to sleep often involves comforting, another maternal occupation that will be discussed in the next section of this chapter. Additionally, feeding is intimately connected to night-time wakings. So, in effect, the co-occupations of getting to sleep and sleeping are intricately related to other co-occupations.

ʕ⇁ Comforting and Self-comforting

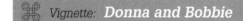

🏵 *Vignette:* **Donna and Bobbie**

As mentioned previously, Donna and Bobbie were able to work out their sleep-related issues within a short period of time after a telephone intervention with an infant mental health specialist, who had merely to confirm how important a mother's need for sleep and rest are to her ability to handle the demands of a very young child. She further suggested that Donna consider asking a family member or friend to come over to the house two nights a week and take her place on the couch next to Bobbie while Donna got some sleep herself. Fortunately,

Donna's sister was working nights as a waitress and felt that it would be no problem at all for her to come to stay with Bobbie after her evening shift two nights a week. Within a week, Donna was feeling much better.

But now Donna had to face Bobbie's seemingly inconsolable crying. Bobbie cried often and was nearly impossible to console. Donna had tried everything: rocking; walking; singing; quiet talking; a baby swing set to a slow, even pace; and white music. Nothing seemed to calm Bobbie. Donna wondered if his crying was related to eating problems. She had abruptly terminated breast-feeding when Bobbie outgrew the one feeding position that she had been taught was comfortable for her, a particular "football hold" that avoided stress on her back and her stomach. This position was no longer possible because of Bobbie's increasing size. So she began bottle-feeding with a commercially available formula.

Bobbie did not tolerate this first formula well. He became quite sick, with projectile vomiting and blood-stained diarrhea. Donna called her pediatrician, who advised staying with this formula for a while longer to see if Bobbie would adjust to it. Donna, however, was not able to follow this advice. She could not tolerate Bobbie's crying and the additional problems. So she switched to another formula. Unfortunately, this second formula resulted in constipation. Again Donna called her pediatrician. This time, she reached another partner in the pediatric group practice. This new doctor suggested yet another regimen: add corn syrup to the formula. Donna was concerned about this suggestion because she had heard that young babies should not be given substances like honey and corn syrup. Again, she did not follow the doctor's recommendation. Instead, she returned to the first formula, and the profuse spitting up and blood-stained diarrhea returned.

By now Donna was confused and angry. Bobbie was crying continually. Donna tried to console him, but was unsuccessful. As mentioned previously, Donna remembered her own childhood and the need for an immediate response to her father's smallest request. Otherwise, he would yell uncontrollably. Was Bobbie going to be like her father? Had she exchanged the tyranny of her father for the tyranny of a baby? Donna was painfully aware that she

had escaped from her unhappy childhood by running away to live with an aunt. She could not run away from Bobbie.

With the support of her infant mental health specialist and her husband, Donna changed from the pediatric group practice to a pediatrician in private practice. Bobbie was diagnosed with lactose intolerance and provided with a special formula that he tolerated. His incessant crying subsided. Donna and Bobbie began to establish some reasonable routines for their daily activities. They even began to have fun with each other. ⌘

⌘ *Vignette:* **Laura and Lana**

Another mother, Laura, just knew that she was carrying a very active baby. It was not that this activity caused Laura pain, but carrying this baby felt so different from her first pregnancy that it caused her some concern. She felt that something was different. Laura talked about this with her obstetrician, who brushed her off with patent reassurances that there was no need for concern.

Laura's birthing experience supported those early feelings of concern. For when her daughter Lana was born, she was blue and was immediately whisked away for intensive medical interventions that Laura felt were not adequately explained to her, and her husband. Laura and her husband were left in the delivery room with no real explanation for what was happening to their baby, and their imaginations went wild! Laura envisioned a seriously damaged child, maybe even a dead child, in those few minutes when Lana was receiving resuscitative interventions. Eventually, Laura was told that Lana had responded immediately to these efforts and would soon be returned to them. But Laura was left wondering: what had happened, and what did this mean for the future? Subsequently Laura received reassurances from her obstetrician that Lana was fine. He speculated that the event had been triggered by the medication that Laura had been given for pain just as Lana had been advancing down the birth canal.

Laura had decided to breast-feed Lana, but their first nursing experience in the hospital was problematic. Lana didn't seem to be able to latch on. A lactation specialist was consulted, and Lana was described as "tongue-tied." Laura had no idea what this meant, but she was provided with instructions and supervision for breast-feeding. She and Lana persisted together and became a reasonably successful feeding team.

However, it was really Lana's inconsolable crying that Laura could not understand. It seemed that Lana cried all the time and that nothing could console her. Laura wondered if Lana had colic. She consulted her pediatrician regularly after Lana's birth, in person and by phone calls. She was determined to understand Lana's distressing crying. Finally, after repeated calls to her pediatrician, she was given an answer. The pediatrician said that it was Lana's temperament. Now, Laura wondered, what's temperament?

Meanwhile, Lana screamed for hours every day. She was inconsolable despite many creative efforts at comforting. Lana had to get so exhausted from crying that she cried herself to sleep. Laura was, by nature, a very quiet person, and all of this crying and screaming had interrupted the peaceful household that she had worked hard to create. Loud or hysterical outbursts of either joy or sadness were not part of this household, where the practice was everything in moderation. In fact, Lana's crying was physically painful for Laura. As Lana grew older, this loud inconsolable crying evolved into tantrums that caused Laura to wonder if Lana were possessed. Despite its physical effects on her, Laura was deeply struck by the persistent and clearly distressed nature of Lana's crying. The inability to console a child who was obviously so distressed was incredibly painful for Laura. She became involved in an infant mental health program, which helped her to understand that Lana was an intense responder and simply had a different intensity of response from Laura's own less intense style of responding

Comforting: A Mothering Co-occupation

Crying has multiple manifestations that include fussing, yelling, screaming, and whimpering. What is common to each, however, is that they all require some type of sensitive and contingent response from mothers. It is a tacit understanding within our culture that mothers must discover the meaning of a cry and eliminate the discomfort or offending element.

For mothers, crying initiates an almost ritualized sequence of events (Barr, 1990). The first consideration is usually hunger. If some type of feeding/eating routine has been established, the timing of the cry may signal hunger. If there is no routine, then crying is often met with an offer of a feeding. Crying may arise from the discomfort of wetness or soiling. A sequence of physical activities then ensues that includes changing diapers, disposing of the diapers (disposition method depends on the use of cloth versus disposable diapers), and resettling. Of course, by now, all possible causes of physical distress should have been examined: a pin that is delinquently open, clothing that is too constricting; clothing that is too warm, too tight, wet, or soiled. There is always the possibility that there is no reason at all for the crying. This sequence of activities is important to mothers because it demonstrates their desire to comfort their infant by finding the cause of his or her distress and eliminating it.

This need for mothers to respond to crying is universal. The pattern of responding, however, is culturally and individually dependent. Again, looking to studies of the !Kung San babies provides an illustrative comparison for North American and Northern European comforting routines. !Kung San babies do not necessarily cry less often, but they are soothed more quickly. !Kung San babies remain in continuous skin-to-skin contact with their mothers because they are carried about throughout the day, feeding about every 15 minutes and co-sleeping with their mothers at night, with no expectation of sleeping through the night. Their slightest cry is responded to immediately. On the other hand, in North American and European routines, the caregiving response involves more separation from the infant both during the day and at night, larger and more widely spaced feedings, and a response to crying that depends on the degree of distress (Shonkoff & Phillips, 2000).

Some research has indicated that responding readily and consistently to infant crying reduces the amount of crying. Crockenburg

(1981) found that babies who received more sensitive responses to their distress because of a more accurate reading of the reason for the distress shifted more to routines of noncrying communication. Further, she found that these infants were happier during more of their first year of life and in less-stressed states.

Donna's story is an example of the complexity of co-occupations. In Donna's situation, there were three interacting co-occupations: feeding, comforting, and readying for sleep. These co-occupations were complicated further by what Fraiberg, Shapiro, and Cherniss called "ghosts in the nursery" (1980). These ghosts are actually troublesome events from the mother's past that intrude on the present life of a mother and her young child. Fraiberg et al. have written: "the ghosts, we know, represent the repetition of the past in the present" (1980, p. 166). Bobbie's crying evoked memories of Donna's past experience with a demanding and loud father who had to be responded to immediately so that further yelling could be avoided. A normal infant occupation, crying, then becomes connected to the mother's difficult past, thus exacerbating the emotional stress of the present.

What both these mothers of young children shared, however, was feeling inadequate to the task of comforting and consoling their infants. Somehow this inconsolability is shrouded in an incomprehensible term for Laura—temperament.

Being Comforted and Eventually Self-comforting: The Infant's Co-occupation

Bobbie and Lana were difficult babies to comfort. Were they colicky? In American culture, the phenomenon of infant colic is always raised when a distinctive pattern of crying can be identified during very early childhood. The pattern is that of early evening distress that peaks in time and duration around age 2 months and often resolves during the third or fourth month. Of course, there is great individual variation in these times. This type of crying is different from other crying in that it seems that nothing can be done to soothe a colicky infant. Because the duration of the cry-

ing can vary from 1 1/2 hours to 3 or even 6 hours, it sometimes feels as if all that the infant does is cry. Sometimes this crying requires medical consultation because it still is commonly believed that colic may be related to digestive problems (Shonkoff & Phillips, 2000). No matter the cause of colic, its implications for the perceptions of who this infant is and how this infant affects family life, and perhaps even who this infant will become, are strong. Often the term "difficult" is attached to infants with colic. This seems to suggest that there is a biological predisposition to being difficult.

Although Lana did not have colic, as her crying was not consistent with the typical pattern of colic, her pediatrician raised the issue of temperament, which is related to individual differences in ways of reacting to events, general mood, capacities for self-regulation, and activity level. These are often clustered together in the term temperament (Shonkoff & Phillips, 2000). Temperament is visible in behavior and is related to regulation of emotions.

As mothers feed, bathe, and comfort, thereby attending to the basic physiological needs of their infants, they are concurrently engaging in the emotional development of the young child and playing an essential role in the infant's development of self-regulation. Emotions are "the observable [public] expressions of feelings and affects through movement, postures, and facial displays" (Rochat, 2001, p. 130). Emde (1987) has written that emotions are by their very nature relational. That is, emotions result from interactions with others. The earliest interactions are those of the infant and his or her primary caregiver.

🖎 Co-occupations and Temperament: Their Contribution to Emotional Development and Self-regulation

Babies begin their lives as totally helpless beings who rely on their caregivers to protect and nurture them. The early co-occupations of feeding, sleeping, and learning to self-soothe, and others not discussed in this chapter, reflect those activities that require mothers to help in the transition from complete dependence to ultimate independence. The early childhood and psychological literature refers to this as acquiring self-regulation. Self-regulation refers to the infant's growing capacity to master tasks that were previously accomplished by the mother alone, or at least in concert with the mother, but that now need to be accomplished by the child (Shonkoff & Phillips, 2000). Though this capacity starts with simple tasks like conforming to the day-night rhythm, it leads later to the powerful capacity to manage oneself by acquiring the behavioral, emotional, and cognitive self-control that will allow competent functioning throughout life. Self-regulation is acquired through and in the daily life co-occupations of young children and their mothers.

In this section of the chapter, self-regulation and some of the recent neuroscience information that impacts the co-occupations of mothers and young children will be discussed. I will begin with a discussion of temperament, which bridges the space between the psychological and the biological because it is grounded in both.

Temperament

Temperament in young children is generally considered an individual characteristic that is rooted in biology (Bates, 1989) and that results in different behavioral tendencies. Some of these tendencies are actually present early in life and remain relatively stable throughout the life span. A constitutional feature implies an expectation of consistency over time (Rutter, 1994). Therefore, the significance of temperament is that it is likely an enduring characteristic that will influence individuals' interactions with their environments for their lifetime (Huntington & Simeonsson, 1993).

There is no universal agreement on a definition of temperament or even of those criteria that comprise temperament. Nevertheless, there are certain ideas that most would agree constitute temperament. These ideas are that temperament involves behavioral features that an individual typically brings to a variety of situations and that are identifiable as that

person's style. Also, features of temperament have been found to be inherited, but no more so than other characteristics (Plomin, 1986).

Additionally, no universal list of traits that denote temperament exists. Thomas and Chess (1986) have derived a selection of traits that resulted from their clinical experiences that were meaningful to the child and that actually differentiated between children. Some of these traits include: difficult/easy, activity level, negative or positive mood, low or high adaptability, reactivity (excitability/arousability), and self-regulation (inhibition).

In the 1980s, Rothbart and Derryberry (1981) wrote that there are two dimensions of autonomic system patterning that determine, at least to some degree, infant temperament. They posited that the limbic system had two physiological modes: excitatory and inhibitory. These two modes determine the traits of reactivity and self-regulation or inhibition.

Kagan summarized Rothbart's definition of reactivity as the "...ease of arousal to stimulation and the ability to modulate that arousal . . . ." (1994, p. 46). When stimulation easily provokes motor activity, crying, other vocalizations, smiling, and autonomic and endocrine responses, we say that the child is reactive. The degree of reactivity can be measured by the length of response time, the intensity of the reaction, and/or the time it takes for the reaction to reach its peak. Those processes that modulate reactivity, such as attention, approach/withdrawal, and self-soothing combine to become self-regulation (Kagan, 1994).

Kagan (1994) cautions us that there are problems with Rothbart's claims. First, infants who react with frequent vocalization and those who react with smiling would both be classified as reactive. Kagan's research indicates that young children inherit two different qualities: ease of arousal indexed by motor activity and vocalization and valence (or quality) of the affective state that succeeds arousal (1994). He found that highly reactive infants are those who are easily aroused, and this heightened arousal is usually followed by distress. Rothbart also considers both autonomic responses and vigorous limb movements as representing reactivity. Kagan alerts us to the difference between children who as infants responded to challenge with an increased heart rate without concomitant motor reactivity and children who as infants were vigorous while autonomically unreactive. Finally, Kagan points out that Rothbart failed to consider the impact of context on reactivity. He posits the notion that reactivity can be too general a construct and therefore should be divided into types based on specific reactions to specific situations. Although I have shared Kagan's cautions, there is still merit in Rothbart's notion of reactivity.

In regard to Rothbart's broad presentation of the notion of self-regulation, Kagan again urges caution (Kagan, 1994). Withdrawal and approach responses are all self-regulating responses. But the more important consideration is which forms the self-regulation routinely assumes: crying, freezing, turning away, or turning toward the new environmental challenge. Infants who are highly reactive assume a joyful response filled with vocalization and smiling, whereas others, although highly reactive, cry when aroused. Kagan has shown that these two types of infants become quite different children later in life.

Kagan (1994) offers a different view of temperament, which he defines as "an inherited profile of behavior, affect, and physiology that is best discovered by observing directly the young child's psychological and biological reactions to specific incentives and charting how these initial biases lead to distinctly different envelopes of behavior and mood that are moderately stable over later childhood and adolescence" (Kagan, 1994, p. 264). He provides two categories, or two hypothetical genotypes, for consideration: the uninhibited and the inhibited. Both are inferred from certain features displayed in early infancy: in particular, high or low reactivity at age 4 months and high or low sympathetic tone during the first 2 months. The uninhibited temperamental category ". . . refers to the appearance of bold, sociable, outgoing behavior in two-year old children" (Kagan, p. 265). The inhibited temperamental category ". . . refers to the actualization of a shy, timid, fearful profile in the second year" (Kagan, p. 265). From his research, Kagan has learned that these two categories have different physiologies and that

each has implications for the actions of the amygdala (a brain structure) and its projections, but direct evidence of the excitability of these anatomical circuits needs to be obtained. Until that is done, Kagan posits the use of behavioral and affective constructs for his temperament profiles. In conclusion, he states his firm belief that there is no determinism that proceeds unchangeably from an early temperamental bias.

Temperament is an individual characteristic that affects the daily co-occupations of mothers and their young children. In particular, those functions that are biological in nature, such as sleep-wake states, for example, clearly demonstrate a relationship to temperament. In a study of young children and nighttime awakening done by Carey (1974), a low sensory threshold emerged as the temperamental characteristic of young children with awakening difficulties when compared with children without such sleep problems. Based on the notion of temperament, professionals offering any interventions to the families of young children need to consider the possible influence of temperament, in particular in the instance of sleep and sensory threshold. This is not to suggest that temperament is the only factor affecting sleep. As we are aware, developmental maturity and context must also be considered.

Keener et al. (1988) had found that infant sleep continuity at 6 months was correlated to mothers' and fathers' questionnaire ratings of temperament, with results stronger for fathers than mothers. Halpern et al. (1994) tried to replicate Kenner's results while further investigating the correlation between maternal ratings of infant temperament and the infant's sleep-wake characteristics. They found instead that measures of infant sleep-wake continuity and organization were more closely connected to behaviorally derived dimensions of temperament than to maternal ratings of temperament. This finding suggests that sleep-wake characteristics and temperament dimensions that are derived from behavior may be mirroring the same aspects of the young child's biological maturity and organization.

In the vignettes of Barbara and David and

Donna and Bobbie we see the potential for temperament to be a factor that is contributing to the co-occupations of settling for sleep and getting to sleep. In Donna and Bobbie's story we also see the complicating interaction between another maternal co-occupation, namely consoling. We have no assessment information with respect to sensory threshold or temperament profile; therefore we are left to wonder whether either Bobbie's or David's sleep difficulties could have been related to their own temperament profile.

What we do know is that in the study from which this chapter's vignettes were drawn, the infant mental health programs were offered for families with "fussy" babies—another term that often connotes an infant with temperament traits that are intense and often interpreted as negative.

Crying and its multiple manifestations are observable behaviors of the temperament characteristic of reactivity in very young children. Crying is often the stimulus for the co-occupations of soothing and being soothed. Reactivity can range from strong to low, with infants with low reactivity often considered the good babies. Yet, in the study by Halpern et al. (1994), a surprising finding was that infants with larger percentages of quiet sleep were rated by their mothers as dull. This dullness reflected a lower level of activity and social responsiveness. Infants with vigorous and excessive crying that is determined to be inconsolable are often perceived as difficult. In the story of Laura and Lana, a pediatrician actually used the concept of temperament to explain Lana's inconsolable crying. However, this conceptual explanation did nothing to help Laura. The complexity of the interactions involved in mother-infant co-occupations should compel interventionists to investigate all the factors affecting both mother and infant in order to construct a useful understanding of what is occurring when problems are identified. It is equally important to communicate this understanding to families in a meaningful way.

Neuroscience Contributions

Greenough and Black conceptualized the brain as experience-dependent (1992).

Specifically, they postulated that the dynamic communication between the mother (the primary caregiver) and the infant generates positive affective states and high levels of the neurochemicals that are the chemical substrate for the optimal environment in which self-regulation develops. Schore (1994) has further postulated that primarily affective experiences account for the brain spurt of the first 2 years. He posits that, from late pregnancy through the second year of life, the young child's brain is in a critical period of accelerated growth. This process requires large quantities of nutrients and interpersonal experiences that are affectively positive. Affective interchanges developed within the crucible of every day co-occupations actually influence the infant's psychobiological systems, resulting ultimately in self-regulation.

In the last 20 years, there has been a major expansion in our understanding of how the brain organizes itself and how genes and the environment interact to affect the brain. Using those recent conceptualizations of child development based on systems thinking and transactional models that were described earlier in this chapter, brain organization can be understood to result from transactions "... between (a) genetically coded programs for the formation of structures and connections among structures and (b) environmental influences" (Fox, Calkins, & Bell, 1994, p. 681). How this information can contribute to our discussion of the co-occupations of mothers and their young children will be explored in this section of the chapter.

The development of new brain cells and neural plasticity have now been shown to be lifelong processes. The most dramatic development, however, takes place within the first few years of life. Brain development from the prenatal period through school entry involves ". . . the development and migration of brain cells to where they belong in the brain, embellishments of nerve cells through the sprouting of new axons or by expanding the dendritic surface; the formation of connections or synapses, between nerve cells; and the postnatal addition of other types of cells, notably glia" (Shonkoff & Phillips, 2000, p. 185).

In early development there is great and redundant synaptic formation, followed by reorganization, elimination, or stabilization of these connections in order to fine-tune these connections for mature needs (Huttenlocker, 1979). These processes, in combination with current evidence that synapses that are used are kept and those that are not used are eliminated, are all part of normal development (Shonkoff & Phillips, 2000).

Experiences are incorporated into developing synaptic connections in the brain through an experience-dependent mechanism (Greenough, 1987; Greenough & Black, 1992). "Experience-dependent synaptogenesis, in contrast, refers to encoding new experiences that occur throughout life, foster new brain growth and the refinement of existing brain structures, and vary for every individual" (Shonkoff & Phillips, 2000, p. 190). Therefore, individual differences in brain development result from the idiosyncratic experiences of an individual. Synaptogenesis is also linked to this experience-dependent mechanism, but all we really know now is that experience allows for more abundant neural connection. Whatever the exact mechanism, this experience-dependent concept allows for the plasticity and adaptability of the brain to the demands of everyday life.

In addition to our increasing understanding of the development of the brain, knowledge of the neurochemistry of the brain is increasing. Shonkoff and Phillips (2000) have noted that the neurochemical systems of the brain are affected not only by activity within the brain itself, but also by activity within the body but outside the brain, as well as input from the external environment. They have written about the evidence from animal research: "For example, the licking and grooming that the mother rat does of her pups (infant rats) appear to enhance the production of serotonin and thyroid hormone, both important in the neurochemistry of brain development (p. 193)." Evidence linking neurochemical activity to caregiving activities in animal models is exciting, but we cannot as yet translate findings from animal research into concrete recommendations for intervention with human children.

Having said that the information available from neuroscience is not currently translatable to intervention with young children, there are some issues related to early experiences and the brain that have been triggering much debate. Two such issues are:

1. The right experiences that should be provided to young children
2. The nature of the timing of experiences; that is, are there sensitive periods?

Both of these issues affect the co-occupations of mothers and young children and will be considered here.

The developmental science of early childhood prefers the use of the concept of "sensitive period" to that of "critical period." "Sensitive periods can be defined as unique episodes in development when specific structures or functions become especially susceptible to particular experiences in ways that alter their future structure or function" (Shonkoff & Phillips, 2000, p. 195). The concept of a sensitive period, when applied to early childhood development, implies:

1. That certain early experiences are necessary to ensure that capacities develop at a time when development is most plastic and most responsive
2. That without certain essential experiences, young children may be at risk for later problems (Shonkoff & Phillips, 2000).

There is evidence from animal research about timing effects, but again, these studies are extremely limited in their ability to translate to the human experience. For example, Greenough and his colleagues (Black & Greenough, 1998; Greenough and Black, 1992) have determined that there are differences in the brain and behavior of rats in different early environments. The brains of rats reared in more complex environments show greater development. An important note here is that this greater development characterized rats that either had been in complex environments early in life or that had been exposed to such environments as adults. Therefore, both early and late exposures were beneficial, but the greater effect was for the early-exposed animals. It is also important to recognize that the effects of exposure to enriched environments diminished with time if the rats were removed from the environment. Shonkoff and Phillips (2000) provide a very useful analogy for us to understand this diminishment. The complex environment is like the tetanus vaccine in that it requires boosters regularly rather than the smallpox vaccine, which prevents disease with a single intervention. Although such animal studies are exciting and enticing, it is a major leap to use such research in respect to human beings.

Within the past 10 years there has been an increasing interest and concern about the impact of stress in the early caregiving environment from ages 0 to 3 years. In this discussion, stress will be defined as in Selye's work (Selye, 1973, 1975) as the ". . . set of changes in the body and the brain that are set into motion when there are overwhelming threats to physical or psychological well-being" (Shonkoff & Phillips, 2000, p. 212). In effect, stress produces shifts in the body's priorities. Stress produces neurochemical changes beginning in the brain that restrains future-oriented tasks, such as learning and preventing colds, in order to shift resources to an immediate threat. In particular, the adrenal glands produce adrenaline and cortisol. Adrenaline works with the sympathetic nervous system to ". . . support vigilance, focus attention, increase heart rate, shunt blood to muscles and away from the digestive system, break down fat stores making energy available to cells, and dampen activity of the immune system" (Shonkoff & Phillips, 2000, pp. 212-213). Cortisol is a steroid hormone that ". . . helps to break down protein stores, liberating energy for use by the body. It suppresses the immune system, suppresses physical growth, inhibits reproductive hormones, and affects many aspects of brain functioning, including emotions and memory" (Shonkoff & Phillips, 2000, p. 213).

Documentation from rodent research has shown that stress hormones adversely affect brain development, particularly that of the hippocampus, which is important for learning and memory (McEwen et al., 1992). Elevation of cortisol dampens the activity of the hippocampus. In addition, other areas of the limbic system and frontal brain are rich in receptors for the steroid hormones. Little is so far known about the impact of these substances on these areas, but there is the potential for the effect to be similar to that in the hippocampus. Lastly, in rodent studies, there is evidence that stress hyporesponsiveness is maintained by maternal contact (Sushecki et al., 1993). Evidence to describe the role of stress-producing hormones, such as cortisol, on human children is only beginning to be collected. Gunnar's work has been with cortisol levels and their influences on the development and functioning of the brain. She has found a negative correlation between cortisol and hippocampal activity (Gunnar & Nelson, 1994) in 12-month-old human infants. She has also found preschool-aged children with cortisol levels that are in the top third of the sample distribution are perceived by their parents and teachers as having the poorest effortful control or self-regulatory abilities (Gunnar et al., 1997).

For human infants, the adrenal system at birth is highly variable and responds to stimulation, such as that found with activities like undressing or weighing. Such activities are known to elevate cortisol (Gunnar, 1998). During the period between ages 3 and 12 months, there seems to be a reduction in cortisol reactivity to stress. If, in nonhuman contact, the mother or a responsive mother substitute serves to buffer a child from increasing stress, then we can hypothesize that human infants may also be so buffered. This is being documented (Nachmias et al., 1996; Gunnar et al., 1996). When this information is considered together, it suggests that ". . . sensitive, responsive, secure caretaking plays an important role in buffering or blocking elevations in cortisol for infants and young children" (Gunnar, 1998, p.210). Hence, safe, secure and supportive caregiving environments for very young children are beginning to be supported by compelling evidence from the hard sciences of neurobiology and neurochemistry. The caveat remains, however, that we are only at the beginning of exploring these issues in young children, and further research is needed.

Implications for the Development of Co-occupations

Joseph (1999) has indicated that "If [children are] reared under neglectful, stressful, or abusive conditions the amygdala, septal nuclei, and the hippocampus may atrophy or develop seizure-like activity, referred to as kindling" (p. 197). But the question that still must be addressed is: what is a stressful environment? I highlighted the neuroscience information that has implications for the developmental period covered in this chapter, that is, the earliest years of life. It is during this time that the co-occupations of mothers and young infants that have been described in this chapter are developing. I suggest that the affective environment that surrounds these co-occupations is as important to development as the actual performance of the co-occupations.

Young children are incapable of regulating their emotions. However, in social interactions with their caregivers, they learn to manage their emotions. Initial experiences with emotion regulation are found within the context of the daily occupations of dressing, playing, being comforted, and others (Schonkoff & Phillips, 2000). These experiences within the caregiving environment have taken on enhanced significance since we have learned that the maturation of the brain itself is experience-dependent (Dobbing & Sands, 1973; Greenough & Black, 1992).

When the interactions between mothers and their young children are repeatedly conflictual, coercive, or abusive, young children are faced with an overwhelmingly demanding emotional environment. Additionally, if mothers are experiencing this same overly demanding emotional climate and are experiencing their own difficulties because of it, infants and young children are without the benefit of a mother who can help them with these difficult emotional environments. Because young children rely on their caregivers for understanding and managing their emotions, if the mother-child co-occupations are experienced within a troubled climate, then both actors are daily grappling with constantly stressful emotional environments that cannot possibly contribute to optimal emotional development and self-regulation.

The stories highlighted in this chapter are of mothers who sought intervention for issues embedded in their co-occupations. With the exception of José's heart problem, neither the mothers nor their young children were being treated formally for any physical or mental health diagnoses. Yet there is a palpable emotional climate surrounding these co-occupations that indicates stress for both the mothers and their young children. I postulate, as Gunnar (1998) has suggested, that mothers provide a buffering function for their young children. When mothers cannot provide this function, the emotional environment surrounding the daily co-occupations is not supportive of optimal child development. Therefore, support for mothers and their young children in the development of their co-occupations within positive affective climates should be available from various mental–health-related professionals.

❧ Conclusion

In this chapter I have discussed three of the co-occupations of mothers and their young children: feeding/eating; getting settled for sleep/sleeping, and comforting/self-comforting. This discussion has been neither inclusive of all the co-occupations possible nor complete in identifying all the factors that could affect them. These co-occupations are important because they form the crucible within which the young child develops emotionally and learns to self-regulate.

This chapter has highlighted the three components of occupational performance: the occupation itself, the individual, and the environment. The stories that were presented were used to make the co-occupations concrete and to demonstrate their contribution to the psychosocial-emotional lives of mothers and young children. In so doing, some of the factors impacting the development of co-occupations have been illuminated. These include: physical characteristics of the individual infant, as in the story of José; contextual implications as found in discussions of feeding and sleeping behaviors; and the psychosocial-emotional needs environment surrounding the performance of occupations.

Furthermore, within the context of these pages, I have just begun to explicate the experiences of mothers and young children in their co-occupations and to understand their significance in light of what we are beginning to learn about brain development in the young child while adding to the growing body of literature about the experiences and activities of mothers (Arendell, 2000). I have shared the experiences of real women who are mothering, and in so doing, supported Forcey's definition of mothering as "… a socially constructed set of activities and relationships involved in nurturing and caring for people" (1994, p. 357). It is in the crucible of co-occupations that are based in the relationship between a mother and her young child that mothering itself is created.

Discussion Questions

- The concept of co-occupations is defined and illustrated in this chapter and also in Chapter 4. Compare and contrast the use of the term "co-occupations" in these two chapters.

- The contributions of nature and nurture to early childhood development have continually been debated. Take a position on the nature/nurture debate and use the information provided in this chapter to support your position.

- In this chapter, you were provided with some insights from current neuroscience research. What did you take away from this presentation, and how do you envision using this information in your clinical practice with young children and their families?

- Imagine yourself as a therapist who will be working with Laura and Lana. How would you explain the concept "temperament" to Laura? Further, if Laura wants to know how you can be helpful if it is true that Laura's temperament is biologically determined, what would you say?

References

Anders, T. F., Halpern, L. F., & Hua, J. (1992). Sleep through the night: A developmental perspective. *Pediatrics, 90,* 554–560.

Arendell, T. (2000). Conceiving and investigating motherhood: The decade's scholarship. *Journal of Marriage and the Family, 62,* 1192–1207.

Barr, R. G. (1990). The early crying paradox: A modest proposal. *Human Nature 1*(4), 355–389.

Bates, J. E. (1989). Concepts and measures of temperament: Applications of temperament concepts. In G. A. Kohnstamm, J. E. Bates, & M. K. Rothbart (Eds.). *Temperament in childhood* (pp. 3–26; 321–355). Chichester, England: John Wiley.

Black, J. E. & Greenough, W. T. (1998). Developmental approaches to the memory process. In J. Martinez & R. Kesner (Eds.). *Neurobiology of Learning and Memory* (pp. 55–88). New York: Academic Press.

Bronfenbrenner, U. (1979). *The ecology of human development.* Cambridge, MA: Harvard University Press.

Bronfenbrenner, U., & Morris, P. A. (1988). The ecology of developmental processes. In R. Lerner (Ed.), *Handbook of child psychology* (pp. 993–1028). New York: John Wiley & Sons, Inc.

Carey, W. B. (1974). Night waking and temperament in infancy. *Journal of Pediatrics, 84,* 756–758.

Coltrane, S., & Adams, M. (2001). Men's family work: Child-centered fathering and the aring of domestic labor. In R. Hertz and N. L. Marshall (Eds.). *Working families* (pp 72–99). Berkeley: University of California Press.

Crockenburg, S. (1981). Infant irritability, mother responsiveness, and social support influences on the security of infant-mother attachment. *Child Development, 54,* 199–1210.

Davidson, R. J. (1994). Temperament, affective style, and frontal lobe asymmetry. In G. Dawson and K. Fischer (Eds.). *Human Behavior and the Developing Brain* (pp. 518–536). New York: Guilford Press.

Davies, D. (1999). *Child development: A practitioner's guide.* NY: Guilford Press.

Dawson, G., & Ashman, S. (1997). On the origins of a vulnerability to depression: The influence of the early social environment on the development of psychobiological systems related to risk for affective disorder. In C. A. Nelson (Ed.). The effects of adversity on neurobehavioral development: Minnesota Symposium on Child Psychology, 31 (pp.245–279). Hillsdale, NJ: Lawrence Erlbaum Associates.

Dawson, G. H., Panagiotides, L., Grofer Klinger, and Hill, D. (1992). The role of frontal lobe functioning in the development of infant self-regulatory behavior. *Brain and Cognition, 20,* 152–175.

Dawson, P. (1992). Should the field of early child and family intervention address failure to thrive? *Zero to Three, 12*(7), 20–24.

Dettwyler, K.A. (1987). Breastfeeding and weaning in Mali: Cultural context and hard data. *Social Sciences & Medicine, 24*(8), 633–644.

Diamond, A. (1991). Frontal lobe involvement in cognitive changes during the first year of life. In K. R. Gibson & A. C. Petersen (Eds.). *Brain maturation and cognitive development: Comparative and cross-cultural.* (pp. 127–180). New York: Aldine DeGruyter.

Dickstein, S., Siefer, R., Magee, K. D., Mirsky, E., & Lynch, M. M. (1998). Timing of maternal depression, family functioning, and infant development: A rospective view. Paper presented at the Biennial Meeting of the Marce Society, June, 1998, Iowa City, Iowa.

Dobbing, J., & Sands, J. (1973). Quantitative growth and

development of the human brain. *Archives of Diseases of Childhood, 48,* 757–767.

Dunlea, A. (1996). An opportunity for co-adaptation: The experience of mothers and their infants who are blind. In R. Clarke and R. Zemke (Eds.). *Occupational science: The evolving discipline.* (pp. 227–242). Philadelphia: F. A. Davis.

Emde, R. N. (1987). The infant's relationship experience: Developmental and affective aspects. In A. J. Sameroff & R. N. Emde. (Eds.). *Relationship disturbances in early childhood* (pp. 33–51). New York: Basic Books.

Fiese, B. (2002). Routines of daily living and rituals in family life: A glimpse at stability and changes during the early child-raising years. *Zero to Three, 22(4),* 10–13.

Forcey, L. R. (1994). Feminist perspectives on mothering and peace. In E. N. Glenn, G. Chang, & L. R. Forcey (Eds.). *Mothering: Ideology, experience, and agency* (pp. 355–375). New York: Routledge.

Fox, N. A., Calkins, S. D., & Bell, M. A. (1994). Neural plasticity and development in the first two years of life: Evidence from cognitive and socioemotional domains of research. *Development and Psychopathology, 6,* 677–696.

Fraiberg, S., Shapiro, V., & Cherniss, D. S. (1980). Treatment modalities. In S. Fraiberg (Ed.). Clinical studies in infant mental health: The first year of life (pp. 49–77). New York: Basic Books.

Frankel, K. A., & Harmon, R. J. (1996). Depressed mothers: They don't always look as bad as they feel. *Journal of the American Academy of Child and Adolescent Psychiatry, 35(3),* 289–298.

Gelfand, D. M., Teti, D. M., Seiner, S. A., & Jameson, P. B. (1996). Helping mothers fight depression: Evaluation of a home-based intervention program for depressed mothers and their infants. *Journal of Clinical Child Psychology, 25(4),* 406–422.

Greenough, W. T. (1987). Experience effects on the developing brain and the mature brain: Dendritic branching and synaptogenesis. In N. A. Krasnegor, E. M. Blass, M. A. Hofer, & W. P. Smotherman (Eds.). *Perinatal development: A psycho biological perspective* (pp. 195–221). Orlando: Academic Press.

Greenough, W. T., & Black, J. E. (1992). Induction of brain structure by experience: Substrates for cognitive development. In M. Gunnar & C. Nelson. (Eds.). *Developmental Behavioral Neurosciences: The Minnesota Symposia on Child Psychology, 24,* 155–200. Hillsdale, NJ: Erlbaum.

Greenspan, S. I. (1997). *The growth of the mind.* New York: Addison-Wesley.

Gunnar, M. (1998). Quality of early care and buffering of neuroendocrine stress-reactions: Potential effects on the developing human brain. *Preventive Medicine, 27,* 208–211.

Gunnar, M., Brodersen, L., Krueger, L., & Rigatuso, J. (1996). Dampening of adrenocortical reactivity during early infancy: Normative changes and individual differences. *Child Development, 67,* 877–889.

Gunnar, M., & Nelson, C. (1994). Event-related potentials in year-old infants predict negative emotionality

and hormonal responses to separation. *Child Development, 65,* 80–94.

Gunnar, M., Tout, K., de Haan, M., & Pierce, S. (1997). Temperament, social competence, and adrenocortical activity in preschoolers. *Developmental Psychobiology, 3(1),* 65–85.

Halpern, L. F., Anders, T. F., Coll, C. G., & Hua, J. (1994). Infant temperament: Is there a relation to sleep-wake states and maternal nighttime behavior? *Infant Behavior and Development, 17,* 255–263.

Hrdy, S. B. (1999). *Mother nature.* New York: Pantheon Books.

Humphrey, R. (1991). Impact of feeding problems on the parent-infant relationship. *Infants and Young Children, 3(3),* 30–38.

Huttenlocher, P. R. (1979). Synaptic density in human frontal cortex-developmental changes and effects of aging. *Brain Research, 163,* 195–205.

Huntington, G. S., & Simeonsson, R. (1993). Temperament and adaptation in infants and young children with disabilities. *Infant Mental Health Journal, 14(1),* 49–60.

Imms, C. (2001). Feeding the infant with congenital heart disease: An occupational performance challenge. *American Journal of Occupational Therapy, 55(7),* 277–284.

Joseph, R. (1999). Environmental influences on neural plasticity, the limbic system, emotional development and attachment: A review. *Child Psychiatry and Human Development, 29(3),* 189–208.

Kagan, J. (1994). *Galen's Prophecy.* New York: Basic Books.

Keener, M. A., Zeanah, C. H., & Anders, T. F. (1988). Infant temperament, sleep organization, and nighttime parental interventions. *Pediatrics, 81,* 762–771.

Kimball, J. (1999). Sensory integration frame of reference: Postulates regarding change and application to practice. In P. Kramer & J. Hinojosa (Eds.). *Frames of reference for pediatric occupational therapy* (2nd Ed.) (pp. 169–204). Philadelphia: Lippincott, Williams & Wilkins.

Kubicek, L. (2002). Fresh perspectives of young children and family routines. *Zero to Three, 22(4),* 4–9.

Law, M., Polatajko, H., Baptiste, S., & Townsend, E. (1997). Core concepts of Occupational Therapy. In E. Towsend (Ed.), *Enabling occupation : An occupational therapy perspective.* (pp. 29–56). Ottawa, ON: Canadian Association of Occupational Therapists.

McEwen, B. S., Angulo, J., Cameron, H., et al. (1992). Paradoxical effects of adrenal steroids on the brain: Protection versus degeneration. *Biological Psychiatry, 31,* 177–199.

McKenna, J. J., Mosko, S., Richard, C., Drummond, S., Hunt, L., Cetel, M. B., & Arpaia, J. (1994). Experimental studies of infant-parent co-sleeping mutual physiological and behavioral influences and their relevance to SIDS. *Early Human Development, 38,* 187–201.

McKenna, J. J., Thoman, E. B., Anders, T. F., Sadeh, A., Schechtman, V. L., & Glotzbach, S. F. (1993). Infant-parent co-sleeping in an evolutionary perspective: Implications for understanding infant sleep development and the sudden infant death syndrome. *Sleep, 16*(3), 263–282.

Nachmias, M., Gunnar, M., Mangelsdorf, S., Parritz, R., & Buss, K. (1996). Behavioral inhibition and stress reactivity: Moderating role of attachment security. *Child Development, 67,* 508–522.

Obermeyer, C. M., & Castle, S. (1997). Back to nature? Historical and cross cultural perspectives on barriers to optimal breastfeeding. *Medical Anthropology, 17,* 39–63.

Olson, J. (1998). *A phenomenological study of infant mental health interventions: The mothers' perspective.* Unpublished doctoral dissertation, Wayne State University.

Plomin, R. (1986). *Development, genetics and psychiatry.* Hillsdale, NJ: Lawrence Erlbaum.

Rochat, P. (2001). *The infant's world.* Cambridge, MA: Harvard University Press.

Rothbart, M. K., & Derryberry, D. (1981). Development of individual differences in temperament. In M. E. Lamb & A. L. Brown. (Eds.). *Advances in developmental psychology* (Vol. 1) (pp. 37–86). Hillsdale, NJ: Lawrence Erlbaum.

Ruddick, S. (1980). Maternal thinking. *Feminist Studies, 6,* 343–367.

Rutter, M. (1994). Temperament: Changing concepts and implications. In W. B. Carey and S. McDevitt (Eds.), *Prevention and early intervention* (pp. 23–34). New York: Brunner/Mazel.

Sadeh, A. (2001). *Sleeping like a baby.* New Haven: Yale University Press.

Sadeh, A., & Anders, T. (1993). Infant sleep problems: Origins, assessment, interventions. *Infant Mental Health Journal, 14,* 17–34.

Sameroff, A. J. (1993). Models of development and developmental risk. In C. H. Zeanah, Jr. (Ed.). *Handbook of infant mental health* (pp. 3–13). New York: Guilford Press.

Sameroff, A. J., & Chandler, M. J. (1975). Reproductive risk and the continuum of caretaking casualty. In M. Horowtiz, M. Hetherington, S. Scarr-Salapatek, & G. Sigel (Eds.) *Review of Child Development Research, Vol. 4* (pp. 187–244). Chicago: University of Chicago Press.

Schore, A. N. (1994). Affect regulation and the origin of the self: *The neurobioloby of emotional development.* Hillsdale, NJ: Erlbaum.

Selye, H. (1973). The evolution of the stress concept. *American Scientist, 61*(6), 692–699.

Selye, H. (1975). Confusion and controversy in the stress field. *Journal of Human Stress, 1*(2), 37–44.

Shonkoff, J. P., & Phillips, D. A. (2000). *From neurons to neighborhoods: The science of early childhood development.* Washington, DC: National Academy Press.

Stern, D. & Bruschweiler-Stern, N. (1998). *The birth of a mother.* NY: Basic Books.

Teti, D. M., O'Connell, M. A., & Reiner, C. D. (1996). Parenting sensitivity, parental depression and child health: The mediational role of parental self-efficacy. *Early Development and Parenting, 5*(4), 237–250.

Thomas, A., & Chess, S. (1986). The New York Longitudinal Study: From infancy to early adult life. In R. Plomin & J. Dunn. (Eds.), *The study of temperament: Change, continuities and challenges* (pp 39–52). Hillside, NJ: Lawrence Erlbaum.

Tronick, E. Z., & Weinberg, M. K. (1997). Depressed mothers and infants: Failure to form dyadic states of consciousness. In L. Murray and P. J. Cooper (Eds.). *Postpartum Depression and Child Development* (pp. 54–81). New York: Guilford Press.

Vergara, E. R. (2002). Enhancing occupational performance in infants in the NICU. *OT Practice, 7*(12), 8–13.

Vygotsky, L.S. (1978). *Mind in society: The development of higher psychological processes.* Cambridge, MA: Harvard University Press.

Weatherston, D., & Tableman, B. (1989). *Infant mental health services: Supporting competencies/reducing risks.* Lansing, MI: Michigan Department of Mental Health.

Wright, P., MacLeod, H. A., & Cooper, M. J. (1983). Waking at night: The effect of early feeding experience. *Child Care and Healthy Development, 9,* 309–319.

Zeanah, C. H., Boris, N. W., & Larrieu, J. A. (1997). Infant development and developmental risk: A review of the past 10 years. *Journal of the American Academy of Child and Adolescent Psychiatry, 36*(2), 165–178.

Zemke, R., & Clarke, F. (Eds.). (1996). *Occupational science the evolving discipline.* Philadelphia: F. A. Davis Co.

CHAPTER 3

The Physical Day-to-Day Care of Young Children: Methods and Meanings

Susan D. Griffin, PhD, MA(Hons), BAppSc(OT), GradDip AppBehSc

 Anticipated Outcomes

I anticipate that, after reading this chapter, readers will:

- Understand the wide range of ways in which mothers go about the day-to-day care of their young children and how they structure their daily mothering occupations into routines
- Understand the effect of the meanings of mothering occupations on how they organize their daily routines and go about mothering occupations
- Understand the ways in which mothers lift and handle their children and the reasons for these choices
- Understand the relevance of these themes and ideas to their own professional practice

Introduction

Mothers organize the physical day-to-day care of young children into routines that are meaningful to them in a variety of ways. This organization is influenced by the meanings of these occupations for the mothers and their families. They physically lift and handle their children in ways that are consistent with these meanings. This chapter explores these concepts and ideas from the perspective of Australian mothers who participated in a number of qualitative research projects. The ideas are explored using a description of "Mary's Day" and the routines of other mothers to practically illustrate the key ideas that have emerged from my research to date. I hope this chapter broadens your understanding of mothering occupations for mothers of young children and causes you to think carefully about your own attitudes toward "normal" ways of getting the physical day-to-day care of young children done.

The chapter includes an introduction followed by a brief description of the research design of the studies from which this chapter draws. This is followed by a detailed respondent profile that illuminates the major ideas discussed in the remainder of the chapter.

The themes from my research are discussed in the context of other research in the area. Professional implications are discussed in the various sections of the chapter and then reviewed in the conclusion. The conclusion also highlights areas of future research and the scholarly implications of the studies.

When my first child was 12 weeks old, I met with a group of friends whose firstborn children were of a similar age to my son Dennis. My answer to the question of "How are you?" was that I was in mourning. Deep creases furrowed their brows as they asked what had happened. No person had died, but my old life had. I had come to realize over the preceding week that I was in a state of mourning for my old life—the one in which I had been able to please myself about what I did, when I did it, and how I did it. I was exhausted from lack of sleep, having been breast-feeding my large son every 2 1/2 hours, 24 hours a day. My nipples were cracked and sore. I felt I had no time for myself, and on some days all I could do was sleep when he slept. On other days I would sit on my front step with my "bundle of joy" on a rug on the front lawn, hoping the trees in the wind would distract him long enough for me to read the chapter of a book, waiting desperately for his father to come home so I could go for a run or walk on my own. As our group of friends moved through that first few months and then the first year of our children's lives, I became increasingly interested in how the choices I made about how I would care for my son on a day-to-day basis affected my well being, both physical and mental. My initial decision to "demand feed" had led to my sense of having no time because I seemed to be always feeding. My choice of a stroller meant I much preferred to walk on my own because the handles were too short and my back ached if I walked too far with the stroller. I found myself avoiding some activities because physically getting there with the stroller was quite difficult. I became aware of the fact that I did things in ways that were at times quite different from the ways of other mothers in my network. Even things that we did the same way were perhaps done so for very different reasons. Bath time was play time for Dennis and me, whereas it was a settling routine for a friend of mine. So while we both bathed our children in the morning, using similar methods, we did so for different reasons. For me, it was because that's when I had the most energy to play; for my friend, it was because it settled her daughter before a late morning sleep.

It took several years for me to come to the realization that I could combine my curiosity about my mothering experiences with my professional interest in human occupations and how they are executed. As an occupational therapist working in an academic setting, I slowly developed and built up a research program around the occupation of mothering. At the time I began my study there seemed to be an extensive body of research literature about the impact of parenting on outcomes for children. My interest however, is in the experiences of mothers as they go about the day-to-day occupations that make up the role of mothering. I am interested in what they do, how they do it, and why they make their choices. I am interested in occupations in which they are engaged, both inside and outside the home, that they feel are part of their mothering role, and I am interested in their experiences of well-being.

My first son is now 10 years old and has two brothers, ages 8 and 5 years. My research program grows slowly as I combine my part-time academic career with my mothering role. The ideas and themes reported in this chapter come from a number of studies on lifting and handling (Griffin & Price, 2000; Seto, 2002) and mothers' physical day-to-day care of their young children (Griffin, 2002). These studies sought to understand what mothers do, how they do it and why they choose to carry out activities the way they do. I also report on some of the meanings various childcare activities have for the mothers who participated in my studies and how they organized and accomplished their tasks. These meanings influence some of the choices of equipment and methods mothers use to get the tasks done. I believe that this information is relevant to all who work with women who are mothers. The wide variety of methods and the even more extensive number of reasons for the choices women make can provide professionals and others that work with women with a range of strategies to call upon when women are having difficulty accomplishing the day-to-day care of their children. I believe that my studies have the potential to highlight the wide range of "normal" ways in which women care for young children. It can help professionals to understand the reasoning behind the choices women make, and thereby assists in making informed suggestions for alternative methods when needed. It can also help us make suggestions for safe, ergonomically appropriate ways to accomplish tasks (e.g., safe lifting and handling of children) that are consistent with these meanings. The wider the range of "normal" strategies available to women, the more empowered they will be in managing the day-to-day physical care of their young children. The ideas and themes emerging from my research are discussed in the context of other literature in the field.

‎ Design of the Studies

The themes and ideas presented in this chapter are a compilation of the insights gleaned from a number of qualitative research studies. Because my research has focused on mothers' lived experiences as they carry out the occupation of mothering, I believe that qualitative methods are the best way to do this. I have always been interested in what mothers do and how they go about their occupations as well as the meanings they attribute to various occupations and how they come to engage in them in certain ways. This approach has been described by Dowling (2000), who looked at the meaning of car use by suburban mothers as a cultural approach that provides "thick descriptions." "A thick description is generated by paying attention to culture, and in particular to the meanings that surround objects and activities" (Dowling, 2000, p. 346). I have found that the most effective way to gather these thick descriptions has been via semi-structured interviews. In each research project, broad research questions have been developed and a semi structured interview used to explore them. This has ensured a similar topic focus for each interview while still allowing mothers to set the parameters or range

of experiences they discussed. Data have been analyzed in each instance using open and axial coding. In each instance, participants were recruited for the study via advertisements in a parenting magazine or at early childhood centers, or by snowballing, which is when one participant provides the researcher with leads for recruiting other participants. This often takes the form of passing on information about the research to other potential participants. Generally, the participants were middle class women who spoke English fluently, covered a range of ages from early 20s to early 40s, and had from 1 to 4 children. The mothers interviewed were all living in a large Australian capital city (Sydney). Their experiences that have informed this research will necessarily have been influenced by this factor. The fact that they were all middle class will also have influenced the values they hold about mothering and the lifestyles they have been able to develop, including their access to resources and financial stability. A similar access to resources and lifestyles by a mostly middle-class sample has been noted by Kellegrew (2000) in her study of mothers of young children with disabilities.

The largest study (approximately 50 mothers) on which I am drawing for this chapter was concerned with how mothers go about the day-to-day physical care of their children under 3 years. I sought to understand what they did, how they did it, why they did it the way they did, and what meanings various activities they included in their mothering role had for them. For the interviews I used the concept of activity settings from ecocultural theory (Gallimore et al., 1989) as a framework. Ecocultural theory emphasizes that a major adaptive task for each family is the construction and maintenance of daily routines through which families organize and shape their children's activity and development. The theory has been developed initially around the experiences of families with a child with a developmental delay but is applicable to all families in my view. The authors propose that ecocultural effects that influence how a family constructs its meaningful daily routines include family subsistence and finances, the accessibility of health and educational services, home and neighborhood safety and convenience, the domestic task and chore workload for the family, childcare tasks, children's play groups and networks, marital role relationships, social support, father's role, and the sources of parental information and goals. Families go through a process of accommodation, adapting to the needs of their particular children by making adjustments in each of these areas. The model focuses on activity settings surrounding everyday interactions with children as the context in which all ecocultural influences have their effect. Activity settings are composed of five factors, which guided my interviews with the mothers. I sought to explore:

1. Who did the task and who else was there at the time?
2. Exactly what tasks were being performed and how?
3. What were the motives and feelings surrounding or guiding the action?
4. What were the values and goals of doing the tasks?
5. How did the mothers come to do it the way they did (whether any scripts guided the actions)?

The interviews opened with a general request for the mothers to tell me about their day. The five factors above were explored using further probes as the mothers discussed their occupations and routines.

The other two studies were smaller (8 to 10 mothers each) and focused around how mothers lift and handle their young children. They sought to understand how mothers lift their children, how much they knew and were able to apply about lifting principles, why they did not necessarily lift their children safely, and what facilitated or hindered them from using good lifting practices in their everyday childcare.

The themes and ideas described in this chapter represent my insights and ideas that have emerged as a result of these research experiences, rather than a detailed and comprehensive report of each research project. The studies on which I am drawing here have been or will be published elsewhere (Griffin, 2002; Griffin & Price, 2000; Seto, 2002). Similarly,

the research design information presented here is to enable you as reader to place the themes and ideas discussed into context, rather than as a detailed account of the research methods employed. It is not my aim in this chapter to explore in detail the links between my own data and ecocultural theory. What follows is a composite profile of the day of one mother, whom I have called Mary, not her actual name. This profile is used to discuss four themes: daily routine or changeable routine, the meaning of activities, the physical and ergonomic organization of caring, and a wide range of normal, which follow later in the chapter. Other mothers' routines and experiences are also used to illustrate points made. A profile of all mothers and their families (using pseudonyms) used in this way is in Table 3–1.

Vignette: *Mary's Day*

Mary's day begins around 6 AM, when she breast-feeds her youngest child, Holly, while in bed. "They say you should give them solids before a breast feed at this stage," she says, but Mary likes to stay in bed as long as she can. Also, she does not know anyone who gets up to give solid food before a morning feed. After Holly is burped, she leaves her to roll on the floor in the bedroom while she takes a quick shower. She puts Holly down by bending at the waist and keeping her legs straight (a stoop lift). Her other children make their way into her room when they wake up. They play with Holly and talk to Mary while she showers. Before going downstairs, Mary dresses her other two children, Mark and Sarah, and washes their faces. They both like to dress on the landing, and Mary has left their clothes on the landing lounge the night before. She leaves their pajamas in a bag on the bathroom door ready for the evening bath time. She makes the beds before she goes downstairs, taking Holly with her from room to room. The others come and go from where she is to the landing where they are playing. If any pajamas or sheets need washing, she collects them as she heads downstairs. John, her husband, has already left for work by the time she gets up.

Table 3–1 Profiles of the Families Featured in this Chapter

Mary is 35 years old and lives with her husband John, 43, in a leafy Sydney suburb. Her husband works full time while she is at home with their three children full time. The children are Sarah, 6 years; Mark, 5 years; and Holly, 9 months. Sarah and Mark are at school and Holly goes to play group twice a week.

Maggie, 39, lives with her husband Malcolm, 38, in a modest three-bedroom house in an inner Sydney suburb. She has three children: Marcus, 5 years; Laurence, 4 years; and George, 2 years. Malcolm works a shift work job, full time, and Maggie works casually on his days off. The rest of the time she is at home with the children. Marcus is at school and Laurence goes to preschool 2 days per week.

Anna, 25, is a single mother with one son, Adam, 2 1/2 years. She is a full-time graduate student at a university and lives in a small two-bedroom apartment in the inner city. She has a subsidized place at a long daycare center for Adam and receives a living allowance as a full time student and parent support benefits.

Marea, 32; Victor, 32; and Robert, 2 live in a modest two-bedroom house. Marea and Victor both work full time and Marea is also studying at the university as a distance student, part time. Robert attends a long daycare center from about 7:30 AM to 6 PM Monday through Friday.

Sarah, 36, lives in an inner city semi-detached house with her husband Michael, 37, and their two children: Harry, 4, and Elizabeth, 2. Michael works full time while Sarah is home with the children full time. She lives close to a local park, which she visits often during the day with the children. Harry goes to preschool 2 days per week.

Margaret, 35, is home full time looking after Dylan, who is 10 months old. Her husband Peter, 39, works full time and is away for long hours during the day. She lives in a leafy suburb with mostly newer houses and is within walking distance of a small local shopping center. She attends a play group weekly.

Amanda, 37, lives with her husband James, 41, and their two children: Hamish, 4, and Katie, 2. They were expecting a third child at the time of the interview. James is a medical practitioner working in a local general practice quite close to home. Amanda is home full time with the children. Hamish attends preschool 2 days per week.

Rosemary, 36, lives with her husband Patrick and her two children: Annie, 8 months, and Jordan, 2 1/2 years. Patrick works full time at the local hospital as a technician while she looks after the children. Jordan attends long daycare once per week to give her a break.

The requirements for breakfast have been laid out on the kitchen bench the night before. She fills the bowls with cereal and milk, and Mark and Sarah eat at the kitchen bench. Holly is in her highchair and gums a toast finger while Mary unloads the dishwasher from the night before. She quickly goes into the laundry to put in the wash while the children are having breakfast. She eats her own toast in between the other activities. Once breakfast is finished, the children use the downstairs bathroom to clean their teeth and read or play together in the family room while Mary makes the school lunches. She usually leaves Holly in the high chair while she does this. The wash is usually finished before Mark and Sarah leave for school, so Mary hangs it out. She takes Holly outside with her and puts her on the back deck to play. She uses a stoop lift to put Holly down and pick the wash basket up and down. The other two children come and go from the back deck to the family room, playing. The last task before they leave for school is to pack Holly's bag. Mary uses cloth diapers, so she makes sure there is a supply in the bag, together with Holly's morning tea. They will be walking to the local elementary school and attending a play group on the way home, at a local church hall. Mary walks to school by choice because she feels it is good exercise for her and the children. It takes about 15 minutes each way. On wet days she drives to school.

On the way to school Mary puts the colored "car diapers" into the trunk of the car. She uses colored ones for the car and always puts them straight back into the car once they are washed. That way she knows she always has a supply when she uses the car to go out. The regular diapers are white and are used at home or when walking to school or the play group. To manage the washing of diapers, Mary has three diaper buckets going. She soaks eight diapers at a time in each bucket and fills and washes the buckets consecutively. This keeps the loads manageable and means that she always has clean diapers on hand. She keeps the buckets on the laundry floor.

Play group lasts a couple of hours and is a chance for Mary to meet with the mothers of other young children. The children play together while the mothers supervise and chat over morning tea. Mary attends the play group twice a week from about 9:30 AM to 11:30 AM. Holly usually falls asleep on the way home from the play group. She stays in her stroller when they get home so that she will stay asleep. While Holly is asleep in the stroller, Mary does some household chores like mopping, dusting, tidying the family room. She also has her own lunch at the kitchen bench and will use the time to organize household bills or make phone calls. Holly has her lunch in the high chair after she wakes in the early afternoon. Mary uses this time to do some preparation for dinner. She watches Holly eat as she works at the kitchen bench. The rest of the afternoon before she picks up her older children from school is spent doing things around the house with Holly in tow. Mary gets less done on days when Holly is unsettled or upset. She spends more time with Holly directly on days when this happens.

Holly and Mary walk up to collect Mark and Sarah from school about 2:30 PM. Two days a week she collects the neighbors' two children also. They all walk back together, arriving around 3:30 PM. The children all have a snack on the back deck or in the family room. They usually have cut-up fruit and cookies. Mary unpacks their school bags and cleans out the lunch boxes while they eat, and also reads any notes from school. Mary uses a wall calendar to keep track of events at school and any notes or payments she needs to send in for school activities. Once a week Sarah attends a dance class in the early evening from 4:30 to 5:30 PM. They drive to the dance class. Mark takes something to play with and Holly usually falls asleep in her car carrier capsule on the way there. Mary brings the carrier into the dance class so that Holly will stay asleep. They get home about 5:45 PM, and Mary finishes the dinner preparations she started while Holly was having lunch. The children all play together in the family room, then have dinner at the kitchen bench. On some

evenings Mary eats with them; on others she waits for her husband John to return home and they eat together after the children are in bed. Mary sits at the bench and chats with the children while they eat, asking them about their day. They play briefly while she cleans up the kitchen. It is homework time after this, so they all sit at the dining-room table. Holly plays on the floor and comes and goes to and from Mary while she helps Mark and Sarah with homework. One other afternoon in the week, Mark has soccer practice, and the routine is the same. Mary's children rarely watch TV except perhaps a children's program on a rainy afternoon. She is aware that they watch a lot less than some of their friends.

On days when they do not go out in the afternoon, the children change from their school uniforms into play clothes when they get home. They do this downstairs in the bathroom, where Mary has left some clothes waiting the evening before when she sorted the wash. They spend the afternoon playing until it is dinner time. Mary will often set up activities for them and then bring in and sort the wash or do some other task that needs to be done. They come and go to and from her, often talking about what they are doing, asking for help. Holly plays around on the floor wherever Mary or the older children are.

Once the homework is finished, the children all go upstairs for a bath. They undress in the bathroom, making a pile of dirty clothes. They all get in together. Holly gets out last because Mary needs to know where she is. The other two dry and dress in the bathroom with Mary's help, using the pajamas that have been in the pajama bag on the door of the bathroom. Once they are in pajamas, they clean their teeth and play on the upstairs landing area. Mary then dries Holly and puts her night diapers and pajamas on while kneeling on the bathroom floor. They all sit on the lounge on the landing for stories before they go to bed. This takes about half an hour. By this time, John is usually home, and he reads the stories while Mary goes down to check on the dinner that she and John will eat when the children are settled. During this time, she also cleans up the bathroom.

Mary goes back upstairs to see the children to bed once story time is over. She is back downstairs with John for dinner between 7:30 and 8 PM. They chat over dinner for a while and then she cleans up the kitchen, stacks the dishwasher to run, and sets out the cereal and other breakfast things for the morning. She then sorts clothes if she has not had a chance to do so earlier in the evening. She may then do the next day's ironing while she watches some TV. She often mops the floor last thing at night so that it has a chance to dry without anyone walking on it. Mary gets into bed around 10 PM and is usually glad to lie down because her back is often quite tired and aching by the end of the day.

On days when Mary does not go to play group, she is often out in the car, grocery shopping or paying bills in the morning. Some days she uses the time to garden or do other big jobs around the house. She fits her activities in around Holly's naps (late morning and late afternoon). She thinks that the routine helps Holly not to become overtired and fractious in the evenings.

This description of Mary's day highlights a number of themes that have emerged from my research: the idea of a daily routine or changeable routine, the meaning of activities, the physical and ergonomic organization of caring, and the wide range of "normal" ways to care for children. These are discussed in the sections that follow, together with other relevant literature.

ꙮ Daily Routine

The description of Mary's day reveals a highly organized daily routine. She does things in much the same way and order each day, relying a great deal on preplanning and preparation to get things done. She has systems in place to deal with diaper washing, bathing and dressing, getting homework done, and a bedtime routine. For Mary, this level of organization and structure to her daily routine means that she can accomplish the tasks she wishes to get done with the greatest ease. The systems she has in place mean that she does not have to think a great deal about what needs to be done or how to do it because she has established a routine that she follows automatically.

She describes the way this enables her to get more done in the time she has and the fact that her children are at home with the routine because they know what to expect and when to expect it.

Mary's day is an example of a highly structured and routinized day. The mothers that I interviewed varied in the extent to which they structured or routinized their day-to-day care of their children. Most mothers had some routine or structure to their day, with children's sleeping patterns being the major determinants of the routine. Many described fitting shopping and housework around the naps of their children. This was particularly the case with mothers of only one child. Most of these mothers organized the majority of their day around the sleeping patterns of their child. For many mothers of younger children who were breast-fed, the pattern for the day was established with the timing of the first breast-feeding and when subsequent sleeping and feeding would follow in the day. Mothers in this situation often described their frustration at not being able to make appointments ahead of time because they would not know when they would be available for an appointment on any given day. Not interrupting the sleep of their child, particularly an only child, was very important to these mothers. For many, this was because of their bad experiences with unsettled evenings if their child did not get enough sleep. For some, it was the chance to catch up on sleep or to have some time out for them when their child slept. In order to get things done, many described preparing to go out while the child was asleep so that they could leave as soon as the child woke and had been fed. This would maximize the time they spent out and about before the next feeding or sleep was due. For mothers with more than one child, sleep was still important, but because of the activities of the older children, younger ones had often developed their sleep routines around the outings and activities of the older children. They would sleep on the way home from play group or on the way to preschool to collect their siblings. For mothers of one child, it was often the child's routine that dictated how the rest of the day would fall into place. When mothers had more than one child, particularly three or more, they were often more prepared to fit the younger child into their routines or those of the older children and theirs combined.

Changeable Routines

Although the majority of mothers had some form of routine, a few did not feel the need for each day to follow the same pattern. One mother like this was Maggie. She had three children, one at school and two others at home, one of whom was still breast-feeding. Maggie had organized sharing of the school drop-off with another mother who lived locally. On days when she was doing the drop-off, the whole family was up, dressed, and ready to leave the house at about 8:30 AM. On other days, she and the younger children would often stay in pajamas, puttering about at home until quite late in the morning. They often did this on weekends. Maggie did not feel that her children needed exactly the same routine each day. She observed her younger children and put them down for sleep when they seemed tired, and this varied from day to day. Some days her toddler would take himself off to sleep when he was tired. They also ate meals at different times during the day when they felt hungry. Maggie felt that this gave her more flexibility about her routine and meant that her children could adjust quite well to whatever the day brought. There was also some flexibility in the time the children went to bed.

Although many mothers had adapted their day to a greater or lesser extent to fit in with the needs of their children, particularly sleeping and feeding needs, a few did not. An example of a mother whose child fitted in with her daily routine was Anna, a single mother with one son, Adam, who was 2 1/2 years old. Anna was a university student working toward a postgraduate (research) degree and using a daycare center part time for Adam. She liked to sleep in and encouraged Adam to do the same. Adam would often be up until around 11 PM while Anna was working on her research, and sometimes they would go out for dinner quite late. They would often sleep until around 10 or 11 AM, and Adam would not get to the daycare center until late morning. As a full-time graduate student, Anna had a subsidized place at the daycare center, and described the less-than-positive reactions she got from the staff when she was "late" in getting Adam there. She lived in a small two bedroom apartment and had created "spaces" in the apartment for Adam and herself. Adam understood about her space and that when she was there, she wanted to be alone for a while. He would go to his space then and play or watch a video. Anna could see Adam from her space and kept an eye on him while she studied. Anna would sometimes spend a couple of nights a week at her grandmother's, which meant Adam's evening routine was often different from night to night.

Another example of a family in which the parents' needs dictated their child's routine was the family made up of Marea, Victor, and Robert. Robert was about 2 when I talked to his mother Marea about their day. Marea and her husband Victor worked full time and Marea was studying part time. They needed to leave home by around 7:30 each morning. To manage this, Robert showered the last thing at night with his father. He was then dressed in the clothes that he would wear the next day and went to bed in them around 8:30 PM. This streamlined the morning routine so that he needed only his diaper changed when he got up. He had breakfast at his own table-and-chair set in the living room while Marea got herself showered and had breakfast. She packed all their bags and lunches each evening after dinner. Each evening she fed Robert his dinner as soon as they got home, around 6 PM. This was possible because each evening she made extra dinner when she cooked for herself and Victor around 7 PM. She could feed Robert at their dining room table while she got started preparing their evening meal or did other chores such as unloading the dishwasher. She put laundry out in the evenings so she would not have to do it in the busy mornings. Marea kept a diary for a week as part of the research and recorded all the things she did with Robert. Her reflections after doing this were that they did not spend any time doing activities that were specifically for Robert. He spent all of his time doing things with his parents that they needed to get done. She commented that she felt she needed to build in some activities such as play times or visits to the park that were focused more around Robert.

The examples of the daily routines of Mary, Anna, Maggie, and Marea show how different levels of structure and repeated daily patterns are built into the mothers' day-to-day care of their young children. All four mothers whose daily routines have been described here were generally happy with the structures of their day. For some, the daily routine was strongly influenced by the sleeping and feeding needs of their children and the mothers' belief in the importance of routines. For others, the routine was organized around their own personal preferences and time needs, such as the demands of work. For Maggie, each day varied, and she did not have a strong need or belief in a similar daily routine. She liked the flexibility of each day being different. While Anna's routine suited her, people from another organization she interacted with, namely the daycare center, did not appreciate what for them was "lateness," repeated on many occasions, because they felt that, if she was not going to use the care place fully, she should give it up for someone else. Each of these mothers and the other mothers I interviewed had constructed a daily routine around the activities that were important for them and were congruent with their values and beliefs about routines for children. This is consistent with ecocultural theory, which proposes that an important issue for families is constructing and sustaining a daily routine of life that has meaning for members (Gallimore, Weisner, Kaufman & Bernheimer, 1989). The process of constructing a daily routine has been referred to as orchestration in occupational science and refers to the "ideation, composition, execution, ordering, and qualitative aspects of occupation through the course of one's day" (Larson, 2000, p.269). Larson overviews the components of orchestration as an informational dimension where choices, decisions and actions are taken depending on the information available; the decision making involves a balanced consideration of all important factors and the envi-

ronment, including the social environment, in which the decisions are being made. Constructing the daily routine means taking into account the abilities and preferences of the members of the family, in this instance the mothers and their perceptions of other family members' needs, as well as the social or organizational context in which the family lives such as support networks. This also raises the issue of organizations outside the family.

Mothers of quite young children who did not interact with outside organizations were able to exercise the most flexibility with their daily routines if they chose to. Once their own activities or their children's activities were linked to outside organizations such as preschools, schools, play groups, or places of employment, fixed time commitments led them to adopt at least some daily routines that were similar and structured from day to day. This is consistent with the research of Dyck (1992), who used time and space maps in her analysis of mothers' daily routines. She found that mothers' interactions with outside organizations for their children influenced the way in which they structured their routines. Similarly, in studies on transportation planning, Kutter (1981, cited in Primeau, 1996) found that participation in certain occupations such as school or work requires compliance with its temporal or time requirements and that these temporal expectations set a daily schedule and routine.

One mother who had not chosen any particular routines or time structures around meal times described her difficulty settling her son into preschool. Sarah had decided she did not want meal times to be an ordeal for her. She simply offered food at various times during the day and often left it out on a small table for her two young children to come to and go from during the day, eating when they wished. She cooked an evening meal, but not necessarily at the same time each day, and the meal would often be carried, hot, down to the local park at the end of her street. She would spoon-feed her children as they swung back and forward on a swing. While she was not interacting with another organization, these arrangements were fine. She described the difficulty her son was experiencing on the 2 days a week he had started to attend a local preschool. Breaks and snacks happened at specific times in the preschool, and her son Julian was having trouble sitting at a table to eat when it was time to eat according to the preschool schedule. Sarah reflected that she was not sure now if her approach had been a good thing, and she was thinking of introducing a bit more structure to the children's routines for meals at home. She felt this might help Julian's and later her daughter Renée's adjustment to preschool.

A number of mothers spoke to me about how disruptive it was, particularly to their morning routines, when someone who was not familiar with the routines got involved. Most often this person was their husband or partner. They described how "he" tried to do things differently from the normal routine or way of doing activities and that this created conflict with the children, who had their own ideas about how things should be done. The mothers often did not view this "help" as very helpful at all. The routines they had constructed suited them and the children, and they preferred to change them only when their children's needs and developmental stages changed.

Whatever choices mothers made about their daily routines, the choices seemed to have been made based on what was important to the mothers. For some who had older children or worked in paid employment, the need to fit in with the time constraints of outside organizations often dictated how their routines would be constructed. Getting everything done in the easiest and smoothest way possible was important for others. For some mothers, getting some time out was important and a regular routine, especially when children's sleep time enabled them to do this. For other mothers, their well-being was enhanced by less rather than more structure, and they maintained this lack of structure actively, even when the outside organizations became part of their lives. Having settled and happy children was important to some mothers, and for some this meant a structured routine, whereas for others it meant being flexible and relaxed. This leads to the next issue I would like to discuss, the meaning of activities.

☙ The Meaning of Activities

As described in the previous section, the motivation behind the different daily routines of mothers varied. So too does the meaning associated with various activities. The meaning of specific activities for the mother and the family will influence how the activity is done, who is involved, where it is carried out, and when it is done. Activities that demonstrate this idea well are *meals or feeding, naps,* and *bathing.*

For mothers like Mary, meals fulfill two purposes. The first is to get children fed, preferably with nutritious food. She is interested in the quality of food her children eat and how much. For this reason, they sit to eat where she can see them, and meals are structured and always in the same place—at the kitchen bench. Although Mary does not always eat with her children, the second purpose of meals is social. She uses the time to talk with them about their day. They talk and interact with one another and with her. De Vault (1991) summarizes the views of some parents in her study: "The parents who spoke about the importance of family meals recognize that meals do more than provide sustenance; they are also social events that bring family members together" (p.39).

Mary is also interested in minimizing the "mess" associated with meals, so they are in the kitchen at the bench, on a surface and floor that are easily cleaned.

Although the social purpose of meals is often more evident in families with slightly older children, it can still be seen with quite young children. Another mother, Margaret, always ate lunch with her 8-month-old son Dylan. In fine weather, she would sit out on her porch with Dylan beside her in his highchair. She would eat her sandwich while she fed him his mashed-vegetable lunch. They would "chat" while they ate. Again she chose an easy to clean place. A similar routine for a mother with a very young child is described by deVault in her study of thirty American families (1991). The evening meal for Margaret was a chance to catch up with her husband Peter. Dylan always ate his evening meal early, and then she and Peter would eat together once he was in bed. Many mothers of young children I interviewed did this in the evening. The extent to which they sat with their children while the children ate, as a social event, varied. For some, their children's eating time was a chance to get other chores done in the kitchen. Some did all three—supervised eating, chatted, and did chores. These mothers had space in the kitchen for their children to sit and eat so that they could get other things done at the same time. For others, it was time to sit and chat without doing other chores. For yet others, it was a social event to sit, eat, and chat. This tended to be more the case when there were also older children in the family. De Vault (1991) also reports the importance of meal times for family conversation for participants in her study. She also reports, however, that this was more of a middle-class practice and occurred less often in working-class families. For some families in my study the routine varied: some evenings included a meal that was a social event for the whole family, but on other evenings the meal was more utilitarian for the children and a social event for the parents on their own. Meals that were family social events were more likely to occur in the evening during the week and to be at a dining table of some sort. Meals that were less social were often in places that were easier to clean, like a kitchen bench or table. Social meals on weekends could be any meal, depending on what the family was doing for the day. Some families rarely used meals as social occasions; their purpose was for eating, which could happen in a variety of places. DeVault (1991) reports that families in her study had sometimes given up family meals when both parents worked outside the home because they were difficult to organize around work schedules. For some families who had valued these family meals, there was distress because they could not be organized easily. Because children in my study were older, if eating was not a social event, the mother would often do other things while her children were eating, and many mothers chose settings for meals that minimized mess and were easy to clean. Breakfast was the least social meal during the week, eaten under loose supervision once the children needed less help. This is consistent with the finding of De Vault (1991, who found that breakfast was the least likely meal to be eaten together by a family. She found that more than half of the 30 families in her study fed their children breakfast while the parents went on with other work.

The meaning of children's daytime sleeps or naps influences how mothers go about facilitating these. If the only purpose of the sleep is for children to get needed rest, then it does not matter as much where or how the sleep occurs. Mothers in this situation are often happy for children to go off to sleep in front or back packs while they go about other activities. The timing of these naps is also less monitored by some mothers and tends to be more flexible. If the sleep or nap represents a time out for the mother to do things for herself or that are harder to do with a child around, she may be more likely to try to establish a routine of the child "going down" in his or her own space, for example a cot or stroller. If the mother's activity is not time dependent, then the timing of the nap can be flexible. Mothers who want to sleep themselves may be happy to lie down with their child, often in the bed they share with their husband or partner.

Often mothers time outings for sleeps. They maximize the child's waking time, going out early while the child is fresh and coming home when a nap is due. Alternatively, they may go out when a nap is due and use the sleep time to accomplish the activity. To a certain extent, this depends on the nature of the away from home activity to be accomplished and if sleep represents child-free time. Mothers who see sleep time as child-free time are more likely to time coming home with sleep time. They aim for their children to fall asleep on the way home and stay asleep once they are home. To facilitate this, mothers often leave a child asleep in a car carrier capsule, which they carry inside. Mothers who walk home will leave their child in a stroller. Outings are often timed around young children falling asleep in strollers before the main activity, such as lunch out, happens. This means that travel has a meaning itself rather than being just a means to an end or a way of getting to and from other meaningful activities (Primeau, 1996). Dowling (2000) found similarly that, for some families, car travel had other meanings than getting children and parents around to activities and events. One activity described in her study was the use of car travel time as "family time" when the mother could chat with her children. This contrasts with research indicating that most travel is a means to an end (Levin & Louviere, 1981, cited in Primeau, 1996). Some mothers use it to get their children to sleep when they want this to occur. For other mothers it may involve changing the travel route to one that is longer to give their child more time to drop off to sleep. For some going out locally, it may mean deciding to walk to get their child to sleep rather than making a short car trip, which would not be long enough for the child to go to sleep. On odd occasions, mothers may drive with the express purpose of getting their child off to sleep and the drive has no other intended purpose.

Although for many mothers daytime sleep means a less grumpy child or baby in the evening, the timing of the sleep is important. Many mothers try to avoid a late afternoon sleep because this often makes settling the child at night difficult. Some effort often goes into ensuring that this does not happen. Days when it is facilitated are those when mothers need children to stay awake longer in the evening, such as for a dinner out. The extent to which mothers vary children's sleep time for their own purposes differs. Mothers who have a strong belief in the need for routines for children do it less often than those whose day-to-day routines are more flexible anyway.

Bathing is another example of an activity with different meanings. Bathing can be simply a means of getting children clean, with no other purpose. For very young children, this means that the timing of the bath can vary according to what is most convenient for the mother. For my first child, I timed his bath for the morning, when I felt I had the most energy. I would often be more tired in the evening and found giving him a bath much more effort at that time. At other times, bathing can have a settling purpose, so the timing of the bath matters. For settling purposes, it usually occurs just before a nap, and often before the child "goes down" at night. It

should be done in a calming way, with stimulating activities such as playing kept to a minimum. As children get older and can sit by themselves, it often becomes a supervised play activity. Mothers may time it to be a distraction when their child is getting fractious. This means it is often in the evening.

If bathing is play time, with mother present, it will often go on for a period of time. If it is not play time, but just to get clean, but the child still needs supervision, it will be very quick. Mothers of children who were a bit older, and who felt that their children were safe in the bath without close supervision, often used bath time to get other activities done. One mother, Amanda, described how she used the time to clean up the dinner things in the kitchen. She could see her two children, Katie (age 2 years) and Hamish (age 4 years) from the kitchen while she worked. They stayed in the bath for as long as she needed to get things done. This meant it could go on for quite a while. Occasionally her husband James came home in time to do the bath. For him it was leisure. He pulled a dining room chair into the doorway of the bathroom and sat down with a glass of wine to watch the children play. When they had had enough, he dried and dressed them. These are examples of enfolded occupations. For the mother, childcare is enfolded with a kitchen task; for the father, childcare is enfolded with his relaxation time. A mother I interviewed also saw it as relaxation time for her. She used to sit on a small stool in the bathroom watching her children play, interacting when it was appropriate. For very young children, the length of the bath was often dictated by how comfortable the mother was while doing the task. If it was awkward for her and made her back ache, she would often make it quite short. One mother got around this problem by finding a stool that meant she could sit at a comfortable height to bathe her 3-month-old child. This meant that the bath could go on longer if she wanted it to. Further discussion of enfolded and unfolded occupations as described by Bateson (1996) occurs in a later section of the chapter.

Although all mothers saw the bath as having a cleaning purpose, the frequency of baths varied. One mother, Sarah, lived in a house with a very big spa bath that was hard to bathe children in. Her children, Harry and Elizabeth, had a full bath only once every 7 to 10 days. The rest of the time they had a "top and tail" wash in the evening when getting ready for bed. Another mother, Rosemary, bathed her younger daughter, Annie, who was about 8 months old, only 3 times a week. She timed these baths to be when another adult was in the house because bath time had become very difficult with her older child, Jordan, age 2 $\frac{1}{2}$, around. He would be very demanding when she was tied up bathing his sister. The timing of her baths became dependent on when someone else was around at convenient times and this only happened about three times a week. Mary, as described previously, bathed all her children together, leaving the youngest, who needed the most close supervision getting out of the bath, to get out last. Some parents bathed with their young children for ease and comfort, sometimes in the shower and sometimes in a bath. Mothers would often try to minimize mess on clothes by bathing their children after dinner in the evening. This meant they could put the day clothes in which their children had eaten dinner straight in to the wash and keep pajamas clean. For some families, bath time signaled the beginning of the going-to-bed routine. If this was the case, it was always at about the same time each evening and would be followed by teeth cleaning and other evening rituals like story time. If the bath was not part of a going-down routine, timing was more flexible, and if the mother was not worried about dirty pajamas from dinner, it even occurred before dinner and the children would then spend the evening in pajamas.

Enfolded Activity

Enfolded activity has been described by Mary Bateson (1996). She suggests that many women are able to get as much done as they do because they enfold other activities with childcare occupations. My research indicates that the meaning of activities influences the extent to which activities for and with children are enfolded with other activities. This also varied according to the extent to which the mothers

felt their children needed to be supervised during the activity. The closer the supervision required, the less likely it is that the activity will be enfolded with another one. If the activity had more than one meaning for the mother, such as meals being a social event or baths being a chance for joint play, the mother was less likely to enfold that activity with another one. Time pressures also influenced the extent to which activities for and with children were enfolded. Marea, who worked full time, enfolded almost all the activities she did with her son Robert to make sure she got everything done that she needed to. This is consistent with Backett (1982), who has described carrying out several activities at once as a necessity to enable mothers to accomplish all the activities they need to get done. For other mothers, there was more time to do some activities just with their children without enfolding them. The meanings of the activities for the mothers influenced how often some activities would or would not be enfolded.

For a few mothers, activities were enfolded, not because of time pressures, but because of a lack of enjoyment doing activities that were just for and with their children. These mothers rarely spent time just playing with their children or walking to the park for their children's enjoyment. Any time spent with their children was enfolded with something they needed to do. These mothers also tended to try to structure in as much child-free time as possible. Boulton (1983) reports findings in Britain of a study of 50 women, half of whom found providing childcare a predominantly irritating and frustrating experience. They found that preschoolers often interrupted what would otherwise be enjoyable activities, and they felt guilty as a result.

For many mothers, enfolded activities were a way to get through some household tasks and childcare tasks more quickly and to free up time for interesting activities that both they and their children enjoyed. A number of mothers described how they adapted the household activities they did so that their children enjoyed helping and participating in these activities with them. Walkerdine and Lucey (1989) describe this as a primarily middle-class way of dealing with increasing demands on mothers' time and the expectation that they be available to their children. They suggest that working-class women are more likely to maintain a distinction between housework and childcare.

Activities that children did not enjoy or could not help with were often not enfolded but left to a time when the children were asleep or when someone else such as a partner or grandparent could look after the children. This is consistent with deVault (1991), who found that some meal preparation that was time consuming and difficult to do with young children around was completed while the children slept.

The foregoing descriptions of how meanings of activities influence the way in which mothers go about doing them for and with their children show how varied the meanings of activities can be. The importance of the meaning of activities for mothers has been highlighted by other authors (Anderson & Gale, 1992; Dyck, 1989, 1990). Dyck (1989, 1990) describes cultures of mothering that include the beliefs, attitudes, and symbols of mothering that in turn influence the practices of mothers. Clearly, my research indicates that these meanings do indeed influence the actual practice of motherhood, with a task such as bathing being done in very different ways depending on the meaning for each mother. In addition, other researchers (Walkerdine & Lucey, 1989) have found that class influences the way activities will be combined or enfolded.

Helping mothers who may be having difficulty accomplishing mothering occupations requires the worker to explore these meanings with mothers to sort out the best way for them to get them done. Providing assistance to enable mothers to enfold some activities with other household tasks may be relevant for some mothers who are having difficulty fitting in all they want to do.

Another component of mothering occupations that emerges from my research and with which mothers may need some assistance is the physical and ergonomic organization of those occupations. In the next section of the chapter, I will explore the physical and ergonomic aspects of the day-to-day care of

young children and the way the meanings of activities can influence how these are done.

❧ The Physical and Ergonomic Organization of Caring

Ergonomics is the "study of people in relation to their work environment" (Mandell et al., 1989, p.159). From a paid employment perspective, the practice of ergonomics is about the "design and modification of the work environment to match human characteristics and capabilities" (King, 1995, p.117). In a home context for mothers of young children, it may be considered the study of how suitable this environment is for conducting the physical day-to-day care of their young children. It also involves the factors that influence the way mothers organize this environment.

Where and how the physical management and care of young children occurs is influenced by a number of factors. The way a mother structures her daily routine will influence where activities such as diaper changing and dressing occur. The place in which the activity occurs will influence the way it is done physically. For example, Mary bathes her children and dresses them in pajamas the last thing at night before a bedtime routine. This means that she dresses and changes diapers in the evening while on the bathroom floor. Her method may be one that is good for her back if she supports herself on one bent-up knee. It is likely to strain her back if she kneels and leans over Holly. She reports that she stoop-lifts each time she puts Holly down or picks her up.

The meaning of activities will also influence how they are carried out physically. For example, if changing time is also play time or a chance to kick around on the floor without diapers, the changing is more likely to happen on the floor in a living space, particularly if there are older children in the family. A mother who views bath time as play time may have spent time thinking about how to do the activity most comfortably for her because it extends over a longer period of time. Someone who sees it only as a way to get clean only may not spend much time making the activity comfortable. It may also be that in those situations when it is impossible to do the activity comfortably over a longer period, the mothers do not use it as play time. The relationships between the meanings of activities and physical location and ergonomics need to be further explored.

"Lifting technique refers to an individual method of performing a lift under given task and environment" (Hsiang et al., 1997, p.64). The most common lifting techniques are *stoop lifting* (Figure 3–1A and B) and *squat lifting* (Figure 3–2 A and B). Most mothers interviewed about how they lift and handle their children used stoop lifting (Griffin & Price, 2000; Seto, 2002). Stoop lifting, which involves keeping the knees straight and bending from the hips, has a much higher likelihood of causing back injury than squat lifting, which involves bending the knees and lifting using the large muscles of the thighs (Anderson & Chaffin, 1986; Wilmarth & Hereker, 1991). The principles of good lifting include squat lifting with a flat back (Delitto, Rose & Apts, 1987); creating a wide base of support by placing the feet apart (Anderson & Chaffin, 1986; Gardener & McKenna, 1999); keeping the load close to the body when carrying (Anderson & Chaffin, 1986; Gardener & McKenna, 1999); and lifting the load in a slow and controlled manner (Anderson & Chaffin, 1986; Gardener & McKenna, 1999).

Mothers often said they did not think about how they were lifting and that stoop lifting was easiest for them to manage quickly (Griffin & Price, 2000). This is consistent with research by Hsiang (1997) that found stoop lifting is performed more frequently because it provides more upper body control and balance as well as more knee clearance. It also requires less energy and therefore may be preferred by mothers who lift children frequently during the day. It does, however, expose mothers to increased risk of back injury. Many mothers know about good lifting and handling principles but are unable to apply them to mothering occupations (Seto, 2002). The information they received in prenatal and postnatal classes focused on the safety of the baby and did not provide much information about looking after their own backs (Seto, 2002). Seto (2002) found that for mothers to adopt lifting and handling methods that looked after their backs, they needed first to appreciate the risks involved in lifting poorly and then to receive information that enabled them to ap-

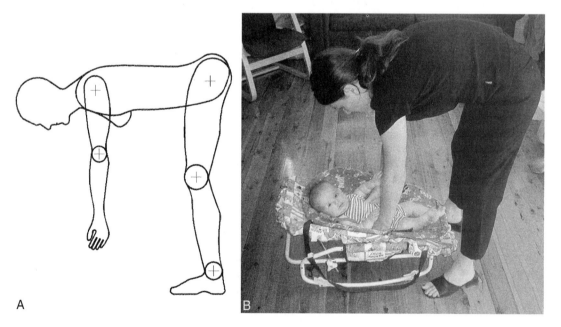

A   B

Figure 3–1 *Stoop lifting.*

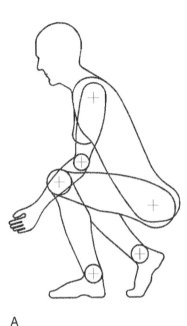
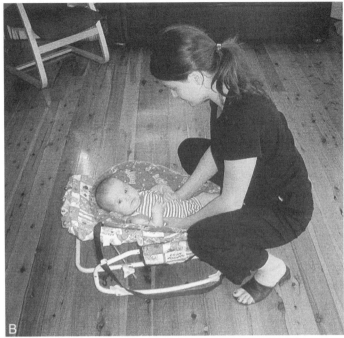

A   B

Figure 3–2 *Squat lifting.*

ply good lifting principles to the mothering occupations they performed. Awareness without practical advice did not lead to behavior change. Similarly, practical advice, even if available, was not heeded unless the mother perceived a threat from poor lifting. The factors that influenced whether or not they perceived a threat from poor lifting included:

- Past or present experience of back injury or recurring pain

- An awareness that their child was growing and, as he or she became heavier, would be harder to lift without discomfort if their methods were poor

- Information they received about the risks of back injury from poor lifting when they were ready to "hear" the information

This is consistent with the Health Belief Model (Rosenstock et al., 1988; cited in Innes, 1997), which indicates the need for individuals to perceive their own susceptibility to injury or pain and believe that it will affect their well-being before they will make behavioral changes. Innes (1997, p.227) recommends

that back care programs provide information as well as "identifying and exploring individual susceptibility and the perceived barriers to behavioral change."

My interviews with mothers about the day-to-day care of their young children support this. Mothers who always used a changing table tended to be the ones who had experienced back pain, either before or since having children. They had incorporated the use of the changing table into their daily routines. Some who had older children in diapers had abandoned the changing table for the same reasons. They described how heavy their 2- to 3-year-old was to lift and how awkward it was to keep the child still on the changing table, so they had moved to the floor. Other research indicates that often these moves were focused around the child's safety rather than the mother's comfort or safety (Griffin & Price, 2000; Seto, 2002).

Mothers often did not receive information about selecting equipment that was the best for them. They found that changing tables were too low; baby baths were too heavy to lift and the stands too low; cots were difficult to get children in and out of; strollers were heavy to lift, with handles that were too short to push comfortably; and car carrier capsules were awkward to get in and out of the car (Griffin & Price, 2000). Because most mothers buy equipment before the birth of the baby, this information needs to be provided in practical ways during the prenatal period (Seto, 2002). Ergonomic considerations such as the height of work surfaces (Carson, 1994), workplace design (Workcover Authority of NSW, 1995), and design of equipment (Brown & Gerberich, 1993) can decrease the experience of back pain for mothers.

Information about lifting and handling is best given in the postnatal period once mothers have settled into a routine with their new babies. In the first few days and weeks after birth, they are overwhelmed with caring for the baby and establishing feeding and sleeping routines. They may not be open to other information until later (Barclay, Everitt, Rogan, Schmied, & Wyllie, 1997; Seto, 2002). Once they have established some sort of routine, they are more aware of how various mothering occupations affect their backs and therefore more open to receiving practical information about how to manage lifting and handling occupations more safely for them. "As posture would seem to be an important factor in the development of long term back ache, there should be greater efforts to make mothers more aware of their posture" (Russell *et al.*, 1993, p. 1302). In an Australian context, this information could be provided via early childhood centers. These are centers that mothers can attend to receive advice on the care of their new babies. These centers often run group programs for new mothers about caring for their children. The information about safe lifting and handling could be incorporated into these programs. In other settings short courses could be offered through doctors' surgeries, health centers, or other education providers.

My experience indicates that this information is best provided for mothers in a very applied way. They need to understand the principles of good lifting and handling and how to look after their backs, in the specific context of mothering occupations. They need to be given very practical examples of how the principles are applied to their everyday occupations. They also need to be able to make changes in the way they carry out these occupations, while still taking into account the meanings that these occupations have for them. They need a chance to practice the techniques in their own homes or situations and to get feedback and assistance with any occupations they are finding difficult, and to be shown ways to make these easier and safer. This is consistent with the education principles required for change in the workplace described by Innes (1997). She suggests that education should take place in real settings and that participants should have time to practice and develop new habitual techniques. This can be achieved in back care education for mothers by assisting them to apply the principles to their own situations, encouraging them to try out the practices and then report and discuss their success or problems in subsequent sessions. Innes (1997) also recommends ergonomic interventions such as job redesign to complement back-care education. In the context of mothers who lift and handle children, this can be achieved by discussing equipment selection and the ways they use their home environment to conduct mothering occupations. For example, various postures that can be used to bathe children that allow more back protection can be discussed and demonstrated via slides or videotape. A wide range of methods is often possible for mothering occupations, and exploring which best suits each mother will enable her to adopt the "best practice" for her situation. Further exploration of the wide range of "normal" ways mothers use to accomplish mothering occupations is discussed in the vignette that follows. This vignette is an illustrative example compiled from composite data. Its subject was not a research participant.

Vignette: *Freda*

Freda is the mother of two young children, Henry, age 4, and Isabelle, age 2. She lives with her husband Michael in a three-bedroom house that they own. She has strained her back while gardening and suffered a disc injury that causes pain whenever she "overdoes" things. She is the primary caregiver for their children while Michael works Monday through Friday as an accountant. Her routine involves caring for her children at home most days except when she goes to play group on Monday and Wednesday mornings. She shops at the local shopping mall once a week, usually Thursday. The children spend time at home playing with each other both inside and outside the house. They also play with two children of similar ages who live down the street. Sometimes they play with these children at home and some times they go down to their friends' house. Because Michael works long hours, Freda is responsible for most of the care of the children. Michael arrives home around 7 PM after the children have had their dinner and a bath. He spends time reading to the children between 7 PM and 7.30 PM, when they go to bed. Freda comes to see you to get advice on how to go about organizing her day so that she can still care for her two young children as much as possible without overdoing things to a point where she may experience more pain.

Reflective Questions:

- How would you go about deciding what suggestions to make to Freda about managing her routine?
- What factors would you need to consider?

⅔ A Wide Range of "Normal"

The descriptions and discussion of mothers' day-to-day care of their young children in the preceding sections points to the very wide range of ways in which mothers go about accomplishing these tasks. There isn't just one way of getting them done or of organizing them. This is consistent with David, who states, "there is no one version of motherhood. What little evidence there is suggests enormous variation in mothering practices" (1984, p.192). Repeatedly, when I interviewed mothers, they would use phrases like "they say" when describing some aspect of childcare and how

their method differed from what "they say." "They" could refer to midwives, early childhood center staff, written materials, or any other person in the position of giving advice to mothers. Many mothers found the advice of these professionals helpful for some of their mothering occupations. Those who seemed to feel most comfortable with their routines, however, were those who had filtered the advice and adapted it to their own situation.

Assisting mothers who may be having difficulty with some aspect of the day-to-day care of their young children will be most effective when the worker is able to present a range of options for mothers to consider in the context of their own needs and circumstances and when the worker can help mothers sort out what activities mean for them and therefore how best to organize them within their daily routines. A fixed approach advocating one way of going about mothering occupations will be successful for those whose values "fit" the approach, but not for others. Our strengths in this area as professionals, I believe, must lie in a varied and individual approach that offers mothers a wide choice of methods and ways of organizing their routines that are personally meaningful. My experiences in interviewing mothers indicate that the degree of structure to their day and the patterns of their activities varied enormously from highly structured routines to very loose routines and that in both instances the occupations of the mothers are accomplished to their satisfaction. The extent to which activities are enfolded also varies according to the meaning of the various mothering occupations to the mother and the family. The meanings of activities were varied, and so too must the ways of accomplishing these be varied to fit in with these values.

This information also highlights the importance of ensuring that those who come to the attention of welfare agencies are not judged against unfair standards of what is "normal." My research indicates a very wide range of what is normal for middle-class mothers of young children. We need to be vigilant that those who are less able to articulate the reasons for their choice of methods or routines are not discriminated against. An example of this is a young mother with an intellectual disability who was part of a study done by colleagues of mine (Mayes, R. Personal Communication, November 10, 2002). She had one young child and was being "watched" by welfare agencies. She and her child had experienced a very busy weekend, and the following day she decided what the baby and she needed was a good sleep. She concluded their evening routine very early that afternoon, and she and the child went to bed at about 4:30 PM. That same afternoon, a welfare agency visitor arrived and, finding them in bed, made notes in the mother's record later about her "inappropriate" behavior. In fact, what this mother had done in this exceptional circumstance was make a good decision based on what her child and she needed. However, because she was unable to make her reasons clear to the visitor, her behavior was labeled inappropriate. We also need to be aware as professionals who are middle class that the meanings of mothering occupations for those who are working class may be different from our own, and we need to ensure that we fully explore these meanings to make appropriate suggestions to these mothers.

✍ Conclusion

Four main themes have been explored in this chapter. These are the variable routines that mothers orchestrate to carry out their mothering occupations. There is wide variability in the extent to which these routines are structured or unstructured. The meaning of occupations for the mothers also varies considerably and influences the way they set up their routines. These meanings also influence the way mothers manage the ergonomic and physical dimensions of their occupations. My studies highlight the wide range of ways that are "normal" for mothers to go about their mothering occupations.

The professional implications of my research include the need to ensure that all mothers are judged fairly when it comes to determining the adequacy of their mothering skills and practices. We need to be mindful that those who come under the scrutiny of wel-

fare agencies are not judged unfairly against some standard that does not take into account the wide range of "normal" ways to accomplish these occupations. We need to ensure that we assist women who may struggle with these occupations by helping them to determine their own values and meanings surrounding their mothering, so that we can better suggest ways of accomplishing these occupations that are consistent with each mother's beliefs and meanings. We need to be aware that each mother will have her own "culture of mothering" that is influenced by a number of factors including class. To encourage mothers to lift and handle their children in the safest ways possible, we need to offer learning that takes into account their real-life situations and allows them opportunities to practice in their own environments and then seek specific advice if they are having problems. We also need to assist them to identify their own risks for injury and fatigue and work with them to establish ways of doing their occupations that are safest but still take into account the meanings of the occupations for them. We can help them to construct routines that are meaningful to them and that enable them to provide adequate care for their children, while simultaneously considering their own physical and ergonomic needs.

My research contributes to furthering our understanding of the nature of mothering occupations, most particularly the importance of meaning in determining how these occupations are orchestrated into routines. Further research is needed to better determine the best and safest ways to lift and handle young children that allow mothers to conduct their occupations safely, in ways that are consistent with their beliefs. The ergonomics of the home in relation to mothering occupations need to be further explored.

Factors that affect the meaning of mothering occupations for mothers need to be further defined. The way the meanings of these occupations affect the other roles and occupations of mothers needs to be explored for women across all socioeconomic groups. Indeed, there is a life's work ahead for me should I choose to travel this professional road. I certainly ponder these issues daily in my own mothering and look forward to the challenges to me personally, as I construct my meaningful routines, and professionally, as I continue to investigate this very interesting area of study. I am forever grateful to the women in the past and the women in the future who give so freely of their time for my research. Your generosity of spirit is wonderful—I thank and salute you.

Discussion Questions ☙

■ Consider a young mother with three children whose eldest is starting school in 2 months' time. She has come to see you because she is concerned about the child's readiness for school. You think it would be good if she did a home program with the child to further develop his fine motor skills. How could you go about introducing this to the mother, taking into account the meaning she ascribes to the various activities in her daily routine? What information would you need to get from the mother? How would you ensure that the home program was meaningful for her and that it fitted into her daily routine in a meaningful way? How would you prepare her for her upcoming interaction with an organization outside her current experience, namely the school and school routine?

■ Consider your own work with clients, your own experiences as a mother, or those of someone you know who is a mother. Think about how the daily routines of mothering were structured in these instances and the meanings of some of the activities that led the routine to be structured this way. What implications would these meanings and routines have if you were working in these situations to improve the skills of those concerned or to help them manage their everyday care of young children?

References

Anderson, P. A., & Chaffin, D. B. (1986) A biomechanical evaluation of five lifting techniques. *Applied Ergonomics, 17,* 2–8.

Anderson, S. C., & Gale, F. (1992). Introduction. In K. Anderson & F. Gale (Eds.). *Inventing Places.* Longman: Melbourne.

Backett, K. C. (1982). *Mothers and fathers.* Basingstoke: Macmillan.

Barclay, L., Everitt, L., Rogan, F., Schmied, V., & Wyllie, A. (1997). Becoming a mother —An analysis of women's experience of early motherhood. *Journal of Advanced Nursing, 25,* 719–728.

Bateson, M. C. (1996). Enfolded activity and the concept of occupation. In R. Zemke & F. Clark. *Occupational Science. The evolving discipline.* Philadelphia: F. A. Davis, pp 5–12.

Boulton, M. (1983). *On being a mother.* London: Tavistock.

Brown, M. Z., & Gerbrich, S. G. (1993). Disabling injuries to childcare workers in Minnesota, 1985–1990: An analysis of potential risk factors. *Journal of Occupational Medicine, 35,* 1236–1243.

Carson, R. (1994). Reducing cumulative trauma disorders: Use of proper workplace design. *American Association of Occupational Health Nurses Journal, 42,* 270–276.

David, M. (1984). Women, family and education. In S. Acker (Ed.). *World year book of education 1984: Women and education.* London: Kogan Page, pp.191–201.

Delitto, N. K., Rose, S. J., & Apts, D. W. (1987). Electomyographic analysis of two techniques of squat lifting. *Physical Therapy, 67,* 1329–1334.

DeVault, M. L. (1991). *Feeding the family. The social organization of caring as gendered work.* Chicago: University of Chicago Press.

Dowling, R. (2000). Cultures of mothering and car use in suburban Sydney: a preliminary investigation. *Geoforum, 31,* 345–353.

Dyck, I. (1989). Integrating home and wage workplace: Women's daily lives in a Canadian suburb. *The Canadian Geographer, 33,* 329–341.

Dyck, I. (1990). Space, time and renegotiating motherhood: an exploration of the domestic workplace. *Environment and Planning D: Society and Space, 8,* 459–483.

Dyck, I. (1992). The daily routines of mothers with young children: Using a socio-political model in research. *The Occupational Therapy Journal of Research, 12,* 16–34.

Gallimore, R., Weisner, T. S., Kaufman, S. Z., & Bernheimer, L. P. (1989). The social construction of ecocultural niches: Family accommodation of developmentally delayed children. *American Journal of Mental Retardation, 94,* 216–230.

Gardener, L., & McKenna, K. (1999). Reliability of occupational therapists in determining safe, maximal lifting capacity. *Australian Occupational Therapy Journal, 46,* 110–119.

Griffin, S. D. (2002). A bath to get clean or to settle for sleep: The meaning of every day mothering activities. Poster presented at the World Federation of Occupational Therapists Congress, Stockholm, Sweden.

Griffin, S. D., & Price, V. J. (2000). Living with lifting: Mothers' perceptions of lifting and back strain in childcare. *Occupational Therapy International, 7,* 1–20.

Hsiang, S. M., Brogmus, G. E., & Courtney, T. K. (1997). Low back pain (LBP) and lifting technique—A review. *International Journal of Industrial Ergonomics, 19,* 59–74.

Innes, E. (1997). Education and training programs for the prevention of work injuries: Do they work? *Work: a journal of prevention, assessment and rehabilitation, 9,* 221–232.

Kellegrew, D. H. (2000). Constructing daily routines: A qualitative examination of mothers with young children with disabilities. *American Journal of Occupational Therapy, 54,* 252–259.

King, P.M. (1995). Employee ergonomics training: Current limitations and suggestions for improvement. *Journal of Occupational Rehabilitation, 5,* 115–123.

Larson, E. A. (2000). The orchestration of occupation: The dance of mothers. *American Journal of Occupational Therapy , 54,* 269–280.

Mandell, P., Lipton, M. H., Bernstrein, J., Kucera, G. J., & Kampner, J. A. (1989). *Low back pain: an historical and contemporary overview of the occupational, medical & psychosocial issues of chronic back pain.* Thorofare, NJ: Slack Inc.

Primeau, L. A. (1996). Human daily travel: Personal choices and external constraints. In R. Zemke & F. Clark (Eds.). *Occupational Science. The evolving discipline.* Philadelphia: F. A. Davis, pp. 115–124.

Russell, R., Groves, P., Taub, N., O'Dowd, J., & Reynolds, F. (1993). Assessing long term backache after childbirth. *British Medical Journal, 306,* 1299–1303.

Seto, D. T.W. (2002). An evaluation of the sufficiency of safe lifting and back care information given in antenatal/postnatal classes. Honours Thesis, Bachelor of Applied Science (Occupational Therapy) Honours, University of Sydney.

Walkerdine, V., & Lucey, H. (1989). *Democracy in the kitchen.* London: Virago.

Wilmarth, M.A., & Herreker, R. (1991). Lifting ability and leg strength. *Journal of Orthopaedic and Sports Physical Therapy, 14,* 24–30.

Workcover Authority of NSW (1995). *Backpack: A Guide to Manual Handling Regulation.* Sydney, NSW: Workcover Authority of NSW.

Maternal Management of Home Space and Time to Facilitate Infant/Toddler Play and Development

Doris Pierce, PhD, OTR/L, FAOTA, and Amy Marshall, BS, OTR/L

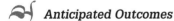

Anticipated Outcomes

We anticipate that, after reading this chapter, readers will:

- Appreciate the importance of the relatively invisible and indirect work of mothers as they create developmental play opportunities for infants and toddlers in the home

🐾 Understand that the efforts a mother makes to create each day's sequence of experiences for her child require a complex series of judgments regarding conflicting priorities, developmental progressions, and choreographic style

🐾 Identify the variety of strategies and factors involved in the maternal work of supporting infant/toddler play in the home

🐾 Explore the concept of co-occupation

🐾 Conceptualize how an understanding of the maternal work of staging infant/toddler play in the home might support intervention

🐾 Introduction

Mothers value, and work to support, the developmental play experiences of their infants and toddlers. Their work entails specific practices and judgments regarding the management of the spaces and objects of the home, as well as the temporal flow of child experiences. The substantive description in this chapter provides an understanding of the complexity of factors and conditions considered by mothers of typically developing infants and toddlers as they do the behind-the-scenes work of staging and choreographing the developmental environment of the home. We believe that this description is relevant to the practice of therapists and others who are concerned with either mothers or their young children.

For many reasons, mothers value childhood play. Within western culture, mothers view play as providing important developmental opportunities. The challenges of play are seen as necessary to the child's gradual transition from a dependent newborn to a skillful, self-directed, and independent young adult. Victorian notions of childhood as a carefree, playful time of life influence mothers' perceptions of themselves as good mothers to the degree that they provide a rich and play-filled childhood. Mothers also value play because of the evident interest of children in play activities and the joy children obviously experience during play. This view of play as joyful and developmentally important is further amplified by the toy industry's powerful promotion of the importance of commercial toys in the lives of children. In addition, moth-

ers are freed to perform household work by engaging their children in play activities.

To support the play of infants and toddlers, mothers engage in a wide array of tasks required to create and maintain the physical and temporal context of play in the home. They obtain, make available, and maintain playthings. They schedule the day around playtimes. They monitor safety with the space of the home. And they constantly revise their strategies to match the fast-developing infant and child. Because the work of creating and maintaining the home play context is unpaid and indirectly supportive of play, rather than directly interactive, it has been widely overlooked even within feminist research on maternal work.

Overviews of Maternal Work

As a mother, Doris Pierce (co-author of this chapter) remembers the long-ago play of her now teen-aged daughter as a time of laughter; joy; conflicts and wrestling with cousins over toys and inclusion/exclusion issues; the fun of picking out new toys for her child; pride in the chaotic and playful environment of her child's room; and constant picking up, cleaning up, and sorting out of toys. Many moments felt like classic glimpses of the joyful play of childhood, that deep engagement in momentary experience and sensation. Sometimes, play was disappointing: there never seemed to be enough time for those Hollywood play moments, mother and child head to head in fascination with play. Reality got in the way a lot. Sometimes her daughter's quiet play with a fresh toy felt like freedom: a release from the demands of joint attention and an opportunity to at last get a shower or start dinner. From the perspective of a new mother, the reality of child's play was quite different from the romantic view offered up in child development classes and toy commercials.

Both Amy Marshall (co-author) and Doris have experienced the usefulness of play in intervention. In their training as occupational therapists, they were exposed to classical play theorists, such as Piaget and Vygotsky, and to play theorists in occupational therapy. It does not take a seasoned therapist to appreciate a child's intrinsic desire for play, or to evoke one's own playfulness in order to facilitate a child's engagement in a treatment session. In home-based practice with infants and toddlers, a novel play object goes far toward creating motivation in the child to work on intervention goals. There is little worse than a boring session in which neither therapist nor child is really engaged.

For Doris, her fascination with play began with a childhood conviction that when she was at school, she learned most on the playground. Her family was playful to a driven extent: boats, planes, painting, gems, photography, stained glass, model planes, model trains, and a series of collections called for every free moment of family time as her father fought off job stress through fervent engagement in adult play. A younger brother with a learning disability lit up during play. Amy's childhood play often required careful planning on the part of her parents because the weekly lineups of various after-school sports (tennis, soccer, horseback riding, bowling, cross-country skiing) was complex and always changing. Countless hours were spent exploring her neighborhood on roller skates; playing kickball or Frisbee on the dead-end street in front of her house; or, if she was lucky, swimming in the pool next door.

As a mother, Doris found that her fascination with her daughter's play, and the amount of work required to support it, fueled her master's thesis on infant object rules. Watching the Sesame Street Muppets sing "Cooperation makes it happen," Doris coined the term "co-occupation," or the way in which two individuals' occupational patterns can require

and be shaped by each other. The term quickly became popular within occupational science and continues to resonate especially with authors when they are describing the dynamics of maternal work. Later Doris collaborated with Gelya Frank in a study of the work of one mother over 5 years of care for a chronically ill child (Pierce & Frank, 1992). In her occupational science dissertation, she returned to study the interactions of infants and toddlers with the physical environment of the home and the work of mothers who supported that developmental play (Pierce, 1996, 2000). In further research, she completed a study of extremely low–birth-weight premature infants using the same design, with the 18 typically developing infants and their mothers in the dissertation study as a comparative sample. Now Doris is the Endowed Chair in Occupational Therapy at Eastern Kentucky University. This role supports her research in several areas, including maternal work, infant/toddler play, occupational therapy program development for at-risk youth, and occupation-based practice. Amy is working on her post-professional master's degree in occupational therapy at Eastern Kentucky University, and is Doris' graduate assistant.

The Unrecognized Work of Mothers

Historically, the ability to procreate has been used to justify limitations on women's freedom (Martin, 1987; Rich, 1986). However, women are "mothers" only to the degree to which they are committed to meeting the demands of maternal work (Ruddick, 1989). In urban middle-class cultures, mothers assume the primary task of providing opportunities for and nurturing the child's emotional and intellectual growth in accordance with demands from society and culture (1989). Therefore, a mother's responsibility for providing these opportunities for her child is enormous. Yet, because this work takes place within the home, it is not understood and is usually unrecognized, at times even by mothers themselves. Studying mothers' work to support the play of their infants and toddlers in the home holds potential for increasing the understanding of occupational therapists, developmentalists, and women's study scholars of this valuable, yet largely unrecognized, work done by mothers.

Spatial and Temporal Dimensions of the Home

The ways in which people negotiate the spatiotemporal context of their homes have been little researched in the social sciences. The significance of basic routines, family therapists Kantor and Lehr (1975) believe, should not be overlooked. Through naturalistic observations of 19 separate households, these researchers developed a framework for better understanding of family processes and behaviors. They argue that individuals and families can be better understood after examining their management of commonplace, habitual events within the surroundings of their homes. It is through this interaction of space, time, and energy, they believe, that people can attain wider meaning within their lives.

Graham Rowles (1991, 2000), a geographer, believes that occupational therapists underestimate the amount of influence that the environment has on one's well-being. He describes environment as including not only the physical but also the social, cultural, and historical meanings that are ascribed to a particular setting. An increased understanding of and sensitivity to this sense of place can be achieved only through examination of the meanings and values that define one's experience of his or her home and personal space (1991). By acknowledging these personally defined perspectives of place, he states, "occupational therapists . . . [can] identify intervention strategies more attuned to the experiential worlds of those they seek to serve" (p. 269).

◆ The Link Between Play and Development

Mothers value the play of their infants and toddlers. The work of mothers to support the development of their children through play opportunities in the home is complex, reasoned, and constantly revised to fit the changing child. That work includes choosing and securing play objects to match developmental

change, facilitating and controlling access to play space within the home and its immediate vicinity, furnishing the home with childcare equipment, positioning the child and objects for play, supporting the continuity of unfolding play sequences, fitting the child's playtime into the priorities and schedules of daily family life, managing disruptions in play, and planning the child's place in the birth order of the family.

Mothers are the stage managers who support the play of their children at home through management of the home's physical space and the objects it contains. The arrangement of the home and the selection of objects it offers influence the child's developmental progress because transactions with the physical environment are necessary for growth and maturation (Piaget, 1962; Wohlwill & Heft, 1987). Play, the primary occupation of children, is the means by which these interactions take place. According to Piaget (1952, 1962), infants and toddlers from birth to age 2 years are at the sensorimotor stage of development, in which play is characterized by its concrete, tangible interactions with objects in the world around them. During this time, object explorations increase in complexity, from the simple action of mouthing or handling an object to the inclusion of other sensory systems such as vision, sound, and touch, which are more specifically responsive to the properties of an object (Palmar, 1989; Rochat, 1989; Ruff, 1984). Belsky & Most (1981) observed object play in children from ages 7 to 21 months and found progressions in manipulative skills, in the use of objects in ways appropriate to the function, in object combinations, and in the beginnings of complex pretend play.

Several studies have shown the negative effects on child development of restrictions in floor freedom through the use of playpens and other infant care equipment (Ainsworth & Bell, 1974; Elardo, Bradley, & Caldwell, 1975; Tulkin & Covitz, 1975; Wachs, 1976, 1979). The factors within the home that seem to evoke the greatest developmental progress are the characteristics of environmental objects and degree of access to the physical environment. Positive relationships have been found between infant development and in-home object complexity, variety, and responsivity (Bradley & Caldwell, 1984; Clarke-Stewart, 1973; Elardo et al., 1975; Jennings, Harmon, Morgan, Gaiter, & Yarrow, 1979; Wachs, 1976, 1978, 1979; Wachs, Uzgiris, & Hunt, 1971; Yarrow, Morgan, Jennings, Harmon, & Gaiter, 1982; Yarrow, McQuiston, MacTurk, McCarthy, Klein, & Vietze, 1983). A factor analytic study of a home physical environment inventory's predictive validity for intelligence showed the highest dependence on measures of the learning materials provided and the mother's facilitation of her child's development (Stevens & Bakeman, 1985). Research indicates that differences in socio-economic status and culture shape the daily experience of infants, especially through the pattern of the mother-infant relationship (Bornstein, Azuma, Tamis-LeMonda, & Ogino, 1990a; Bornstein, Toda, Azuma, Tamis-LeMonda, & Ogino, 1990b, 1991; Rubin, Maioni, & Hornung, 1976). Infants of specific groups of mothers, such as teen-agers or women with depression, are also at high risk for compromised development (Coll, Vohr, Hoffman, & Oh, 1986; Lyons-Ruth, Zoll, Connell, & Grunbaum, 1986).

Research has shown that the spatial awareness of infants develops during free play in familiar environments (Gibson, 1986; Neisser, 1976). However, the majority of infant play development research is implemented in a standardized and restricted laboratory setting, in which predetermined play objects are passively handed to the infants and their interactions with those objects quantitatively analyzed. Little research has studied self-directed infant action of free play in the home (Haith, 1990; Hendricks-Jansen, 1996).

Play is the predominant waking occupation of children. It is the primary means by which children gain multiple developmental and social skills. Mary Reilly (1962, 1974) hypothesized that children learn rules of people, objects, and movement during play. Play lays the foundation for the increasingly complex interactions with the world that a mature individual must make on a daily basis.

✒ The Primary Study

Design

The findings reported here are one portion of a study of the development of interactions of children aged 1 to 18 months, with their everyday physical and temporal environments, and the work of their mothers in creating those home play settings (Pierce, 1996, 2000). The design combined grounded theory (Glaser & Strauss, 1967), which categorizes phenomena by way of in-depth qualitative examination of data, and natural history (Goodall, 1986), which depends primarily on longitudinal observation of individuals in their natural environments and is frequently used in studies of nonhuman primates. The study produced a substantive descriptive theory, detailed enough to support clinical application, but not so specific as to prevent generalization to a variety of settings (Glaser & Strauss, 1967).

Participants

The participants in the study were divided into three groups: a pilot sample of four mother/infant dyads, a comparative sample of videotaped chimpanzee mother/infant dyads, and a primary class-stratified sample of 18 typically developing Caucasian infants and their mothers that included nine male and nine female infants. Caucasian infants were used simply to obtain a homogeneous sample.

Data Collection

In the primary sample of 18 mother-infant dyads, data were collected monthly in the home, from 1 through 18 months of age, yielding a total of 313 data collection visits. Data included:

- 313 brief written observation records that addressed types of play observed, methodological issues, researcher reflections, and early points of analysis
- 313 maternal interviews, each lasting approximately 45 minutes and totaling approximately 6000 transcribed pages, focused on changes in the infants' and toddlers' object play interests, use of

home space, play sequencing, developmental changes in play, and maternal work to support play

- 313 videotaped free play samples, totaling 180 hours, of the infants and toddlers interacting with the typical play objects of their homes, yards, and neighborhoods

Data Analysis

Data analysis occurred concurrently with data collection and use of multiple methods. A computer-assisted video analysis system, modeled on a prototype developed for Jane Goodall's video archive at the University of Southern California, was used to examine and code the videotapes of infant/toddler play. Qualitative text analysis software was used to analyze the maternal interviews, observation records, and topical memos. Analysis included extensive memoing, compilation of an audit trail to document the emergence and construction of the theoretical description, and regular peer debriefing sessions.

☙ Mothers: Stage Managers and Choreographers of Infant/Toddler Play in the Home

The day's activities in the 18 homes in the study did not simply unfold in a sequential, predictable pattern. Mothers acted as behind-the-scenes stage managers and choreographers to provide their infants and toddlers with a safe and stimulating play environment. They were constantly involved in infant positioning, toy selection, play space set-up, safety monitoring, and controlling access to different spaces of the home, yard, and immediate neighborhood. The ways in which mothers coordinated the temporal flow of activities in the home included moment-to-moment decisions, general and constantly revised guidelines to the daily schedule, and long-term conceptualizations to which the mother aspired. Decisions made by mothers about the space and time of infant/toddler play in the home required fine judgments within the conflicting priorities of supporting infant/toddler development, in-

suring infant/toddler safety, maintaining a sense of order in the home, and retaining maternal sanity. Each mother created and maintained a home environment that reflected her own values, experience, and efforts to deal with the demands of her family's particular situation. Throughout this chapter, we have placed several cameo descriptions of particular mothers in the study and the unique play settings they created for their children. By doing this, we hope to more clearly illustrate the theoretical description of the work that mothers do to support the play opportunities of their children.

☙ Stage Management: The Maternal Work of Managing Play Space in the Home

⌘ *Vignette:* **Joanne—Setting the Stage at Home**

Joanne, a pediatric occupational therapist as well as a Discovery toy distributor, stayed home to raise her infant daughter, Leslie, while her husband worked as a lawyer. Leslie had one brother, 22 months older than she, an active and competitive fellow who struggled hard to deal with the amount of attention the baby received during the video data collection sessions. The space of their home was relatively large. A fenced and grassy backyard with a large cement pad opened off of the back-sliding glass doors. A sandbox, plastic slide, and children's plastic picnic table were kept outside. However, the living room and dining room portions of the house were barred from the infant by baby gates. In addition, the house had two stories, necessitating a gate near the bottom of the stairs and one at the top. The den and kitchen area seemed to be the most often-used play spaces. They were furnished with couches and chairs, a small table and chairs in the kitchen, a television and mini-trampoline in the den, and bins of toys and shelves of books at a low level for access by the two children. A great variety of high-quality developmental toys were available, some from the mother's inventory of Discovery toys. Upstairs, Leslie and her sibling both had their own rooms.

As a pediatric occupational therapist, Joanne often had observations that were not as typical as those of the other mothers, especially concerning aspects of motor and sensory development. The play of her daughter was unique in her early development of motor skills, the variety of high-quality developmental toys with which she was interacting, and the constant interruptions of her object play from her older brother. She also seemed markedly more interested in climbing activities than most of the other infants, although this may have been modeled after her brother's play interests or facilitated by her mother's allowing her to climb.

The Material Culture of Play

For humans, material objects within one's environment are required for one to function and adapt to everyday life experiences. In anthropology, these objects, or artifacts, are studied to derive meaning from the culture. The physical objects of human material culture include tools, shelters, furniture, vehicles, foods, domesticated animals, vessels and cookware, clothing, toys, recorded information, and artistic and symbolic objects. Interpreting meaning through physical objects has also been used in other fields, such as history and psychology (Berger, 1992; Csikszentmihalyi & Rochberg-Halton, 1981; Schlereth, 1985). Similarly, within the culture of childhood, toys and other physical household objects that children seek out and play with can be examined to aid understanding of that particular culture because these are their "tools" of play (Cross, 1997). This examination is especially appropriate for infants and toddlers, who have not yet left the concrete stage of development and commonly play with toys and other objects (Piaget, 1952, 1962). Throughout history, toys have changed dramatically in relation to the changing attitudes toward the nature of play itself (Cross, 1997; McClary, 1997). In western cultures, in particular, children possess a wide variety of toys from which to choose. Mothers create and maintain this selection of objects designed for play.

Choosing Play Objects
Availability

The mothers' choices of play objects provided children with the opportunity to develop through their playful interactions with these objects. First-time mothers were more influenced by the market and what they "ought to buy." The more experienced mothers usually based their choices on the expected developmental progression of their infants. Many of the mothers in the study were regular consumers of commercial toys, although some, frequently those who had limited financial resources, stated that they did not believe that commercial toys were important. It is a middle-class value within the United States to consider toys as tools for physical and mental development (Cross, 1987); not all parents feel that providing numerous toys is necessary for their child's growth. The following quotes from my (Doris Pierce's or DP's) research illustrate the varying availability of commercial toys within two separate households.

Mother (M): When I was little, I had the best parents as far as like making sure that I had every developmental toy. It's funny, because Rick [her husband] didn't do that as much. His belief on children and having developmental toys isn't as strong as mine. But I know where it comes from, it comes from the fact that my mom always, I mean, I had everything. And they always worked with me... (Interview [I], Belle, 8 mos.) (Pierce, 1996, p. 268).

The mother was pretty direct about saying that the baby doesn't really have any toys. Things have been tight and her children mainly just play with household objects and use their imaginations. (Observation Record [OR], Julie, 2 mos.) (Pierce, 2000, p. 293)

Developmental Considerations

Some mothers recognized, when toys no longer engaged their children, that the children had lost interest in the toys because of their progressing development. This was especially true when the infant had no siblings to distract him or her or with whom to play, and the mother suddenly found it more difficult to find the time to cook dinner or complete other household work. The motivation for mothers to continue making frequent trips to the toy store to buy new play objects was inspired not only by their desire to continue their infant's developmental progression, but also by a desire to free themselves to do household tasks. In this segment, one mother described different strategies that she used to keep her toddler occupied while she worked in the kitchen.

> M: The big key is, is the room safe and blocked off? And then I'll just let her have at it. And, you know, like if I need her to be occupied while I'm in the kitchen, I'll just hope that she'll— you know, I might direct her to here, to there. So far, she'll actually sit and watch videos, but I don't succumb to her yet and I try to avoid it for both of them. Sometimes I might open a cupboard and just go, "Hey, look at this," you know. The other thing that's a definite diversion is she'll eat crackers any time. (I, Leslie, 14 mos.)

Household Object Play

By 8 months of age, the infants desired a large quantity of novel objects for play, which posed a difficulty for mothers of low socioeconomic status. Some met this challenge by providing infants with a multitude of household objects for play. Also, as infants became increasingly mobile, they constantly sought out interesting objects in the house. Anything within arm's reach held possibilities. The degree to which the mother allowed access to the home and its contents either restricted or expanded the child's developmental opportunities. If allowed, toddlers would climb over and under furniture, rip magazines, carry objects around, empty containers and storage sites (such as shelves, drawers, and toy boxes) onto the floor, play with family clothes and shoes, and simply travel down hallways and in and out of rooms. Kitchen cupboards were a primary play space in the study. Mothers encouraged cupboard play, not only because it offered a multitude of objects for manipulation and interaction, but also because the cupboards were typically within view of the areas in which they performed most of their household work. However, although some mothers encouraged play with household objects, oth-

ers discouraged it, especially in upper socioeconomic status homes where formal rooms contained many breakable objects.

As infants grew into toddlers, mothers began to be more concerned with selecting toys that offered educational concepts, such as shape sorters, picture and talking books, and puzzles. However, these objects, most common in the upper socioeconomic status homes, were usually used for social interaction between mother and child, rather than as solitary play independently initiated by the toddler.

Social Routes by Which Play Objects Enter the Home

The routes by which toys entered the home showed some primary influences of western culture on the work that mothers do in supporting the home play environment. The toy industry exerted a powerful influence on the types and number of play objects within the home. Beyond the mother's personal selection of toys from a toy store or offering household objects for play, there were also several ritual events that typically drew developmentally appropriate objects into the homes. In the study, these were called "import events," and they included baby showers for firstborns, gift-giving holidays, birthdays, extended family gifts and loans, and commercial routes.

Baby Showers

At least one baby shower was held for each of the first-time mothers in the study. Female relatives, friends, co-workers, or church group members hosted these events. This ritual included providing the "tools of the trade" to new mothers. Gifts were of a practical nature, including clothing, infant-care equipment such as bathtubs or highchairs, and small toys. The following interview excerpt describes the variety of gifts that were given to one mother.

> ***Doris Pierce (DP):*** Did you have a baby shower?
> ***Mother (M):*** Uh-huh, I had a couple of them.
> ***DP:*** What did they give you?
> ***M:*** There were a lot of clothes and our room we're doing in Winnie-the-Pooh, so a lot of the Winnie-the-Pooh stuff . . . . A lot of little things. A lot of bath things. I got a lot of bath stuff, the bathtubs and all the stuff that goes with it and

the towels and shampoos and lotions and soap, I got a lot of that. Little rattles and big stuffed animals. And then we got other things. A lot of bath things.

DP: What about the other shower? Same things?

M: One was with work and also there was one from the church here. Kind of a ladies' group, kind of most of the same things. A lot of little infant things, little gowns and receiving blankets and that, because I didn't have a lot of those.

DP: So it was mostly stuff for coming home?

M: Yeah. I had one that gave me older things. More books. Most of them were mothers and things that they used. Yeah, and they give like all the little nail clippers, all those kind of things that you wouldn't have. Medicines they use.

DP: They were mostly experienced mothers?

M: Uh-huh. Mostly the mothers that already know . . . Oh, yeah, like his little medicine things. And a lot of people gave those little shock things, things that you put in the outlets.

DP: The safety things, yeah.

M: Those kinds of things and the door latch things for your kitchen. And those kinds of little things.

DP: Did anybody make things for the baby?

M: An afghan.

DP: Someone made it just for him?

M: A friend. Yeah. And then we got one from the nurse, because he was born on Christmas day. The labor nurse had finished an afghan while they were waiting for me to deliver. They gave us a big poinsettia and lots of little diapers and gift certificates and I walked down and there's this big basket full of stuff. Little teddy bears and diaper service and they gave us a bunch of stuff. (I, Kevin, 1 mo.) (Pierce, 1996, p. 256)

Holidays

Holidays, especially Christmas and Hanukkah, were also routes for importing play objects into the home. The type of objects given to infants on these occasions tended to be commercial and gender-stereotyped toys. The following quote describes the abundance of playthings in one home after Christmas morning.

The toys in this home are incredible. Lots of importing going on here, especially from the maternal grandmother. Such items as a doll that names its body parts when you touch them, a big soft Velcro Mr. Potato Head, a big table that converts into a Duplo table, a train that the infant can ride around a track by depressing a large button in front of the seat, a plastic dishes set with goblets, and soft books that have parts you can move from one page to another. Nice discussion by Mom of the infant's experience of Christmas, opening one toy after the other, then going right to bed absolutely exhausted. (OR, Belle, 16 mos.) (Pierce, 1996, p. 258).

Birthdays

Another primary import event was the infants' first birthdays. Once again, the number and type of gift varied according to the economic level. A large riding toy was usually included, and girls typically received baby dolls. The following observation record describes a child who did not receive the usual first birthday gifts.

A terrible session. This child seems discontented with anything in the house, only happy playing with either the researcher's equipment or going outside. Frankly, I think she is incredibly bored. For her birthday, she received Bible music for infants, a couple of small music-making toys, but no big riding toys like the other 1-year-olds, no big push or pull toys. We couldn't even get through the interview. (OR, Alison, 13 mos.) (Pierce, 1996, p. 258)

Relatives

There were also several routes whereby extended family members introduced play objects for the infants. Visiting relatives frequently brought gifts such as stuffed animals, which were used (with varying degrees of success) as a catalyst for shared play with the infant. Grandmothers or aunts often made the infant special gifts, usually of a soft, comforting cloth material such as infant quilts, afghans, cloth books, and stuffed animals. Relatives with children just older than the infants would pass on or loan outgrown toys and infant-care equipment. Some grandmothers or mothers also brought out of storage objects that had been their own as children, passing them on to the infants. The symbolic meaning seemed to refer to the temporal cycles of family generations, as well as a sharing among the mothers of their feelings about raising a daughter, as seen in the following quote:

> M: My parents brought these rattles that I had from when I was a child, which is fun because like this one is real, real light. So we actually stuck it in her hand. Of course she was uninterested. They're kind of delicate and pretty. They're very light. So that was pretty fun 'cause she could hold on to it. I mean she wasn't particularly interested. Yeah, these four are old. And this is old. This was mine too. It looks like somebody made it, in fact. I don't know if they did. Looks like beads somebody put together. (I, Alison, 2 mos.) (Pierce, 1996, p. 259).

Commercial Influences

Examining these cultural routines of gift-giving to infants and toddlers demonstrates the degree to which the provision of play objects in the home is influenced by an ever-present commercial culture. Parents made frequent and enthusiastic forays through toy stores, bringing home new play items to engage and entertain their child. Of the 18 infants in the study, 6 also received developmental toys at 6-week intervals from a toy club presented in *Parent Magazine.* One infant belonged to a first book club also. The toy industry exerted a powerful and omnipresent influence on the mothers. This observational segment questions the degree of influence that mass media and the rise of developmental toy companies have on parents in their selection of toys.

> A shot of a rattle collection given to the child by his grandmother, several rattles of increasing developmental complexity. His mother said she thought her mother found them in a baby catalogue. They are just into the first rattle of the collection now. I am constantly impressed by the degree to which the toy manufacturing industry influences what these infants have for interaction and the types of large equipment with which they are managed. The toy club is one of these examples, although it may differ somewhat because it is based in the Johnson & Johnson toy series. This company is well known for a series of monographs on play and other

aspects of child development that are fairly scholarly. I wish there was some way in which I could gain insight into the perspective out of which these toys are being created within the toy industry. How much is child development research, how much parent purchasing attitudes research, how much just the economics of manufacturing and mark-up? (OR, Kevin, 2 mos.) (Pierce, 1996, p. 259)

Vignette: *Norah—Directing Play*

Alex was the first son and second child of a young couple who had just moved from Texas to the far eastern end of greater Los Angeles. The family fell into low levels of socioeconomic status. Alex's father was an automobile factory worker who worked the night shift at the end of a long commute. Norah stayed home with the two children. They lived in two small two-bedroom apartments successively during the study. They were excited to be about to move to a just-purchased mobile home at the conclusion of the study. Neither apartment had play space outdoors, although the second apartment did have a very small patio that was enclosed by a low wall and overshadowed by the upstairs apartment's porch. The two children shared a bedroom. Toys were not kept in the living area, but brought out to the children. Norah did not make much effort to offer or encourage Alex to interact with particular play objects once he outgrew the less mobile stage of being placed in the bouncer or below an overhead gym. She also frequently took objects from him until he was about 16 months of age, at which time he began objecting to her confiscation of his objects and forcibly resisting her.

Both Alex and his sister played with a moderate number of toys. They experienced some difficulty using push toys within such a small space. Alex seemed to receive quite a few vehicle toys, which held meaning to his family regarding his special value as a boy. He received a collection of hand-sized cars that his grandfather had been saving for a grandson, and his father would model car noises for him to make when he was on his riding toys. Despite this attention, Alex appeared to exhibit a rather impoverished repertoire of actions.

Facilitating and Controlling Access to Play Objects

Infancy

In the early months of their infants' lives, mothers set up blankets on the floor with play objects within reach. Once the infant was more mobile, mothers typically positioned them near toy shelves to encourage their independent retrieval of desired toys, although some enclosed them in a confined play area to prevent them from wandering off. In later months, rather than positioning the infants themselves, mothers used verbal cues to direct their children to these desired objects. This next mother describes how she positions toys away from the baby to encourage her independent retrieval.

> *DP:* When you're setting up the play area there, how do you put the toys? Do you put them . . .
> *M:* I don't put them right next to her, yeah. I put them like 6 inches to a foot away from her, usually, and then she'll take them to random places. (I, Belle, 5 mos.) (Pierce, 1996, p. 270)

Toddlers

With mobile toddlers, mothers changed the environment to promote independent play. For example, they re-arranged kitchen cupboards, placed toys on low shelves in the living area, and brought in toy boxes. Furthermore, many mothers used "novelty-maintaining" strategies. For instance, they would store toy boxes out of sight and then rotate them in and out of the play areas every few weeks. Or they would store away the new gift toys, bringing them out only when they felt their child needed something new with which to play.

> M: I've never quite figured out how to put them away. I started at night kind of rearranging stuff and making it nice in the morning because I've noticed that she's happier if they're kind of put in place and she can discover them. If they're all left in the mess she left them in the day before, she gets tired of it really fast and comes to me kind of bored. So if I put them out, even if it's the same toys but they're in slightly different spots arranged a little bit differently, then she'll go to it first thing. (I, Alison, 17 mos.) (Pierce, 1996, p. 271)

Mothers of multiple children typically stored all the toys together, which provided the infant/toddler with a larger choice but with a less accurate developmental fit. Some mothers promoted independent initiation of play by setting out favored toys at the eye level of the infant, such as on a coffee table, where it was likely to be noticed. The floor plan of the home was sometimes modified to reduce work of replacing and putting away toys. For example, some mothers switched their child's bedroom into the living room.

Spatial Considerations

Two of the single mothers in the study who lived with their parents had less ability to modify the home, resulting in different play experiences for their infants and toddlers. In these situations, they spent more time redirecting and repositioning their children away from taboo objects within the child's reach. The following observation records the challenge of the diminished sense of control over her child's play space that this mother felt while living with her mother:

> [Michael's grandmother's] house is becoming a poor fit too, lots of furniture and knick-knacks in a small space. Michael spends a lot of effort trying to reach baskets of magazines on the floor, little end tables with lamps delicately balanced on them, vases of prize roses, and cords running to electrical outlets. Today, Michael played with a few new toys. Some container play, some supported standing play at the coffee table. The mother has the doorway to the rest of the house beyond the living room blocked with the playpen. This was the first time that she was able to list any points at which Michael is being told no. When I left, Michael was climbing up the stairs with his mother, complete with back pain [from a recent car accident], crawling along behind him. (OR, Michael, 12 mos.) (Pierce, 1996, p. 272)

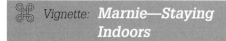 *Vignette:* **Marnie—Staying Indoors**

Marnie and her husband, both accounting majors at a small private college, were the parents of a single child named Belle. She was cared for entirely at home. Well into the study, a nanny was engaged several mornings a week to assist the parents in completing very heavy course loads before graduation.

During the first months of data collection, the family lived in a small student housing apartment on campus. The living room/kitchen area abutted onto a busy outdoor sidewalk, so the blinds were kept closed at all times. There was no yard with the apartment. Marnie reported going for stroller walks and, later, walks around the commons with Belle. Belle insistently requested to go outdoors many times during the study, but Marnie explained that she did not like her to play in the grass outdoors because it was full of burrs. The interior of the apartment was crowded with their small amount of furniture: a couch, large rocker, dining set, computer desk, coffee table, and video center. There was a master bedroom, which was off limits to Belle; a bathroom; and the infant room. The infant room appeared to be little played in, but was equipped with frilly, new infant furniture set (crib, chest of drawers, lamp table, bassinet).

After graduation, the family moved into a larger and brighter apartment, complete with a small back yard. A room off the living room was designated the playroom. There the toys were beautifully arranged: riding and pushing toys along the wall; two large shelves of stuffed animals, books, and other toys displayed as in a toy shop; dolls and large stuffed animals in play chairs, cradles. and highchairs; a large child's table that converted to an interlocking block surface in the center of the room; and a large riding train and track circling half of the room. In fact, the playroom contained a larger number of expensive developmental toys than was seen in any of the other participants' homes. Although the parents were of a low socioeconomic status, the maternal grandmother, a neuropsychologist, was often mentioned as the source of this remarkable variety of toys. Although the richness of toy selection may not typify lower social status homes, the cramped quarters, press for time, and lack of access to outdoor space did.   ⌘

Furnishing and Positioning in Play Space

Mothering an infant in the Caucasian suburban sample of this study included the use of an amazing variety of tools that were designed for this work. Devices for carrying and positioning an infant included slings, snuggles, baby backpacks, bouncers, carriers, car seats, swings, playpens, and strollers. Most of this infant management equipment was in all of the homes, especially those of the higher socioeconomic status families.

In order to correctly position the infant in the equipment, mothers were required to make several considerations. Most important was whether the positioning device would interest and occupy the infant enough to free the mother for other household tasks. The infant was usually positioned with a view of his or her mother. Infant access to objects of interest for gaze and contact were also considered. Sometimes infants were repositioned from one piece of equipment to another when they appeared bored. In public spaces, strollers served as the primary positioning device.

Safety was a primary concern to mothers when choosing equipment. For example, the correct positioning of the car seat in the car and the timing of the change from an infant to a toddler car seat occupied the mother's judgment. Infants with close-aged siblings were more frequently placed in various types of equipment to keep them out of their siblings' reach. Older infants, who desired more movement, were frequently put in walkers or jumpups. Playpens were used only in environments that were unsafe or in which it was inconvenient for a baby. Mothers in the lower socioeconomic status homes expressed more concerns over infant safety and exercised more restraint of the play of their children. However, although the more expensive homes of the higher socioeconomic status families were also larger, toy stocked, and complete with manicured lawns, there were many areas of the homes—offices, formal living and dining rooms, pool areas, detached garages, laundry rooms, and live-in housekeeper quarters—that were off limits to the infant. This resulted in approximately the same amount of space available to them as to babies of lower socioeconomic status homes. In fact, the lower socioeconomic status mothers used the greatest amount of creativity and flexibility in accommodating spaces to fit the needs and desires of their children.

Other management tools were designed for specific activity sites. The mothers used infant bathtubs, and then sitting rings for the family bathtub. For sleeping, there was the infant swing and the bouncer in the early months, a bassinet beside the bed for infant sleep, a crib for later months, and possibly a toddler bed by 18 months of age. An adult-sized rocking chair was in almost every home. Several homes had children's rockers. A changing table, located in the infant's room, was in every home, although it was not always used. Every home had a highchair for the infant. One mother had a bike trailer to tow her children along when out for a ride. The variety of infant-care furnishings that were used in these homes and the thinking that mothers do in making use of these tools support the notion that the spatial arrangement of tools and devices in the infant's environment composes a large portion of the mother's infant care practices.

Access to Outdoors

Mothers were especially vigilant about access to outdoors, although the back yard was also managed as a play space when closely supervised. This was understandable, given that there were many risks in the outdoor environment that could not be controlled. In some of the homes in the lower levels of the socioeconomic status, however, the back-yard space was small to nonexistent. Those who did have yards tended to keep larger toys there, such as swing sets, riding toys, and sandboxes. The space was also conducive to push toy and riding toy play.

Spatial Ties Between Mother and Infant

The mothers' occupations of managing the home were in a dyadic interplay between their own occupations and those of their infants: this is co-occupation. Both mother and infant appeared to be linked in space by an invisible rubber band. At times, it was difficult to discern who was following whom. Especially in the first few months of the infants' lives, mothers kept quite close to their newborns, and frequently engaged in face-to-face games such as peek-a-boo. If the infant was not being held, he or she was nearby in a swing or another piece of positioning equipment.

> Mother did not expect my visit and seemed very tired. It continues to be difficult to get shots of the child separate from his mother. It is even difficult to get the mother to stop goo-gooing in the baby's face long enough to answer the interview questions! It is evident that she thinks the proper place for the baby is in her arms at all times. It is also evident in her comments that this effort is wearing on her considerably. The baby is the focus of attention for the whole family: two grandparents and Mom in the house, extended family nearby, including his uncle, who was the birth coach. (OR, Michael, 3 mos.) (Pierce, 1996, p. 250)

Infants progressed from being constantly in their mothers' arms to playing just within arm's reach, to exploring the house independently. Co-occupation patterns were linked across time and space, such as when a toddler would bring toys out of the toy box to play with them and later the mother would return the toys to the box. The emerging mobility of the infant changed the mother's management patterns. The mother's actions in choosing toys and allowing access as the child's abilities changed shaped the child's opportunities for play.

Although some mothers seemed to spend more time following their infants, other mothers seemed to take the lead. The independent self-directedness that the infant displayed influenced the degree to which he or she led the mother throughout the house or neighborhood. Mothers who tended to allow the infant to lead and control the spatial tie were frequently mothers of only children, who had time to indulge the infant and were commonly of upper socioeconomic status. Mothers with more than one child were more likely to be leaders of the mother/child dyad. The following is an excerpt from an interview with a mother with only one child, who spent an hour daily in following her infant as she explored the neighborhood.

> ***M:*** I think that if there wasn't the street and I could just let her go she kind of looks at me and if I go one way, she goes the other, so she would go a long way.
> ***DP:*** She doesn't seem worried about where you are.

M: See, she doesn't even look back, it's like if I look back there, I know you're gonna come. (I, Alison, 17 mos.) (Pierce, 1996, p. 251)

🐾 Choreography: The Maternal Work of Managing Play Time in the Home

The daily activities in the homes of the study never fit a predictable, typical pattern. Each mother choreographed the family's day differently. Of course, for mothers employed outside the home, a portion of the infant's day was delegated to the routines of a day-care center. The transition of a mother returning to outside employment greatly affected the infant's day. The ways in which mothers coordinated the flow of activities in the home operated at many levels: moment-to-moment decisions, general and constantly adjusted guidelines for the day's activities, and long-term conceptualizations of how the day should go and to which the mother aspired.

Safety

The practices of the mothers in the study as they shaped the play environment in which their infants/toddlers developed were various and demanding. They emanated from a variety of motives, including desires to keep the infant safe, to facilitate the infant's development, to maintain order in the home, and to allow the mother to engage in other household labor beyond infant care with the infant present. In order to reach these ends, the mothers created and maintained infant space. This required judgment and decision making, selection and use of play objects and infant-care equipment, and constant manipulation of the objects that made up the physical environment of the home. They were especially concerned about the safety within the home, which held many dangers for their infants. They controlled for these hazards by investing in baby latches, plug protectors, coffee table corner pads, toilet locks, and "choke-proof" measuring cylinders. Furthermore, mothers used their own bodies to block or carry their infants away from unsafe places. Mothers who were less financially secure appeared to be more concerned about the safety of their infants within the home. The following segment describes the concerns of a mother as she redesigns her new home to fit the needs of her child.

> Aaron's family is now happily ensconced in their new Claremont home and Aaron, apparently, is spending a lot of time in his little playpen as his mother unpacks. He is playing with toys found during the move, new to him, but developmentally young for him mostly. Mother is concerned with safety hazards of the pool (new fence installed; only she knows the combination), cupboards (father beginning to install baby latches), and walker tipping at meeting of carpet and floor (walker temporarily retired). The house seems a lot larger than their previous home. Aaron is now in the room with his immediately older brother, instead of with his sister, much to her relief. (OR, Aaron, 9 mos.) (Pierce, 1996, p. 274)

As the infant matured and gained mobility, the size of the space over which the mother was required to maintain control expanded. Initially, it was only the peri-personal space of the infant that was of concern, but as the infants of the study got older, their mothers were actively altering the physical space of the home to accommodate their child's development. This mother expressed her frustrations with her toddler's increasing territory and the danger it posed:

> As I was leaving, the mother admitted that her neighbor had to stop his car the day before because Bruce was in the middle of the street. His mother was working on the new computer. She said, "He is so fast now!" Evidently, Bruce does not yet have a sense of boundaries to his home setting. Or he does, but violated them. Mother says that her father is dying now, any day, so a lot of things have to be let go, such as sorting toys and dragging out another sandbox. (OR, Bruce, 14 mos.) (Pierce, 2000, p. 293)

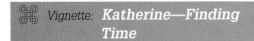 🎗 *Vignette:* **Katherine—Finding Time**

Aaron was the fourth child in a family falling into high levels of socioeconomic status. Katherine was a doctorally trained developmental psychologist, working part-time, and her husband was in the aerospace industry. When Katherine was at work, the children were watched in their home by their grandmother. During the study, the family moved from a moderately sized single-level home to a larger single-level home. In the early months, this infant experienced a large degree of spatial restriction because of the mother's concerns about his safety in the presence of his very active brother, who was close in age. In the larger home, he appeared to have more freedom and less conflict with his brother. As in most of the higher-status-level homes, there was a portion of this home that was clearly set aside for adults, a formal living room. A door was kept closed to keep Aaron from entering this area at one end, and a baby gate was at the other. Most of Aaron's play occurred in the den, in the bedroom that he shared with his immediately older brother, and outside. The outdoor area of this family's second home was perhaps the largest in the study, and was furnished with a large variety of riding toys, climbing objects, sandbox, and other large playthings. Inside, there was a good selection of developmental toys that appeared to have already been used by the older children. The infant also frequently played with kitchen plastics and pans.

Katherine's management of the family's activity pattern appeared to be a full but well-organized schedule. She did not appear to feel much time pressure except during their move, even though this was also the largest family in the study. The older sister, who was 11 years older than Aaron, enjoyed helping her mother with baby care and would play with the infant along with her girlfriends.

In the early months of Aaron's participation in the study, he seemed to be spending a greater portion of time in a playpen or walker than any of the other infants in the study. Throughout the study, he experienced a larger portion of observation of sibling play, as opposed to self-directed object interactions, which seemed to typify the infants in this study with close-aged older siblings.   ⌘

Multiple Schedules

Unlike the mother just described, some mothers in the study reported that sometimes they felt as if they were simply "maintaining"

their infant rather than actually interacting with him or her. They were concerned that they were asking too much of the infant by re-arranging sleep or feeding schedules to fit into the family routine. Furthermore, they worried that their infants were so easily entertained as to be ignored or neglected by the rest of the family. The following mother expresses her frustrations with the lack of time in her day:

> M: I've come up with a new awareness, though, that, I mean, aside from the fact that they're going to scream if they're going to scream. I mean, they're kids. She's 2, that's what she's going to do, so be prepared. But, we were taking on too many activities—too many big activities in a given day. And then by the end of the day I've gotten—you know, I've gotten all these chores done and trying to get them to the park or this or that and we're just all fit to be tied. Bill comes home and it's like, aaah! And we're just all too agitated. And I realize it's because I've had them out doing too many things. So, I've been trying this new approach where we're only going to do one major activity a day and then try to do some home time and then the other thing is, if we have to be out and I have no, you know, it's my fault and I have to let them scream or, you know, it's kind of helping diffuse my reaction to their playing. We had to go to the grocery store in spite of everything and it was so hysterical, because they were slowly—they just slowly edge up to the explosion point. And then Billy dumped my coupon package all over the floor and there was just a sea of coupons and I said, "Okay, this is my fault, I brought you here. That's life." (I, Leslie, 14 mos.) (Pierce, 1996, p. 281)

Maintaining Play Sequences

Mothers intervened in their infants' play in order to initiate the play with an object, to discontinue an interaction, to support the continuity of an interaction the infant was attempting, to distract the infant, or to entertain the infant for a length of time required by the mother within the larger pattern of the day. To do this, the mother would often demonstrate the toy's potential for interaction by pushing it, bouncing it, or otherwise showing its possibilities. Less experienced and more directive mothers appeared to do this more often, disregarding the infants' occurring interactions with other objects as they did so.

Discontinuing play most often had to do with the mothers' previously discussed concerns with safety and maintaining order in the home. Attempts to engage the infant in extended play were usually related to the mothers' desire to do some household work, talk on the telephone, or take a shower. The most challenging situation in which mothers needed infants to remain engaged with play objects was during travel. They kept toys stored in the car that were played with only during driving and bought fresh objects for long trips. They took an assortment of infant management devices and play objects with them on trips to visit relatives.

⌘ *Vignette:* **Kelli—Composing a Routine**

This mother was home with her infant son, Zeke, for the first 4 months, then back to work part time briefly, and finally full time. The infant was enrolled at the same developmental preschool as was his 3 1/2-years-older sister when Kelli returned to work.

Kelli's home space included a large home of two floors and a yard rarely observed to be used. The garage was used for riding and driving toys. A sunporch off the family room was filled with toys, and the two children were encouraged to play in that area. In addition to a couch, chair, and exercise machine, the sunporch contained a play kitchen, small riding toys, and a wide variety of bright developmental toys in good condition stored in laundry baskets. Kelli was fairly permissive in allowing Zeke's use of space, even assisting him in learning to use the stairs with supervision.

This home was unique in the degree to which Kelli used organized strategies for storage and rotation of toys. She kept different types of toys in large clear boxes and would switch them with those kept in a closet, in order to keep interest in the toys high through novelty. She also stored away all Christmas and birthday gifts in order to save them for opening gradually as situations needing a fresh object arose. She was very receptive to Zeke's desire to move within the downstairs areas of the house, simply following him from room to room.

The temporal context of this home also appeared fairly routinized. Kelli and her children usually went upstairs after dinner for bath, story, and perhaps a little evening play time. The family's shoes were kept together inside the door to the garage, and Zeke would go get his shoes and bring them for help in putting them on, as an indication that he wanted to leave. The mother's work schedule, complemented by the preschool's schedule, structured most of the weekdays. Kelli appeared to be relatively sensitive to the sequences of her infant's play, pulling out new objects for engagement only when interest in other activities waned.   ⌘

Establishing Infant/Toddler Routines

Mothers used routines to lessen their constant negotiation of infant activities. The core components of the daily routine were feeding, sleeping, and the mother's personal responsibilities. Play periods were fitted conveniently between sleep and feeding, often paired with the mother's attempts to accomplish household work, which made the child's independent play especially important.

Feeding

Feeding was the earliest routine to emerge. The infants quickly began to recognize the feeding position and became visibly frustrated if expected actions did not occur when they were placed in that position. During the interviews, mothers often commented on how they were trying to shape the feeding schedule to establish a mealtime that included the whole family. They would avoid positioning the infant in order to postpone feeding, or pick up and settle the infant at the chosen site for feeding if that was what they wished to initiate. By 6 months of age, the infants became sensitive to the chosen feeding site, and by the time they were 1 year of age, the mothers began to synchronize infant mealtimes with that of the father and the rest of the family, such as in this family:

M: She knows when it's mealtime. And it's amazing, now that I'm weaning her, you sometimes forget—

DP: Does she sit with you at dinnertime and eat, or does she eat at a separate time?

M: Well, they both—the times we've tried to all sit down together is sort of funny. I don't know why, but they're hungry as soon as Bill gets home and I find that I'm always trying to give them something to eat—when I'm just starting to cook. So, we all try to sit. Even if they've already eaten separate. (I, Leslie, 12 mos.) (Pierce, 1996, p. 279)

Sleeping

Developing a schedule for sleep required the mother to consider the changing biotemporality of the infant, her own chores that needed to be accomplished during the day, and the nap schedule of other siblings. Several mothers of multiple children observed differences in the greater degree of flexibility required to shape a sleep schedule for a second or later child than was required for the first. Sleep schedules that were synchronous with those of other siblings carried the added benefit of a welcome break for the mother to attend to other chores.

> M: There goes the morning nap. She may fall asleep in the car on the way to our playgroup. With Billy, I was rigid with naps and I am trying to provide her with the sleep. I'm almost trying to push her into napping with brother in the afternoon and take cat naps in the morning so that they can both be down for my sanity and they can both have the comfort of a quiet place instead of snagging short naps. (I, Leslie, 4 mos.) (Pierce, 1996, p. 280)

Household Tasks

In the later months of the study, mothers were successfully teaching toddlers to assume some of the routines the mothers had established for them. Besides the bedtime routine, they learned routines for leaving the house, for feeding pets, for self-care, and for participating in household work. One of the most common activities in which toddlers began to participate in household work was laundry. The youngest child reported as participating

in laundry was a 10-month-old girl. By the age of the child in the following excerpt, toddlers had multiple household routines in which they participated.

> *DP:* Is he still interested in helping you?
>
> *M:* Right, he gets things in the dishwasher. The other day there's some bowls in the dishwasher, the silver bowls, and he took them out of the dishwasher for me, and put them in the cupboard. In his cupboard. And if I'm ever cooking now, or doing anything, if I'm mixing up something, he'll go get a bowl, or a little strainer, or something like that and hand it to me. I gotta take it from him. He puts his laundry in the washer and he pushes the laundry down the hall. He's got to get the basket for me. He pushes that. (I, Kevin, 14 mos.) (Pierce, 1996, p. 280)

Disrupters

There were three factors that disrupted the temporality of the infant's independent play: the presence of playing siblings, a television in the same room, and the issue of toy ownership.

Siblings

When siblings played with an object, the infant was attracted to the same object. When the sibling was close in age, this frequently resulted in a conflict over the item. Older siblings tended to fill more of a caregiver role. The infant with the closest-aged sibling, only a 14-month span between them, had the greatest degree of play disruptions. He experienced constant acts of aggression from his brother, which were only marginally controlled by his mother. Many of his interactions were disrupted by his brother snatching the object from his grasp as the older sibling walked past. Infants did not seem to understand the loss of these objects in the early months. At approximately 8 months of age, however, they began to loudly protest the loss of objects to a sibling. Mothers struggled to devise ways of preventing and reacting to this inter-sibling aggression and competition over play objects.

> *DP:* How is Oscar's play, as a second child, compared to how his brother's was at this age?

M: Everything is interrupted. You know, whereas Jeff could sit there and do something for a long time, there would be no one to interrupt him. Oscar is constantly being interrupted all the time. You know, he'll be playing with his toy and then it's gone. You know, he'll be in the walker and then he's pushed across the room. Or, you know, its like, I think he's going to deal better with change, I don't know. I think that probably the biggest difference is the interruption and the loud noise. It's loud, you know, where with Jeff it was quiet. But as far as what affects Oscar is the interruptions, constant interruptions. And the disruption of his schedule. He's constantly being woken up when he's not ready to get woke up. And falling asleep when he's lying on the floor over here and I'm in the kitchen, I turn around, he's asleep. Oscar isn't on a schedule yet. Where Jeff was on a schedule by 4 months old. And also too, I run more errands and stuff and figure, oh, Oscar will just sleep in the car or whatever, whereas with Jeff, oh, no, it's Jeff's nap time, we have to stay home now. But I'm anxious to get Oscar on a schedule, it's just not happening yet (I, Oscar, 4 mos.) (Pierce, 1996, p. 254)

Close-aged infants and siblings were often encouraged by mothers to play in separate areas, especially if the older child was interacting with objects considered unsafe for the infant. Close-aged siblings were sometimes placed beyond access to infants, such as up at a table or beyond a baby gate. When playing near the infant, the close-aged sibling was required to follow behavioral guidelines from the mother. This was irregularly successful. Mothers also used mediation techniques such as making sure there were two popular play objects, keeping special objects belonging to the sibling off limits to the infant, and teaching the older child to trade objects with the infant.

Toy Ownership

The reason for some of the competition over play objects seemed to be an issue of ownership: all the toys that had previously belonged to the sibling were passed on to the new baby. Different mothers handled this issue differently. In some homes, all toys belonged to everyone. In others, there were certain toys that belonged to just one child. In homes with multiple children, toys tended to belong to everyone, although some toys that were considered unsafe were kept away from the infant. Some siblings quickly realized where in the house they could place their favorite toys out of reach of the infant. These special object storage places moved higher and higher during the study, as the infant's ability to penetrate vertical space increased over 18 months. Having an older sibling also introduced certain objects into the infant's environment at an earlier age. Mothers of close-aged siblings also reported that infants were exposed earlier to books and to play with objects with small pieces, such as a collection of hand-sized cars or a block set. Of course, there are also conflicts, as the following segment shows.

M: She—there was some conflict. She likes to just draw. She kind of goes and draws all over his trains [his chalk drawings on the back patio]. And he gets upset. So I said, "Well, Billy, you know, let's just give her a different place to draw." It used to be—I think a month ago I would have said, "Well, you know, she doesn't know any better." She's starting to show that she knows. And so we say, "Leslie, you have to draw over here." And, you know, "This is Billy's," and really trying to teach her now that, "This is yours and that's his."

(I, Leslie, 16 mos., brother 3 yrs.) (Pierce, 1996, p. 254)

Television

The infants and toddlers in the study, although showing only passing interest in television watching during the early months, became easily mesmerized by television as they matured. By about 1 year old, they frequently were seen carrying videotapes around to request that they be started, and by age 2 years, were able to use the remote control to turn on the television. Only one home did not have a television; many had it on constantly, although all the mothers expressed their displeasure with this. It was tempting, however, to use "the one-eyed babysitter" to obtain a break from the demands of managing the infant's activities.

M: Usually, I demand that, you know, they pretty much know that they're supposed to only eat in there, but this is like a real privilege. Plus, they just, it's amazing—and Barney comes on next. And we don't usually watch. But the few times I've needed—I've started to realize that if I really need that moment of peace and then I'll try to make sure that they're not just there forever and that the one-eyed babysitter really helps, especially in the evening dinner hour. (I, Leslie, 16 mos.) (Pierce, 1996, p. 282)

Vignette: *Susan—Shaping the Setting*

Susan lived with her retired parents in a condominium community, where she raised her son, Michael. He was the center of attention for the three adults in the home. He was a very large child and sought an unusually high amount of physical holding. Early in his infancy, both mother and grandfather separately and in several different sessions offered enthusiastic explanations to me of how the world would be improved if adults were just more child centered. As Michael matured, however, he engaged in more self-directed explorations of the physical setting. When he was old enough to roam the house, his mother became equally enthusiastic about a child-rearing philosophy that addressed the child's need to be out of the center of attention and observing, rather than being at the center of family activity. This led to increased independent time for him in his playpen, playing with a provided selection of toys.

The spatial and temporal contexts of this setting were unique in several ways. First of all, the space was quite small for three adults and an infant. It was crowded with furniture and a lifetime of precious objects displayed on low tables and shelves. Susan felt that she had very limited control over the arrangement of the space and spent a great deal of time in limiting Michael's movements toward the display of attractive objects once he became mobile. The toys available to him were not large in number. He was encouraged to play with them in limited spaces. Unlike most of the young children who had riding toys by 1 year of age, Michael did not receive any until nearly the end of the study. His

motor development appeared a bit slower in comparison to that of the other infants, which could be because of his large size or the setting.

Choreography: The Maternal Work of Managing Time in the Home

Maternal differences in the management of temporal context were evident because of factors such as time required to work outside the home, presence of other children in the home, variable degrees of maternal control over the home setting, and amount of maternal experience. Mothers working outside the home often expressed concerns about the limited amount of time that they could spend with their infants. They tended to stay very close and were more directive with their infants' play during the data collection sessions. Mothers of multiple children and full time college students also reported this time pressure, but appeared to respond by becoming less involved in the infant's play. Mothers in situations in which they had little control in shaping the setting to their infants' needs experienced great pressure in the moment-to-moment supervision of their infant's play.

The following video script describes the actions of Susan's son, Michael, at home with his mother and grandparents. The home was filled with furniture, mementos, and treasured objects displayed all around. At this recording, this small town home was also filled with a Christmas tree and many different Christmas displays, including an electric train and a snowy village scene. The following description shows how this setting required the mother to constantly reposition the infant away from desired, but forbidden, objects in her parents' home.

> The baby crawls to the Christmas tree, where his mother promptly removes him and positions him in a toy boat. He immediately crawls out of the boat and back to the tree, and Mom removes him again. After he has been crawling halfway up the stairs, Mom brings him down and positions him in supported standing at the

coffee table. Once again, he begins to crawl up the stairs and Mom brings him back to the coffee table. This time, he picks up a ball, carries it up the stairs, and grabs the television remote. Mom brings him back downstairs. He crawls into the kitchen; Mom brings him back into the living room, positioning him at the coffee table once again. He crawls to a shelf of cookbooks, and Mom brings him back. He crawls to the mini-blinds in the kitchen and attempts to manipulate them; Mom brings him back. (Video, Michael, 13 mos.) (Pierce, 1996, p. 283).

℘ Conclusion

Play is the medium by which infants and toddlers develop. Valuing the development of their children, mothers act as the stage managers and choreographers behind the play scenes of the home. They choose, maintain, and provide play objects to match the child's evolving developmental capacities. They manage the child's access to the spaces of the home and the immediate outdoor surroundings. They furnish spaces with childcare equipment and monitor those spaces for safety. They manage the child's day within the complex priorities of the needs for the child's development and safety, the need for order in the home, the mother's need for peace of mind, and the multiple schedules of family members. They support the child's efforts to maintain play sequences and defend the child's play from common disruptions. They work to establish temporal routines within the child for feeding, sleeping, and playing. This indirect and out-of-sight work, although central to the development of the child and the creation of a home and family, is generally unrecognized.

This substantive description of the co-occupations of developing infants and toddlers at play and mothers doing the work of supporting play provides us, as therapists, with needed insight into the daily experiences of mothers. By examining the ways in which mothers view their responsibilities to the child, analyzing the daily care mothers provide, and understanding maternal work in terms of the spatial and temporal routines that

mothers manage, occupational therapists can better provide assistance to mothers and caregivers of children within the home (Pierce & Frank, 1992). Exploring the individual phenomenology of women's experiences with their infants and toddlers at home can provide important insights to the therapist that might not be so apparent in a clinical setting.

If we are providing interventions to mothers, an understanding of the work of creating the home play setting can provide us with the basis for offering mothers well-informed, occupation-based, and client-centered care. For example, consider now the maternal work faced by multiple-birth mothers, heading home from the neonatal intensive care unit with one or more at-risk infants. Certainly, anyone could appreciate the challenges ahead for such a mother. This study details those potential challenges in a way that could support a discussion with such a mother of priorities, supports, needs, and pressing decisions, a way that would be only vaguely understood without this description. For mothers with disabilities, the study highlights possible issues of importance: the mother's desire to control and shape the home play space and play experiences of her infant or toddler to fit the child's developmental level, possible adaptations to the spaces and routines of mothering work, significantly more complex sets of conflicting priorities in managing her child's development in the home, and factors that may limit her ability to establish childhood routines and fend off disruptors of infant/toddler play.

For therapists focused on goals for children with disabilities, an understanding of how the maternal work of supporting infant/toddler play in the home occurs provides insights into how positive effects of intervention can be extended into the daily life of the family. Seeing the complex spatial and temporal management of the home enables the therapist to better design appropriate and effective intervention for the child. A better understanding of the home helps the therapist to alter routines as well as objects within the environment to establish developmentally appropriate play. This might be done by introducing new objects to the child, facilitating play between child and mother, or initiating changes in the child's access to the surrounding environment. To provide excellent occupation-based care, it is critical that occupational therapists have more research on the dynamics of the occupations with which, or in hope of which, we intervene.

Discussion Questions 🐾

- Compare similarities and differences between any two mothers in the study regarding their management of home space and play objects.

- How does the toy industry influence and shape infant/toddler development through maternal choices of play objects? Is this a good influence or a bad influence?

- The mothers and their children in this study illustrate the dynamics of a co-occupation, or one person's occupational pattern shaping and being a required part of another's. If the toddler had not carried toys from the toy box all over the house, the mother would not be picking up toys and carrying them back to the toy box at the end of the day. If the mother had not placed toys out on the blanket of the prone noncrawling infant, the infant would not be playing with toys while lying on the blanket. What co-occupation patterns can you identify in your own life?

- How much time each day do you think a mother of a toddler spends in the indirect work of creating, maintaining, monitoring, sequencing, and making judgments about the play opportunities available to her child in her home?

- Given this description, what factors (beyond disabilities of mother or child) should be considered red flags for potentially preventing a mother from providing a high quality developmental environment for her child in her home?

- List as many ways as you can in which an occupational therapist might assist a single mother who has paraplegia and uses a wheelchair to fully engage in the maternal work described here of creating developmental opportunities in the home for her child.

References

Ainsworth, M. D. S., & Bell, S. M. (1974). Mother-child interaction and the development symbol of competence. In K. J. Connolly & J. S. Bruner (Eds.). *The growth of competence.* New York: Academic, pp. 97–188.

Belsky, J., & Most, R. (1981). From exploration to play: A cross-sectional study of infant free-play behavior. *Developmental Psychology, 17,* 630–639.

Berger, A. A. (1992). *Reading matter: Multidisciplinary perspectives on material culture.* London: Transaction Publishers.

Bornstein, M. H., Azuma, H., Tamis-LeMonda, C., & Ogino, M. (1990a). Mother and infant activity and interaction in Japan and in the United States: I. A comparative macroanalysis of naturalistic exchanges fo- cused on the organization of infant attention. *Interna-tional Journal of Behavioral Development, 13,* 267–287.

Bornstein, M. H., Toda, S., Azuma, H., Tamis-LeMonda, C., & Ogino, M. (1990b). Mother and infant activity and interaction in Japan and in the United States: II. A comparative macroanalysis of naturalistic exchanges. *International Journal of Behavioral Development, 13,* 289–308.

Bornstein, M. H., Tamis-LeMonda, C., Pecheux, M., & Rahn, C. W. (1991). Mother and infant activity and interaction in France and in the United States: II. A comparative study. *International Journal of Behavioral Development, 14,* 21–43.

Bradley, R. H., & Caldwell, B. M. (1984). The relation of infants' home environments to achievement test performance in first grade: A follow-up study. *Child Development, 55,* 803–809.

Clarke-Stewart, K. A. (1973). Interactions between mothers and their young children: Characteristics and consequences. *Monographs of the Society for Research in Child Development, 38,* 6–7 (Serial No. 153).

Coll, C. G., Vohr, B. R., Hoffman, J., & Oh, W. (1986). Maternal and environmental factors affecting developmental outcome of infants of adolescent mothers. *Developmental and Behavioral Pediatrics, 7,* 230–236.

Cross, G. (1997). *Kid's stuff: Toys and the changing world of American childhood.* Cambridge, MA: Harvard University Press.

Csikszentmihalyi, M., & Rochberg-Halton, E. (1981). *The meaning of things: Domestic symbols and the self.* Cambridge: Cambridge University Press.

Elardo, R., Bradley, R. H., & Caldwell, B. M. (1975). A longitudinal study of relation of infants' home environment to language development at age three. *Child Development, 46,* 71–76.

Gibson, J. J. (1986). *The ecological approach to visual perception.* Hillsdale, NJ: Erlbaum.

Glaser, B. G., & Strauss, A. L. (1987). *The discovery of grounded theory: Strategies for qualitative research.* Chicago: Aldine.

Goodall, J. (1986). *The chimpanzees of Gombe: Patterns of behavior.* Cambridge, MA: Belknap.

Haith, M. M. (1990). Progress in the understanding of sensory and perceptual processes in early infancy. *Merrill-Palmer Quarterly, 36*(1), 11–27.

Hendricks-Jansen, H. (1996). *Catching ourselves in the act: Situated activity, interactive emergence, evolution, and human thought.* Cambridge, MA: MIT Press.

Jennings, K. D., Harmon, R. J., Morgan, G. A., Gaiter, J. L., & Yarrow, L. J. (1979). Exploratory play as an index of mastery motivation: Relationships to persistence, cognitive functioning, and environmental measures. *Developmental Psychology, 15,* 386–394.

Kantor, D., & Lehr, W. (1975). *Inside the family.* San Francisco: Jossey-Bass Publishers.

Lyons-Ruth, K., Zoll, D., Connell, D., & Grunbaum, H. U. (1986). The depressed mother and her one-year-old infant: Environment, interaction, attachment, and infant development. *New Directions for Child Development, 34,* 61–82.

Martin, E. (1987). *The woman in the body: A cultural analysis of reproduction.* Boston: Beacon Press.

McClary, A. (1997). *Toys with nine lives: A social history of American toys.* New Haven, CT: Linnet.

Neisser, U. (1976). *Cognition and reality.* New York: W. H. Freeman and Company.

Palmar, C. F. (1989). The discriminating nature of infants' exploratory action. *Developmental Psychology, 25,* 885–893.

Piaget, J. (1952). *The origins of intelligence in children.* New York: International Universities Press.

Piaget, J. (1962). *Plays, dreams, and imitation in childhood.* New York: Norton.

Pierce, D. E. (1996). Infant space, infant time: Development of infant interactions with the physical environment, from 1 to 18 months. (Doctoral dissertation, University of Southern California, 1996). *Dissertation Abstracts International, 57,* AAG9705160.

Pierce, D. (2000). Maternal management of the home as a developmental play space for infants and toddlers. *American Journal of Occupational Therapy, 54,* 290–299.

Pierce, D., & Frank, G. (1992). A mother's work: Two levels of feminist analysis of family-centered care. *American Journal of Occupational Therapy, 46,* 972-980.

Reilly, M. (1962). Occupational therapy can be one of the great ideas of twentieth century medicine. *American Journal of Occupational Therapy, 16,* 1–9.

Reilly, M. (1974). *Play as exploratory learning.* Beverly Hills Sage Publications.

Rich, A. (1986). *Of woman born: Motherhood as experience and institution.* New York: W. W. Norton.

Rochat, P. (1989). Object manipulation and exploration in 2- to 5-month old infants. *Developmental Psychology, 25,* 871–884.

Rowles, G. (1991). Beyond performance: Being in place as a component of occupational therapy. *American Journal of Occupational Therapy, 45,* 265–271.

Rowles, G. (2000). Habituation and being in place. *Occupational Therapy Journal of Research,* supplement 1, 52–67.

Rubin, K. H., Maioni, T. L., & Hornung, M. (1976). Free play behaviors in middle- and lower-class preschoolers: Parten and Piaget revisited. *Child Development, 47,* 414–419.

Ruddick, S. (1989). *Maternal thinking: Toward a politics of peace.* Boston, MA: Beacon Press.

Ruff, H. (1984). Infant's manipulative exploration of objects: Effects of age and object characteristics. *Developmental Psychology, 20,* 9–20.

Schlereth, T. J. (1985). Material culture and cultural research. In T. J. Schlereth (Ed.). *Material culture: A research guide.* Lawrence, KS: University Press of Kansas.

Stevens, J. H., & Bakeman, R. (1985). *A factor analytic study of the HOME Scale for infants. Developmental Psychology, 21,* 1196–1203.

Tulkin, S., & Covitz, F. (1975, April). *Mother-infant interaction and intellectual functioning at age 6.* Paper presented at the meeting of the Society for Research in Child Development, Denver, CO.

Wachs, T. D. (1976). Utilization of a Piagetian approach in the investigation of early experience effects: A research strategy and some illustrative data. *Merrill-Palmar Quarterly, 22,* 11–30.

Wachs, T. D. (1978). The relationship of infants' physical environment to their Binet performance at $2\frac{1}{2}$ years. *International Journal of Behavioral Development, 1,* 51–65.

Wachs, T. D. (1979). Proximal experience and early cognitive-intellectual development: The physical environment. *Merrill-Palmar Quarterly, 25,* 3–41.

Wachs, T. D., Uzgiris, I. C., & Hunt, J. McV. (1971). Cognitive development in infants of different age levels and from different environmental backgrounds: An exploratory investigation. *Merrill-Palmar Quarterly, 17,* 283–317.

Wohlwill, J. F., & Heft, H. (1987). The physical environment and the development of the child. In D. Stokols & I. Altman (Eds.). *Handbook of environmental psychology.* Malabar, FL: Krieger, pp. 281–328.

Yarrow, L. J., Morgan, G. A., Jennings, K. D., Harmon, R. J., & Gaiter, J. L. (1982). Infants' persistence at tasks: Relationships to cognitive functioning and early experience. *Annual Progress in Child Psychiatry and Development, 1,* 217–229.

Yarrow, L. J., McQuiston, S., MacTurk, R. H., McCarthy, M. E., Klein, R. P., & Vietze, P. M. (1983). Assessment of mastery motivation during the first year of life: Contemporaneous and cross-age relationships. *Developmental Psychology, 19,* 159–171.

CHAPTER 5

Toys for Shade and the Mother-Child Co-occupation of Play

Susan A. Esdaile, PhD, MAPS, AccOT, OTR, SROT

Anticipated Outcomes

I anticipate that, after reading this chapter, readers will:

- Have an increased understanding of the importance of play in mother-child interaction

- Have an increased understanding of how mothers contribute to enabling and enhancing their child's play

- Have an increased understanding of what constitutes play as a mother-child co-occupation

- Have further insights regarding the relationship between research and professional practice

- Have further insights regarding societal, expert, and experiential influences that shape and determine individual and generational shifts in professional practice

Introduction

When I first started working with a community-based, child- and family-focused program in the western metropolitan region of Melbourne, Australia, one of the nurses mentioned a program that sounded really interesting. It was run by a community nurse for mothers who were on court orders for child abuse. This meant that the mothers were required to report weekly to a designated community health worker. This nurse had developed various strategies for encouraging the mothers to stay with the program, so that she could engage them in discussions that could assist with child-rearing issues. She found that the mothers did not like to talk about their problems, but enjoyed making or doing things such as potting plants, tie-dying, cooking, or going on outings with a small group. Further, she had observed that the incidence of inappropriate, coercive, or aggressive parenting was less frequent after one of these activity groups. The women seemed to be happier, more relaxed, and better able to handle their children.

This gave me the idea that involving mothers of preschool children in toy making could be a useful way to approach mothers who were "at risk." The idea of using the process of making toys as a conduit for learning about child development and enhancing mother-child interaction through play seemed logical. The program that I worked with part time, as an occupational therapist-consultant, had very broad altruistic aims. These were to:

- Foster child development through personal involvement of families in an educational context
- Provide programs to enrich the social, emotional, and physical environment and to ensure that children with special needs have these needs met optimally
- Provide for the early detection and health assessment of children who are more vulnerable to developmental limitations because of adverse social influences
- Provide a home-centered, parent-child support service for families of children with special needs.(Best & McCloskey, 1978).

So I had the opportunity and was successful in applying for funding to develop and evaluate a series of toy-making workshops for parents (mainly mothers) of toddlers. That was the beginning. I continued to work with this program on a sessional basis for 12 years while also working as an educator. (Esdaile, 1996; 1994; 1987; Esdaile & Greenwood, 1990; 1995, a, b, and c; Esdaile & Sanderson, 1987a and b).

The premises of this chapter are that:

- Play is an important part of child development.
- Mother-child interaction is an important part of mothering.
- Play is an important part of the mother-child interaction because it facilitates and enhances the interaction while contributing to the child's development.

I have focused on two broad themes and discuss these from the perspective of mothers and professionals. The one that I discuss first is *the importance of play* in child and later development and in mother-child interaction, including the contribution of mothers in facilitating play opportunities for their children and engagement in play with their children as a mother-child co-occupation. The other theme is *professional practice* and the way in which different theoretical understandings, professional expertise, personal skills, and life experiences influence its honing. Although discussed separately, these themes are always interrelated because what we do and how we do it occur simultaneously. Working with mothers was what I did, and this led me to realize how mothers struggle to do the best they can, often feeling inadequate, unsupported, and criticized (e.g. Hardyment, 1983). So I came to realize that it was important to create a space in which mothers could find their strength and improve their parenting skills. Using and making toys was part of how I worked because it was an effective way of providing the "shade" in which mothers could grow to claim their agency. As we, the mothers and I, jointly engaged in an enjoyable, emotionally undemanding task, problems could unfold without strain and be addressed more gently, under the shade of the toys the mother was making for her child.

🦆 Play: An Important Occupation

Play and Child Development

Play is important at every stage of life. The development of a healthy capacity to play is a life task, not just a childhood one, and relates to the growth of self-knowledge and creativity (Reilly, 1974). The central elements of true play are self-forgetfulness and absorption in the occupation itself. Work has an outside goal; play is an end in itself. A high level of play throughout the life cycle is a distinguishing human characteristic that fosters cultural creativity and learning, and is therefore essential to human survival (Huizinga, 1950). The fundamental humanness of play was summed up by Schiller (1882), who wrote: "man only plays when in the full meaning of the word, he is a man, and he is only completely a man when he plays" (p.319). The complexity of play cannot be described in terms of a single concept. Levy (1979) suggested a dialectical view of play that encompasses all the intrinsic and extrinsic elements of nature-nurture issues as well as the cultural and historical context. The elements of self-motivation, fun, and pleasure are essential to play and are also its more elusive elements. Exploration through play leads to the development of competence, which is the precursor of achievement. This applies to adults as well as children (Reilly, 1974), which makes play interactions between mothers and their children particularly important.

My clinical work and research using play as a child or parent-child occupation was initially influenced by concepts and theories that described the importance of play in terms of child development. This perspective has been and continues to be an important area of concern for professionals who work with children and their families (for example, Bundy, 1993; Knox, 1996; Parham & Primeau, 1997; Takata, 1974). Briefly, these development-related areas include:

- The adaptive function of play, a characteristic of biological immaturity in the young of humans and other species, that emphasizes the practice of behaviors needed for survival (Bruner, Jolly & Sylva, 1976; Groos, 1896/1976; Wood, 1997).
- Social learning through play, and its relationship to the practice of skills for later work (Montessori, cited in Hardyment, 1983), as well as social learning through play that differs from work (Erikson, 1963; Florey, 1981).

- The mastery and wish-fulfilling elements of play that are expressed through the use of fantasy, make-believe, and symbolic play (Freud, 1959; Singer, 1973). These elements also contribute to cognition and learning, creative problem solving, and the ability to manipulate ideas and direct a play narrative (Piaget, 1962; Slade & Wolf, 1994; Stagnitti; 1998; Stagnitti & Unsworth, 2000; Vygotsky, 1976).
- Physically active, exploratory play that enhances neuromuscular coordination and perceptual motor skills and can be applied to purposeful occupations that include problem solving and cognition (Cratty, 1986; Reilly, 1974; Sutton-Smith, 1970).

In considering all these elements of play, it was important to remember that, above all, play needs to be intrinsically enjoyable and spontaneous (Smith, 1986). The central elements of play, self-forgetfulness and absorption in the activity itself, transcend the critical aspects of self-scrutiny (Barnett, 1991; Florey, 1981; Reilly, 1974). As Bundy (1993) observed: "without playfulness, all activities can become work" (p.217).

Play and Mother-Child Interaction

The importance of interaction with others to facilitate learning through play has been highlighted in various studies (Bruner, 1986; Strom, 1984; Uzgiris, 1979). Through interaction with an adult caregiver, often the mother for infants and toddlers, children experience trust, learn to express affection, learn about communication and reciprocal interchange, have the opportunity to explore in a safe environment, and learn through modeling of behavior from the caregiver and through positive reinforcement of achievement. Parental knowledge about, and attitudes toward, play are important factors in child development (Bronfenbrenner, 1986). Play is also an important factor in enhancing positive mother-child interactions. Through play, the consequences of real-life experiences are suspended and opportunities can be provided for increasing the elements of social cohesion related to nonwork experiences, thus promoting spontaneously joyful interactions between parents and children (Barnett, 1991; Florey, 1981; Lear, 1993; Slade & Wolf, 1994; Sylva, 1993).

Early childhood researchers continue to be interested in promoting and evaluating mother-child interaction, for example, Feldman and Greenbaum's study (1997) of affect regulation and synchronicity in mother-infant play, in which they found that synchronicity and attunement had a positive effect on the development of symbolic competence. Other studies have continued to demonstrate that maternal warmth and responsiveness is an important factor in the development of social skills (Steelman et al., 2002). These studies underscore the importance of early intervention that aims to reduce neglect in mother-child interaction and to foster positive engagement (Fagan & Dore, 1993; Girolametto, Verbey, & Tannock, 1994; Rubin et al., 1998). Occupational scientists have also explored mother-child interaction in terms of child development, for example, the occupation of play, parent-child interaction and social competence (Larson, 1995). Another example is Pierce's (2000) study of maternal management of home as a developmental play space for infants and toddlers that is discussed further by Pierce and Marshall in Chapter 4 of this text.

Finding ways to enhance mother-child interactions is especially important when coercive, abusive relationships have been identified or when there is a risk factor that these may develop. Numerous programs have been developed and evaluated to address these problems (e.g., Goff Timmer, Borrego & Urquiza, 2002). A number of health professionals working in the early childhood field, such as nurses and occupational therapists, have developed special programs to facilitate parent-child interactions for special groups such as toddlers born pre-term (Magill-Evans & Harrison, 1999), or for infants who have disorders of self-regulation, manifest in irritability, poor self-calming, sleep and feeding patterns and hypersensitivity to sensory stimulation (DeGangi et al., 1997). Other studies have reported engaging mothers in play interaction with children who have disabilities (e.g. Hinojosa & Kramer, 1997: Humphry, 1989).

In a recent Cochrane review of parent training programs that aimed to improve maternal psychosocial health (Barlow & Coren, 2002), it was found that parenting programs could make a significant contribution to the short-term psychosocial health of mothers. However, these investigators found little evidence to support the idea that the results are maintained over time, partly because the follow-up data are scarce and limited. I think that it is also important to note that this study included only 23 randomized, controlled trials in which participants had been randomly allocated to an experimental and a control group, the latter being a waiting-list, no-treatment, or placebo-control group. Because study 4, discussed below, had parenting stress as a component and was classified as a randomized controlled study, I was asked to contribute to this Cochrane review.

The importance of play in parent-child interaction and its facilitation through the use of age-appropriate toys has been recognized and utilized by professionals working in the early childhood field over an extensive period (e.g. Benjamin, 1947). Similar basic philosophical tenents echo central concepts imparted in advice to parents over countless generations:

> Do not train boys to learning by force and harshness, but lead them by what amuses them, so that they may better discover the bent of their minds (Plato, The Republic, VII, cited in Bettelheim, 1988, p. 55).

Educating parents about child development through the use of play and toys has been a key element in a number of early intervention programs for socially disadvantaged groups. For example, Slaughter (1984) successfully used mother discussion groups and toy demonstrations in her work that was a part of *Project Head Start* (Slaughter, et al., 1989, United States Department of Health, 1975). I had used similar principles (Esdaile, 1996; Esdaile & Sanderson, 1987). Donoghue (1986), an early childhood educator in the United Kingdom, and Daly Smith (1982), an occupational therapist in Western Australia, had also focused on play and toys in early intervention, and incorporated a home-visiting component in their programs. The importance of creating play opportunities for children at risk because of social disadvantage, and educating parents about play and play materials is underscored by the fact that in situations of poverty and social disadvantage, play is often diminished. For example, Polakow's (1993) studies of families living in poverty, on the edge of an affluent society, provide poignant examples of the ways in which the struggle for survival robs children and their families of the opportunities to play and be playful. The importance of providing opportunities to play, and the relevance of play in child development, has been discussed extensively in *Project Head Start* reports. In her recent work with mothers receiving infant mental health intervention, Olson (1998) found a disturbing absence of play, or playfulness. Facilitating play and involving parents in play situations with children with disabilities has been an important area of professional involvement for occupational therapists (e.g. Bundy, 1993; 1997; Burke & Shaaf, 1997; Florey, 1981; Hinojosa. & Kramer, 1997; Humphry, 1989: Knox, 1996; Parush et al., 1987).

In my own work with mothers, I incorporated a number of concepts about play and toys that included enabling and facilitating the mother-child occupations of play and playfulness, as well as play as the mother-child co-occupation of play. The occupation of facilitating a child's play includes creating space in the home where play can occur spontaneously, having toys and play materials available, making sure that these are developmentally appropriate for the child, providing challenge and opportunity to explore, but avoiding frustration. The latter can occur when there are too many toys available at any one time, or when toys are not age appropriate. My references for these aspects of play and mothering occupations were from developmental psychology, early-childhood education and occupational therapy (e.g. Bruner, Jolly & Sylva, 1976; Florey, 1981; Strom, 1984; Sutton-Smith, 1970). Creating play situations within household work and encouraging playfulness within this context were other important aspects of the mother-child occupation of play that I considered. Often this was as a parallel

occupation, for example, when the mother was cooking and her child also cooked on a "stove" constructed from an upturned box, with small pieces of apple she stirred with a wooden spoon. A broad range of literature about play could be appropriately cited to support how mothers can create play opportunities for their children in the context of their housework (e.g. Barnett, 1991; Bundy, 1993; Donoghue, 1986).

Another aspect of the mother-child occupation of play is play as a co-occupation. This is a reciprocal, synchronized interaction between mother and child that is, at best, child directed. Bruner (1986) describes it in terms of communication and language development. It is also frequently a part of the child's make-believe play (e.g. Singer, 1973; Vygotsky, 1976). These were my major theoretical sources for conceptualizing this aspect of play. It involves allowing the child to initiate the play, and being cued by the child's direction. This interactive play behavior can be readily observed in mother-infant play of give-and-take, or peek-a-boo. The infant initiates the game, and ends it by looking away when she becomes bored or when the mother is not following her cues appropriately. Play, as a co-occupation, is developmentally important, as the child tests his or her skills and limits and his or her ability to control an interaction. Play can also be challenging to an adult caregiver who has difficulty interpreting the child's cues. The co-occupation of play is often easier to sustain with infants than toddlers.

More recently, occupational scientists have contributed rich insights to various strategies mothers use in facilitating their children's play (e.g., Larson, 1995; Larson, 2000; Pierce, 2000) and playfulness in the context of family work (e.g. Primeau, 1998). Chapter 4 by Pierce and Marshall and Chapter 6 by Primeau in this text add further research data and discussion to this topic.

✍ Working as a Professional

We have been taught that, as professionals, we learn certain skills, and to function effectively, we need to understand the theoretical assumptions on which these skills are predicated. In order to be effective professional practitioners, we need to understand and use theory appropriately. Learning skills is simply not enough (McColl, Law, & Stewart, 1993). Mitcham (2003) has grounded this discourse creatively by describing it in terms of shopping, an occupation with which we are all familiar. So, in order to be good consumers of theories, we need to shop carefully to ensure that we use the correct theories to address our professional concerns and shape our practice. A focus on clinical reasoning and the reflective aspects of practice have been helpful influences in regard to theory-based practice.

Over the past decade or so, an extensive body of literature on clinical reasoning has assisted health professionals to reflect on their practice and identify the elements that delineate advanced practice from novice practice. For many of us, these reflections started with Schön's work (1987) on reflective practice, and continued to evolve as we read the publications that resulted from an ethnographic study of clinical reasoning in occupational therapy (e.g., Mattingly & Fleming, 1994). Clinical reasoning and reflective practice continue to be topics of relevance and interest to health professionals, particularly nurses, occupational and physical therapists, as well as educators and artists (Higgs, 2003; Higgs, & Titchen, 2001a and b).

Influences

It would be fair to say that the above citations related to professional practice are my recent and current influences. However, I started working with mothers and children before these studies and their publication. As a novice therapist, I worked in a large university teaching hospital, where one of my duties was to provide a play group for the children's ward each morning for 2 hours. Many of the children in this ward had rare, complicated, often painful disorders that were not then readily treatable. Often I was the only health professional with whom they had contact who did not do painful things to them. Each morning, I arrived with a basket full of toys and was greeted with shouts of "Here comes the toy lady!" This was my first experience of using "toys for shade," in this case, shade from an

intrusive and painful medical world. I sensed that what I was doing was relevant, and that it mattered, but in terms of what was professionally valued by my peers and other colleagues, it was not ranked highly. So, I was happy to move on to a more advanced level, as the occupational therapist in the cardiopulmonary unit of the hospital. This was where I started working with women who were mothers, and who had difficulties with parenting because of their health problems. These problems constituted the "critical incidents or irritations" (Yerxa, 1994, p.7) that launched me into my first research project, a study of the working problems of women who had heart disease. Working with women, mostly mothers, has become a major occupation of my professional life.

When I embarked on using toys to enhance parent-child interaction and child development, some years later, I was influenced by Rogers' model (1959) of client-centered therapy, the affective education movement (e.g. Castillo, 1978) and Gestalt therapy (Oaklander, 1978; Perls, 1969), and other expressive ways of working with people. So I became aware of the process in therapeutic interventions and how the therapist uses himself or herself in an interaction. The experience of attending a Gestalt workshop on clowning was particularly formative. In this workshop we learned *to be present* without performing, the way a clown comes into a space and is there for the audience before she actually performs. This requires being there for others and passing beyond the self-conscious state of monitoring one's own performance. It is something that all performing artists who succeed in their art have learned; otherwise, they simply lose their audience. However, it is not a requirement for health and other professionals who perform their work for an already captive audience. Learning to be *fully present*, and knowing when I was not, as well as being able to identify the full or only partial *presence* of others in interactions, were very powerful lessons that I learned.

I was also influenced by concepts of community-based practice, health education, and health promotion that incorporated a partnership between the client and professional, a true sharing of initiative and responsibility (Roter et al, 1981). Therefore I "adopted a central theoretical framework in which learning is conceived to be a process of participation and a collaboration that is prompted by the learner's life-long drive for understanding and personal growth" (Esdaile & Sanderson, 1987a, p. 270). I blended my role as a therapist with that of community educator.

The Honing of a Personal Perspective

Soon after commencing my community-based work with families, it became obvious to me that mothers felt uncomfortable about the scrutiny of professionals and direct identification of their problems. They felt at ease with the idea of making age-appropriate toys for their children because this occupational engagement afforded them "shade" from self-disclosure and did not focus on their problems directly. These problems could surface with time, in a seemingly oblique fashion that allowed me the opportunity to continue working with the mothers and their children individually, or to refer them to other practitioners or agencies if required. In fact, many times when a mother was referred to one of my generic play and toy workshops by a community-based maternal and child health nurse, or another professional because of some problem that mother was experiencing, she would call me to say she could not come. Often she added: "I am really okay, I don't want to take up space that some one else may need." These statements confirmed that my low-key approach was acceptable to mothers. This was supported by the evaluations of participants of the programs and by the fact that community agencies (mostly community health centers, preschools, and child-care centers) invited me back to work with them. However, I was not producing impressive empirical data or doing "high-prestige" work. One of the pediatricians I met at the time summed it up by saying, "You are the only occupational therapist I know working with children and families who is not trying to be a pediatric neurologist." This seemed to be true, and I accepted it pragmatically without attributing a value judgment to this status quo. My work seemed to be more

closely allied to that of early-childhood educators, but when we were actually working together, as we often did, as a therapist, I was much more process oriented than my colleagues in education. My coauthor on two publications, Sanderson, was then a preschool teacher working in early intervention.

I went on evaluating what I did, reported it within the agency in which I worked, to other agencies with which I had contact, at local and national conferences, and then in professional journals. Because I had not sought the one right answer to any of the problems I encountered in the community, I was content to go on working in what Schön (1987) had described as the "swamp [where] lie the problems of greatest human concern." As a practitioner, I had chosen not to work on the "high ground" where problems can be readily solved, but to "descend to the swamp of important problems and nonrigorous inquiry." (p. 3).

In hindsight, I would say that what Schön (1987) had described as nonrigorous I would now describe as differently-rigorous. However, I think that following the thread of that discussion belongs to the Reflections and Conclusions section of this chapter. The foregoing description of my professional perspective is what I brought to, and applied in, the years of work that I shall now describe.

Working with Mothers of Preschoolers: Research and Practice

In Table 5–1, I have listed chronologically 8 studies that I conducted over a period of 12 years. Given the processes of publishing in refereed journals, they were not necessarily published in the same chronological order. I also wrote numerous reports and did conference presentations and invited presentations related to this work. The following narrative includes little of the detailed description of the studies, the methods and analyses used or all the outcomes because I believe that all these details would make the reading of this chapter cumbersome. Interested readers may refer to the published articles cited. Also, I have not spent equal time in discussing the studies because some are more directly related to the main themes of this chapter than others.

Pilot Study

This was a community-based exploratory project supported by the state health department (Esdaile & Sanderson, 1987 a). Parents of 2- to 3-year-olds were the target group because this toddler age group received fewer services. Infants were seen more often in community health centers because of mandatory health programs, and children over 3 years

The study	Participants	Key outcomes	Publications
1. A Descriptive Pilot Study	30 mothers of preschoolers	Participants' awareness of the importance of play increased; approval given to continue work: 5 F/T OT employed to do similar work in another region	Esdaile & Sanderson, 1987a British Journal of Occupational Therapy Esdaile & Sanderson, 1987b "Toys to Make," Penguin, Australia
2. Relaxation with Children: Evaluation	66 13 boys, 53 girls, 3 teachers, 11 foster parents, 22 student occupational therapists	Need for stress management with children confirmed and the importance of identifying individual and group expectations pre-program demonstrated	Esdaile, 1987 Australian Occupational Therapy Journal
3. Inter-rater Study of Mothers' and Childcare Workers' Perception of Toddlers	25 mothers of 2–3-year-olds, 3 childcare workers	Low or inconsistent inter-rater reliability found between childcare workers on most variables and low between mothers and childcare workers	Esdaile & Greenwood, 1990 Australian Occupational Therapy Journal
4. Toy-Making and Toy-demonstration Workshops	101 mothers of 2–3 year-olds in the survey 35 mothers in experimental and control groups	Positive evaluations by participants, rich descriptive information, but no statistically significant data	Esdaile, 1996 American Journal of Occupational Therapy
5. Relationships between Mothers and Toddlers	103 mothers of 2–3-year-olds	Mothers' low self-concept as educators of their children was predictive of maternal stress; for some mothers, rating of child temperament resulted in different relationships to mothers' perceptions of stress	Esdaile & Greenwood, 1995a Occupational Therapy International Esdaile & Greenwood, 1995b Journal of Family Studies
6. Follow-up Study of Parenting Stress and Relationships	104 mothers of 2–5-year-olds in the survey part, plus 16 who were interviewed	Additional stress related factors were identified from the interview data	Esdaile & Greenwood, 1995c Journal of Family Studies
7. Comparison of Mothers and Fathers: Parenting Stress and Relationships	53 mothers and 25 fathers of preschool children	Both mothers and fathers of children with disabilities were more stressed than those who had nondisabled children; there were some gender-related differences	Esdaile & Greenwood, 2003 Occupational Therapy International
8. Children with Disabilities: Mothers' and Fathers' Experiences	Seven families of children aged from 2–39 years 19 informants interviewed: 7 mothers, 6 fathers, and 3 siblings	Participants talked about emotional pain, physical and financial burden in caregiving, and how they took control and took care of their problems	Esdaile, 1998a & b Papers presented at the World Federation of Occupational Therapists' Congress, Montreal, Canada

Table 5–1   A dozen years of working with parents of preschool children

were then eligible to attend preschool. Also, because many parents find active toddlers, who often have limited impulse control, challenging to manage, this age group was considered to be most at risk of abuse, neglect, or lack of play opportunities because of parents' limited understanding of their needs. The overall aims of the workshops were to:

- Disseminate information about child development informally
- Assist parents to discover their own skills and resources
- Facilitate socialization and problem-solving within the group
- Enhance child development through play and age-appropriate toys
- Enhance positive parent-child interaction through enjoyable, playful experiences
- Encourage families to become familiar with and use the available community resources

I worked with five groups of participants, in different community locations within the same region, and offered three 2-hour sessions over consecutive weeks. The participants signed up in response to an advertisement in the local newspaper and posters distributed in a local mall. These simply invited people who had preschool children to come and have fun making inexpensive, age-appropriate toys for their children, using mainly recycled materials. Two of the series of sessions were offered in the evening to allow fathers and mothers working full-time to attend. A faculty member of a local community college childcare program worked with me, and before the commencement of the sessions, we hired and trained childcare workers to take care of the participants' children while the parents were engaged in making toys. We enrolled 30 participants on a first-come basis; all were mothers; 2 worked full time and 11 part time.

Each session was predicated on a theme related to play and child development. In the first session, the focus was on exploratory play and learning through play. The pull-out-scarf box, illustrated in Figure 5–1, was made from an ice cream container and scarves tied together. It is an example of a toy, made from

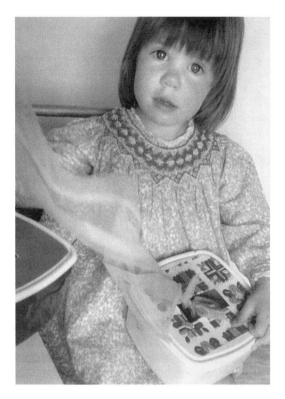

Figure 5–1 *A 30-month-old girl playing with a pull-out scarf box. (From Esdaile, S., & Sanderson, A. (1987). Teaching parents toy making: A practical guide to early intervention. British Journal of Occupational Therapy, 50(8), 268, with permission.)*

scrap materials, that demonstrated concepts of in and out as well as differentiation of textures and colors.

The second session involved puppet making, with a focus on make-believe and symbolic play. I used this as an opportunity to discuss behavior, limit setting, modeling, and the importance of imaginative play. In the third session we made toys that involved more gross motor activity, using large appliance boxes to create tunnels and old tires to make swings. This was an opportunity to discuss the importance of active play and to reassure mothers that toddlers are supposed to be "on the go" and need to move. This session also afforded opportunities for discussing safety issues and toddlers' cognitive limitations in perceiving danger and setting their own limits. Appliance boxes proved very useful because they could

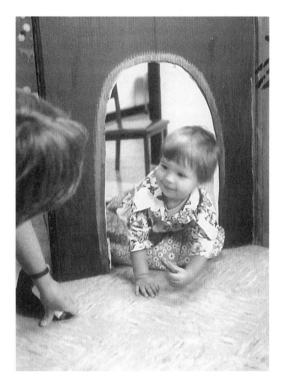

Figure 5–2 *A mother with 18-month-old child crawling through a play screen. (From Esdaile, S., & Sanderson, A. (1987). Teaching parents toy making: A practical guide to early intervention. British Journal of Occupational Therapy, 50(8), 269, with permission.)*

be used to encourage active play and were easily folded for storage at the end of the day. Figure 5–2 shows a child crawling through one of these constructions, with her mother encouraging her.

Participants filled out pre- and post-program questionnaires. Responses provided a wealth of information about the participants' problems and expectations. Two major problems expressed by mothers were a lack of understanding of their child's development and the limitations of their child's cognitions. Another was inability to deal with "acting-out" behavior or shyness appropriately, often imposing too many environmental restrictions—for example, not allowing a child to play with plastic kitchen utensils. Puppets were the most popular toys with the mothers, and they often expressed their own feelings and did their most constructive problem-solving while making puppets. There was consensus that the

workshop's aims had been met, and participants demonstrated an increased awareness of the importance of play in child development. They also suggested having six, rather than just three, sessions to a program. The manager of the agency with which I worked felt that the project was a success; the other agencies with which we collaborated agreed. My report to the health department was also well received. Based on its findings, a half-time occupational therapist was appointed to work in another region in a high-rise apartment complex where many families at risk were already being investigated for parenting problems. I was set to continue with this work and had learned to exploit "toys for shade." I used the toys to protect mothers from being caught in the glaring discomfort of self-disclosure that could result in their running away from the humiliation of a disclosure that they were not yet ready to manage. Messy tables with cups of coffee, cookies, and half-made toys provided a nonthreatening environment in which to work. Figure 5–3 is one such setting where mothers made puppets.

Another outcome of this work was a book on toy making and play development (Esdaile & Sanderson, 1997b), which was predicated on the theoretical constructs and research described in studies 1 and 2 in this chapter. However, the book was written for people in general who live or work with children, not just professionals, so the theoretical constructs that gave it structure were not "spelled out" for the reader.

Relaxation with Children

I continued to work in the community, mainly with health centers, preschools, elementary schools, and childcare centers, often using toys and toy making adapted to suit different needs because I found that this low-key approach was effective. As many of the families with whom I worked were stressed by poverty, unemployment, lack of skills, or other factors, it became clear that they needed some assistance with relaxation. Using relaxation techniques that were turned into games that could be played with children became part of my community program repertoire. Often these sessions were added to programs that

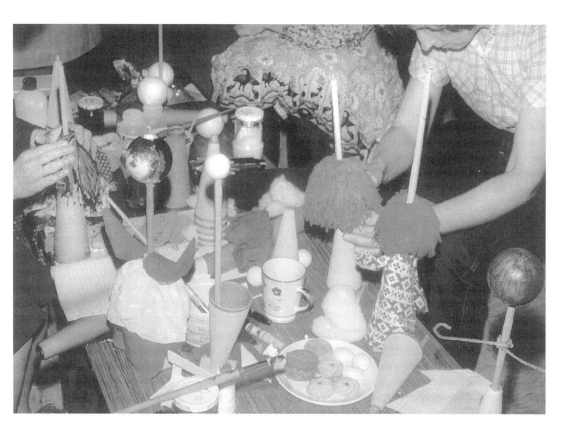

Figure 5–3 *Mothers making puppets at a workshop. (From Esdaile, S., & Sanderson, A. (1987). Teaching parents toy making: A practical guide to early intervention. British Journal of Occupational Therapy, 50(8), 269, with permission.)*

incorporated toy making. I made a point of evaluating the participants' experience of programs, but many of these evaluations did not become part of formal research. The participants in the programs about which I published the evaluation outcomes (Esdaile, 1987) were preschool and elementary school teachers, foster families, and student occupational therapists who took an elective that was part of the experiential course component of the program in which I taught. Evaluating relaxation programs for different groups, using nonparametric statistical analysis of variance, proved to be a useful exercise. I found that although certain basic elements of stress management were common to any program that addressed the subject of relaxation, it was essential to develop each program in collaboration with the participants who were going to use it. This was further confirmation of my be-

lief in sharing the responsibility and initiative with my clients (Roter et al., 1981; Esdaile & Sanderson, 1987a).

Inter-rater Reliability Study

This was part of the larger randomized controlled study using toy making and toy demonstration workshops that I shall describe next. I was interested to know, first, whether the childcare workers who took care of the children in a play group situation while I worked with the mothers agreed in their perception of the children's temperament; and second, to know how their ratings compared with the mothers' ratings. We used both Pearson's product-moment correlations and generalized kappa to assess the degrees of inter-rater reliability (Bartko & Carpenter, 1975). We found a high level of agreement (r=821) between the childcare workers' rating of the children's temperament on the "easy-difficult" scale, and a lower level of agreement for individual temperament factors. Agreement between mothers and childcare workers was low on the "easy-difficult" scale (*r*=262). (Esdaile & Greenwood, 1990). The main point of this study was to demonstrate the inappropriateness of making assumptions about agreement between members of a healthcare team and the clients with whom they work. I believe that it is important to acknowledge the different perceptions that individuals bring to a situation and work within the structure of the differences.

Toy-Making and Toy-Demonstration Workshops

This program was the second study I conducted as part of my doctoral dissertation; it was structured as a randomized control intervention program. Before planning it, I had conducted a pilot study in which I interviewed 19 mothers of 2- to 3-year-olds and three community nurses whose health centers the mothers attended with their children. I did this to find out what mothers felt they needed in terms of programs to assist with their children, and what the nurses thought the mothers needed to enhance their parenting skills. The assessment tools I planned to use in a larger study were administered to the mothers to ascertain their suitability. The outcomes of this pilot study (Esdaile, 1990) and my previous community work informed the conceptual framework that I developed for this intervention study.

My community work and the pilot study already conducted had strongly indicated that mothers often found their toddlers' behavior difficult, and the child's temperament was often contributing to problematic mother-child interaction issues. Many mothers seemed to find the more reactive, less self-regulating "difficult" toddlers hard to manage. I felt that mothers' attributions of responsibility to themselves or their child for positive and negative interaction outcomes and their self-efficacy and sense of competence in assisting their child's development and learning were also related to their experiences of parenting stress. I used five standardized, self-report questionnaires that mothers were asked to fill

out before and after the program, to examine mother and child, and interaction factors discussed above. These were: the Short Temperament Scale for Toddlers (Fullard, McDevitt & Carey, 1984; Prior et al., 1989), the Behaviour Check List, (Richman, Stevenson & Graham, 1982), the Parenting Stress Index (Abidin, 1990), the Revised Parent Attribution Test (Bugental & Shennum, 1984), and the Parent as a Teacher Inventory (Strom, 1984). I also developed a questionnaire to evaluate mothers' perceptions of each session separately as well as the overall 10-week toy making workshop program. I held two groups of weekly workshops, and had a control group that filled out the standardized tests, but did not participate in the program. Each session lasted for 2 to 3 hours and included a play group for the children in an adjoining room of the same building, with childcare staff whom I had trained. This gave mothers and children the opportunity to "consumer-test" the toys.

I assessed outcomes on the standardized tests using a series of single-factor analyses of covariance and found no evidence for changes in any of the variables. To assess the participants' responses to the program, I used a nonparametric test, the Mann-Whitney U (Siegel, 1956). The results were generally positive and the open-ended section included details about aspects of the program that were particularly important or meaningful to the participants. I did a follow-up study 18 months later, and again had no statistically significant results to report.

However, there was a wealth of less direct support for the concept of "toys for shade" and evidence for a ripple effect that was rich and varied. The mothers who had participated in the workshops reported that they continued making toys. I was invited to conduct many more programs in the community. I was asked to speak to various groups, where I often met other professionals who told me stories about mothers who had attended my toy-making programs. Many had started local playgroups and took on leadership in other areas related to children and families. I even met people in unexpected places, such as standing in line in the grocery store, who recognized me and then told me about initiatives that they attributed as starting with someone attending one of my programs. So I felt that using the concept of "toys for shade" was a valid way to practice, although I had no scientific way of demonstrating it (Esdaile, 1996). The following vignettes illustrate how the concept worked in practice for some of the mothers who were participants in study 4.

⌘ *Vignette:* **Tracy, Who Never Missed a Session**

Tracy was a 21-year-old mother of two boys, one nearly 3 years old and the other aged 13 months, who participated in the fourth study and attended the toy-making workshops. Immediately after the first session, she and her family relocated, moving 20 miles out of town, so she had to make a special effort to attend the remainder of the sessions. Tracy liked the "opportunity to talk to other moms, knowing I'm not alone." She also said that she found the sessions very "confidence building." Tracy had little formal education and was an inexperienced mother, but was eager to learn. She felt comfortable in the informal setting of the program, and said it was the only time in her week when she did not have to watch her children. Therefore she made sure she attended every one of the 10 consecutive meetings. This required some effort and organization because she did not have the use of a car. She attended sessions on Mondays, and every Sunday afternoon she packed for herself and her children and traveled by train to her mother's place. She was always ready ahead of time when the community bus called to pick her up at 8:30 AM on Mondays. She was an enthusiastic, involved participant who visibly enjoyed the experiential learning process, kept all her handouts in a ring-binding folder, and made more toys during the week between sessions, as well as after the program. ⌘

⌘ *Vignette:* **Marion, Who Learned to Use Power Tools**

Marion was a quiet mother of two girls aged 3 years and 20 months. She rarely participated in discussions, but was clearly listening to what others were saying. She lived with her in-laws, and although her comments were guarded, it was clear she was not finding this situation easy. It seemed that she had no space and no voice in her family. In the process of making wooden toys, she underwent a transformation. Handling tools, especially power tools, was something from which the men in her family had excluded her. She took to the occupation of woodwork with concentration and creativity, surprising herself, as she said: "It is very interesting, making wooden toys; it can bring out talents that you didn't know you had." At first, her family doubted that she had indeed made such attractive wooden toys. But she convinced them. After making the wooden toys, Marion seemed brighter and was more outgoing in the group, often initiating the discussion. In the follow-up survey 18 months later, she added a little note to say she was still making toys and that she and her family were now living in their own apartment. It seemed that her confidence as a toy maker had carried over to her family life. ⌘

⌘ *Vignette:* **Janice and the Follow-up Questionnaire**

Janice had a 2-year-old son and a 7-month-old daughter. She was an anxious young woman who had a lot of difficulty interpreting her children's cues, and was inclined to view them negatively, attributing mischievous intent to random actions. For example, when her baby made swiping, uncontrolled movements and knocked something over, Janice's reaction was to tell the baby she was "a bad girl" and even to spank her. This was when I used "toys for shade" with careful deliberation. I noted her actions, but instead of commenting on them, I focused on some problem solving in relation to the toy making: "Use a little more glue here," or "Trim this piece." I knew that if I drew attention to her poor parenting, she would feel ashamed and not return. So I waited until the next session, and found a way to talk about child development and play in a way that explained her children's behavior, which she had misinterpreted. I am sure she was aware of her parenting problems, and appeared anxious to be accepted, which she was in this group. Over the time of the program, she did appear to be more relaxed with her children and interacting more positively with them. How important these sessions had been for her was revealed when she completed her follow-up questionnaire and gave it to her husband to drop off at our office. On the way there, he had a car accident in which he was not seriously hurt but had cuts as a result of a broken windshield. Janice was determined to have her say and "rescued" the blood-stained questionnaire from the car and delivered it to me personally the next day.   ⌘

⌘ *Vignette:* **Lisa and Her "Feral" Child**

Lisa was a 22-year-old mother of two boys aged 30 months and 12 months. She had rated her older child, Tim, as very difficult; others were inclined to agree. One of the childcare workers had described him as being like "one of the feral children from *Mad Max III*," a movie about a violent, disorganized society set in the future, which was then being shown. When I was cleaning up after the first session, a large, tough-looking man wandered in, saying he was looking for the "obedience school." I thought he must have been looking for a school where owners learn to handle their dogs. I told him that he had come to the wrong place and offered him a telephone directory so that he could look for the right place. However, further conversation revealed that he was Lisa's brother and that our concepts of child development were at opposite ends of the pole. I later learned from Lisa that the family's favorite strategy for managing Tim was to visit relatives in the country, where there was a large, fenced field, where they would "let Tim loose, out of harm." Lisa was an unmotivated participant in the sessions, and attended only 60 percent of them. I arranged with the driver of the community bus to call her half an hour before she had to be ready, but this did not guarantee her attendance if something more interesting cropped up. Unlike most of the other mothers, Lisa was a somewhat disengaged parent and not particularly interested in the program I was offering. I included her in a vignette

to make the point that although a low-key, non-threatening program suited many mothers, giving them the opportunity grow in confidence in the shade of the toy-making sessions, Lisa needed something different. My professional guess is that she could have benefited from infant mental health intervention, working with a specialist who would visit her at home (Fraiberg, Shapiro, & Cherniss, 1980).   ⌘

Relationships Between Mothers and Toddlers

This study was conducted in the same geographical region as study 4, used the same standardized measures, and also involved mothers and their preschool children (Esdaile & Greenwood, 1995a & b). We used a survey method to explore relationships between child temperament and behavior; mothers' attributions for mother-child interaction outcomes, and mothers' perceived stress and self-concept as educators of their children. We used a variety of multivariate techniques to investigate the relationships between variables, including: correlations, multiple regressions and discriminant function analyses. The results demonstrated that mothers' low self-concept, as educators of their children, was predictive of maternal stress. Also, mothers who had rated their child as "difficult" (reactive and non–self regulating) were less stressed if they attributed responsibility to their child for negative mother-child interaction outcomes. Conversely, mothers who had rated their child as having an "easy" temperament were more stressed if they attributed responsibility to their child for negative mother-child interaction outcomes. This suggested shifting the blame and reduced maternal stress, but possibly put the child at risk of abuse if the child were to be blamed for actions beyond his or her control. Also, taking responsibility for negative outcomes could increase maternal stress. Both scenarios were potentially problematic. Additionally, the finding that mothers' low self-concept as educators of their child predicted perceptions of stress strongly suggested that mother-focused prevention and intervention programs had a place in community health practice.

Follow-up Study of Parenting Stress and Relationships

We conducted this study to find out more about parenting stress and attributions (Esdaile & Greenwood, 1995c). We surveyed more mothers of toddlers, using the same parenting stress and attribution measures used in the previous studies, as well as a modified version of the attribution measure in which the items addressed a mother's own experience more directly. We also interviewed 16 of the participants. The interviews suggested a number of stress-related issues that were not covered in the Parenting Stress Index (Abidin, 1990). They included the sometimes conflicting nature of social support, the need for personal and physical space in the home, the effect of children's illnesses, and the variability of parenting styles. When we added 16 new items to the Parenting Stress Index, 11 of them correlated with existing items, but there were 5 factors that seemed not to be addressed in the original instrument. These related to issues of support, lack of space in the home, the mess created by children and their equipment, concerns about having ideas about parenting that were different from those of others, and lack of sleep, especially when children are ill, a frequent situation with preschoolers prone to upper respiratory and other infections. We also found that mothers' responses to items related to parent-child interaction outcomes differed if they were considering their own child, as opposed to any child with whom they might be interacting, but we were left with uncertainties about the interpretation of these factors. Because this study included a larger percentage of well-educated, more financially secure women than the previous studies, it was interesting to note that their experiences of parenting stress did not differ from those of women with fewer resources.

Comparison of Mothers and Fathers: Parenting Stress and Relationships

By this time, we had quite a lot of general information about mothers of toddlers in regard to parenting stress and parenting attributions for parent-child interaction outcomes. Because parents of children with disabilities are more vulnerable to parenting stress and

its adverse long-term outcomes (Bristol, Gallagher & Holt, 1993), we went on exploring this issue. We were also interested to find out more about fathers because their experience was less frequently reported in the literature, and some studies had indicated that fathers experience less stress than mothers in relation to having a child with a disability (Cameron, Dobson & Day, 1991; Drake & Goldberg, 1992). My community work was mostly with mothers, but it also included fathers. They too seemed to respond to the concept of toys for shade, but differently from mothers. Fathers appeared to prefer focusing on the task itself, and responded to more technically complex constructions, such as making swings and sand pits. They helped each other and chatted about parenting issues obliquely to each other, rather than to me. Mothers were more inclined to talk to me directly about their problems once they felt more at ease, and selected smaller projects, working parallel to rather than with others, sharing and discussing problems directly. These observations are consistent with the male-female differences in communication styles described by Tannen (1991).

We found that having a child with a disability did increase parents' experience of parenting stress, and also revealed some differences in the perceptions for mothers and fathers. For example, mothers were more likely to report experiencing depression and loss of a sense of competence, and for some fathers, restriction of their role was a factor associated with stress. The only statistically significant finding on the attribution variable was that the presence of a disability resulted in higher attributions of credit to the child for positive parent-child interaction outcomes for both mothers and fathers, thus showing acknowledgment of the extra effort children with special needs often have to make in order to succeed at what they do (Esdaile & Greenwood, 2003).

Children with Disabilities: Mothers' and Fathers' Experiences

By this time, I am sure that many readers must be thinking that using qualitative methods would be a more appropriate way to explore complex contextual issues about mothers and children, and maybe wondering when I would get to this. And this is indeed where the insights from my professional practice, the honing of my skills and perspective, and the outcomes of my research led me. Actually, studies 6, 7, and 8 were all done with support from the same grant, so it had not taken quite as long to come to this point of view as it may appear from this chronological account. The interviews with seven mothers, six fathers and three siblings of people with disabilities, across a wide age range, produced rich contextual data about the lived experience and occupational engagement of the families involved. Participants in the study talked about the emotional pain and the physical and financial burden in their caregiving and how they found their agency in order to take control of their lives (Esdaile, 1998 a & b). I still have more work to do to complete reporting their stories, but that is outside the scope of this chapter.

ꙮ Reflections

I think that the outcomes of studies 5, 6, 7, and 8 indicate that mothers, and also fathers, find parenting challenging and often stressful in different ways for different reasons, and this is exacerbated when they have a child with a disability. Mostly, they are aware of the issues that challenge them. I also believe that they can best resolve their challenges if they start with shade from the glare of immediate self-disclosure, because this can be intimidating when faced with experts, especially when these experts are in a hurry. Making toys to learn more about play and child development is just one way of providing the shade that can allow mothers (and fathers) the opportunity to learn new skills, increase their sense of efficacy, enhance parent-child interaction, and promote playfulness. Mothers and fathers need space to overcome their challenges, claim their agency, and participate fully in their chosen occupation of parenting.

When I started working with families in the community, health professionals were focused on being scientific and producing quantita-tive, empirical data to support their practice. In terms of what I was doing, this was difficult; but in principle, I did not disagree with it because I was aware of the pitfalls of the nonscientific: for example, attributing childhood autism to maternal disengagement. By the time I stopped working in the western metropolitan region of Melbourne, scholarly thinking in the health professions had started to shift. What Schön had described as "nonrigorous" could now be framed as "differently rigorous". It was becoming possible to be a scholarly practitioner and work in a contextual, holistic way. This was a generational journey for many of us. We were supported in this journey by scholars like Yerxa (1991, 1994), whose clear vision of ethical practice emphasized the dignity and centrality of meaningful occupation and integrated research and education with practice; and by social scientists like Gergen (1994; 1999), who challenged traditional scientific thinking and argued for a human science as social construction. The rethinking of social science continues in new, exciting, and challenging ways. Flyvbjerg (2001) argues that the strength of the social sciences lies in their rich, reflexive analysis of values and power. A major shift in the way many of us now practice is reflected in the way we have claimed the power of our own voice and acknowledge that we bring our own lives, who we are, what we do, and what we read to the way we practice (Denshire, 2002).

"Although the researcher's voice is present in all research, the researcher is perhaps most visible and audible in qualitative research" (Hasselkus, 2003, p. 7). The increased acceptance of using qualitative methods in health sciences has given professionals the opportunity to legitimately study complex, unquantifiable human concerns. This way of thinking has created its own intellectual challenges and demands for rigor. However, it is encouraging and constructive that there is open discourse about these issues in qualitative research. Addressing the challenges to understanding the creation of meaning about the lives of our research participants, as well as our own practice, is a positive aspect of research collaboration between professionals and their informants (e.g. Lawlor, 2003, Primeau, 2003).

However, despite the shift to acknowledging and valuing the intuitive and reflective, I think that quantifiable data still holds a strong power base. According to the criteria of the Cochrane review of parenting programs (Barlow & Coren, 2002), Study 4, described above, was not effective. This is reasonable, given the criteria of a randomized control trial, and the fact that there were no statistically significant results to meet these criteria. What is not reasonable is the choice of the methodology to evaluate such programs. I am also aware that, on a personal level, I was influenced by economic rationalism, or was it realities? When I offered programs for just mothers or parents who did not need an identified problem to attend, many problems unfolded. I always "found" people who needed follow-up or referral to another health professional. In Study 4 this was the case for 28 percent of the participants or their children. Another factor that gets overlooked is that it is actually cost-effective to provide services to those who are managing quite well because they are able to make positive contributions in their own communities with relatively little support. For example, some mothers who attended my programs went on to set up play groups in their neighborhoods. Given the choice, I would have easily available services for all mothers, fathers, and other caregivers of young children and provide additional services for those with special needs because of a disability or other problem. By the time problems are "officially" identified, much early intervention time may have been lost. Also, I would always want to make sure that there was space with shade so that the sense of playfulness can flourish.

Conclusion

The challenge to anyone who works with mothers and children (and other people) is to be a rigorous, scholarly practitioner without becoming consumed by notions of cost effectiveness or losing the essence of open scientific inquiry amid statistical significance. Being an evidence-based practitioner is important, but it requires skill and reflection to make appropriate and ethical judgments about the evidence. Doing good work is essential but not easy, and it is not always clear how "doing good work in difficult times" (Gardner, Csikszentmihalyi, & Damon, 2001, p.3) can be achieved. Health professionals, educators, and others who work in spheres that serve people use knowledge from both the physical and social sciences. Both are important for humankind. The scholarly, ethical practitioner is the conduit through which knowledge from the physical and social sciences is blended to provide the appropriate prevention, intervention, or treatment. Children represent our future, so we need to care for them and their caregivers. We have known for a long time that play enhances creativity and problem solving (e.g., Groos 1896/1976), so we need to make sure that our work with mothers and children provides the shade in which play and creativity can flourish.

Discussion Questions

- Consider how you could reconcile the demands of both reflective and evidence-based practice in your sphere of work. Discuss this issue with your colleagues and formulate a plan.

- Consider how you might use another occupational engagement with a different client group that could provide participants with "shade" the way this concept worked with toy making for mothers of toddlers.

- Identify cost-effective strategies for working with mothers of preschoolers in your community. How might you combine the resources of professionals and volunteers?

- Identify "differently rigorous" strategies you could use to study complex issues related to mothers and children.

References

Abidin, R. R. (1990). *Parenting stress index manual.* 3rd ed. Charlottesville, Virginia: Pediatric Psychology Press.

Barlow, J., & Coren, E. (2002). *Parent-training programmes for improving maternal psychosocial health.* Oxford, UK: The Cochrane Library.

Barnett, L. A. (1991). Developmental benefits of play for children. In B. L. Driver, P. J. Brown & G. L. Peterson

(Eds.). *Benefits of leisure*. State College, Pennsylvania: Venture Pub. Inc. pp. 216–247.

Bartko, J. J., & Carpenter, W. T. (1975). On methods and theory of reliability. *The Journal of Nervous and Mental Disease, 163,* 307–317.

Benjamin, Z. (1947). *Talks to parents*. London, UK: National Association of Maternity and Child Welfare Centres and for the Prevention of Infant Mortality.

Best, J. B., & McCloskey, B. P. (1978). Early Childhood Development Program-Detection. *Australian Family Physician, 7,* 837–841.

Bettleheim, B. (1988). *A good enough parent*. London, UK: Pan Books.

Bristol, M. M., Gallagher, J. J., & Holt, K.D. (1993). Maternal depressive symptoms in autism: A responsive psychoeducational intervention. *Rehabilitation Psychology, 38,* 3–10.

Bruner, J. (1986). Play, thought and language. *Prospects: Quarterly Review of Education, 16,* 77–83.

Bruner, J., Jolly A., & Sylva, K. (1976). Play. Its role in development and evaluation. Harmondsworth, Middlesex, England: Penguin Books Ltd.

Bronfenbrenner, U. (1986). Ecology of the family as a context for human development: Research perspectives. *Developmental Psychology, 22,* 723–742.

Bugental, D. B., & Shennum, W. A. (1984). "Difficult" children as elicitors and targets of adult communication patterns: An attributional-behavioral transactional analysis. *Monographs of the Society for Research in Child Development, 49* (1, Serial No.205).

Bundy, A. C. (1993). Assessment of play and leisure: Delineation of the problem. *American Journal of Occupational Therapy, 47,* 217–222.

Bundy, A. C. (1997). Play and playfulness: What to look for. In L. D. Parham & L.S. Fazio (Eds.). *Play in occupational therapy for children*. St. Louis: Mosby, pp. 52–66.

Burke, J. P., & Shaaf, R.C. (1997). Family narratives and play assessment. In L. D. Parham, & L.S. Fazio (Eds.). *Play in occupational therapy for children*. St. Louis: Mosby, pp. 67–84.

Cameron, S. J., Dobson, L .A., & Day, D. M. (1991). Stress in parents of developmentally delayed and non-delayed children. *Canada's Mental Health, March,* 1991, 13–17.

Castillo, G.A. (1978). Left-handed teaching. Lessons in affective education. 2nd Ed. New York: Holt, Rinehart and Winston.

Cratty, B. J. (1986). *Perceptual and motor development in infants and children*. 3rd Ed. Englewood Cliffs, NJ: Prentice-Hall.

Daly Smith, P. (1982). *Play—Occupational Therapists' work*. Paper presented to: Australian Association of Occupational Therapists' 12th Federal Conference, Adelaide, August 11–14 , 1982.

DeGangi, G. A., Sickel, R. Z., Kaplan, E. P., & Weiner, A. S. (1997). Mother-infant interactions in infants with disorders of self-regulation. *Physical and Occupational Therapy in Pediatrics, 17,* 17–44.

Denshire, S. (2002). Viewpoint. Reflections on the confluence of personal and professional. *Australian Occupational Therapy Journal, 49,* 212–216.

Donoghue, N. (1986). *Home visiting and toy library project*. London, UK: The Cicely Northcote Trust.

Drake P. R., & Goldberg, S.(1992). Father-infant interactions and parenting stress with healthy and medically compromised infants. *Infant Behavior and Development, 17,* 3–14.

Erikson, E. H. (1963). *Childhood and society*. 2nd Ed. New York: W. W. Norton & Co. Inc.

Esdaile, S. A. (1998a). A child with a disability: Mothers' and fathers' perspectives. Poster paper presented at the World Congress of Occupational Therapists, Montreal, Canada, May 31–June 5, 1998.

Esdaile, S. A. (1998b). Every child has the God given right.... Paper presented at the World Congress of Occupational Therapists, Montreal, Canada, May 31–June 5, 1998.

Esdaile, S. (1996). A play-focused intervention involving mothers of preschoolers. *American Journal of Occupational Therapy, 50*(2), 113–123.

Esdaile, S. A. (1994) Invited comment: A focus on mothers, their children with special needs and other caregivers. *Australian Occupational Therapy Journal, 41*(1), 3–8.

Esdaile, S. A. (1990). A mother focused intervention study examining relationships between two to three year old toddlers' temperament and behaviour and maternal causal attributions, stress and self-concept as educators of their children. Unpublished doctoral dissertation. Bundoora, Victoria: La Trobe University.

Esdaile, S. (1987). Relaxation with children: An evaluation of workshops for teachers, parents and students. *Australian Occupational Therapy Journal, 34,* 4–13.

Esdaile, S., & Greenwood, K. A (2003). A comparison of mothers and fathers of children with and without disabilities. *Occupational Therapy International, 10*(2),115–126.

Esdaile, S. A., & Greenwood, K. M. (1995a) Mother-toddler relationships: An intervention study and exploration of key variables. *Journal of Family Studies, 1,* 142–152.

Esdaile, S., & Greenwood, K. M. (1995b). A survey of mothers relationship with their preschoolers. *Occupational Therapy International, 2,* 204–219.

Esdaile, S. A., & Greenwood, K. M. (1995c) Issues of parenting stress: A study involving mothers of toddlers. *Journal of Family Studies, 1,* 153–165.

Esdaile, S., & Greenwood, K. (1990). Comparison of mothers' and child-minders' ratings of toddlers' temperament—An inter-rater reliability study. *Australian Occupational Therapy Journal, 37,* 137–141.

Esdaile, S., & Sanderson, A. (1987a). Teaching parents toy making—A practical guide to early intervention. *British Journal of Occupational Therapists, 50,* 266–271.

Esdaile, S., & Sanderson, A. (1987b). *Toys to make*. Ringwood, Victoria: Penguin Australia Ltd.

Fagan, J., & Dore, M. M. (1993). Mother-child play in neglecting and non-neglecting mothers. *Early Child Development & Care, 87,* 59-68.

Feldman, R., & Greenbaum, C. W. (1997). Affect regulation and synchrony in mother-infant play as precursors to the development of symbolic competence. *Infant Mental Health Journal, 18,* 4–13.

Florey, L. (1981). Studies of play: Implications for growth, development and for clinical practice. *The American Journal of Occupational Therapy, 8,* 59–524.

Flyvbjerg, B. (2001). *Making social science matter. Why social inquiry fails and how it can succeed again.* Cambridge, UK: Cambridge University Press

Fraiberg, S., Shapiro, V., & Cherniss, D. S. (1980). Treatment modalities. In S. Fraiberg (Ed.). Clinical studies in infant mental health: The first year of life (pp 49–77). New York: Basic Books.

Freud, S. (1959). *The psychoanalytic treatment of children.* London, UK: Image Publishing Company.

Fullard, W., McDevitt, S. C., & Carey, W. B. (1984). Assessing temperament in one to three year old children. *Journal of Pediatric Psychology, 9,* 205–216.

Gardner, H., Csikszentmihalyi, M., & Damon, W. (2001). *Good work. When excellence and ethics meet.* New York: Basic Books.

Gergen, K. J. (1994). *Toward a transformation in social knowledge.* 2nd Ed. London, UK: Sage Publications Ltd.

Gergen, K. J. (1999). *An invitation to social construction.* London, UK: Sage Publications Ltd.

Girolametto, L., Verbey, M., & Tannock, R. (1994). Improving joint engagement in parent-child interactions: An intervention study. *Journal of Early Intervention, 18,* 155–167.

Goff Timmer, S., Borrego, J., & Urquiza, A. J. (2002). Antecedents of coercive interactions in physically abusive mother-child dyads. *Journal of Interpersonal Violence, 17,* 836–853.

Groos, K. (1896/1976). The play of animals: Play and instinct. In J. Bruner, A. Jolly, & K. Sylva (1976). Play. Its role in development and evaluation. Harmondsworth, Middlesex, UK: Penguin Books Ltd., pp. 65–67.

Hardyment, C. (1983). *Dream babies. Child Care from Locke to Spock.* London, UK: Jonathan Cape.

Hasselkus, B. R. (2003). From the desk of the editor. The voices of qualitative researchers: Sharing the conversation. *American Journal of Occupational Therapy, 5,* 7–8.

Higgs, J. (2003). Do you reason like a (health) professional? In G. Brown, S. Esdaile, & S. Ryan (Eds.). *Becoming an advanced healthcare practitioner.* Oxford, UK: Butterworth-Heinemann, pp. 145–160.

Higgs, J., & Titchen, A. (2001a). *Practice knowledge & expertise in the health professions.* Oxford, UK: Butterworth-Heinemann.

Higgs, J., & Titchen, A. (2001b). *Professional practice in health, education, and the creative arts.* Oxford, UK: Blackwell Science, Ltd.

Hinojosa, J., & Kramer, P. (1997). Integrating children with disabilities into family play. In L. D. Parham & L. S. Fazio (Eds.). *Play in occupational therapy for children.* St. Louis: Mosby, pp. 159–170.

Huizinga, J. (1950). Homo Ludens. In E.W. Gerber and W. J. Morgan (Eds.) (1979). *Sport and the body: A philosophical symposium,* (2nd Ed.) Philadelphia: Lea & Febiger.

Humphry, R. (1989). Early intervention and the influence of the occupational therapist on the parent-child relationship. *The American Journal of Occupational Therapy, 43,* 738–742.

Knox, S. (1996). Play and playfulness in preschool children. In R. Zemke & F. Clark (1996) (Eds.). *Occupational science. The evolving discipline.* Philadelphia: F. A. Davis, pp. 81–88.

Larson, E. A. (2000). The orchestration of occupation: The dance of mothers. *The American Journal of Occupational Therapy, 54,* 269–280.

Larson, E. A. (1995). The occupation of play: parent-child interaction in the service of social competence. *Occupational Therapy in Health Care, 9,* 103–120.

Lawlor, M.C. (2003). Gazing anew: The shift from a clinical gaze to an ethnographic lens. *American Journal of Occupational Therapy, 5,* 29–39.

Lear, R. (1993). *Play helps.* (3rd Ed.). Oxford: Butterworth-Heinemann Ltd.

Levy, J. (1979). Toward a science of play in the twenty-first century. *Leisure Today, 2,* 32.

McColl, M. A., Law, M., and Stewart, D. (1993). *Theoretical Basis of Occupational Therapy: An Annotated Bibliography of Applied Theory in the Professional Literature.* Thorofare, NJ: Slack.

Magill-Evans, J., & Harrison, M. J. (1999). Parent-child interactions and development of toddlers born preterm. *Western Journal of Nursing Research, 21,* 292–312.

Mattingly, C., & Fleming, M. H. (1994). *Clinical reasoning. Forms of inquiry in a therapeutic practice.* Philadelphia: F. A. Davis.

Mitcham, M. (2003). Integrating theory and practice: Using theory creatively to enhance professional practice. In G. Brown, S. Esdaile, & S. Ryan (Eds.). *Becoming an advanced healthcare practitioner.* Oxford, UK: Butterworth-Heinemann, pp.64–89.

Oaklander, V. (1978). *Windows to our children. Gestalt therapy approach to children and adolescents.* Moab, UT: Real People Press.

Olson, J. (1998). A phenomenological study of infant mental health interventions: The mothers' perspective. Unpublished doctoral dissertation, Wayne State University.

Parham, L. D., & Primeau, L. A. (1997). Play and occupational therapy. In L. D. Parham & L. S. Fazio (Eds.). *Play in occupational therapy for children.* St. Louis: Mosby, pp. 2–21.

Parush, S., Lapidot, G., Edelstein, P. V., & Tamir, D. (1987). Occupational therapy in mother and child health centers. *The American Journal of Occupational Therapy, 41,* 601–605.

Perls, F.S. (1969). Gestalt therapy verbatim. New York: Bantam Books.

Piaget, J. (1962). *Play, dreams and imitation in childhood.* New York: Basic Books.

Pierce, D. (2000). Maternal management of home as a developmental play space for infants and toddlers. *The American Journal of Occupational Therapy, 54,* 290–299.

Polakow, V. (1993). *Lives on the edge. Single mothers and their children in the other America.* Chicago: The University of Chicago Press.

Primeau, L. A. (2003). Reflections on self in qualitative

research: Stories of family. *American Journal of Occupational Therapy, 5*, 9–16.

Primeau, L. A. (1998). Orchestration of work and play within families. *American Journal of Occupational Therapy, 52*, 188–195.

Prior, M. R., Sanson, A. V., & Oberklaid, F. (1989). The Australian temperament project. In G. Kohnstamm, J. Bates and M. Rothbart (Eds.). *Handbook of temperament in childhood*. Wiley: London, UK, 537–554.

Reilly, M. (Ed) (1974). *Play as exploratory learning*. Thousand Oaks, CA: Sage Publications.

Richman, N., Stevenson, J. E., & Graham, P. J. (1982). *Pre-school to school: A behavioral study*. London, UK: Academic Press.

Rogers, C. R. (1959). A theory of therapy, personality, and interpersonal relationships, as developed in the client-centered framework. In Koch, S. *Psychology: The study of a science*, Vol. 3, New York: McGraw-Hill.

Roter, D. L., Rudd, P. E., Frantz, S.C., & Commings, J.P. (1981). Community produced materials for health education. *Public Health Reports, 2*, 169–172.

Rubin, K., Hastings, P., Chen, X., Stewart, S., & McNichol, K. (1998). Interpersonal and maternal correlates of aggression, conflict, and externalizing problems in toddlers. *Child Development, 69*, 1614–1629.

Schiller, (1882/1979). Von F. Letters XV from Essays and letters volume VII. In E. W. Gerber & W. J. Morgan (Eds.). *Sport and the body. A philosophical symposium*. 2nd ed. Philadelphia: Lea & Febiger.

Schön, D. A. (1987). *Educating the reflective practitioner*. San Francisco: Jossey-Bass.

Siegel, S. (1956). *Nonparametric statistics for the behavioural sciences*. Tokyo, Japan: McGraw-Hill.

Singer J. L. (1973). *The child's world of make-believe. Experimental studies of imaginative play*. New York: Academic Press.

Slade, A. & Wolf, D. P. (Eds.)(1994). *Children at play. Clinical and developmental approaches to meaning and representation*. New York: Oxford University Press.

Slaughter, D. T. (1984). Early intervention and its effects on maternal and child development. Monograph. *Society for Research in child Development, 48* (Serial No. 202).

Slaughter, D. T., Washington Lindsey, R., Nakagawa, K., & Shahariw Kuehene, V. (1989). Who gets involved? Head-start mothers as persons. *Journal of Negro Education, 58*, 16–29.

Smith, P. K. (1986). (Ed.). *Children's play. Research develop-ments and practical applications*. New York: Gordon and Broach Science Publishers.

Stagnitti, K. (1998). *Learn to play. A practical program to develop a child's imaginative play skills*. West Brunswick, Victoria: Co-ordinates Publications, a division of Co-ordinates Therapy Services, Pty., Ltd.

Stagnitti, K. & Unsworth, C. (2000). The importance of pretend play to child development: An occupational therapy perspective. *British Journal of Occupational Therapy, 63*, 121–127.

Steelman, L. M., Assel, M. A., Swank, P. R., Smith, K. E., & Landry, S. H. (2002). Early maternal warm responsiveness as a predictor of child social skills: Direct and indirect paths of influence over time. *Journal of Applied Developmental Psychology, 23*,135–156.

Strom, R. (1984). *Parent as a teacher inventory manual*. Bensenville, Illinois: Scholastic Testing Service, Inc.

Sutton-Smith, B. (1970). *A descriptive study of four modes of children's play between one and five years*. New York: Columbia University.

Sylva, K. (1993). Work or play in the nursery? *International Play Journal, 1*, 5–15.

Takata, N. (1974). Play as a prescription. In M. Reilly, (Ed). (1974). *Play as exploratory learning*. Thousand Oaks, California: Sage Publications. pp. 209–246.

Tannen, D. (1991). *You just don't understand. Women and men in conversation*. New York: Ballantine Books.

United States Department of Health, Education, and Welfare Administration for Children—Youth and Families. (1975). *Head start performance standards*. Washington, DC: Government Publisher.

Uzgiris, E. C. (1979). (Ed.). Social interaction and communication during infancy: New directions for child development. Volume 4. San Francisco: Jossey Bass.

Vygotsky, L. (1976). Play and its role in the mental development of the child. In J. Bruner, A. Jolly, & K. Sylva (1976). *Play. Its role in development and evaluation*. Harmondsworth, Middlesex,UK: Penguin Books Ltd., pp. 537–554.

Wood, W. (1997). Insights from the play of nonhuman primates, In B. E. Chandler (Ed.). *The essence of play in a child's occupation*. Bethesda, MD: The American Occupational Therapy Association. pp. 17–49.

Yerxa, E. J. (1991). Seeking a relevant, ethical, and realistic way of knowing for occupational therapy. *The American Journal of Occupational Therapy, 45*, 199–204.

Yerxa, E.J. (1994). In search of good ideas for occupational therapy. *Scandinavian Journal of Occupational Therapy, 1*, 7–15.

CHAPTER **6**

Mothering in the Context of Unpaid Work and Play in Families

Loree A. Primeau, PhD, OTR, OT(C)

Anticipated Outcomes

I anticipate that, after reading this chapter, readers will be able to:

 Define mothering

 Discuss the literature and research findings related to divisions of unpaid work in families

 Distinguish between traditional and nontraditional gender ideologies and gender practices

 Identify and discuss two types of parental strategies used in mothering in the context of unpaid work and play in families

 Describe parental participation in play within household work

Introduction

> Biology is the least of what makes someone a mother.
>
> —Oprah Winfrey (as cited in Rattiner, 2000, p. 17)

When I was invited to contribute a chapter to a book on "mothering," I asked myself this question: Don't fathers mother, too? According to Webster's dictionary (1984), "to mother" means "to nourish and protect" (p. 459). Given this definition, the literature (Averett, Gennetian, & Peters, 2000; Coltrane, 1996; Deutsch & Saxon, 1998; Dienhart, 2001; Ehrenberg, Gearing-Small, Hunter, & Small, 2001; Ehrensaft, 1987; Gilbert, 1985; Haas, 1992; Kimball, 1988; Lareau, 2000; McKeering & Pakenham, 2000) and my own research (Primeau, 2000a, 2000b) indicates that fathers *do* mother. During my graduate work, I became interested in exploring gender dynamics in families, particularly as they related to household work—that is, both housework and childcare tasks. This interest led to my doctoral research, which examined unpaid work and play within families with equal attention to mothers' and fathers' participation in these occupations. Thus, my conceptualization of mothering is shaped by the following:

- Mothering is an occupation in which both mothers and fathers engage on a daily basis.

■ Mothering, defined as the physical and psychological nourishment and protection of children, occurs in the context of unpaid work and play in families.

This chapter will highlight *how* mothering by both mothers and fathers occurs in this context. To begin, I will briefly review the literature on divisions of household work, especially divisions of childcare between mothers and fathers. Next, I will present four families' stories that illustrate the diverse ways in which they divided unpaid work in their homes. Then I will present findings that describe both mothers' and fathers' mothering of their children in the context of unpaid work and play in their families.

As stated, mothering is defined in this chapter as the physical and psychological nourishment of children in which both mothers and fathers engage on a daily basis in the context of unpaid work and play in families. Data from a qualitative-research, multiple-methods study highlight *how* mothering occurred in this context. The study was grounded in the literature on divisions of unpaid work, including childcare, between mothers and fathers. The stories of four families are presented to illustrate the diverse ways in which mothers and fathers divided the work required to maintain their families. Their stories also demonstrate how divisions of unpaid work, whether traditional or nontraditional, serve as a foundation on which mothering in the context of unpaid work and play in families is based. The study's findings indicate that parents used strategies of segregation and inclusion to organize their time and play with their children, resulting in time and play interspersed with household work and time and play embedded in household work. Parental participation in a specific type of play embedded in household work is presented as an example of mothering that is performed by both mothers and fathers in the context of unpaid work and play in families.

↩ Unpaid Work in the Home

Studies from around the world, including highly industrialized as well as less industrialized nations, indicate that, although women have increased their participation in paid work outside the home, they remain responsible for the majority of unpaid work in the home. This conclusion is based on data collected from 16 countries: Australia (Baxter, 1997; Bittman, 1999; Dempsey, 1997), Canada (Baxter, 1997; McFarlane, Beaujot, & Haddad, 2000), China (Lu, Mame, & Bellas, 2000; Zhang & Farley, 1995), the Czech Republic (Krizkova, 1999), Finland (Bittman, 1999), Jamaica (Rooparine et al., 1995), Japan (Kamo, 1994), Mexico ("Domestic workers," 2000), Norway (Baxter, 1997), Pakistan (Akram-Lodhi, 1996), Slovenia (Cernigoj-Sadar, 1989), Spain (Sanchez & Hall, 1999), Sweden (Baxter, 1997; Roman, 1999), Turkey (Bolak, 1997), the United Kingdom (Wilson, 1999), and the United States (Baxter, 1997; Robinson & Milkie, 1998; Zhang & Farley, 1995). Not only are women responsible for more of the unpaid work in the home than men, but also they tend to complete those household tasks that need to be done more frequently (i.e., throughout the day, daily, or weekly) than men (Beckwith, 1992; Coltrane, 1990; Gunter & Gunter, 1990, Robinson & Spitze, 1992; Shaw, 1988; Shelton, 1992). For example, household tasks typically completed by women, such as meal preparation and clean-up, laundry and clothing care, and tidying or cleaning the house, are generally completed over the course of a day, daily, or weekly, whereas household work tasks typically completed by men, such as car maintenance, yard work, taking out the garbage, and household repairs, are completed on a variable, but usually no more often than weekly, basis.

Childcare tasks are among those household tasks that demand completion on a frequent basis. Despite the current rhetoric of fatherhood that describes the "new father" as a nurturer, an active and involved participant in the care of his children on a daily basis, research suggests that there is a discrepancy between this image of fatherhood and the actions of fatherhood (Atkinson & Blackwelder, 1993; Daly, 1993, 1994; Ehrenberg et al., 2001; Lareau, 2000; LaRossa, 1988; Marsiglio, 1993; McMahon, 1998). Examination of fathers' actions around the world in terms of their time spent caring for their children indicates that, on average, fathers spend approximately 25 percent of the time that mothers do caring for their children (Owen, 1995).

Lamb (1987) separated parental involvement in childcare into three components:

1. Engagement: Time in which there was one-to-one interaction with the child, including physical care or play
2. Accessibility: Time in which the parent was in close proximity to the child and, although doing something else, was readily available to the child
3. Responsibility: Consisting of accountability for the child's health, welfare, and safety through such things as ensuring that the child had clean clothes to wear and attended doctor appointments.

In families in which mothers were not employed in the paid workforce, fathers were estimated to spend an average of 20 to 25 percent of mothers' time in engagement activities and an average of 33 percent of mothers' time in accessibility activities. When mothers were employed outside the home, fathers spent an average of 33 percent of mothers' time in engagement activities and an average of 66 percent as much time as mothers in being accessible to their children (Lamb, 1987). Mothers were responsible for their children an average of 90 percent of the time, regardless of their participation or nonparticipation in paid work.

Barnett and Baruch (1988) also found that fathers' responsibility for childcare tasks, defined as remembering, planning, and scheduling a task, was low. Among 160 fathers, 113 stated that they were not responsible for any childcare tasks; 35 reported that they were responsible for one childcare task, and 12 reported responsibility for two or three tasks (Barnett & Baruch, 1988). Current research supports these findings: Ehrenberg and colleagues (2001) found that the men and women in their study agreed that a greater proportion of responsibility for childcare tasks rested with mothers than with fathers. This study indicated, however, that a task-oriented approach to divisions of childcare was less likely to predict marital satisfaction, perceptions of parental competence, and closeness to children than psychological and relational aspects of shared parenting, such as similar parenting goals, spousal support and praise, and flexibility in division of childcare. The authors hypothesized that mothers in their sample "may be more accepting of the fact that they are responsible for a greater proportion of childcare duties as long as their husbands participate in family-oriented activities, are willing to help out when necessary, and are explicitly supportive of their efforts as wives, mothers, and workers" (Ehrenberg et al., 2001, p. 150). Similarly, although fathers did not exhibit high levels of involvement in the day-to-day aspects of childcare, they were observed to make important contributions to the daily routines of families as initiators of playful interactions and laughter, shapers of the flow of conversation, and teachers of life skills to their children (Lareau, 2000). In summary, the research literature suggests that divisions of unpaid work, including childcare, and play with children in the home are important dimensions of mothering in which both mothers and fathers engage on a daily basis.

✍ A Continuum of Divisions of Unpaid Work in Families: Traditional to Nontraditional

Every family faces the dilemma of how to accomplish the work required to nourish and protect their children. Specifically, parents must decide how best to provide their children with economic support as well as physical and psychological nurturance. Resolutions of this dilemma are as individual and unique as families themselves. Nevertheless, commonalities do exist. Families lie along a continuum of traditional to nontraditional divisions of work, depending on their gender ideologies (what people believe and feel) and their gender practices (what they do) (Primeau, 2000b). Families with traditional gender ideologies expect a woman, even though she works outside the home, to identify primarily with her home activities and a man to identify primarily with his paid work (Hochschild, 1989). Accordingly, traditional gender practices are those in which the woman, even if she works outside the home, is responsible for over 60 percent of the household work, including those tasks typically seen as women's work (cooking, cleaning, laundry, and childcare) and, often, those tasks that are typically seen as men's work (outdoor, indoor, and car maintenance) (Primeau, 2000a). Families with nontraditional, or egalitarian, gender ideologies expect the woman and man to identify jointly with the same spheres: home, paid work, or both (Hochschild, 1989). Nontraditional gender practices are those in which the woman and man both work outside of the home and household work (housework and childcare) are shared within a 60 to 40 percent range or childcare tasks alone are shared within a 60 to 40 percent split (Primeau, 2000a) (Fig. 6–1).

To illustrate how mothering occurs in the context of unpaid work in families, I will present data from a qualitative research, multiple methods study that examined unpaid work and play in 10 two-parent families from the Los Angeles area. Data were collected using participant observations (46 observations; 109 hours), intensive interviews (20 interviews; 43.5 hours), and a questionnaire on divisions of household work. I wrote extensive field notes after each observation in the families' homes, including methodological notes on my actions, thoughts, and feelings while in their homes. The interviews were audiotaped and transcribed verbatim. To preserve the participants' anonymity, pseudonyms are used. The following stories are from four families: Linda and Sam, a couple with traditional gender practices; Susan and Bill, another couple with traditional gender practices; Monique and Stuart, a couple whose gender practices approach nontraditional; and Kim and George, a couple with nontraditional gender practices based on their shared childcare. As Table 6–1 demonstrates, these families were chosen for their representation of the continuum of traditional to nontraditional divisions of work.

Maternal Responsibility and Paternal Assistance

Vignette: *Linda and Sam*

Sam worked full time outside the home as a computer programmer. Linda was studying to be a court reporter and worked full time outside the home as an accounting clerk. When I first started visiting their home, Linda was home during the day with their children, Katlyn, a 3-year-old girl, and Mary Jane, a 1-year-old girl. She attended night school to become a court reporter 3 nights a week for approximately 3 hours a night. This was a recent change, occurring within the previous 2 months. Before that time she had been going to school during the day while the children were at a babysitter's house. Two weeks after my first visit to their home, Linda began a full-time job as an accounting clerk and the children returned to spending weekdays at the babysitter's house.

This family divided their work along traditional gender lines. Although Sam shared the shopping and errands, Linda completed the majority of the household work. She also completed half of the indoor maintenance tasks that are typically completed by men. When I commented on how busy Linda must be with a full-time job and night school three times a week, Sam stated that he tried to "help out," but as he continued to talk, it became clear that he expected Linda to manage their home. Instead of assuming that they had equal responsibility for ensuring that the household work got done, he expected her to be "in charge" and to have primary responsibility for organizing and delegating household work to him.

Traditional gender ideologies underlie Sam and Linda's traditional gender practices. When I asked why Linda had stopped working, Sam replied, "It's just because the mother always stays home when she's pregnant.... I guess that's just the normal thing. The daddy goes to work and the mommy stays home type of thing. I think that's the normal in society." When I asked Linda why she was training to become a

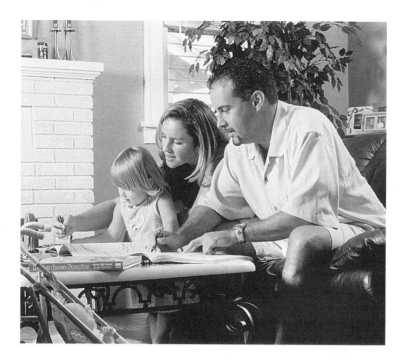

Figure 6–1 *These parents, who have a nontraditional division of work, are both actively engaged in play with their daughter.*

court reporter, she replied, "Well, because that will allow me to schedule my work more around my family. I can work freelance and work when I want to work instead of having a 9-to-5 job where I have to be there Monday through Friday. I'll be able to make good money and schedule the work when I want it." Clearly, Linda intended to fit her job in around her family responsibilities. She was not alone in this approach to managing her participation in paid work and household work in this manner. Women frequently adapt their participation in

Table 6–1 Families illustrating the continuum of traditional to nontraditional divisions of work			
Division of household work	Family	Participation in paid work outside the home	Household work categories in which father crossed gender lines to share work 60/40%
Traditional	Linda and Sam	Father—F/T* Mother—F/T	Shopping and errands
	Susan and Bill	Father—F/T Mother—F/T	Cooking and meal clean-up
	Monique and Stuart	Father—F/T Mother—F/T	Almost shares childcare (37%) Shopping and errands Managerial tasks
Nontraditional	Kim and George	Father—F/T Mother—F/T	Childcare

*Full-time paid work participation

paid work to the demands of their household work participation. Men's participation in paid work is generally seen as distinct and protected from the demands of household work (Bergen, 1991; Shelton, 1992).

Three of the six women from the traditional families in this study were actively working toward obtaining paid work that would allow them to schedule it more easily around the household work within their families. Two other women from traditional families spoke of moving into part-time work once their children reached school age so that they could be home when their children came home from school. The sixth woman had already made the decision to stay at home full time with her children. Only one of the four women from the nontraditional families in this study spoke of adjusting her job to accommodate her household work. She was working part time during the time that she was in the study and told me that she was actively resisting her employer's requests to work full time. She was, however, using some of her time off from paid work to pursue an acting career. One nontraditional couple was working together toward starting a family business that would allow both of them to schedule their paid work around their household work. The remaining two women from nontraditional families made no mention of changing their full-time jobs or the amount of their participation in paid work to accommodate their household work.

Linda and Sam demonstrate a pattern of childcare, or mothering, that has been termed maternal responsibility and paternal assistance (Primeau, 2000a). It was observed in three of the four traditional families in this study. Fathers' abdication of responsibility for the children when mothers are present is characteristic of this pattern. During an observation with Sam and the children while Linda was absent, I noticed that he immediately changed his focus from the children to a television show as soon as she arrived home. He went "off duty" the moment she walked through the door.

Sam frequently spoke of his wish that Linda would communicate to him what it was that she wanted him to do around the house. He

said," She doesn't communicate as well as I do. And I've told her, 'I won't help until you ask me.'" Sam's resistance to helping Linda with the household work without being specifically asked to do so was not unique. Passive resistance, waiting to be asked and hoping not to be, is a strategy frequently used by men to avoid participation in household work (Hochschild, 1989; Komter, 1989). Nor was Linda alone among the women in the study in the assumption of almost sole responsibility for the work with little complaints and few requests for help. Many women do not like to ask their husbands for help (Berk, 1985; Hochschild, 1989). ⌘

Shared Ideologies and Negotiated Practices

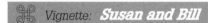

⌘ Vignette: *Susan and Bill*

Susan and Bill both worked full time for the same computer technology company, he in the technical division and she in customer service. Susan was also taking night classes at a university. They had a 3-year-old boy, Michael, and Susan gave birth to another boy as we were nearing the completion of data collection. Their son went to preschool during the day. They had a traditional division of household work. Although they shared the cooking and meal clean-up, Susan was responsible for the majority of the household work.

When I asked Susan how she and Bill divided the housework and childcare, she replied:

> There's no set schedule. Whatever needs to be done, needs to be done. If neither Bill or I are doing anything at that particular time and Michael needs something, I'll usually go do it with him. ... The housework, we usually work together. ... Bill usually does most of the cooking and I do the dishes. ... I'm usually the one who does the laundry more than him. Anything else, we set aside one day when we're going to straighten up and we'll just do it together. Or one day, if I have a lot of time, I'll do everything, and if he has time, he'll do it.

During his interview, Bill offered a similar sentiment:

> There's a rule in marriage. . ... Each person does 100% of the work at any given moment in time. This business of 50/50, I think is absolute baloney. Because that doesn't work. It's never 50/50. It's each person does what needs to be done at the point it needs to be done. If I can do all of the cooking because I'm good at it, or most of the cooking, that doesn't mean that if I don't come home, she doesn't cook. . ... Let's say she more often would do the laundry and I've got the time to do it, I'm not going to sit there and say, "Well, I don't have to do that. That's her job."

Both Susan and Bill seemed to be saying that they were equally invested in the completion of household work. They saw it as work that needed to be done and that could be done by whomever was available to do it. Their division of household work was based on equity rather than equality. Under a system of equity, fairness is judged on the basis of one's relative contributions or merits (Thompson, 1991). A system of equality dictates a 50/50 split of responsibility for household work, and each person has equal status within the system (Schwartz, 1994; Thompson, 1991). Equality is easy to measure; each person shares equally. Under a system of equity, "one person's definition of fair is often another person's definition of exploitation" (Schwartz, 1994, p. 155). Egalitarian couples have been found to mix equity with equality to ensure that justice is being served within their divisions of household work. The danger of reliance on equity alone is that what seems to be "fair" can result in a situation of inequality, as can be seen in Susan's and Bill's case.

As their interviews continued, Susan and Bill shared additional information about their division of work. At one point, while talking about who did what around the house, Susan said:

> In general, I don't want to say I do more. [Long pause] Well, maybe I do, but not begrudgingly. Because he's trying to get a business going and a lot of times he's working on the computer for a client or something, then I need to do stuff around the house more than he does. But also the other way around

too. When I'm doing my studies, then he picks up the slack. But, in general, my time with Michael is more affected by taking care of him and the household stuff than for Bill, I think. ... Yeah, so I think, in general, women do more.

Bill reached the same conclusion. He said, "It really does fall into what needs to be done. That's the overriding concern. She will tend to do certain things more than I do, but not 100 percent. But definitely over 50 or 60 or 70 or even 80."

When Susan compared herself to Bill, she acknowledged that she carried a greater responsibility for household work than he did. This acknowledgment did not result in a sense of injustice on her part because she saw the time that he was released from household work as time he spent in paid work participation. Thus, he was still contributing to the overall good of their family. Women rarely use 50/50 split comparisons with their husbands as evidence of unfairness in the division of household work (Thompson, 1991). They tend to recognize injustice when men get personal care and service when they do not. Susan stated that Bill allowed her time from household work to pursue a college degree; therefore she did not perceive injustice in their division of household work even though she completed the majority of it.

In this case, Susan and Bill had negotiated a compromise in their division of work based on their shared traditional gender ideology, leading to their traditional gender practices. Bill appeared to be accepting of Susan's wish both to be a "good mother" and to have a career, yet still expected her to be primarily responsible for the work at home. Susan expressed boredom with her job and a desire to stay home with her children, but also stated that she intended to have a career as a teacher. Both of them, however, put Bill's work at building a consulting business ahead of his involvement in household work and, therefore, ahead of her career plans. Although, at first glance, Susan and Bill seemed to share an equalitarian gender ideology, in reality, they actually shared a traditional gender ideology in which they both expected Susan to identify primarily with her home activities and Bill to identify primarily with his paid work.

Reluctant Participants

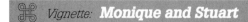
Vignette: **Monique and Stuart**

Monique worked outside the home full time as a secretary from 6:30 AM to 3:00 PM every weekday. Stuart was a sales manager who worked out of their house. By his estimate, he participated in paid work approximately 2 hours a day. They had a 3-year-old girl, Bridget, and a 6-month-old boy, Richard. The children spent weekdays from 9:00 AM until 3:30 PM at a babysitter's house. Although this couple's division of household work was traditional, it approached nontraditional in that Stuart almost shared childcare within the 60 to 40 percent range. He and Monique estimated that he completed childcare tasks 37 percent of the time. Stuart also crossed gender lines to share shopping and errands and managerial tasks, which are typically completed by women, and Monique crossed gender lines to participate in outdoor maintenance tasks.

They shared a traditional gender ideology that supported their gender practices. When I asked Monique why she worked outside the home. She said, "Because Stuart doesn't make enough money. It's our house payments and we have two cars, two insurance payments, and we don't have as many bills as we used to, but a majority of it is just the financial situation. Believe me, if I didn't have to work, I would not be there." Monique stated that she did not want to work outside the home any longer than she needed to. During her interview, she made many statements that revealed that she was a reluctant participant in paid work. Often her voice was veiled with sadness when she talked about not being able to be home during the day with her children. She was clear, however, about Stuart's role: she expected him to have a financially stable job and make enough money to support their family comfortably.

Stuart also had traditional beliefs that led him to think that Monique should have primary responsibility for the children. He wanted her to be there when the children came home from school without seeming to recognize that his job allowed him to be home all day and available to his children in the after-school hours. He stated that he couldn't be a primary caregiver and would not want to be because he would "lose it." When I asked Stuart how he and Monique divided the housework and childcare, he replied, "Well, there's really no divide. She does everything. And then she'll delegate something to me. I mean, unless she says, 'Do that' or 'Help me out with Bridget. Go in there and watch her.' I don't really do, as far as responsibilities like that, I don't do anything, unless I'm told."

During her interview, Monique revealed that Stuart had only recently begun to get up during the night to care for Richard, their 6-month-old son. Given that Monique got up each day at 4:30 AM to be at work at 6:30 AM and Stuart typically didn't get up until 7:30 or 8:00 AM, the fact that he had not gotten up with Richard before this point in time provided a significant piece of information about this couple's gender practices. As I listened to this couple talk about Stuart's lack of help with the care of the baby and with the housework, I wondered how Monique could have managed to do all the work involved in caring for the children and maintaining the home without more help from him. I also questioned why it had taken her so long to ask Stuart to get up during the night with the baby. Clearly, his failure to do so earlier was indicative of his reluctance to participate in the care of his son. Monique's answer to my question of how she felt about Stuart's not sharing the caregiving, even though she participated in paid work, provided some insight into this puzzle:

> It's OK. I need help. And he is starting to help me more than he was. Especially when I first went back to work. I was just a mess. I was just losing my mind. And he wasn't helping me at all. And I just flat out told him, 'Look, I need help. Emotionally I need some support and, just around the house, I need a break from the baby every once in a while. ... You're off being able to go play with Bridget and have a good time and I can't. I need that special time with her too, as much as you do.

And you need to do some bonding with the baby.' But little, fragile things, it makes him very, very nervous. And I understand that, but he's got to look at it from my point of view too where I need some support. ... So I said, 'I need your help.' And he is getting a lot better. And, as I said, Richard's getting older and I know it's just going to improve. But even him getting up in the night last week for the first time was a tremendous help. And a lot of it may be my fault. I didn't know if I could trust him or if he could calm Richard. ... And I think my biggest fear is I just felt like I was always the one that had to do it. I was the only one that could do it. I was just so tired last week and when I asked him and when I saw that he could do it, it was like, wait a minute. And he can go back to bed at 4:30 and maybe get an extra 2 hours, 3 hours sleep. Where me, I have to get up. So I always felt guilty like, well, I know Stuart needs his sleep and I know this and this and this. Now I'm thinking, yeah, but I need my sleep just as much as he does. And he can go back, like he went back to bed at 4:30 this morning, he slept for another 2 $1/2$, 3 hours, where I was out of the house in an hour and a half. So a lot of it, where I never thought I could count on him or that he could do it, and when he just did it that one time last week, I never really pushed it, but now where I felt bad asking him to do it, it's like, well, I need it just as much as he does. I still feel kind of bad, like when I asked him to get up this morning, but then I thought, it's okay. He can do his part too. So I feel a little bit more confident.

This lengthy quote from Monique's interview illustrates four features of traditional gender ideologies that lead to traditional divisions of childcare within families. First, Monique asked for Stuart's help only when she was emotionally and physically exhausted and could no longer do it on her own. Men and women frequently perceive men's participation in household work as a response to women's personal needs (Thompson, 1991). Instead of seeing their childcare as part of the process of providing care in an equitable way, men view it as their response to their wives' need for respite. Thus, men get credit from their wives for doing some of the childcare as a personal favor to them.

The second point concerns Monique's reference to Stuart's fear of handling what he perceived to be a tiny, fragile baby. Stuart also referred to his lack of skill and comfort with babies during his interview. His incompetence was used as a justification for his lack of help with the childcare tasks. This justification was gender specific in the sense that it was acceptable for him to use that particular excuse, but it would not have been acceptable for Monique to excuse herself from childcare for that same reason (Thompson, 1991). As a woman, she is expected, by virtue of the social construction of gender expectations, to have an acceptable level of competence in caring for a baby (Komter, 1989; Major, 1993; Thorne, 1992).

The third point is related to Stuart's justification for his lack of participation in childcare. Monique lacked confidence in and harbored fears about Stuart's ability to provide adequate care for the baby. Other mothers and fathers in the study who held traditional gender ideologies echoed these beliefs and feelings. They referred to the mother's greater ability to provide for the infant's or young child's care, her lack of faith in the father's ability to do so, and the father's decreased skills and comfort in this area. By accepting their husbands' justifications, the women perpetuated a traditional division of household work within their families (LaRossa, 1988; Thompson, 1991). This mixture of thoughts and feelings about men's competence in caregiving and women's confidence and trust in men's ability to be dependable parents is a common experience. Men frequently point out obstacles in their own homes to their participation in childcare, citing their wives' insistence that care be provided according to the women's way of doing things. In response, women state that men's reluctance to get involved and prove themselves as parents leads to their lack of trust and confidence in the men's parenting abilities (Gibbs, 1993). Clearly, the data show that Stuart was a reluctant participant in childcare.

The fourth point portrayed in Monique's quote was her admission of feeling guilty about asking Stuart for help. Even after convincing herself that she was justified in asking him to help out, she still felt "bad" and needed to remind herself that it was okay for her to ask. This point highlights how several of the women in the study held deeply ingrained beliefs that household work, and particularly childcare, was their primary responsibility. Many studies have demonstrated the strength of these socially constructed beliefs in perpetuating gender inequality in divisions of household work (Ferree, 1991b; Major, 1993; Thompson, 1991).

Some of the men who participated in the study indicated that change may eventually occur, albeit slowly, within their families' divisions of household work. For example, Stuart said, at the end of his interview, that answering the interview questions made him think about things, such as "what things I'm doing right and what things I'm doing wrong." He stated that the process of putting his actions into words made him more aware and gave him the opportunity to think about what he was doing. At the end of her interview, Monique confirmed Stuart's newfound awareness when she commented on their participation in the study, "I think we enjoyed it. I even think that it did Stuart some good. Just different little things. Like he made a comment to me, 'You really do carry a lot on your shoulders, Monique.' And I [thought], maybe his talk with Loree did some good the other night. So that was kind of neat. For him to make a comment like that I thought, good, maybe it did open your eyes a little bit. So after he made that comment, then I said to him, 'Get up. Richard's crying.' [laughs]. ... I definitely think it put some thoughts into his head." Here we can see how Monique's assessment that Stuart had begun to recognize the inequity in their division of household work bolstered her sense of entitlement to his participation in the work and led her to increase her expectations for his help.   ⌘

His Work, Her Work, Their Work

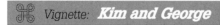

⌘ *Vignette:* ***Kim and George***

Kim and George both worked full time outside the home. She was an insurance sales manager for a rental car company and he was a painting contractor. They had two children, a 5-year-old boy, Christian, and a 2-year-old girl, Julia. The children went to preschool and a babysitter's house, respectively. This couple had a nontraditional division of work. They shared childcare within a 60 to 40 percent range. With the exception of cleaning the house, where the majority of the tasks were completed by paid help, Kim and George divided the rest of the household work along traditional gender lines. Kim had primary responsibility for cooking and meal cleanup, laundry and clothing care, shopping and errands, and managerial tasks, all of which are typically completed by women. George's areas of responsibility fell within those traditionally seen as men's work, that is, outdoor, indoor, and car maintenance. Even so, their division of household work was nontraditional because George crossed gender lines to share childcare.

George's feelings about Kim's participation in paid work indicated that he held a traditional gender ideology about divisions of household work. He said, "My Utopia would be for Kim to not have to work. ... That would be my utopia. I would love to live in 1953. She stays at home and I'm the father that goes and works ... that would be what I would like. ... But she couldn't do that. I can't afford it. I mean I couldn't pay for us to do that." He explained that it was also Kim's choice to work outside the home, "It's a choice, oh, yeah. She's a very motivated person and she needs to have challenges and staying around the house wouldn't challenge her at all."

George accommodated Kim's desire to participate in paid work by sharing childcare. The remainder of the household work, however, was completed according to traditional gender expectations. When I commented on the cleanliness and neatness of their home, George said that Kim was always cleaning. The differences between his standards for cleanliness and hers are illustrated by his statement that he preferred to clean when it was dirty and he could see the results of his work, but that she cleaned when it was hardly dirty. George's statement resonates with research indicating that women's levels of identification with housework and men's expectations that their work will not meet their wives' standards are associated with less participation in housework on the men's part (Coltrane, 1990; Ferree, 1991b; Major, 1993). These findings translate into a situation in which the more a woman cares about having a clean house, the less her husband will complete tasks typically seen as women's work. This dynamic seemed to be operating in Kim's and George's case. George's justification that Kim's need for a clean house was greater than his need and her acceptance of this justification transformed the necessary housework into her personal need and robbed her of the right to his help (Thompson, 1991). Kim's high standards for having a clean house placed the demands of the work upon her (Coltrane, 1990; Gunter & Gunter, 1990; Ferree, 1991b; Major, 1993).

Although Kim expected to be able to participate freely in paid work and expected George to do the same, she did not expect him to participate equally in household work, indicating that she held a traditional gender ideology. She acknowledged inequity in their division of housework tasks, but she didn't perceive it as unfair. Even under very lopsided divisions of household work, many women do not perceive unfairness in their primary responsibility for household work (Baxter, 2000; Berk, 1985; Major, 1993; Thompson, 1991). In contrast, Kim stated that their division of childcare was "probably leaning more towards George doing more than I am right now." But the fact that her job was a primary source of income, and therefore necessary for the good of the family, most likely led to her feelings of entitlement to George's participation in childcare, if not in other areas of household work (Ferree, 1991a; Thompson, 1991).

George's shared responsibility for childcare and his unique point of view on mothering arising from the interactions between his traditional gender ideology and his nontraditional gender practices were evident in his response to my question about their decision not to have any more children. He compared it to basketball: playing two-on-two basketball versus three-man basketball requires a change from man-to-man coverage to zone coverage. He said that moving from parenting two children to parenting three children requires going from one-to-one coverage to zone coverage, as in, "You cover that area, I'll cover this area." George's sports analogy demonstrates how men are able to incorporate their ways of knowing and being into mothering when they increase their participation in child-

care. Men's full participation in the care of their children will require not only completion of their fair share of the work of childcare, but also their discovery and acknowledgement of their own mothering beliefs and practices, thereby rendering justifications of lack of training, experience, and competence in childcare obsolete.   ⌘

The stories of these four families illustrate the diverse ways in which mothering occurs in the context of unpaid work in families. Each couple's gender ideologies and gender practices interacted within the reality of their daily lives to generate their own unique solution to the universal dilemma facing every family, that is, how to accomplish the work required to nourish and protect their children. The division of unpaid work in a family, wherever it may fall on the continuum from traditional to nontraditional, provides the foundation for mothering in the context of unpaid work and play.

⮞ Mothering in the Context of Unpaid Work and Play

Mothering in the context of unpaid work and play in families relies on parents' use of two types of strategies: segregation and inclusion. Strategies of segregation lead to time and play with children interspersed with household work; strategies of inclusion result in time and play with children embedded in household work, which are manifested as either parental participation in play within household work or scaffolded play within household work (Primeau, 1998). When parents used strategies of segregation to intersperse time and play with household work, family routines emerged sequentially throughout the day. Parents with a typical schedule of paid work (weekdays on, weekends off) almost unanimously stated that they were least likely to spend time playing with their children on weekday mornings and that weekday evenings and weekends were their most likely times to spend with their children (Primeau, 1998). For those mothers who were home on weekdays, early mornings were unlikely times for play with their children, whereas late mornings and early afternoons were more likely to be times in which they would play and interact with their children.

All parents in the study used strategies of inclusion to combine time and play with their child with their completion of household work. When asked about their play with their children or their favorite things to do with them, all mothers and half of the fathers described play embedded in household work, that is, either parental participation in play within household work or scaffolded play within household work (Primeau, 1998). Of particular interest to mothering in the context of unpaid work and play in families is parental participation in play within household work.

⚓ Parental Participation in Play within Household Work

All parents in this study, both mothers and fathers, employed parental participation in play within household work as a strategy of inclusion to embed time and play with their children in their household work. Here is an example of George engaged in play with his children within household work. As I drove my car onto their street, I saw Julia and Christian running along the sidewalk in front of their house. They were in their bathing suits and George was sprinkling them with the hose as he watered the lawn. I parked the car across the street from their house. Julia stopped running away and watched as I walked over to their front yard and greeted George. He had turned the hose back onto the grass while he greeted me. I laughed as I watched the kids. They had run away from George and the hose during his last sprinkle and were now stopped just outside the immediate reach of the hose. They were baiting their father by saying, "Neener, neener, neener, Daddy! You can't get me!" as they started to slowly walk back within range of the hose. George pretended not to notice them and then suddenly lifted the hose from the grass to sprinkle them. This action sent the kids running down the sidewalk again out of the water's reach.

Linda also played with her children while engaged in household work. I observed her one day while she was cleaning the house. She was dancing and swaying to music turned up loud on the stereo system as she was vacuuming and keeping a close eye on her daughters. While still engaged in her work, she initiated play with her 3-year-old daughter, Katlyn, who had picked up a leather belt from the floor. Linda said, "Oh, that's Daddy's belt. Can you take it upstairs and put it in his closet?" Katlyn walked over and tried to give the belt to me, leaving it on the stairs when I wouldn't take it. Linda picked up the belt and snapped it in the air toward Katlyn a couple of times, asking her if Daddy had taken it off to spank her with it. She tapped Katlyn's bottom with it a time or two and then told her to take it upstairs and put it away or she was going to get her with it. Katlyn squealed with anticipation as she grabbed the belt and headed over to the stairs with it in her hand. Linda chased after her, telling her that she was going to get her and use the belt on her if she didn't go and put it away now. Katlyn got partway up the stairs, turned around, and snapped the fully-extended belt in Linda's direction. Linda said, "Oh, you're not going to get me with that. I'm going to get you! I'm going to get you!" She made a small charge up the stairs after Katlyn, who turned and ran farther up. Linda continued to tell her that she'd better get going or she was going to get her. Both Linda and Katlyn were laughing and it was obvious that they were playing a familiar game.

As I watched this play episode, I noted that Linda's play with Katlyn was directed toward getting her to comply with her request to put the belt away. As such, it was embedded in Linda's work of cleaning the house. The instrumental use of pretend play by mothers in the context of household chores and caregiving to proactively manage their children's behavior and to negotiate problematic interactions has been documented (Haight, Masiello, Dickson, Huckeby, & Black, 1994). Kim explained her rationale for using play in this manner:"I think sometimes I'll use play to diffuse a situation. I'm not sure that that's really appropriate, but that's what happens. Obviously, their attention spans are the big key to a lot of things, and the longer you are somewhere, the harder it is to keep them focused.… [The other day] I took them out to lunch.… They had the best lunch, but then, towards the end, I was waiting for the check and they were finished with their food and they wanted to get out of there. We took the sugar packets and we were building things. I mean you just have to make stuff up sometimes. Otherwise, they would have probably kicked us out of the restaurant because we were being so obnoxious… You make it a game like that and that seems to work a lot better."

Parental participation in play embedded in household work occurred during both housework and childcare, but it occurred most often while parents were engaged in childcare tasks. I observed examples of play embedded within childcare occupations throughout the daily routines of the families. Although most parents said that play with their children did not occur in the early mornings, I observed Susan introduce play in what seemed to be an attempt to wake up her 3-year-old son, Michael, during a weekday early morning visit. It was 5:45 AM when she woke him up and brought him out to the living room. After a few minutes, she turned on the television as she said, "Should we see if there are any cartoons on? Do you think there will be cartoons on this morning?" With Michael watching closely, she started at Channel 2 and flipped up through the channels. Channel 9 had cartoons, but Susan went right past it to Channel 10. Michael gasped. She kept changing the channels, saying, "Oh, those aren't cartoons." Michael shouted, "Cartoons!" She laughed, "Oh, were those cartoons?" as she flipped back to Channel 9.

Later, when Michael had awakened, he was ready to initiate play on his own. But the time was approaching when they had to leave the house, and Susan had a different agenda. Michael was engrossed in the cartoons on TV and had not eaten his cereal. Susan said, "You need to eat. Do I need to turn off the TV so that you can eat?" He replied quickly, "No," and began to eat his oatmeal. Later, as Susan rushed to get out of the house, already behind schedule, she again intervened in his attempts to play. Michael was reaching for a toy as Susan was putting on his shoes and brushing his hair. She took it from him just as he was getting

ready to play with it and pushed it farther back on the coffee table. She told him in an almost pleading tone that they needed to go now and that he could play with it tonight when they got home.

During this observation, I noted that Susan participated in play with Michael within the work of preparing him for preschool, but each time this play interfered with her agenda of getting him ready for school, she set limits on it. Susan was clearly using play to facilitate the accomplishment of her mothering work. This early-morning visit underscored the parents' statements that there was little time for play during workday early mornings. One exception to this general rule occurred within a nontraditional family in which the husband worked in real estate sales. His early mornings were less hectic than other parents' mornings because his days started later and he was usually not required to start work at a specific time. Here is an example of his participation in play embedded in childcare. As David, the father. brushed his daughter Kristin's hair, she watched a children's show on television. The television characters were singing a song about working for a mean boss who told them to push buttons all day long. The song had five choruses and progressed to pushing the button with the right hand, the left hand, the right foot, the left foot, and the tongue. Both Kristin and David sang along with the song and completed its required actions. David's participation interrupted his work with her hair. The song became quite silly, and they laughed as they moved their arms, legs, and tongues as if pushing buttons on a machine. When the song was over, David and Kristin stopped their various gyrations and he returned to styling her hair.

Among families in which both parents participated in paid work, once the children and parents were ready to leave the house, the next childcare occupation was the commute to day care or preschool. Seven parents, six mothers and one father, mentioned commuting time when I asked about their play with their children. Four mothers specifically stated that it was one of their favorite things to do with their children. Although Haight and colleagues (1994) found that mothers frequently engaged in pretend play while in the car with their children, the majority of the play embedded in commuting identified in this study consisted of verbal play or talking with the child, listening to music, singing, and playing learning and memory games. Stuart and Monique both described participating in verbal play and singing while taking their daughter Bridget to and from her day care.

Susan talked about what she enjoyed during her commuting time with Michael: "The time we drive back and forth to school is real nice. I ask him how his day was and what he did, that kind of stuff…. Because it's our time. It's just he and I… And it's when he's relaxed, I'm relaxed. And it's 15 minutes, we can just listen to music or just talk about things and what we're going to do that night and stuff like that. It's nice." Another mother, Carol, expressed similar sentiments about commuting with her son, Greg, "Riding in the car with him! Oh! It's so much fun. Oh, my gosh, I love being in the car with him. I think because I'm away from my house. Okay, oh, major revelation: my best play times with him, I think, are when I'm away out of the house. I have no phone calls. I have no laundry staring at me. No dusting. In the car when it's just the two of us, and Paul's even said the same thing, it is so awesome just to hear what he says about the cars or the people. We talk just so much more in the car. There's something about it. I guess it's kind of cozy."

In contrast to play embedded in commuting with their children, which seemed to be relaxed and enjoyable to the parents because of the absence of other demands besides driving and playing, play embedded in many physical mothering tasks seemed to have a facilitative purpose. Parental participation in their children's play was a way of accomplishing the work inherent in these tasks. Generally, most parents did not encourage or participate in play with their children during mealtimes except in their efforts to get them to eat. Here is an example of Linda's participation in play with her daughter during mealtimes. Katlyn started to make roaring noises. Linda told her that she was getting good at that and asked her if she could take a big roaring bite for her. She made the same roaring sound that Katlyn had

been making. Katlyn picked up her sandwich and roared as she took a big bite of it. Linda said, "Oh, that was a big one!" (Fig. 6–2)

Sometimes I observed a situation in which the parents looked as if they wanted to suppress their children's play during mealtimes, but did not because it facilitated their children's eating. During one of my visits, Carol stopped short of telling Greg not to play while eating his dinner, but reminded him to watch his manners. Greg picked up a piece of pasta, stuffed it into his mouth, and chomped on it with his mouth open. He picked up a second piece of pasta and held it up to his mouth. It looked as if Carol was getting ready to caution him about eating with his mouth open when he said, "Watch me take a monster bite!" He bit the pasta piece in half and chomped on it. He stuffed the remaining piece in his mouth. Carol smiled as she reminded him not to chew with his mouth open.

In another example from my field notes, Jennifer introduced play in what seemed to be an effort to avoid eating her lunch. Her father, Mike, appeared to be an unwilling participant in her play as he tried to ensure that she ate more of her sandwich. Although their play was mutual, it was at cross purposes. Jennifer became more resistant to eating than she had been before. As Mike offered her the sandwich, she turned her head away from him. When he moved so that the sandwich was in front of her mouth again, she pressed her lips together and giggled through them. She refused to open her mouth to take a bite. Her refusals to eat seemed to be almost play or teasing. Mike also seemed to play for a moment by laughing with her as she giggled, but then he became intent upon getting her to take a bite. He would tell her to open her mouth wide and she would do so, only to close it just as he tried to put the sandwich inside it. She giggled each time they did this. During this play sequence, he affectionately called her "Goofy" a couple times as he tried to get her to comply with his requests to eat. Mike continued to try until he was able to get her to take another bite of the sandwich.

A particularly playful sequence occurred during Linda's attempts to clip Katlyn's fingernails. Katlyn had been playing in the water at

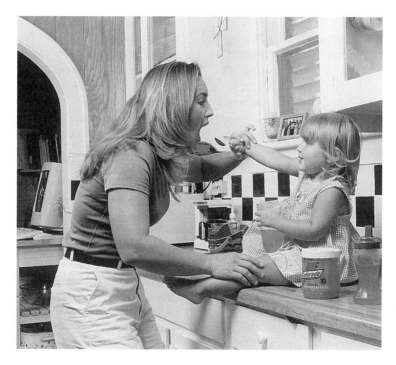

Figure 6–2 *This mother is using a strategy of inclusion to embed play with her daughter in the childcare occupation of feeding.*

the kitchen sink and was resistant to having her fingernails clipped. Similar to Jennifer, she seemed to be using play to avoid doing what her mother wanted her to do. Katlyn was trying to grab the nail clippings from her mother, giggling nonstop as she did so. Linda joined in Katlyn's play, racing with her to see who would get custody of the clippings. When Linda had finished with Katlyn's left hand, she tried to start cutting the fingernails on her right hand. Katlyn refused to let her have her hand and kept pulling it away from her mother while she giggled heartily. Linda protested loudly and in a playful manner. Katlyn laughed as she hid her hand behind her back. Linda poked at Katlyn's stomach as she commented on how giggly she was. She teased her, "Why are you so giggly? Did you have giggle juice this morning?" Katlyn didn't reply as she giggled uncontrollably.

Bath time was one childcare occupation in which the parents' participation in play was not as subject to their ulterior motivations as others were. Eight parents, four fathers and four mothers, talked about bath time with

their children as being a fun experience. Two fathers and one mother identified play embedded in bath time as one of their favorite things to do with their children. I observed David bathing his daughter Kristin on two separate occasions. Both times he embedded play in the work involved. Here is an example. Kristin asked David if he would make her a mustache and a beard. He took the funny foam soap and squirted it on her so that it formed a beard and mustache. Kristin asked him to get a mirror for her so that she could see what she looked like. He finished his artwork on her face and brought her the mirror. He said, "Oh, I think you need some eyebrows." He told her to put her head back and he squirted some eyebrows on her. As she continued to look at herself in the mirror, David asked, "Should we put a horn on you? Let's give you a horn." He squirted a dollop of soap on her head. He said, "Now, you look like a unicorn." She laughed as she looked at herself in the mirror. After a few more minutes, David told Kristin that it was time to wash her up and get her out of the tub.

Most of the families in this study had familiar bedtime rituals, which often included reading a story to the children. A couple of families incorporated television or videotapes into the occupation of settling their children into sleep. Some of the families' bedtime rituals were elaborate or lengthy; some were not. A few parents waited until the children were sleepy to put them into their beds and then sang a lullaby before leaving them to sleep. Some children were allowed to fall asleep in "Mommy's and Daddy's bed," watching television or videotapes. One child was tucked into his bed with a book and a read-along cassette tape and player and was left to settle himself into sleep. All of the children were kissed goodnight and given some type of night light to allay any fears of the darkness that they might have.

One family's bedtime ritual included "10 kisses" that were exchanged every night. I overheard this ritual, as it occurred in the child's bedroom upstairs, from my post at the bottom of the stairs. Paul (the father) said, "Ten kisses! 1, 2, 3, 4, 5, 6, 7, 8, 9, 10!" with a kiss falling on the number 10. Greg giggled and shouted, "No! No! No!" Paul counted again, this time loudly kissing Greg on numbers 9 and 10. This game continued for a couple of minutes, with Paul stopping short of giving Greg his 10 kisses each time. Greg's protests were vocal and the play eventually degenerated into noisy kisses and loud giggling from both father and son.

Playful interactions such as this one that occurred in the context of housework and childcare are examples of the ways in which both mothers and fathers mother their children. Parents used strategies of segregation and inclusion (Primeau, 1998) to intersperse time and play with their children throughout their daily routines of unpaid work and to embed play with their children in their unpaid work.

♪ Conclusion

Mothering is defined as the physical and psychological nourishment and protection of children. Both mothers and fathers engage in mothering on a daily basis in the context of unpaid work and play in families. Families' divisions of unpaid work, traditional or nontraditional, provide a foundation upon which mothering in the context of unpaid work and play in families is based. In the literature on divisions of household work, it is clear that women are still completing the majority of unpaid work in the home, including childcare, regardless of whether or not they participate in paid work. Findings from my study, however, indicate that families lie on a continuum of traditional to nontraditional divisions of work, depending on parents' gender ideologies and gender practices. Families along this continuum divide the work required to nourish and protect their children in many different ways, which leads to diverse patterns of mothering.

Linda and Sam, who shared a traditional gender ideology, demonstrated traditional gender practices and, specifically, a mothering pattern of maternal responsibility and paternal assistance. Fathers' abdication of responsibility for their children when mothers are present, their strategy of passive resistance to participation in household work—waiting to be asked and hoping not to be—and mothers' assumption of almost sole responsibility for household work with few requests for help are characteristic of this pattern of mothering.

Although, at first glance, Susan and Bill seemed to share an equalitarian gender ideology, their sole reliance on equity, rather than a mix of equity and equality, required them to negotiate a compromise in their gender practices and, thereby, their pattern of mothering. They shared a traditional gender ideology in which they both expected Susan to identify primarily with unpaid work in the home and Bill to identify primarily with paid work. While Bill did not abdicate his responsibility for mothering, his primary identification with paid work frequently released him from mothering.

Monique and Stuart also shared a traditional gender ideology in which they each expected Stuart to have primary responsibility in paid work and Monique to have primary responsibility at home. Their circumstances, however, required them to be reluctant participants: Monique in paid work and Stuart in unpaid work. Their story elucidated four key features of gender ideologies that lead to traditional gender practices and patterns of mothering. First, women and men often perceive men's participation in household work as a response to women's personal needs and a personal favor to them. Second, men's incompetence in caring for children, when compared to women, is often used as a gender-specific justification for their decreased participation in mothering. Third, women's acceptance of this gender-specific justification perpetuates traditional gender practices in their families. And, fourth, many women hold deeply ingrained beliefs that household work, and particularly childcare, is their primary responsibility. The strength of these socially constructed beliefs also perpetuates traditional gender practices and patterns of mothering.

Kim and George shared a traditional gender ideology, but, unlike Monique, Kim had a strong desire to participate in paid work outside the home. George accommodated her desire by sharing childcare; therefore their pattern of mothering differed significantly from that of the other couples presented here. George's use of a sports analogy to describe his experience of mothering demonstrated how men are able to incorporate their ways of knowing and being into mothering. Men's discovery and acknowledgment of their own mothering beliefs and practices will render justifications of lack of training, experience, and competence in childcare obsolete and lead to the celebration of men's ways of mothering as different and distinct from women's ways of mothering.

When we consider mothering in the context of unpaid work and play in families, we find that parents use strategies of segregation and inclusion to spend time and play with their children. Parents used strategies of segregation to intersperse time and play with their children with household work, leading to sequential family routines throughout the day. Parents used strategies of inclusion to embed time and play with their children within household work. Interestingly, all the parents in my study, both mothers and fathers, engaged in parental participation in play within

household work. This type of play occurred in both housework and childcare tasks, but was seen most often during childcare tasks. Frequently, play was used by the parents to facilitate their accomplishment of the work, particularly the physical tasks, involved in mothering. I often observed parents playing with their children during feeding, dressing, bathing, and putting the children to bed at night. These data demonstrate that mothering, by both mothers and fathers, occurs in the context of unpaid work and play in families. (Fig. 6–3)

We can draw two major conclusions from this chapter that will expand our understanding of mothering and enhance our work with families. First, families resolve the dilemma of how to accomplish the work required to nourish and protect their children in diverse ways. Each family's division of unpaid work in the home is unique, depending on their gender ideologies and gender practices. Second, because mothering occurs in the context of

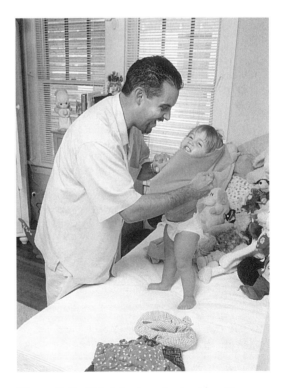

Figure 6–3 *This father's mothering is readily apparent in his play with his daughter, which is embedded in the physical work of getting her dressed.*

unpaid work and play, all fathers, whether traditional or nontraditional, mother in some
way, shape, or form. Fathers' mothering is
most readily apparent in their play with their
children while engaged in childcare tasks.
Thus, I have answered the question with which
I began this chapter: Don't fathers mother
too? Yes, indeed, they do!

Discussion Questions 🐛

■ To which gender ideology do you subscribe:
traditional or nontraditional/egalitarian?

■ How is your gender ideology enacted in your
gender practices and/or your pattern of mothering?

■ How does your understanding of mothering in
the context of unpaid work and play in families affect your thinking about or your work
with families?

References

Akram-Lodi, A. H. (1996)."You are not excused from
cooking.": Peasants and the gender division of labor in
Pakistan. *Feminist Economics, 2,* 87–105.

Atkinson, M. P., & Blackwelder, S. P. (1993). Fathering in
the 20th century. *Journal of Marriage and the Family, 55,*
975–986.

Averett, S. L., Gennetian, L. A., & Peters, H. E. (2000).
Patterns and determinants of paternal child care dur-
ing a child's first three years of life. *Marriage & Family
Review, 29,* 115–136.

Barnett, R. C., & Baruch, G. K. (1988). Correlates of fathers' participation in family work. In P. Bronstein &
C. P. Cowan (Eds.). *Fatherhood today: Men's changing role
in the family* (pp. 66–78). New York: John Wiley & Sons.

Baxter, J. (2000). The joys and justice of housework.
Sociology, 34, 609–631.

Baxter, J. (1997). Gender equality and participation in
housework: A cross-national perspective. *Journal of
Comparative Family Studies, 28,* 220–247.

Beckwith, J. B. (1992). Stereotypes and reality in the division of household labor. *Social Behavior and Personality,
20,* 283–288.

Bergen, E. (1991). The economic context of labor allocation: Implications for gender stratification. *Journal of
Family Issues, 12,* 140–157.

Berk, S. F. (1985). *The gender factory: The apportionment of
work in American households.* New York: Plenum.

Bittman, M. (1999). Parenthood with penalty: Time use
and public policy in Australia and Finland. *Feminist
Economics, 5,* 27–42.

Bolak, H. C. (1997). When wives are major providers:
Culture, gender, and family work. *Gender & Society, 11,*
409–433.

Cernigoj-Sadar, N. (1989). The other side of employed

parents' life in Slovenia. *Marriage and Family Review,
14,* 69–80.

Coltrane, S. (1996). *Family man: Fatherhood, housework,
and gender equity.* Oxford, UK: Oxford University Press.

Coltrane, S. (1990). Birth timing and the division of labor in dual-earner families: Exploratory findings and
suggestions for future research. *Journal of Family Issues,
11,* 157–181.

Daly, K. (1994). Uncertain terms: The social construction
of fatherhood. In M. L. Dietz, R. Prus, & W. Shaffir
(Eds.). *Doing everyday life: Ethnography as human lived experience* (pp. 170–185). Mississauga, ON: Copp Clark
Longman.

Daly, K. (1993). Reshaping fatherhood: Finding the models. *Journal of Family Issues, 14,* 510–530.

Dempsey, K. (1997, Spring/Summer). Women's perceptions of fairness and the persistence of an unequal division of housework. *Family Matters, 48,* 15–19.

Deutsch, F. M., & Saxon, S. E. (1998). Traditional ideologies, nontraditional lives. *Sex Roles, 38,* 331–362.

Dienhart, A. (2001). Make room for Daddy: The pragmatic potentials of a tag-team structure for sharing
parenting. *Journal of Family Issues, 22,* 973–999.

Domestic workers take day off. (2000, July 23). *Houston
Chronicle,* p. 31A.

Ehrenberg, M. F., Gearing-Small, M., Hunter, M. A., &
Small, B. J. (2001). Childcare task division and shared
parenting attitudes in dual-earner families with young
children. *Family Relations, 50,* 143–153.

Ehrensaft, D. (1987). *Parenting together: Men and women
sharing the care of their children.* New York: Free Press.

Ferree, M. M. (1991a). Gender, conflict, and change:
Family roles in biographical perspective. In W. Heinz
(Ed.), *Theoretical advances in life course research* (pp.
144–161). Weinheim, FRG: Deutcher Studien Verlag.

Ferree, M. M. (1991b). The gender division of labor in
two-earner marriages: Dimensions of variability and
change. *Journal of Family Issues, 12,* 158–180.

Gibbs, N. R. (1993, June 28). Bringing up father. *Time,*
52–56, 58, 61.

Gilbert, L. A. (1985). *Men in dual-career families: Current realities and future prospects.* Hillsdale, NJ: Lawrence
Erlbaum.

Gunter, N. C., & Gunter, B. G. (1990). Domestic division
of labor among working couples: Does androgyny
make a difference? *Psychology of Women Quarterly, 14,*
355–370.

Haas, L. (1992). *Equal parenthood and social policy: A study
of parental leave in Sweden.* Albany, NY: State University
of New York.

Haight, W. L., Masiello, T., Dickson, K. L., Huckeby, E., &
Black, J. E. (1994). The everyday contexts and social
functions of spontaneous mother-child pretend play
in the home. *Merrill-Palmer Quarterly, 40,* 509–522.

Hochschild, A. (1989). *The second shift: Working parents
and the revolution at home.* New York: Viking.

Kamo, Y. (1994). Division of household work in the
United States and Japan. *Journal of Family Issues, 15,*
348–378.

Kimball, G. (1988). *50-50 parenting: Sharing family rewards
and responsibilities.* Lexington, MA: D. C. Heath.

Komter, A. (1989). Hidden power in marriage. *Gender & Society, 3,* 187–216.

Krizkova, A. (1999). The division of labour in Czech households in the 1990s. *Czech Sociological Review, 7,* 205-214.

Lamb, M. E. (1987). Introduction: The emergent American father. In M. E. Lamb (Ed.), *The father's role: Cross-cultural perspectives* (pp. 3–25). Hillsdale, NJ: Lawrence Erlbaum.

LaRossa, R. (1988). Fatherhood and social change. *Family Relations, 37,* 451–457.

Lareau, A. (2000). My wife can tell me who I know: Methodological and conceptual problems in studying fathers. *Qualitative Sociology, 23,* 407–433.

Lu, Z. Z., Maume, D. J., & Bellas, M. L. (2000). Chinese husbands' participation in household labor. *Journal of Comparative Family Studies, 31,* 191–215.

Major, B. (1993). Gender, entitlement, and the distribution of family labor. *Journal of Social Issues, 49,* 141–159.

Marsiglio, W. (1993). Contemporary scholarship on fatherhood: Culture, identity, and conduct. *Journal of Family Issues, 14,* 484–509.

McFarlane, S., Beaujot, R., & Haddad, T. (2000). Time constraints and relative resources as determinants of the sexual division of domestic work. *Canadian Journal of Sociology, 25,* 61–82.

McKeering, H., & Pakenham, K. I. (2000). Gender and generativity issues in parenting: Do fathers benefit more than mothers from involvement in child care activities? *Sex Roles, 43,* 459–480.

McMahon, A. (1998). Blokus Domesticus: The sensitive new age guy in Australia. *Journal of Australian Studies, 56,* 147–157.

Owen, K. (1995, February 20). U.S. dads lag in child-care duties, global study finds. *Los Angeles Times,* p. A5.

Primeau, L.A. (2000a). Divisions of household work, routines, and child care occupations in families. *Journal of Occupational Science, 7,* 19–28.

Primeau, L. A. (2000b). Household work: When gender ideologies and practices interact. *Journal of Occupational Science, 7,* 118–127.

Primeau, L. A. (1998). Orchestration of work and play within families. *American Journal of Occupational Therapy, 52,* 188–195.

Rattiner, S. L. (2000). *Women's wit and wisdom.* Mineloa, NY: Dover Publications.

Robinson, J. P., & Milkie, M. A. (1998). Back to the basics: Trends in and role determinants of women's attitudes toward housework. *Journal of Marriage and the Family, 60,* 205–218.

Robinson, J. P., & Spitze, G. (1992). Whistle while you work? The effect of household task performance on women's and men's well-being. *Social Science Quarterly, 73,* 844–861.

Roman, C. (1999). Not from love alone: Power and the division of housework. *Sociologisk Forskning, 36,* 33–52.

Roopnarine, J. L., Brown, J., Snell-White, P., Riegraf, N. B., Crossley, D., Hossain, Z., & Webb, W. (1995). Father involvement in child care and household work in common-law dual-earner and single-earner Jamaican families. *Journal of Applied Developmental Psychology, 16,* 35–52.

Sanchez, L., & Hall, C. S. (1999). Traditional values and democratic impulses: The gender division of labor in contemporary Spain. *Journal of Comparative Family Studies, 30,* 659–685.

Schwartz, P. (1994). *Peer marriage: How love between equals really works.* New York: Free Press.

Shaw, S. M. (1988). Gender differences in the definition and perception of household labor. *Family Relations, 37,* 333–337.

Shelton, B. A. (1992). *Women, men, and time: Gender differences in paid work, housework, and leisure.* Westport, CT: Greenwood Press.

Thompson, L. (1991). Family work: Women's sense of fairness. *Journal of Family Issues, 12,* 181–196.

Thorne, B. (1992). Feminism and the family: Two decades of thought. In B. Thorne & M. Yalom (Eds.), *Rethinking the family: Some feminist questions* (rev. ed., pp. 3–30). Boston: Northeastern University.

Webster's II new Riverside dictionary. (1984). New York: Berkley Books.

Wilson, F. (1999). Genderquake? Did you feel the earth move? *Organization, 6,* 529–541.

Zhang, C., & Farley, J. E. (1995). Gender and the distribution of household work: A comparison of self-reports by female college faculty in the United States and China. *Journal of Comparative Family Studies, 26,* 195–205.

CHAPTER 7

Teenage Mothers: Roles, Occupations, and Societal Challenges

Doreen Y. Head, MS, OTR and Susan A. Esdaile, PhD, MAPS, AccOT,

OTR, SROT

Introduction
> *The Authors*
> *Teenage Mothers: A Social Context*

Background Information
> *Societal Issues*
> *Education and Poverty*
> *Health Issues*
> *Race and Class*

The Interviews
> *What We Did*
> *What We Found*
> *Interviews With Staff Members*
> *Limitations and Implications*

Conclusion

Anticipated Outcomes

We anticipate that, after reading this chapter, readers will:

- Have an increased understanding about societal attitudes and prejudices regarding teenage mothers
- Have considered the significance of educational disadvantage associated with poverty in relation to teenage mothers
- Have an awareness of the health risks associated with teenage pregnancy and motherhood in the context of social deprivation
- Be able to contribute to program development to assist teenage mothers and teenagers at risk of becoming pregnant

Introduction

In this chapter we present an overview of social, educational, and health issues that affect teenage mothers in affluent western cultures, in particular the United States. We focus on the experience of single teenage mothers who are at risk of continuing social disadvantage and health problems because of poverty and limited education. We describe a small, exploratory, phenomenological study, conducted in an urban school for pregnant teenagers and teenage mothers to illustrate the issues raised. In conclusion, we invite the reader to consider the implications for future research and practice and consider how affluent societies may help to bridge the gap of disadvantage that exists for many single teenage mothers.

The Authors

I (Doreen Head) became interested in this topic because of several life experiences. I was raised in the urban area of Detroit, Michigan, in a neighborhood where many of my childhood friends became parents during their teenage years. As I began my career as an occupational therapist, I worked with adolescents in a long-term mental health treatment facility where pregnancy and other reproductive health issues were major treatment themes. As a graduate student working on my Master of Science degree in occupational therapy, I developed a resource guide for pregnant teenagers (Pritchard, 1995). This was a part of my clinical work, which involved assisting parenting adolescents who were at a higher risk for physical, mental, developmental, educational, and socioeconomic problems.

I (Susan Esdaile) am interested in this topic as an extension of my feminist, phenomenological perspective and the value that I place on giving voice to socially and economically disadvantaged women who are frequently at risk of being marginalized and trivialized (e.g., Olson & Esdaile, 2000; Polakow, 1993). The research participants whom we describe in this chapter are all African-American, a cultural heritage shared by one of us, Doreen Head. However, both of us are relative newcomers and novices in regard to the rich and complex body of African-American feminist scholarship. We acknowledge that this chapter is exploratory and preliminary both in terms of the research, and the knowledge we bring to examine it.

Teenage Mothers: A Social Context

Research data related to adolescent development suggests that there is role conflict associated with teen mothering. In industrialized societies, adolescents are expected to focus on the development of their vocational roles and delay parenthood until they are financially able to support a child (Brooks-Gunn & Chase-Landsdale, 1995; Herrmann, 1989). Teenage mothers are most often represented in the context of an emphasis on the fact that they are a financial burden to the community. The United States has the highest teenage pregnancy rate in the western world. The rates are especially high among black adolescents of low socioeconomic status. Race is not necessarily a factor; rather, the persistence of poverty, joblessness, and lack of hope are the contributing factors (Innocenti Report, 2001). In the United States, more than half the Federal Welfare budget goes to women who were teens during their first pregnancy (Pierre & Cox, 1997). Being perceived as a financial burden is a contributing factor to negative attitudes about teenage mothers. Therefore, the positive qualities of many teen mothers tend to be disregarded and their individual situations or capabilities may be ignored or submerged by overall pessimistic presentation of their situation (Kelly, 2000). This negative stereotyping has a detrimental influence on the health, as well as the physical and psychosocial development, of teen mothers. There are long-term risk factors for the teen mother, who may not be able to move beyond a cycle of poverty and educational disadvantage that will further curtail the future welfare of her child and subsequent children. Therefore it is important to focus health and educational efforts not only on prevention of pregnancy, but also on assisting teenage mothers to become skilled, responsible, healthy adults (Flanagan, 2001; Kelly, 2000).

✒ Background Information

Societal Issues

In western cultural traditions, single teenage mothers, have always been regarded with disapproval and perceived as a threat to morality and a drain on community resources. Their treatment has been both harsh and punitive unless the father of the child could be identified and was willing to marry the mother (Ulrich, 1990). These historically discriminatory attitudes and what we would now consider unlawful practices continued to traumatize single teenage mothers into the 1970s. Coercing mothers to give up their children for adoption and not even allowing them to see their infants was common practice up to the 1970s. Many of these mothers lacked the resources and support to withstand medical and social coercion. The long-term mental health problems that resulted from their traumatic birthing experiences and forced separation from their infants is now documented and better understood (Bye, 2001).

Although single teenage mothers in the 21st century are less likely to be forced into having their infants adopted against their will, they remain disadvantaged and experience prejudice regardless of their level of personal competence. The case of Amanda Lemon, a student with a 3.8 grade point average, illustrates this point (Kelly, 2000). Her scholastic abilities and

… community volunteer work caused her to be invited to join the local chapter of the National Honor Society, but that decision was reversed on the grounds that the graduating senior was also a mother. The existence of her child was proof that Amanda Lemon had engaged in sex, which was reason enough for her teachers who made up the honor society selection committee to rule her inadequate in the character department (Kelly, 2000, p. 1).

Kelly (2000), who is a feminist ethnographer and educator, argues in favor of inclusive schooling, in which the additional services that teenage mothers need are offered within the structure of the mainstream school system. She considers it discriminatory to group students for different instruction based on pregnancy and parenthood. This is a point of view the reader may want to reflect on after reading the account of the interviews in this chapter because the participants involved were students and teenage mothers in a special school. Kelly also provides an illuminating analysis of the insidious nature of social discourse about teenage mothers that obscures the real issues of unequal power based on age, gender, class, and race. People who are poor, young, female, and undereducated are most often disempowered.

Education and Poverty

Two recent reports from the United Nations Children's Fund Innocenti Research Centre on teenage births in rich nations (Innocenti, 2001) and educational disadvantage in rich nations (Innocenti, 2002) provide extensive empirical data to support the fact that teenage

parenthood is "a significant disadvantage in a world which increasingly demands an extended education, and in which delayed childbearing, smaller families, two-income households, and careers for women are increasingly becoming the norm." (2001, pp. 5–6). The United States teenage birth rate of 52.1 million per year is the highest in the developed world, and about four times the European Union average, despite some decrease in the incidence of teenage births during the past decade. Giving birth as a teenager is strongly associated with disadvantage in later life because the "statistics suggest that a teenage mother is more likely to drop out of school, to have no, or low qualifications, to be unemployed or low-paid, to live in poor housing conditions, to suffer from depression, and to live on welfare" (2001, p. 3). For these reasons and because the children of teenage mothers are at greater risk of continuing to live in poverty becoming the victims of abuse or neglect, and later becoming involved in crime or drug abuse, teenage births are viewed as a burden on society. This is one of the main reasons why great effort is made to prevent teenage births in the majority of advanced countries. In countries such as the Netherlands, where sex education is comprehensive, and contraceptives are freely available, teenage births are among the lowest of the 28 rich countries included in the Innocenti Report (2001). Other factors such as the free availability of abortion, for example, in Japan, also contribute to low teenage births.

"For some time, a significant section of public and political opinion in the United States has argued that sexual abstinence is the only appropriate sex-education message for unmarried teenagers. Contraceptive advice, the argument runs, carries the inevitable subtext that it's all right to start having sex" (Innocenti Report, 2001, p. 24). Since 1996, $ US 400 million have been spent in the United States on abstinence campaigns, and one in three American high schools has an "abstinence only" policy on sex education. In a national survey it was found that the proportion of teenage girls having sex had declined between 1991 and 1997, from 52.6 percent to 51.5 percent. Some have attributed this to the abstinence campaign. However, this is not a statistically significant decrease, and so it needs to be considered within the context of other factors. Another major influence may be the overall effect of HIV/AIDS and other sexually transmitted diseases. In the meantime, teenagers are exposed to overt sexuality from all levels of the media, which creates conflict and paradox in regard to the abstinence campaign.

It has also been argued that welfare payments to unmarried mothers encourage teenage pregnancy. The fallacy of this assumption is evidenced by the high proportion of single mothers represented in the 32.9 million people in the United States who, according to the 2001 Census, lived below the poverty threshold (Reeves & Graydon, 2003). The issues of welfare and welfare reform are discussed fully in Chapter 18 of this text. The Innocenti Report (2001) states that "Reducing teenage births provides an opportunity to reduce the likelihood of poverty, and its perpetuation from one generation to the next" (p. 2), and recommends a multipronged approach that includes comprehensive sex education and the availability of contraception and health care.

However, educational disadvantage continues to exacerbate the problems of teenage mothers. Examining relative educational disadvantage is a powerful indicator of overall education in a country. Reading, math, and science literacy of 15-year-olds and math and science achievement of 8th grade students were used to assess levels of education across 24 rich member countries of the Organisation for Economic Co-operation and Development (OECD) (Innocenti, 2002). Countries were ranked by the extent of the difference in achievement between children at the bottom and the middle of each country's achievement range. Countries at the top of the range, such as Finland, Spain, Portugal, and Canada, are doing relatively well in containing inequality by not allowing their low achievers to fall too far behind average performance in the nations' schools. Countries such as the United States, Germany, New Zealand, and Belgium, at the bottom, have much wider educational gaps between low achievers and the national average. The students whom we interviewed

represent a group at the low end of this gap. They are in high school, and some are on the verge of graduating, but poverty and social disadvantage ensure that their educational achievement is below that of their peers who are not disadvantaged.

Health Issues

The health risks associated with teenage birth in the context of poverty and low educational achievement compound the problems of teenage motherhood. Many teenagers experience pressure to become sexually active, and may become sexually involved to comply, before they are emotionally or physically ready. They are at risk of becoming victims of physical and psychological abuse and contracting sexually transmitted diseases (Wiseman, 2002). "Every year some 3 million American teenagers contract a sexually transmitted infection (about 1 in every 4 sexually experienced teenagers). Approximately a quarter of all new cases of HIV/AIDS are diagnosed in young people under the age of 22." (Innocenti Report, 2001, p.17). Ignorance about contraception and the lack of availability of contraception appear to be major contributing factors to these dismal statistics.

Concerns about the health problems of adolescent girls have been voiced repeatedly over the past decade. Robinson (1991) called it a health crisis, pointing out that "adolescents are the only age group in this country whose mortality rate has *increased* over the past thirty years" (p. 243). The statistics she listed included several factors already mentioned, such as sexually transmitted diseases, pregnancy, poverty, abuse, including substance abuse, and low level of education. She also lists adolescents who are the victims of homicide, are injured by guns, commit suicide, or are killed in automobile accidents. The physical risks for adolescents, especially if they are already disadvantaged, are serious and extensive. Psychological damage and long-term consequences of mental illness are equally damaging and pervasive (Gilligan, 1990). We have already noted that depression is associated with teenage birth (Innocenti, 2001). Low self-esteem can also have serious long-term implications (Connolly, 1989) and act to exacerbate long-term outcomes for the teenage mother and her child or children.

Because a higher percentage of teenage mothers are already at risk because of social disadvantage, the health risks for their children are also compounded. However, the biological risk factors only apply to very young teenage mothers, 14 years and under. The risks include low birth weight and increased risk of infant mortality (Geronimus & Korenman, 1993). Poor birth outcomes for teenage mothers appear to be less directly associated with developmental status than family status, race, and ethnicity. "The findings do not support the stereotypical view that poor, black teenage mothers are the most prone to engage in unhealthy behaviors [such as smoking and drinking] during pregnancy" (p. 222) that may compromise the health of their infants. "Such behaviors were more commonly reported by white mothers and older mothers" (p. 222). A major compounding factor is that many teenage mothers, like those we interviewed, have few healthcare services available to them.

Race and Class

Although our focus is on teenage mothers, not race, because all the participants in our study are African-American, it is appropriate to include some comments about race and class. The students came from socially deprived families, and the health care personnel who worked with them are representative of middle-class, educated, professional black women. Disadvantaged black teenagers have been described in numerous reports dating back to Moynihan's controversial report published by the Office of Policy and Planning Research in the United States Department of Labor (Rainwater & Yancey, 1967). The report claimed that segregation and discrimination had not been legislated away. Although Moynihan's intent had been to draw attention to the perpetuation of inequality of resources and opportunities for black families, he has been severely criticized for presenting an idealized picture of white family stability and for his lack of scientific rigor. But, racist narratives about motherhood, poverty, and welfare continue to represent idealized myths of mother-

hood as essentially white and within nuclear families and, in contrast, represent negative images of mothering by other ethnic groups (Connolly, 2000). The birth rate for black teenagers in the United States remains high; relatively, it is twice as high as for white teenagers, and thus contributes to social and educational disadvantage (Innocenti, 2001). The fact that class and educational disadvantage, not race, are the major contributing factors to the higher incidence of births among black teenagers has been stated in many studies. However, we need to emphasize that low-income African-American adolescents can and do have the insight and agency to rewrite their negative scripts, take responsibility, focus on education for their future, and avoid early pregnancy. An important aspect of the conditions that enable girls to claim their agency is the support and involvement of parents and strong role models from the African-American community (Martyn & Hutchinson, 2001).

The inclusion of mothering in feminist discourse owes a major debt to the scholarship of black women. Patricia Hill Collins (1994) is prominent among them. She has stated that: "For women of color, the subjective experience of mothering/motherhood is inextricably linked to the sociocultural concern of racial ethnic communities—one does not exist without the other" (p. 47). In our study, the teenage mothers experienced two very different communities that are geographically linked. One is their home, where they may face struggles with poverty, crime, and abuse, in neighborhoods that are not safe. The other is their school, where they can be safe; receive education, childcare, and health care, and have positive role models. In common with many black women, the students in our study have multigenerational role models for mothering; these include grandmothers, aunts, and other caregivers (Jenkins, 1998). In the next section of this chapter, we describe our exploratory study and discuss its implications.

✍ The Interviews

Given the importance of ensuring that teen mothers develop into healthy, skilled adults who are able to take care of their child (or children), we believe that it is important to increase knowledge about the lived experience of teenage mothers. This information has the potential to enhance the formulation of appropriate programs that can ensure the healthy development of teenage mothers and their children. The purpose of our exploratory study was to ascertain, for illustrative purposes, the mothering experiences of teenage girls who are also students. We also wanted to get information from healthcare professionals who work with the teen mothers in an educational setting in order to increase our understanding about their views regarding programs to assist teenage mothers.

To start this line of inquiry, we planned an exploratory, phenomenological study (Fontana & Frey, 2000) in which we interviewed teenage mothers attending a special school and the healthcare professionals who worked with them. We were particularly interested in their occupations and roles as high school students and parents/ caregivers. The school we selected was built in 1960 as an elementary school, and converted to its current use 3 years ago. It is located in an inner-city urban area. There are 140 students enrolled, and it is free to female residents of the city in grades 7 to12. It is one of three schools that offer specialized programming for pregnant teenagers and mothers. These schools were established to keep pregnant teenagers and teenage mothers at school so that they can complete their high school education. Students are able to complete basic graduation requirements, take academic electives, and receive diplomas. In addition, classes are available that focus on childbirth preparation, mother-infant nutrition, and infant care and child development. Enrolled students may also receive meals including breakfast and lunch, prenatal care, family planning and counseling services. Day care is provided for their child or children while they attend classes. However, the school does not involve students in the range of organized, after- school, sporting, and social activities that are frequently associated with high schools. The neighborhoods surrounding the school include both ends of the economic spectrum with low-income, single homes and apartments and middle-class, moderately high-income homes.

To obtain a range of potentially relevant information for further research, we decided to use a semi-structured interview format (Fontana & Frey, 2000) and also to administer the Adolescent Role Assessment (ARA) (Black, 1976) to the teenage mothers. We chose to add this instrument to the interview questions we developed because it is congruent with the occupational focus of our perspective. In regard to the teenage mothers we planned to interview, we were interested in ascertaining if they were able to select, plan, and carry out their daily activities and getting an idea of their sense of achievement in their occupations as mothers and students. (Herrmann, 1989; Yerxa et al., 1989). In her earlier work (Pritchard, 1995), Doreen (Head) had found that, in congruence with Herrmann (1989), who had conducted a study of teenage mothers using the ARA, the teenage mothers with whom she worked demonstrated role conflicts between the developmental tasks of adolescence and their maternal roles. Another aspect of Herrmann's findings that resonated with Doreen's experience was the fact that teenage mothers had more conflict with older infants than younger ones. Because of the limitations of the ARA, and its lack of methodological robustness, Hermann had recommended using qualitative methods as well for future studies of teenage mothers.

The ARA is a semi-structured instrument that yields both quantitative and qualitative data. It is based on an occupational behavior model developed by Ginzberg (1972) and Reilly (1974). It is designed to identify movement through three stages of occupational choice and outline a progression of decision-making stages from childhood to adulthood related to worker role development. Black (1976) identified three developmental stages of occupational choice: childhood—play, adolescent—socialization, and adulthood—work. The instrument is designed to ascertain if the adolescent has acquired stage-specific skills in the occupational choice process.

The six domains of functioning (in bold type below) are identified in the ARA in four sections. The second domain, adolescent—socialization, has three subdomains (Black, 1976). The respondent is asked to answer questions related to a total of 21 items (italicized below). The domains are:

I. **Childhood—Play**, which has six items related to activities: *rules, interactions, fantasy, role models*, and *interests*

II. **Adolescent—Socialization**, which includes three subdomains:

A. Family, with three items: *interactions, responsibilities*, and *economics*

B. School, with five items: *consistency, responsibility, feedback, role models*, and *activities*

C. Peers, with three items: *activities, time,* and *community*

III. **Adolescent—Occupational Choice**, which has two items: *work* and *choice stage*

IV. **Adult—Work**, which has two items: *goals* and *fantasy*

The ARA is administered as a semi-structured interview, through casual-dialogue, which facilitates its use in conjunction with other interview questions. "To score each item, two to four structured interview questions are asked. For example, under the childhood—play domain, scoring of the 'interests' item is based on two questions: What kinds of interests did you have as a kid? How do those interests compare with current interests?" (Huebner et al., 2002, pp. 203–204). The responses to the items are contingent on the subjective judgment of the person administering the assessment. Responses are scored as a plus (+), which indicates appropriate behavior; zero (0), which indicates marginal or borderline behavior; or minus (-), which indicates inappropriate behavior.

Black (1976) stated that performance and goals and expectations are part of the "evolutionary acquisition of skills in the occupational choice process" (p. 75). She stressed that if skills are not acquired at an age-appropriate stage, later developmental stages may be adversely affected. She suggested that the ARA should be used as "an initial step in attempting to identify crucial variables for adaptive adolescent role performance" (p. 79). In our study, the ARA was used to identify the level of understanding that each girl had for her various responsibilities as a mother, daughter, student, caregiver, and teenager. We were mindful of that fact that the questions are intended to be subjective and to diminish value judgments, and that familiarity with the questions and the rating scale is essential to understanding the perception the teen mother may have of role expectations.

The ARA is not a standardized instrument, and despite its potential usefulness, there are few reported studies in which it has been used. In a recent study, Huebner, Emery, and Shordike (2002) examined the responses of 101 adolescents aged 12 to 17 years to explore the psychometric properties and theoretical usefulness of the ARA as a measure of career adaptability. They found that the internal consistency of the ARA was low, with few age-related differences. However, identified factors such as developing aspirations, self-efficacy, interpersonal competencies, and autonomy, as consistent constructs of career adaptability, differentiated between high and low scorers in congruence with related literature. In conclusion, they suggested major changes to the content and scaling of the ARA, as well as development of a new assessment of career adaptability. However, Huebner et al. acknowledged that their study should be interpreted cautiously for several reasons. These included the small sample size in comparison to the number of items in the instrument, the homogeneous nature of their subjects, and the possibilities of interviewer bias and error. They also stressed the importance of further assessment development and research related to this topic.

What We Did

Doreen Head, co-author of this chapter, interviewed the six teenage mothers at the school they attended for approximately 30 minutes each, using a semi-structured format. The mothers ranged in age from 15 to 18 years and had been recruited through the social worker at the school, with whom Doreen had professional contact through the community service component of her academic position. The questions that the students were asked are listed in Table 7–1.

After the students responded to the ques-

Table 7–1 Questions for semi-structured interviews with teenage mothers

Students were first asked to provide demographic information about their age; the age of their child or children; their living arrangement; whether they attended school; and, if so, which school, their grade, their employment status, and childcare arrangements.

Question 1.
  a. Can you describe a typical day?
  b. Can you describe an ideal day?

Question 2.
  a. Tell me about your baby.
  b. Do you find your role as a mother easier now that the baby is older, or was it easier when he or she was younger?

Question 3.
  What do you think others expect from you as a teen mom?
  Your parents?
  Other family members, grandparents, siblings, foster parents, or others with whom you live?
  Your peers?
  Your boyfriend/spouse?
  Your teacher?
  Your employer?
  Society?

Question 4.
  What are some of the ideas that you have about being a mom?

Question 5.
  Thinking about the past, present and future:
  a. Do you think that your life has changed since you became a mom?
  b. What are your plans for the next 6 to 12 months?
  c. What are your plans for the more distant future, say in 5 years?

---

tions listed in Table 7–1, Doreen administered the ARA (Black, 1976) as part of the interview schedule, using casual dialogue as recommended by Black. Scoring of the instrument took place after the interview was completed.

Doreen subsequently interviewed three health professionals (two nurses and a social worker) who work with the teenage mothers for approximately 10 to 15 minutes each, at the special school where they work. The questions they were asked are listed in Table 7–2.

The interviews were audiotaped, transcribed, and analyzed. We did this as a three-stage process of unitizing, categorizing, and forming themes (Lincoln & Guba, 1985; Morse & Field, 1995; Strauss & Corbin, 1990). In our first level of analysis, we looked for the content of what the teenage mothers and health professionals were saying, and listed it. In the next stage, we re-examined the data and looked for commonalities within each of the categories to create unifying themes that retained the meaning of the respondents' statements. We then looked for relationships and patterns among the themes and quotes from the interviews to illustrate them. Last, we examined the themes and quotes in relation to our background reading and clinical experience (Ryan & Bernard, 2000). We conducted each stage of the analysis separately, then checked with each other and fine-tuned our findings to achieve consensus. In this exploratory study, we had decided not to do member checking with the participants, but will consider doing that in further research. We had already identified the limitations of the study at its onset, but at the end of the analysis process, we clarified them again and reflected on its relevance to possible program development and future research. In the next section, we first present the demographic information about the participants and the results from scoring the ARA (Black, 1976), then

---

Table 7-2 Interview with professional staff members working with the teenage mothers

Professional staff members were asked to provide demographic information about their current role/job title, their professional qualifications and level of education, their work setting, the nature of the service they provide, whether their work with the teenage mothers was the major focus of their work, and whether they served other groups in their professional capacity.

Question 1.
  In what capacity do you work with teen mothers?

Question 2.
  Do you provide any special programs or services for teen mothers?

Question 3.
  What do you think are the most important issues to consider for people who work with teen mothers?

Question 4.
  Do you find that there are any obstacles or problems associated with working with teen mothers?

Question 5.
  a. How do you think society views teen mothers?
  b. Do you share this view?

---

proceed to present and discuss the results of the analysis we have described.

What We Found

As presented in Table 7–3, the teenage mothers' children were all toddlers or babies under 3 years old, one of the 18-year-old mothers had 2 children, and another 18-year-old was 9 months pregnant. Two of the 18-year-olds were about to graduate from school; one of the graduating seniors also worked in paid employment and the other had worked previously and wanted to work again.

Ms. Young is a clinical social worker who is responsible for the health and welfare of some of the teenage mothers. She starts to work with them while they are still pregnant, and after the birth of their babies, she makes home visits until they are ready to return to school. Ms. Smith is a nurse and educator whose primary responsibility is child health. She works in the on-site day care center of the school. There are 12 childcare providers who work with the center, and she ensures that the babies and older children stay in the system and have their immunizations up to date. She also mon-

Table 7-3 Demographic information about the teenage mothers

Teenage mother	Age in years	Child/children's age in months	Living arrangements	Education	Employment status
Nancy	15	22	With mother	Grade 9	Unemployed
Mary	18	13	With mother	Grade 10	Unemployed
Joan	18	35	Teen Support Housing Program	Graduating	Working at a school for girls
Sharon	17	17	With aunt	Grade 9	Unemployed
Diane	18	12 and 9 months pregnant	Teen Support Housing Program	Grade 12	Previously employed, currently unemployed
Marsha	18	First child 24, second child 9	With grandmother	Graduating	Unemployed

Table 7–4 Demographic information about the healthcare professionals		
Healthcare professional	Job description	Qualifications
Ms. Young	School social worker	Clinical Social Worker (CSW) Master of Social Work
Ms. Smith	School nurse	Registered Nurse BSN Master's degree in Education
Ms. Brown	School nurse	Registered Nurse Master's degree in Education

itors mother-child interaction. Ms. Brown is also a nurse and educator, and her primary responsibility is the health of the teenage mothers. She helps them with issues related to their healthcare providers and any other health issues. She and Ms. Smith often work together, and in the summer, when only one of them is employed, she takes care of the children's as well as the mothers' health concerns. Demographic information about the three healthcare professionals working with the teen mothers, whom we interviewed: Ms. Young, Ms. Smith, and Ms. Brown, is described in Table 7–4.

In Table 7–5 we present the teenage mothers' scores on only the positive response scores of the ARA (Black, 1976).

Although the girls had many positive responses and were able to verbalize role expectations related to work and parenting and to identify work goals and aspirations for the

future, several negative responses were identified. For example, in Section I, Childhood—Play, Nancy's responses were scored positively for four out of six items (4/6) and two items, not noted above, were scored negatively. Neither Nancy (4/6) nor Joan (4/6) were able to identify engagement in fantasy play and childhood interests. Nancy was also unable to identify specific social interactions with her family (2/3). Both Nancy and Mary had difficulties engaging in school activities (4/5), and Sharon had difficulty maintaining consistent behavior and grades, taking responsibility for study habits, and having assignments ready (3/5). Both Nancy and Mary had difficulty identifying time engaged in activities with peers (1/3). Being able to identify goals and expectations is part of the "evolutionary acquisition of skills in the occupational choice-process" (Black, 1976, p. 75), and if skills are not acquired at early stages, later stages may

Table 7–5 Teenage mothers' scores on the ARA (Black, 1976)						
Categories	Nancy	Mary	Joan	Sharon	Diane	Marsha
Section I Childhood—Play	+ 4/6	+ 6/6	+ 4/6	+ 6/6	+ 6/6	+ 6/6
Section II Adolescent—Socialization						
a. Family	+ 2/3	+ 3/3	+ 3/3	+ 3/3	+ 3/3	+ 3/3
b. School	+ 4/5	+ 4/5	+ 5/5	+ 3/5	+ 5/5	+ 5/5
c. Peers	+ 1/3	+ 1/3	+ 3/3	+ 3/3	+ 3/3	+ 3/3
Section III Adolescent—Occupational Choice	+ 2/2	+ 2/2	+ 2/2	+ 2/2	+ 2/2	+ 2/2
Section IV Adulthood—Work	+ 2/2	+ 2/2	+ 2/2	+ 2/2	+ 2/2	+ 2/2

be affected. Engaging in fantasy and childhood play are important aspects of development. If these experiences are absent or limited, there can be detrimental long-term effects on cognitive and language development and problem-solving abilities (Stagnitti & Unsworth, 2000).

In the first level of our analysis of the interviews, we identified the content related to the questions asked in the interviews. These included:

- Descriptions of their day
- Expectations of others (including family, school, and society)
- The girls' views on mothering and how their lives have changed since they became mothers
- Their plans for the immediate and more distant future
- What was involved in taking care of their children, including things that may be easier or harder as the children grow
- Memories of their own childhood activities
- Their thoughts on friends and other peers, school, teachers, work, and their leisure pastimes

In the second level of analysis we identified six major themes: *the ups and downs of family life; taking care of the baby; the future; work and school; friends, associates and society*; and last, *the disconnections*, to express some of the contradictions and missing connections expressed by the teenage mothers.

The Ups and Downs of Family Life

The teenage mothers described many of the positive and negative aspects of family life. Nancy talked about the way she and her sister, who also had a similar-aged toddler, shared childcare and resources: "We don't have to go clothes shopping as much because if (my child) can't fit into something, then my niece can fit into something, so we take turns." Nancy also expressed her regret about the fact that her mother works and is not there when she and her sister get home from school. "We don't see her until the weekend... that kind of hurts me a bit, because my baby don't get to see her grandmother. When she gets bored or

frustrated and stuff, she calls 'Grandma' and Grandma is not there." Then she added: "And my father, I really don't care much about" but didn't elaborate further. Mary was able to articulate the importance of a supportive family when she said, "I think it is important to know what is going on in your daughter's or son's life, because you want them to be able to come to you ... and tell you anything." She described her mother's support during her pregnancy, and described their relationship as "great... because we can talk, we can do anything."

Others were not so fortunate; for example, Joan's mother had been on drugs for 9 to 10 years. "While she was on drugs, I was left in the house by myself for 2 weeks. She like abandoned us and we had to go through Child Protection Services and all that stuff." However, Joan also identified positive aspects of her relationship with her parents. She said that during her early childhood, before her mother became a drug addict, she was there for them, but her father was not around, he was "always on the road. Now, even though he is not physically there, he's there mentally and financially, so he's there to help me. He's there, coming up to spend time with me and my baby." Joan lives in a home, which is part of a church-sponsored teen support program.

Sharon was ambivalent about living with her aunt because she felt that her aunt was very critical of her and refused to babysit during the weekend so that she could go out sometimes. However, what hurt Sharon most was the fact that she had lost her parents and grandmother, as well as two aunts. "I was 7 when my father died. I was like 10 when my mama died. I was 12 when my grandmother died. I was like 13 when my aunt died and I had an aunt that died ....it will be a year next month, on the 30th. I was 15." She went on to talk about how she frequently cries when people say that her baby looks like her mother, adding: "I wish my mama was there so she could see this baby."

Diane, who also lived in a special home for teenage girls, said that she had not respected her parents or taken any notice of their attempts to curtail her behavior. She added: "I also go to therapy for my family problems so it's like, has improved." She didn't elaborate.

Marsha, who had two children, lived with her grandmother and explained that her parents were both in jail. She said that having children had steadied her. "I am not gonna say that having my kids at a young age was good, but if I didn't have them, I know by now I would have dropped out of high school. If I dropped out of high school, I would not be living at home. I would probably be out on the streets somewhere. Before I had my kids I was just like wild. I have changed totally." She added: "They settled me down real good. I was just out there real bad, smoking and drinking. I don't do none of that now."

All the teenage mothers spoke about the fact that the family members with whom they live, or staff members in the home, expect them to take care of their babies' needs. They accepted this as part of what they had to do. They also talked about the way their siblings and cousins play with their baby but can be annoying to them. Mary's comment about her younger brothers, who seemed to love their niece and spent time with her, was typical. She said with a chuckle: "They drive you crazy, yes! (Chuckle). We try to get them out of the house."

Taking Care of The Baby

All the teenage mothers talked about taking care of their babies as part of their daily routine. Nancy said, "My mother expects me to look after her and clean up after her. Everything she messes up, I gotta clean up after her, be a mother to her." She then chuckled, as if acknowledging and accepting this. Sharon's comment was similar: "Feeding them, changing them, making sure they are clean at night, making sure they eat, they go to the doctor." For most, childcare included a very long day, getting up at 5 or 5:30 in the morning to be ready with their child for the 7 or 7:30 AM school bus. For various reasons that ranged from taking time to spend with friends and family, especially if they worked late like Marsha's grandmother, the mothers seemed to be up until around 11 at night or later. Being tired and wanting more time to sleep was mentioned by all the teenage mothers. As Mary said, "It [motherhood] is physically, emotionally, and mentally straining. It's not

that bad, but it's there, because you know you get no sleep." She went on to say that now her daughter was 13 months old, she got more sleep, but it was not enough, and her life was restricted. "I can't do the things I want to do. Things I used to do... So, it's like I can't go nowhere ..."

Although all the teenage mothers seemed to be clear about the importance of feeding their children and keeping them clean and safe, as well as playing with them, they appeared to have little understanding about developmental needs or stages of child development, or what constitutes age-appropriate play. Nancy was even quite vague about the age of her child, first describing her as a 1-year-old, then adding later that she would be 2 in less than a month. They often used words like "cute" or "mean" to describe what their children did, attributing intent to the child's actions that would not have been age-appropriate. Children's activity levels and curiosity were often described in terms of individual traits rather than seen as typical behavior for the child's age. However, they showed pride in their children, and though they found having them so young difficult, they accepted them as part of their life, and talked about having more.

Joan's comments about her 35-month-old daughter show that she was gaining insight and learning to understand her child. "One minute (A) is cool, she'll be nice and say 'Hi' to everybody, like give them a hug. The next minute she's like 'leave me alone!' But, before, like 2 months ago, she used to fight, hit people, hit kids, anything. ... The reason she was doing it is because I was aggressive with her, like when she was 6 months, I used to be real aggressive with her. That made her aggressive." Joan then went on to describe how watching another mother's abusive behavior with her 2-year-old and this mother's 4-year-old child's attempts to assist the abused toddler made her realize that she needed to be more nurturing with her own child.

The Future

The teenage mothers were clear about wanting a better life for their babies, and they saw this in terms of their own achievement, in being able to have well-paid jobs and their own houses. Joan said, "I plan that 5 years from now ... to have a house, a good job, a good family, and I'm living good." She acknowledged the relevance to this plan of continuing with her education, and added: "From now until 6 months, I hope I learn to read better." Mostly, they knew what kind of work they wanted to do in the future. Joan wanted to be a pediatrician and work with premature babies, and saw her reading difficulty as a problem she had to overcome. Others also mentioned medicine, psychology, and nursing as future career choices. Mary, who had also described the richness of her childhood fantasies, which included raining money in December for Christmas, and when she was 8 years old, planning to be the first black President of the United States, or a star basketball player, had plans that were pragmatic as well as ambitious. She identified her immediate plans quite succinctly. "My immediate plan is to get a job so I can help my mama maintain our family. For like 2 years, or a year or two from now, I plan on being out of school. ... I plan on attending college, but that's a little iffy, because, you know, I don't know that much about it." But she had not lost sight of her earlier, high aspirations, and added: "If I do get the chance, I am gonna go [to college]. I plan on going to study psychology, or law, or something, so that I can buy my mama a house."

Joan's major concern for the future was to move out of the city and be safe, away from the threat of drugs and AIDS. She saw herself in the future as married, "living in a nice big house with a car.... Show my kids that I am going to make them a happy family." She reiterated a number of times, "I just want to have a happy family." Diane also expressed concerns for her future family when she said that what she wanted was "to mold my child to be somebody better. You know what I am saying? I want better for her than I can [have]." Diane also wanted to be "a lawyer, doctor, or child psychologist." She added her reasons: "because I enjoyed working with kids all my life and kids like me cause I have a lot of patience. And for a lawyer, [because] I like to argue my point."

Only Nancy, the youngest of the teenage mothers, was vague about her future plans. She talked about watching *ER* on television and thought she might like to be a nurse. Her comment, "I go with the flow. Whatever happens, happens at that particular time," summed up her attitude.

Work and School

Most of the teenage mothers talked about working, possibly part time while they were still in high school. Immediate plans mentioned included working in a supermarket, or drug store. As Mary said: "Right now I'll do Walgreen's, McDonald's, or CVS, or something like that. But, in the future I will not be working there. I will have my law degree or my psychology degree or ... be a chef, something like that." Reflecting on the idea of being a chef, she added, "I am going to go to school to cook." But, on further reflection, she favored psychology, because "I like listening to people's problems and giving them advice that they could go by." However, her attitude toward study was unclear. She said that she spent 2 or 3 hours a week on study, "if it is an important class that I know I want to pass," but she also said, "I watch TV all the time."

Mostly, the student-mothers felt that they were doing all right at school and described their grades as As, Bs, and Cs, with some Ds. Generally, they were not failing, and most seemed to be trying to attend regularly. They also talked about making an effort to be there on time. Some of them, like Joan, were on the school honor role, but they were often ambivalent about school. As Marsha said, talking about school, "I don't know. I just lost my focus. I loved school at first, and then I am like 'It's almost time to graduate and I am just tired of school and ready to get out.' I just lost it. I don't want to do no work. I am like, I look at my progress report and it's all A's and like one B. [Now] it's all D's and C's. It ain't me at all. I can do it. But, I just don't." Wanting to do more schoolwork, but somehow not being able to push themselves to do it, was a common experience. However, they were positive about the school they were attending, especially about the special programs on nutrition and parenting that helped them with their babies.

As Diane explained, work is "necessary cause you need money." She described what she liked about work. "You be with people. I mean it's fun. If you have a job that you like, you want to go there every day. That's how it was mostly with all my jobs. I want to go there every day just to see people that you work with. So, it's good. I would like to work half-time, just to see my friends at work. I didn't [just] go to get money." However, she didn't like hard jobs such as working in a restaurant, or difficult customers. Her vocational plans for the future were to go to technical school and train to become a nursing assistant. Family members influenced her career goals: "[in our family] I have an RN [Registered Nurse], we have a doctor in the family. My auntie is an LPN [Licensed Practical Nurse]. Yeah, I got three or four people I know....I think we got one dentist."

Friends, Associates, and Society

Some of the teenage mothers made a clear distinction between friends and associates; they showed some wariness in referring to someone as a friend, which raised issues of trust. They seemed less involved with friends and peers than teenagers who participate in more organized after-school activities. As Marsha said, "I have more associates than friends." Their social sphere included family, school, and sometimes work, and often very limited contact with their immediate neighborhood. They did not feel safe outside. Joan summed it up succinctly.

> "I really don't associate with my neighborhood. You, they barely catch me outside. If I am outside, I am going to the store and I am right back. But I know for a fact that there is drug dealing going on over there and all that stuff and that kind of bothers me. I am sitting by my window watching them sell drugs on the park and there will be kids over there .... and they [the drug dealers] have kids of their own ... and I be thinking 'how can they sell drugs in front of the kids and in front of everybody else's kids?' They be out there, crack heads walking up there trying to buy drugs, and I'll be just sitting there watching. I know what they doing. But, it's like the police so shady these days, they don't care either."

Marsha's comments show the ambivalence about friends and associates and why none of the teenage mothers interviewed was familiar with the parks or other recreational facilities in their neighborhoods.

The teenage mothers were well aware of societal ambivalence about them. Mary's comment seems to speak for all the teenage mothers interviewed. "Society is awful. It's awful, and I say that because a lot of people don't understand what we go through. I mean, unless they was a teen mother... they don't understand what we are going through. Then they place a lot of blame ... 'Well, look at how young she is! Look, she got a child!' They think 'Well, is she on welfare or something and I got to pay for her?' You ain't got to pay for me! I ain't worried about you... There are good programs out there to help you out, but society expects an arm and a leg and it's too much drama for me". They understood that in the society in which they lived, you were respected for being able to take care of your own needs, especially financially, and wanted to show "them" that they could do it—take care of their child or children and themselves, doing what society expected of them. They did not want anyone to look down on them for not taking care of their own needs.

The Disconnections

In analyzing these data, one had a sense of disconnectedness that emerged like a subscript to other comments and experiences described in the interviews. Most of the teenage mothers seemed to have no daydreams. Mary was an exception, and had lots of dreams and ideas, but even for her, especially considering that she was 18 years old, there was little connection between her goals and a process for achieving them. They spent little time studying and almost none reading for pleasure. Their career aspirations were often high, wanting to be lawyers, doctors and psychologists. The possible impact of having a reading problem and studying to become a pediatrician was something that Joan seemed to understand only partially. She talked in terms of achieving her goals, both professionally and financially, and having a happy family and a large house (and even owning several houses) 5 years from now.

Disconnectedness was also expressed in the lack of trust they seemed to have in relationships. Marsha talked about the fact that the father of her two children is helpful, and supports her in taking care of them. However, she also mentioned that she had another boyfriend, wanted to make her own way, and didn't want a permanent relationship at present. She wanted first to achieve her career goals. Sharon and her aunt looked out for each other, but seemed to need some level of discord to keep a distance between them. Perhaps all the early deaths in their family made them wary of a commitment in caring. The extent of the teenage mothers' disconnectedness from what it might actually take for them to achieve their goals was made even clearer when the professionals who worked with them were interviewed.

Interviews with Staff Members

The interviews with the school staff members, who were described in Table 7–4, were subjected only to the first level of analysis because they were quite short. However, it was clear that these people worked hard to take care of the basic health needs of the mothers and babies, and that they were achieving positive outcomes with limited resources. Ms. Young described some creative ways in which she managed to find resources to assist the teen mothers with their basic child care needs when their families are not able to do it. Ms. Brown described the way in which she created opportunities to assist the teen mothers through her own involvement with other organizations. "We work with the Black Caucus, and I work as a committee member related to their teen parent conference [held recently].... We have a partnership with [B] health center, and I serve on some committees with them. They are actually trying; they have some money set aside for teen pregnancy prevention."

Doing what they can to protect the girls from abuse at home and from other associates is also a major role for the staff. Because the teen mothers are legally minors, looking out for them needs to be done with care. Ms Young said, "...because of my law enforcement background, I do try to take care of those

things and partner with the police department to get people in here to provide extra services for the students." Sometimes the abuse comes in the form of prejudice. Ms. Young gave an example. "The bus driver would not stop for the girls with their babies. They would keep going and the girls would come in late. They wouldn't allow them to bring the strollers on the bus...Comments were made by people ... 'you are too young to have a baby'."

All three of the school staff interviewed stressed that it was essential to develop trust with the teen mothers and not to be judgmental. As Ms. Young said, "I try not to judge them because I don't know what—if I were put in the same situation and same family situation— what would happen to me? And so I try and listen to their stories. I sit there and let them tell me the whole story and then we work on ways that they are comfortable with in trying to change something. ... I hope that I have enough compassion for them and the baby." Ms. Brown expressed similar sentiments: "Just understanding that this is the road that she has traveled, not necessarily a negative or positive one, but we want to help her from this point on to be able to reach all the goals and aspirations that she may have and in some cases help her make decisions as far as making some positive changes in her life." Ms. Smith expressed her acceptance of the teenage mothers and her concern for them in negotiating on their behalf, or helping them negotiate when, as teenagers attending a medical clinic, they were not taken seriously. She said, "I think people should be more understanding, more helpful, and more supportive."

Helping the teen mothers to develop basic skills in child- and self-care and life skills was another important aspect of the work done by staff in the school. Ms. Smith said, "I provide the teen moms with any type of referral that needs to be made; I assist them with making doctors appointments, interpreting prescriptions for their babies. Many of the babies have a lot of respiratory conditions such as asthma, a lot of colds, maybe bronchitis, things of that nature, so I assist them with whatever they need in regards to their baby's health." She also described helping the mothers learn how to interact positively with their babies, adding, "You need to assist them to improve their parenting skills without actually taking over because if you take over then they resent it." Ms. Brown seemed to speak for all three staff members when she said, "Most of the students, once they get here and understand that the majority of the people here are in their corner, it kind of makes a difference in their lives."

However, it was clear that they did not have enough time to do what they felt was needed. But their strong commitment kept them going. Ms. Brown said, "I think, number one, you really have to be committed and realize that there are some ups and downs and you have to want to make a difference in their lives and their children's lives."

Limitations and Implications

Limitations

We acknowledge the many limitations of this exploratory work. The interviews were short, and participants were interviewed only once. So, many issues were not explored in depth. A major issue that was only superficially addressed in the interviews was sexuality. Therefore, we really cannot say what the teenage mothers who were interviewed thought about any aspect of sexuality, including relationships, contraceptives, and sexually transmitted diseases. The time spent with the professionals was particularly limited. Therefore we again acknowledge the exploratory nature of our study. However, we also believe that this preliminary work has the potential to inform further research, and we plan to conduct more interviews with teenage mothers and staff members who work with them. We also have been encouraged by others, such as Laliberte-Rudman and Moll (2001), who recommend doing pilot interviews in preparation for more in-depth ones. We also think that the development of programs for teenage mothers and those "at risk" of becoming mothers needs to be given careful consideration to ensure that the programs are appropriate to a particular group, not based on a generalized, one-size-fits-all view of adolescents.

Implications

In the third part of the analysis, we reexamined the themes and quotes in relation to our background reading and clinical experience (Ryan & Bernard, 2000). Some overarching issues or themes that emerged were the teenage mothers' goals to have a *better future for their children* and to have a *happy family*. They also saw themselves as achieving their goals through their own work in well-paid jobs. *Extended family* and *community support* were clearly seen as very important by all the teenage mothers. Nancy described how she was sorry that her mother, who worked long hours, saw her baby only at weekends. Mary praised her mother for helping to keep the family together, and wanted to be able to buy her a house. Joan spoke of her father, who was not physically there, but was emotionally and financially supportive. Sharon deeply regretted the loss of her family and was hanging in there with her aunt, whom she respected despite some difficulties. Diane described her family influences of nurses and other health professionals on her own career choice. Marsha spoke of the steadying influence that having children had brought to her life. The positive role modeling provided by the school staff members was also an important aspect of their community (Martyn & Hutchinson, 2001). Their comments seemed to be in congruence with the opinions of black feminist scholars such as Hill Collins (1994) and Jenkins (1998), who stated that the family, including extended family and community, is considered important by women of color.

It was also evident that these teenage mothers are *doing what they have to do*. They are acknowledging their responsibilities, taking care of their babies, and knowing that society expects them to be independent. They admitted that being a teenage mother is hard, but they want to succeed. Maybe they don't always know what to do, as illustrated in the interviews with staff members in particular, but most are trying. *Doing what they had to do* is a theme that we have encountered with other women mothering under difficult circumstances, who have also, like Marsha, spoken about the steadying influence of having their children (Olson & Esdaile, 2000).

Health issues, fatigue, and *sometimes not being able to manage* also emerged as overarching themes, especially when the interviews with the teenage mothers and health care professionals were considered together. However, these problems are not unique to teenage mothers. Older, better-educated mothers, who have more financial resources, also complain about fatigue, especially because of lack of sleep; have health problems; and sometimes cannot manage. These issues are also raised in other chapters of this text, for example Chapters 3 and 6, and have been recurring topics in studies that included older, professional mothers (Esdaile & Greenwood, 1995).

There were some issues that are frequently discussed in the literature related to teenage mothers for which we did not find support in these interviews. The first was *role conflict*. The conflicts discussed were related to lack of resources, restricted time, especially for leisure activities, and fatigue, the common complaints of all mothers of young children, as we discussed previously. Is it possible that adolescent role conflict is an affluent middle-class construct that may not be experienced by young people whose lives have always held many survival challenges?

Low self-esteem, frequently described in relation to teenage mothers, was not evident in the interviews we have described. The teenage mothers had high aspirations and ambitions, but unclear ideas about ways to achieve their goals. But they envisioned themselves as achieving. We also did not find any support for literature that states that teenage mothers find their *older children more difficult than younger.* This didn't emerge from what they said; rather the contrary, for example, when Joan talked about being more understanding with her 3-year-old than she had been when her child was 6 months old.

✒ Conclusion

Teenage mothering is a complex phenomenon that, in a societal context, includes families, communities, schools, and the agencies

and services with whom a teenage mother has to interact. In this chapter, we have focused on these broader societal issues, and have attempted to give voice to the teenage mothers interviewed as they discussed childcare and school, seeking employment, surviving in tough neighborhoods, and learning new skills as mothers and students. We observed the fact that they had little time or opportunity to engage in self- and peer-focused social occupations typically seen as a major part of adolescent development in western cultures. On the other hand, we also noted that they had much in common with other, older, more affluent women who are mothering babies and toddlers.

Many important questions that are relevant to the future welfare of teenage mothers and the future of their children remain unanswered. We, as a society, need to know what educational systems can best retain teenage mothers until they complete high school. In order to break a cycle of poverty, they need to be able to attain the level of education necessary to earn realistic wages that support them. To know how this can be done, more programs need to be developed to support teenage parents, and these programs need to be carefully evaluated and modified on an ongoing basis to meet the needs of diverse individuals and communities. Doing all of this is beyond our scope; however, we look forward to exploring this topic further and learning more about the individual experiences and motives of teenage mothers because we believe that they have been the subject of much age- and gender-related generalization.

Finally, we want to thank Dr. Judy Olson for her contribution to this chapter. She provided thoughtful reflections, carefully considered advice, and encouragement in the preparation of this chapter that went well beyond her role as a coeditor of this text.

Discussion Questions 🕊

- Can you suggest any strategies that would help the teenage mothers described in this chapter to realistically reach their goals?
- What do you think about special schools for

pregnant teenagers and teenage mothers versus inclusive schooling where the resources they need are provided within a regular school system?

- How do you think that teenage mothers could be better supported to increase their knowledge about children's development and needs?

- The issue of teenage sexuality is frequently discussed in the literature. Although it did not emerge in our interviews, it is an important topic. What are your views about this issue? Support your position with unbiased, empirical evidence.

References

Black, M. M. (1976). Adolescent Role Assessment. *American Journal of Occupational Therapy, 30,* 73–79.

Brooks-Gunn, J., & Chase-Lansdale, L. (1995). Adolescent parenthood. In M.H. Bornstein (Ed.). *Handbook of parenting, Vol. 3. Status and social conditions of parenting.* Malwah, NJ: Lawrence Erlbaum, 113–149.

Bye, C. (2001). Kidnapped at birth. *The Sun Herald-Tempo,* April 1, 2001, 8–9.

Connolly, D. (2000). Mythical mothers and dichotomies of good and evil. Homeless mothers in the United States. In H. Ragoné & F. Winddance Twine (2000). *Ideologies and technologies of motherhood. Race, class, sexuality, nationalism.* New York: Routledge, 263–294.

Connolly, J. (1989). Social self-efficacy in adolescence: Relations with self-concept, social adjustment, and mental health. *Canadian Journal of Behavioural Science, 21,* 258–269.

Esdaile, S. A., & Greenwood, K. M. (1995) Issues of parenting stress: A study involving mothers of toddlers. *Journal of Family Studies. 1*(2), 153–165.

Flanagan, P. (2001). Teen mothers. Countering the myths of dysfunction and developmental disruption. In C. G. Coll, J. L. Surrey, & K. Weingarten (Eds.). *Mothering against the odds. Diverse voices of contemporary mothers.* New York: The Guilford Press, 238–254.

Fontana, A., & Frey, J. H. (2000). The interview. From structured questions to negotiated text. In N. K. Denzin & Y. S. Lincoln (Eds.). *Handbook of qualitative research (2nd Ed.).* Thousand Oaks, CA: Sage, 645–672.

Geronimus, A. T., & Korenman, S. (1993). Maternal youth or family background? On the health disadvantages of infants with teenage mothers. *American Journal of Epidemiology, 137,* 213–225.

Gilligan, C. (1990). Joining the resistance: Psychology, politics, girls and women. *Michigan Quarterly Review, 29,* 501–536.

Ginzberg, E. (1972). Toward a theory of occupational choice: A restatement. *Vocational Guidance, 20,* 169–176.

Herrmann, C. (1989). A descriptive study of daily activities and role conflict in single adolescent mothers. *Occupational Therapy in Health Care, 6*(4), 53–69.

Hill Collins, P. (1994). Shifting the center: Race, class, and feminist theorizing about motherhood. In E. N. Glenn, G. Chang, & L. R. Forcey (1994). *Mothering, ideology, experience, and agency.* New York: Routledge, 45–65.

Huebner, R. A., Emery, L.J., & Shordike. A. (2002). The adolescent role assessment: Psychometric properties and theoretical usefulness. *American Journal of Occupational Therapy, 56,* 202–209.

Innocenti Report Card (2001). A league table of teenage births in rich nations. Issue number 3. United Nations Children's Fund (UNICEF), Florence, Italy: United Nations Children's Fund Innocenti Research Centre.

Innocenti Report Card (2002). A league table of educational disadvantage in rich nations. Issue number 4. UNICEF, Florence, Italy: United Nations Children's Fund Innocenti Research Centre.

Jenkins, N. L. (1998). Black women and the meaning of motherhood. In S. Abbey & A. O'Reilly (Eds.). *Redefining motherhood. Changing identities and patterns.* Toronto: Second Story Press, 201–213.

Kelly, D. M. (2000). Pregnant with meaning. Teen mothers and the politics of inclusive schooling. New York: Peter Lang.

Laliberte-Rudman, D., & Moll, S. (2001). In-depth interviewing. In J. V. Cook (Ed.). *Qualitative research in occupational therapy.* Albany, NY: Delmar Thomson Learning, 25–51.

Lincoln, Y. S. & Guba, E.G. (1985). *Naturalistic inquiry.* Newbury Park, CA: Sage.

Martyn, K. K., & Hutchinson, S. A. (2001). Low-income African American adolescents who avoid pregnancy: Tough girls who rewrite negative scripts. *Qualitative Health Research, 11,* 238–256.

Morse, J. M., & Field, P. A. (1995). *Qualitative research methods for health professionals (2nd Ed.).* Thousand Oaks, CA: Sage.

Olson, J., & Esdaile, S. (2000) Mothering young children with disabilities in a challenging urban environment. *American Journal of Occupational Therapy, 54*(3), 307–314.

Pierre, N. J., & Cox, A. (1997). Teenage pregnancy prevention programs [Review]. *Current Opinion in Pediatrics, 9,* 310–316.

Polakow, V. (1993). *Lives on the edge. Single mothers and their children in the other America.* Chicago: The University of Chicago Press.

Pritchard, D. Y. (1995). Resource guide to community services for pregnant teens. Unpublished master's project. Department of Occupational Therapy, Wayne State University, Detroit, Michigan.

Rainwater, L. & Yancey, W. (1967). The Moynihan report and the politics of controversy. Cambridge, MA: MIT Press.

Reeves, S. & Graydon, R. (2003). Welfare, low-wage work offer single mothers few alternatives. *Habitat World, December 2002/January 2003,* 18–19.

Reilly, M. (1974). *Play as exploratory learning.* Beverly Hills, CA: Sage.

Robinson, C. R. (1991). Working with adolescent girls: Strategies to address health status. In C. Gilligan, A. G. Rogers, & D. L. Tolman (Eds.). *Women, girls and psychotherapy. Reframing the resistance.* New York: Harrington Park Press, 241–252.

Ryan, G. W., & Bernard, R. (2000). Data management and analysis methods. In N. K. Denzin & Y. S. Lincoln (Eds.). *Handbook of qualitative research (2nd Ed.).* Thousand Oaks, CA: Sage, 769–802.

Strauss, A. & Corbin, T. (1990). *Basics of qualitative research: Grounded theory techniques and strategies.* Newbury Park, CA: Sage.

Stagnitti, K. & Unsworth, C. (2000). The importance of pretend play to child development: An occupational therapy perspective. *British Journal of Occupational Therapy, 63,* 121–127.

Ulrich, L. T. (1990). *A midwife's tale. The life of Martha Ballard based on her diary 1785–1812.* New York: Vintage Books.

Wiseman, R. (2002). *Queen bees and wannabees. Helping your daughter survive cliques, gossip, boyfriends and other realities of adolescence.* New York: Crown Publishers.

Yerxa, E. J., Clark, F., Frank, G., Jackson, J., Praham, D., Pierce, D., Stein, C., & Zemke, R. (1989). An introduction to occupational science, a foundation for occupational therapy in the 21st century. *Occupational Therapy in Health Care, 6,* 1–17.

CHAPTER 8

Mothering across the Lifecourse

Elizabeth Francis-Connolly, PhD, OTR

Anticipated Outcomes

I anticipate that, after reading this chapter, readers will:

- Have "heard" the voices of women describing their mothering experiences and the meaning those experiences have for them

- Be able to describe how the occupation of mothering evolves and changes over time

- Be able to explain mothering as a social-cultural construct that changes over time as women and their children age

Introduction

Motherhood has been glorified throughout time and has become sacrosanct in American culture. It is a common subject of artists like Cassatt and Monet, who often portray mothers and children beautifully. Motherhood has also been vilified. Archaic fairy tales such as *Cinderella* and *Snow White* continue to provide powerful negative images of stepmothering (Salwen, 1990). Current media often portray negative images of teen mothers and single mothers because they do not fit the image of the two-parent family. Thus, they are depicted as financially dependent on society and as bad mothers. Many of the current heated American political debates are based on assumptions about a mothering ideal. Discourses on welfare reform, adoption policies, The Family Leave Act, and the pro-choice debate are all examples of how a motherhood ideal influences public policy.

Motherhood is a ubiquitous phenomenon. It is written, portrayed, and debated. This is not surprising, because we all have (or had) mothers. Motherhood is also a major life role for more than 85 percent of adult American women (U.S. Bureau of the Census, 1997). However, the commonness of this phenomenon masks its importance and complexity.

Motherhood is an intricate phenomenon. There is much more to mothering work than is initially revealed in literature, the arts, and polarized in political discourse.

It is just within the last 20 years that researchers have begun to focus on the subject of motherhood. It had previously been marginalized as being unworthy of study, a phenomenon taken for granted because of its commonness. Indeed, a fourth grader, after listening to his mother and me discuss my research, turned indignantly to his mother and said, "I know all about mothers; how come she got a doctorate for this?" This fourth grader's attitude is still held by many because we see mothers all around us. Fortunately, a series of social changes has shifted the research focus to parenthood and specifically to motherhood. These social changes include the second-wave feminist movement, the entry of women into the paid work force, and decreasing family size (Lupton & Barclay, 1997).

I have completed several research studies that have explored motherhood across the lifecourse, using in-depth interviewing and focus groups with over 60 women (Francis-Connolly, 1998, 1999, 2000). This chapter will discuss the findings from these studies and will illuminate how mothering evolves and changes as women and their children age.

ℒ Past Research on Motherhood

First-person accounts of motherhood emerged in the late 1960s and 1970s from second-wave feminist scholars. As more women entered the paid work force they struggled with issues of motherhood and work in a patriarchal society. Further, with women entering academia, they began to research and write about issues important to them. Betty Friedan's *The Feminine Mystique* (1963) was influential in exposing the myths of glorified housework and motherhood. Her book set the stage for reflective mothering accounts by other female writers and researchers.

Rich's book, *Of Women Born: Motherhood as experience and institution* (1976) is a classic example of the early feminist motherhood literature. Much of her book is based on self-reflection and personal journals. She describes the conflicting emotions of anger and tenderness she felt as a new mother. Oakley's book, *The Sociology of Housework* (1974), is another example of this genre. Here Oakley exposes three "Myths" of motherhood: that children need their mothers, that mothers need their children, and that motherhood is the most natural and greatest achievement in women's lives. These early first-person accounts and exposes on motherhood suggest that there was variation of motherhood images and practice. These early accounts provided the impetus to further explore motherhood. Subsequent researchers examined the perspectives of teen mothers, lesbian mothers, and motherhood from various ethnic backgrounds. Inclusive in this body of literature is a look at changing motherhood practices throughout history (Coll, Surrey, & Weingarten, 1998; Knowles & Cole, 1990).

Thurer (1994) traces images of motherhood from the prehistoric Stone Age to the present. She examines how idealized images of motherhood are reinvented as each age or social group defines motherhood anew. In tracing changing images of motherhood, Thurer notes that throughout history (with the exception of the post-World War II era) mothers seemingly had other obligations in addition to raising their children. Much of the childcare responsibilities were delegated to older children and servants.

The work of other researchers (McMahon, 1995; Knowles & Cole, 1990; Polakow, 1993) has shown the diversity of mothering practices and images. This illustrates the multiple influences (ethnicity, sexual orientation, marital status, social economic status, and cohort) on motherhood practice, suggesting that the motherhood image is fluid and changeable. Missing from the literature is an exploration of mothering beyond the early years of a child's life. Past research has focused on the early years of parenthood, with little attention paid to parenting beyond children's adolescence. Rossi and Rossi (1990) also observed the lack of research examining parenthood over the lifecourse. They noted that research is conducted at two ends of the continuum:

the transition to parenthood and adult children providing care to elderly parents. A recent book chapter entitled *Parent-Child Relationships in Adulthood and Old Age* argues that "parent-child relationships are a lifespan issue" (Zarit & Eggebeen, 1995, p. 119). Interestingly, the authors identify the "critical issues" as all relating to adult children's caregiving to aging parents. There is no discussion of parenting experience, activities involved in parenting adult children (beyond financial exchange), or how the occupation of parenting evolves and changes as children age.

My interest in examining motherhood stems from my becoming a mother at age 31 and finding the experience much different than my expectations. This was in spite of the fact that I had spent much time taking care of nieces and nephews and had even worked briefly in a neonatal intensive care unit. When I returned to graduate school and started reading the family literature, I was not only surprised to find little research on motherhood, but quite puzzled to find absolutely nothing on mothering adult children. It was as if motherhood ended after children reached adolescence and left home, and then was reestablished when parents became elderly and needed assistance from their adult children. However, from informal conversations with colleagues and observations of friends and family members, I knew that mothers of young adult children were still very much a part of their children's lives and that they still felt very much like mothers. Thus, my research has been an attempt to fill a gap in the family literature and to begin to build an understanding of how motherhood evolves and changes over the lifecourse.

↜ Perspectives on Motherhood

If we agree that motherhood is a complex phenomenon, defining this construct is not an easy task. In the literature, motherhood is defined in several different ways. In research publications dating back 20 years and more, there tends to be a traditional view of motherhood. This body of research links women's reproductive capabilities directly to motherhood. Although this biological construct is seen as outdated by current social scientists, the biology argument is often used in political discourse. Family-leave policies and adoption issues are examples of political discussion that employ a biological stance.

Another view of motherhood is from a social-learning perspective. A major emphasis of this approach is to understand the ways in which individuals think about their social experiences and how those thoughts influence behavior (Coltrane, 1998). An underlying assumption of this perspective is that if specific mothering skills are learned, mothers will then have the desired outcome of a well-behaved and happy child. A visit to any bookstore will show the enormous number of parenting books and videos. Parenting classes are common offerings at hospitals and community education centers. This social-learning perspective simplifies the work of mothering and the diversity of mother work. It implies that all mothers and children have similar needs and that mothering is done in similar contexts.

Currently, many family researchers view motherhood as a social construct (Thurer, 1994; Glenn, 1994; Phoenix, Woollett & Lloyd, 1991). Social construction refers to the process by which motherhood (and mothering) is culturally defined within social, economic and historical contexts (Apple & Golden, 1997). Motherhood as a social construct is embedded in both micro (mother-child relationships) and macro (social, cultural, economic) relationships (Sommerfeld, 1989). This micro/macro view acknowledges the complex social factors that contribute to motherhood. Social construction is the process by which people develop an understanding of the world and themselves (Coltrane, 1998). Thus, the goal of social construction is to understand the phenomenon from the standpoint of those who live it. This approach provides a basis to explore the multiple realities of motherhood for the women in my studies.

I, too, view motherhood as a social construct learned through social interactions rather than implied through biological links. I believe that motherhood is constructed within layers of micro and macro variables such as intrafamily dynamics, economic and social resources, ethnicity, and culture. These variables provide diversity to the role of motherhood. Women continually refine their definition of motherhood through daily interactions with others (friends, family, co-workers, and so forth). Further, this construction process is affected by the environmental and social contexts in which women live.

The occupation of mothering is also a social construct with historical and cultural variation. It is defined in the literature as the work that women do in caring and nurturing children (Glenn, 1994). Ruddick's (1980; 1989) classic research frames mothering within this caring and nurturing construct. She uses the concept of "maternal practice" to describe mothering. She argues that mothers are concerned with protecting, preserving, and fostering their child's growth and development. Further, Ruddick (1980) notes that mothering must be done within acceptable parameters of the social group. At times, satisfying mothering demands may be at odds with the social group. Mothers need to solve and negotiate these conflicting demands and this is not always an easy task.

Arendell (2000) observes that "Mothering is often associated with women, because it is women who do the work of mothering" (p. 1192). However, this does not imply that all women mother nor that all women are innately qualified for the job. As Howard and Hollander (1997) point out, polarized gender ideology can be harmful in several ways. First, by viewing parenting as something only women do, men are not allowed to "experience sustained involvement and commitment to parenting" (p. 34). Assuming that women are more caring and nurturing sets women up to do all the parenting. They are assumed to know how to mother and to enjoy mothering. This gendered parenting stereotype contributes to a hierarchy that disadvantages both men and women.

Gender ideology has remained intact despite women's entrance in the paid labor force (Hochschild, 1989). Male participation in household and childcare tasks will increase only when there is a shift in the belief system,

for example, when both men and women are viewed as capable of caring and nurturing.

It is important to note the broad definition of mothering in the literature. What does it mean to care for and nurture children? What does it mean to foster their growth? The specific activities that women do in caring for children is underexplored and underdefined in the literature. This concept of mothering will be further examined within this chapter.

ℒ➤ My Research

Wasserfall (1993) suggests that it can be empowering for informants to participate in a research study. In essence, they become experts in that they share their knowledge of a particular phenomenon. The women whom I contacted were quite amenable to being interviewed about their mothering experiences. Because mother work has been marginalized as being ubiquitous, instinctual, and natural, many participants felt my research helped legitimize their work as mothers. Because motherhood was the research focus, it brought mother work out of the margins and made it center place for these women. One older woman of a young adult child thanked me for inviting her to participate, stated that no one had ever asked her opinions about mothering, and was thrilled that someone was finally doing this kind of research. Several women commented that they loved having the opportunity to talk about their children.

I started with a convenience sample of women known to me who fit the criteria identified in my research protocols. I then asked participants if they knew other women who might be interested in being interviewed for this research study. This technique, known as snowballing, is a means to increase the number of participants (Weiss, 1994). When using snowball sampling, it is important to have multiple and different points of entry to obtain participants. Thus, I contacted a friend who worked at a local hospital, my mother-in-law who lives about half an hour from my home, associates at another university, a friend who lives in a farming community west of my home, and people known to me from the church to which I belong. All of these resources led me to other women who were willing to participate.

The mothers interviewed and participating in the focus groups ranged in age from 24 to 83 years of age. Table 8–1 is an overview of the participants. The women, on average, had two children, but this number varied. Younger women just starting their families often had only one child; older women who had become mothers in the 1950s and 1960s often had larger families, which were more typical of that historical period. Thus, the number of children ranged from one to eight.

The women in my studies tended to be well educated; most had received a bachelor's degree and many had advanced degrees. They were all white and were married or in cohabitating, long-term relationships. Two of the older mothers had been widowed. Most of the women were employed outside of the home at least part time. Some of the mothers of adult children described staying at home when their children were young but had returned to the paid work force as their children became more independent. Again, this is a typical pattern for middle-class American families given the historical period (1960s and 1970s) when these women were raising their young families.

Employment was often a topic of discussion during the interview sessions and focus groups. Despite different employment sta-

Table 8–1 Description of participants*

Number of Participants:	61 women
Age Range:	24–83 years old
No. of children:	1–8, M=2.4
Education:	Range from high school diploma to doctoral degree; 42% had an advanced degree
Employment:	82% worked at least part time or more

*All of the participants are white women living primarily in the midwestern area of the United States. Most (92%) were married; the others were in long-term cohabiting relationships.

tuses, each participant seemed to want to find a commonality with my employment and/or student status. The mothers who were students viewed me as a fellow student who could empathize with juggling school and family work. The mothers who were employed outside of the home commented, "Isn't it nice to work and have some separate space from the kids?" The stay-at-home mothers noted that, as a university professor, I have a "flexible work schedule" and "summers off" to be with my daughter. I agreed with all of them. This illustrates that employment is a hot topic among mothers. In the United States and perhaps elsewhere in the world, there is tension between women who work and women who stay home. Of course, this "choice" to work or stay home is not really an option for many women. As is evident, overall my participants are well educated and have economic and social resources. This allows them many opportunities to make the choice to work outside of the home or not. They can afford quality childcare or household help. They have access to good health care and can provide safe, stimulating environments for their children. Further, by being married mothers, these women have more social acceptability; they fit the image of a two-parent household. Many of the women recognized these advantages and openly questioned how much more difficult mothering would be without these resources.

Gaining entrée and developing trust are essential ingredients in most qualitative research methods (Weiss, 1994). Being a mother is the qualification that initially brought me to this research. As a mother, I had some understanding of my participants' lives. Hopefully, this allowed participants to be more open and reflective in their responses. Many of the participants knew ahead of time that I was a mother, and those who did not inquired early in the interview session. The women often interjected answers with "You know what it's like" when discussing some aspect of motherhood. In these instances, I was careful not to make assumptions and pressed the mothers for clarification or elaboration. The mothers of young children often asked for mothering advice or validation because I was perceived as the mothering "expert." I was asked about breast-feeding, sleeping schedules, family beds, potty training, and other mothering dilemmas. I felt comfortable sharing my ideas because it added to the openness of the interviews. However, knowing that there is no right answer to these questions, I tried to preface my comments with "What worked for me" or "Something that you might want to try…" I was careful to not act as though I was the expert or knew the right answer.

Next, I will describe the themes that emerged from the interviews and focus groups with my participants. The reader should note that all names used in this chapter are pseudonyms to protect the identity of the participants.

Mothering as a Lifetime Occupation

What the mothers in my studies have told me loudly and clearly is that mothering does not end when a child leaves home but is a lifetime occupation. Delores, a 74-year-old mother of two daughters, noted:

> It doesn't go away, it doesn't. Those maternal feelings do not go away. In spite of what I was so proud of—I'd say, you know, when they were growing up and you go through all of those stages of childhood—what I would espouse was, well, our goal as parents [is] to teach our children to get along without us. I remember saying that over and over, and I must have looked like a puffed mother hen because I said it so many times, and I believed it. But it's one of the most difficult things that I have done in my life. And it's still; it still lingers, as an ex-mother-in-law, and as a mother of daughters who are now 46 and 48….It still stays.[1]

A 50-year-old mother of three and grandmother of an 18-month-old talked about mothering forever and continuing to learn how to mother.

> Also, that mothering role grows because not only do you have your own children, but I feel very, very attached to my children's spouses. I love them almost as much as if they were my own children. So, it's like your family continues to grow and your mothering continues to grow. It goes on in different ways.[1]

Thus, for these women motherhood continued as their children grew older. How they mothered changed, of course, but the role of being a mother never ended. In some ways this motherhood role became more difficult. Many of the women talked about having to sit back and watch their adult children make mistakes or get hurt. However, they felt that they should not interfere in their children's lives. Rose, a 71-year-old mother of three children and grandmother of five, noted:

> You can wrap them in cotton and sweet little blankets and you wrap them in your love and you hold them close, but you love them just as much when they grow up; just every bit as much. In fact, they've this long history of love then, and you see many times where something is a danger point, and you can certainly draw their attention to it, but also have to recognize that you gave him life and everyone has their own right to live it. Their way to live it may not be the way you want them to, but nevertheless, they have to have their chance. Many times you have to help them put themselves together after they've made some pretty big mistakes.[1]

As noted earlier, there is limited research examining motherhood beyond the children's adolescence. The implication is that motherhood ends when children leave home. However, the participants all voiced the idea that motherhood does not end but continues as children mature into young adults. Gross (1985) aptly identifies the young adult stage of motherhood as the *orbital stage* signifying a child's launch into the orbit of independence. Young adult children (identified in this study as ages 18 to 29 years) are beginning to build separate lives from their parents. They are leaving home to attend college, start a full-time job, launch a new career, move into their own apartment, or get married. They are stretching their wings and flying on their own. However, as children enter this young adult stage, they still need their mothers for instrumental and emotional support. Thus Gross's (1985) metaphor includes an orbit around the mother planet. The mothers interviewed by Gross (1985) were surprised and pleased to be actively mothering young adult children. The mothers in my research also spoke of the pleasure in participating in their child's life. One mother of a 22-year-old daughter and a 27-year-old son noted:

> I think this is a wonderful stage because we're healthy and active and can do things with them. They are at an age when they might want to do a lot of things with us. Once they have their own families, you become immersed in that. Not that you're not going to see each other, but it is a nice stage now because they are sort of grown up and independent and [we] have fun together as people.[2]

This mother viewed time with her "sort of grown up" children as remarkable because they enjoyed each other's company and doing activities together. She described going to cultural events with her children and getting together for lunches and weekly family dinners. She also recognized that when her children marry and have their own children, they will not be as available to do these types of activities. So she and her husband were truly enjoying this young adult stage. Another mother of a 27-year-old son remarked, "This is the best part now, the payoff."

Many of the mothers I spoke with commented on the difficulties of the orbital stage of motherhood. Cara, a 54 year-old mother in one of the focus groups, noted the following when asked about how motherhood changes:

> That's the real hard part of parenting too. When you know, you've seen the writing on the wall; you almost anticipated a matter. And then you're there to pick up their pieces and be their partner and help them through it... That same love is there when, well my oldest is 29, it's the same love then as when they were newborns.[1]

Rose continues this line of thought by adding:

> And then the grandchildren come and you're just as involved with each of them, and my goodness, I go to bed and I have to wait forever to get to sleep because I have so many to pray for.[1]

Contrary to the popular myth that women experience an "empty nest syndrome" when their children leave home, research indicates that in fact many women are happier and less depressed and have increased marital satisfaction after their children have left home, as compared to women of similar age with children at home (Etaugh, 1993). Gross (1985) agrees that the image of a lonely middle-aged mother is a myth, but also notes that women need to develop a new image of this mothering stage because the myth is so culturally ingrained. None of the participants in my studies discussed feeling lonely or having an empty nest after their children left home.

I found that the women in this study feel a close link to their children, offering them various forms of help and support. They feel connected to, provide support to, worry about, and derive happiness from their children forever. This point is exemplified by Cara's comment above when she talked about being a partner to her children and when Rose discussed having to lend support to her children after they have endured a marital crisis. It is evident that, for these women, motherhood is an occupation that does not end.

Several additional themes emerged from the interviews of mothers with young adult children that I will further describe in this chapter. I refer to them as motherhood themes and they are:

- Invested participants
- Wide-angle lens
- Advice givers
- Taboo talk
- Transitional cohort
- Perfect mother image

First, I discuss the tasks and activities that mothers currently engage in while caring for their children. I named this the *invested participant* theme because the mothers remained invested in caring for their children. Next, I found mothers were quite reflective on their experiences of mothering over time. Instead of focusing on one stage of motherhood, they were able to view motherhood through a *wide-angle lens*. I discuss these mothers as *advice givers*, in contrast to the preschool-stage mothers who actively sought out advice. The fourth theme centers on the mothering *taboo talk* described by these women.

After the discussion of the topics, I will discuss the women's perceptions of fatherhood and their husbands' role in caretaking. This view of fatherhood was interconnected with the women's work beliefs. Because the women's views of fatherhood and work seem to be in transition from traditional to contemporary models, I identified this theme as the *transitional cohort.*

It is important to keep in mind that most of the mothers of young adult children were baby boomers, born in the post-World War II era. Most were raised in typical middle-class families during the 1950s and 1960s. They became mothers approximately 20 to 25 years ago during the 1970s, a time of much social change in the United States, and this time period influenced the women's construction of motherhood, fatherhood, and work.

Lastly, I explore how a *perfect mother image* influences the participant's mothering experiences.

Invested Participants

I asked mothers to describe the tasks and activities they currently perform in caring for their children. Naturally, preschool mothers generated a lengthy list of caretaking activities. I was curious to discover the types of activities mothers of young adult children would identify. I was even unsure if they would address this area on the questionnaire that I gave to participants before their interviews. But my fears were unfounded; all the young–adult-stage mothers identified several tasks and activities they engaged in with their children. I use the terms "tasks" and "activities" to identify the smaller aspects of occupation and because most people have a clearer understanding of what these terms mean in contrast to "occupation," which causes confusion.

These mothers *remained* invested in their children's lives. Certainly the mothering tasks and activities have changed as their children have matured, but they continue to care for and nurture their children. They provide instrumental support, emotional support, and a home base to which their children can return. The mothers felt connected to their young adult children and described an emerging interdependent relationship with them.

There were many examples of providing instrumental support to children. Mothers who had children in college spoke of significant financial assistance for tuition, room and board, clothing, and other items. Health and car insurance was also provided by some of these mothers, and several bought cars for their children to use for work or at college. Another mother described buying baby items for the child of her 28-year-old daughter, who was a graduate student:

> Kim and John didn't have money for buggies and this and that and I did. In one sense I need to be looking for retirement, but I also wanted to do that. They didn't ask me ever for anything. It just made me happy to be able to do that, and to make all the crib bumpers and do all those things. I just wanted to.[2]

This mother was clearly pleased that she was able to provide for her daughter, son-in-law, and new grandchild. Others described ways they helped their children, including providing meals and other incidentals. For many, providing instrumental support was still part of their mothering role. When I asked one mother how this stage of motherhood was different from when her children were younger, she replied:

> It's not really any different than when they were children. It's just that they have different needs now than as a child. I think the fact that they had to be fed and clothed and I had to do it all before, but they still have to be fed and clothed and sometimes they don't have the money and you still need to be there.[2]

The mothers discussed in-depth the *emotional support* they provide to their young adult children. At this stage, the mothers provided an "ear for listening" and acted as "sounding boards." One mother wrote, "listen, listen, listen" on her questionnaire in response to the tasks and activities question. Vanessa, a mother of two college-age sons, viewed her current role as a mother as "just being available, nurturing them into adulthood." She described the activities of her role in more detail:

> Hanging out if they need support and hearing where they are going. It's important to be

around to find out more stuff about what is going on with them and to show them I'm available to listen. I look at the kids that are in trouble and I think they need someone to really believe in them, to let them know they are really cool kids.

Vanessa was not intrusive in her sons' lives, but felt it important to be available, to bolster them, and to provide positive feedback. She described a busy household with her sons' summer work schedules and informally designated family time. "It's not like when they are little and you can talk with them at the dinner table about their day." This mother had a career as a college professor, but felt it was important to be available when they wanted to talk, and wanted to know what was going on in her sons' lives. Another mother with four young adult children living at home also spoke of being available to listen:

> I do that [listening] a lot at night. That's hard sometimes when I'm in the midst of studying, but they want to talk. I think my youngest is real good at feelings and real good at saying what he needs, and he can solve his own problems if I keep my mouth shut long enough and let him or reflect back to him. But he gets to a place where he is OK and he leaves.[2]

I found this *availability* component of mothering striking at this stage. I pictured listening as more of a component of mothering elementary and middle school-aged children, for example, the traditional mother greeting the child after school with "How was your day, dear?" But these mothers were consciously listening to their children. Many of the women talked about filling a unique niche for their children by being a sounding board, an understanding and concerned adult. In fact, the children sought their advice on everything from buying a home to handling a colicky child to dealing with a relationship gone bad.

Sociologists have noted the trend of adult children returning home (White & Rogers, 1997; White, 1994). This trend was clearly evident among the mothers I studied. College-age children returned home for extended stays during semester breaks and for summers. Children often came home to live after college

while launching their careers as a means to save money. Other mothers reported their children returned home after a divorce, while building a home, or during a cross-country move. Sometimes these children brought their spouses or their children with them.

For the most part, the mothers reported being pleased to offer their children a home base. Most revealed that co-residence with an adult child was fine for a limited period of time, but not a permanent solution. One mother with four young adult children at home commented that she was looking forward to her eldest child moving out because his presence was disruptive to the household.

Overall, these mothers felt connected to their young adult children. In addition to the interviews, I asked the women to rate the level of closeness they felt to their children on a questionnaire, on a scale of 1 to 10, with 10 being the closest. I also asked them if this degree of closeness was something they anticipated. The mothers' comments were mixed on whether they anticipated the degree of closeness. Some said they had "planned for it," whereas others felt it was a bit less than they had hoped for. None appeared surprised. Although these types of measures are often positively skewed, I believe the written comments clearly support the degree of closeness these mothers felt.

The degree of closeness identified by the mothers of young adult children is less than the mothers of preschool age children. Other researchers have also found a decrease in closeness of the parent-child relationship over time (Hofferth, 1998). Bernscheid, Snyder & Omoto (1989) suggest that child/parent closeness is U shaped, with the highest degree of closeness reported at younger and older ages.

Whether they are actually less close or the closeness is somehow different is difficult to discern. However, this difference in closeness makes sense; children are maturing and separating from their parents. As children grow older, they develop their own network of friends and other close relationships. Young adult children spend less time with and are less dependent on their parents than they were as preschoolers. All of these factors contribute to the degree of closeness reported by these mothers of young adult children. Interestingly, the lowest ratings of closeness (scores of 3 to 7) were from mothers of sons. In fact, the mother of a daughter and two sons rated the degree of closeness differently by gender. Although I am unsure what this gender difference indicates, there is research that suggests daughters provide more support to older parents than sons (Rossi & Rossi, 1990). Researchers Kaufman and Uhlenberg, (1998) noted that "females are more involved than males in maintaining intergenerational relations" (p.927). Further, they note that the mother-daughter relationship is closer than the other dyad types, perhaps because of women's investment in family relationships. Perhaps gender identification is another explanation for the higher levels of closeness reported by the mothers of daughters. Consistent with Chodorow's (1978) explanation of why women mother, she notes the gender identification of daughters with their mothers.

I asked the mothers when they thought about their children. "All the time," was the resounding answer. The following comments from three different mothers were typical:

(1) Oh, many times during the day. I think about what they're doing. Now that they're grown, maybe I don't think about them as much because I'm busy with my own activities. But I always think about them in the morning and evening; I'm anxious to hear from them if I haven't heard. Then I give them a call.[2]

(2) Sometimes when I know that they have a specific thing happening on a given day, like if I know Catherine's in the middle of a particularly important exam. On specific times like that. At other times, I think your mind just occasionally goes one way or another, and you say, "Oh, I wonder what's so and so's doing right now?" When something sparks a thought about that.[2]

(3) All the time. There are pictures all over the house. I think about them every day. So I see them every day [referring to the pictures] when I get my breakfast and lunch and I say hello to them every day. I know Caitlin [her granddaughter] thinks I'm nuts sometimes when I'm standing there talking to the pictures. But I think of them every day. I don't know whether it's because they were my life or what.[2]

These mothers reported being in contact with their children often via the phone, e-mail, or visits. During one interview, the woman's beeper went off. She checked it, smiled, and said, "Oh that's my daughter." I asked if she wanted to use my phone and call her daughter. "No," she responded. "That was our code, she beeps me once a day with 1-4-3, which means, 'I love you."

This connection between mothers and children also had a reciprocal quality. Not only did children seek parents out for instrumental and emotional support; the mothers were starting to view their children as adults. They enjoyed each other's company, going to events together, and sharing family problems. Of her son and daughter, one mother observed, "I see them as adults and as some of my dear friends." Another mother noted,"They talk to you on a different level—it's a normal adult conversation."

When measuring the success of motherhood, this same mother commented, "For me, the success of being a good parent is having your children want your company." These mothers enjoyed their children's companionship and cherished activities together. They talked about going to movies, for walks, to meals, shopping, and even on vacations. According to these mothers, the children initiated these events as often as their mothers did. These mothers also looked to their children for emotional support. A mother whose son was going through a divorce spoke of the emotional support she received from her daughter. The mother was only comfortable sharing these family issues with her daughter. She was truly comforted by her daughter's support.

Sociologists Alice and Peter Rossi (1990) write about "help exchange" between generations. Similar to my findings, they discuss both instrumental and expressive (emotional) support exchanged between parents and children. They discovered several important findings: adult children report giving more help of a personal, supportive nature, whereas parents provide more instrumental support to children. Although I did not measure the amount of expressive and instrumental support exchanged between mothers and their children, it did appear that the young adult children were providing only emotional support at this stage. Young adult children are just starting their careers and do not have the financial and network potential of their parents.

In addition, the Rossis (1990) found that mothers give and receive help to and from children more than fathers. In my study, I did not specifically ask the mothers about the amount of support that fathers provided, nor did I interview fathers. However, many of the mothers used the plural "we" to indicate that both parents were involved in providing instrumental support.

The concept of "help exchange" seems sterile, somehow bound by obligation instead of love or affection. However, the mothers in my study described more than an exchange of help. They provided support to their children, not out of duty but because of their bond with their children.

I named this theme *invested participants* because the mothers remained active in their children's lives. They provided support to their children and were starting to receive support in return. They took pleasure in spending time with their children doing mutually enjoyable activities. They continued to think about their children "all the time." Certainly the mothers of preschool age children could be seen as "invested participants" as well. However, the point is that the mothers of young adult children are still actively mothering their children. Certainly the mothering has changed from earlier stages, but they have not discontinued this important occupation. This finding is surprising given the lack of attention to mothering young adult children. The mothers themselves did not seem surprised that they were still actively invested in mothering. They had mothered these young adult children for many years and certainly were not going to stop being invested in their welfare.

The Wide-angle Lens

I found the interviews with mothers of young adult children more captivating than those with mothers of preschool-age children, perhaps because I have yet to personally experience mothering a young adult child. I found that mothers of young adult children used a wide-angle lens to view their mothering experiences. Most had been a mother for more than 20 years and could reflect on motherhood's many stages. They saw a panoramic picture instead of the close-up view.

They spoke of the intense joy as well as the intense pain of mothering. When asked to describe parenthood, one woman said:

> I would describe parenthood as the most awesome responsibility, which I probably didn't realize when I entered motherhood. It's a wonderful stage of being, but it's a state of caring and worrying and responsibility that never leaves you for an instant. Even though my children are grown up, it stays with you. I think about them all the time. They're just a part of my being. It brings you tremendous joy, but it brings you the most severe pain that you have in your life.[2]

Many of them spoke of the pain and disappointments of mothering when children "stepped off the track," as one mother put it. They described times when their children had problems with drugs or alcohol, went through divorces, left college, or were arrested. They spoke of watching their children make poor choices or when they were "self-absorbed, lied or procrastinated." One mother was disappointed when her children "don't reach as far as I feel they can go" and also "when they don't allow themselves room for mistakes and when they are insensitive to others." Another noted, "I'm disappointed in some of their actions or decisions that could have been better choices." One mother wrote that it was important to "separate my issues from his, my dreams from his dreams."

The joy and pride mothers felt in their children tempered the pain and disappointment. These mothers expressed pride in their children's accomplishments and joy in being mothers. Vanessa, the mother of two college-age sons, noted the joy she felt "just looking at them as bright, young, healthy men as well as their accomplishments in school, athletics, and other extra-curricular activities." This pride was not necessarily for the things typically identified—As on report cards, receiving a full scholarship to Harvard, getting a promotion at work, or being an outstanding athlete. The mothers identified pride when their children exhibited sensitivity to others and worked hard. One mother stated that she felt pride:

> When they interact in caring/respectful ways with others including assertiveness, honesty, responsibility with family, friends and co-workers. When they struggle with and come through adversity or challenges.

Another mother spoke of the personal qualities that brought her joy:

> I think what brings me joy lately is seeing some behaviors that I think are very important. For instance, caring for others, caring for the community, having basic things outward. I've seen things lately in both kids that have just made me feel good. We've got an aunt who is sick. I spoke to her and my son will say, 'What's her phone? I'll give her a call.' And without me saying, you know you really should call. Or they talk to you on a different level. It's not a 'Can I' or 'I want' or 'I need help in the kitchen', It's a normal adult conversation. This is the joy that they just want to talk to you, or that one of them calls and asks you to lunch. You know it is just nice. 'Dad said you had a cold, how are you feeling?' You know just some of that stuff that's so important to me; I don't care how much money they make. I want them to be nice people; happy, nice people.

The mothers at this stage seemed more confident in their mothering skills and abilities. Asked if they felt judged as mothers, they typically replied that they did not. They spoke of feeling judged by others when their children were younger, but now that their children were older, they did not feel judged anymore. One mother said, "I've matured, I don't care what anybody thinks." Several commented that the judging that mattered to them was by their children. These women are not novices at mothering at this stage and are more comfortable in their mothering abilities. This may be partly a result of adult development; as people age, they become less concerned with other's perceptions of them. Perhaps society also holds mothers less accountable at this stage because the children have become young adults and the mothers' job is perceived to be finished.

When asked if they had regrets or would have done anything differently as mothers, I frequently received a resounding "No." One mother stated:

> I like what my father used to say and I think the same thing about being a mother and raising two sons, " did the best I could every day and if I could have done better, I would have."

Mothers at this stage can view the big picture, both the joys and pains of motherhood. They have a wide-angle lens to reflect on their mothering.

Advice Giving

The mothers of young adult children were the mother generation to the preschool-stage mothers that I interviewed. In fact, I had two mother-daughter dyads within my sample. Of course, all of the interviews were done separately and the mothers and daughters did not know each other's responses.

Mothers of preschoolers typically seek advice about mothering dilemmas from trusted others, often their own mothers. Thus, it was not surprising that young adult stage mothers often spoke of giving advice to their children on a variety of topics including mothering. Young adult stage mothers provided emotional support and gave advice to their children.

Not surprisingly, several of the mothers of adult children were also grandmothers. These women provided parenting advice to their children. It was interesting in the two mother-daughter dyads; the daughters spoke of seeking their mother's advice and being reassured by their wisdom. The young adult stage mothers spoke of providing information to their daughters about mothering. They also described their joy in watching their daughters mothering.

Susan, mother of a 27-year-old son and grandmother of an 8-year-old grandson, spoke of receiving advice as a young mother. She has become more vocal as a grandmother:

> Looking back on it, I think I was given some really horrible advice. I didn't speak up as a parent because I just relied on them [her mother and older sisters]. I thought, 'Well, this is how it is.' But now with my grandson I am much more verbal.

Susan had evolved from being the one given the advice to the grandmother who provides the advice.

It makes sense that, with more mothering experience, the young adult stage mothers would be asked by their children to give advice about parenting. With all the advice giving and seeking, it suggests that mothering is learned and not necessarily innate.

Taboo Talk

The issue of a mothering taboo emerged late in my interviews with the young–adult-stage mothers. During my 18th interview, the concept of mothers not speaking about mothering negatives came out. I asked Vanessa, a mother of two college-age sons, what was unexpected about mothering:

> *Vanessa:* I think what was really unexpected for me is that some parents step out of the role. They just say to their children, "Here is the money, here is the car." Parents don't talk about parenting with each other anymore. It makes it a lot harder. Other parents don't support each other and they undermine other parents. Interviewer: Can you give me an example?
> *Vanessa:* Well, around drinking issues. I don't serve other kids alcohol in my house, and I would expect other moms not to serve my [underage] kids at their home. But they don't respect that. They go ahead and serve kids beer and then put me down to my kids.

Vanessa not only spoke of a taboo in discussing parenting issues but also felt undermined by other parents for her rules. I was fascinated by this disclosure, and subsequently asked other young–adult-stage mothers to comment whether they had similar experiences. The next two participants confirmed

Vanessa's feelings. They agreed and also commented that mothers spoke only of their young adult children's achievements and avoided discussing any frustrations of mothering.

Corrine, a mother of two daughters aged 23 and 28, concurred with Vanessa and stated:

> Parents of kids that were compliant and placid, looked at me with my kids who were doing mildly daring things with an attitude of "Well, why are your kids doing that? What are you doing wrong?"

Although the young–adult-stage mothers are more confident in their mothering abilities, a mothering taboo was evident in these three mothers. Corrine identified what is at the heart of the taboo: that if mothers speak of frustrations or difficulties with their children, they must be doing something wrong. Mothers are held responsible for children's behavior, whether it is not sleeping through the night as an infant or acting out as a teenager.

The taboo discussed by these young–adult-stage mothers was different from how it was described by the preschool-stage mothers. For the young–adult-stage mothers, the taboo was discussing negatives about one's children; whereas for the preschool-stage mothers, the taboo was discussing difficulties about mothering in general. They felt that it was not acceptable to discuss the burdens of being a mother because it reflected back on their mothering abilities. Because the young–adult-stage mothers were more confident in their mothering abilities, the taboo was focused on their children. Somehow they felt that it would be disloyal to one's children to discuss them in less than a positive light. It may also be that it would reflect back on their mothering abilities because mothers are often held accountable for their children's successes and failures.

I am uncertain why the mothering taboo did not emerge earlier in these young–adult-stage mothers' interviews. Perhaps because I was not looking for a mothering taboo and did not pursue this line of questioning, it did not emerge. Another possibility is that a mothering taboo was not common among mothers of children at this stage. Perhaps, because of their developmental stage, they are more confident as women and mothers.

However, because it did emerge in all of the last three interviews, I suspect that if I had probed in earlier interviews, it would have been evident.

The Transitional Cohort

The mothers spoke frequently about fatherhood and their husbands' role in caring for and nurturing their children. In fact, I was surprised at the significant amount of interview time used to discuss fathers. I asked only three questions related to this subject: What tasks and activities does your husband perform in caring for the children? Have these changed as the children have grown older? How would you define or describe fatherhood? However, the mothers often elaborated on their husbands' interactions with their children or used the collective "we" or "us" in discussing motherhood.

There was a range of views among these mothers from traditional models of fatherhood as provider to more contemporary models of fatherhood as co-parent. Many mothers talked about their husbands as being the traditional income provider while they stayed at home when their children were young. When I asked how this was decided or negotiated with their husbands, they responded, "It was just how it was done." They also indicated that this arrangement was expected when they started their families.

> I think it was implicit and I have to admit that we come from very traditional farm family backgrounds, both of us. I almost hate to admit this. Our traditional backgrounds are not valued and you almost feel a little like, I don't want to say I'm from a traditional family. But we were raised in that fashion. We both had mothers who stayed at home.

One mother who returned to work when her children were young noted the extra burden on her:

> And of course if they were sick or anything, I always stayed home. But it was always me. It's like I can't say "we" because it was like that was the mother's role. It wasn't just their father, in a sense. He was brought up an old German where the women do this and the men do that. And I was the mother. I took care of the children. It's

not that he didn't try to help a little bit, but not really. He never changed diapers. He barely ever fed them a bottle.

Despite more traditional family structures, the mothers noted the positive changes in parenting roles and the increased sharing of childcare tasks observed of parents today. Many defined fatherhood and motherhood similarly. They viewed themselves as the generation sandwiched in between traditional family structures and contemporary parenting. Three mothers spoke of being influenced by "the women's movement." One described being angry with her husband for not doing more around the house.

> He would read stories to them in the evenings and when he's come home. He'd take them outside with him on the weekends. I think when the women's movement came along; I started being irritated that he wasn't doing as much as I thought he should. We had some conflict around that.

Another woman referred to Betty Friedan's book (1963) as helping to shape her ideas about mothering, being a housewife and working. She described this as posing some difficulty:

> I don't know when Betty Friedan wrote her book, *The Feminine Mystique*, but I remember that was one of the first things I read when I was in school. I don't remember the book completely, but I think I was in the generation where I thought I had to do everything. I thought I not only had to be a good mother and wife, I had to be out in the career world and I had to be successful in a career. So I think I got the expectation somewhere that I had to be good at everything. That's what this was about, this women's liberation for me. I guess I had to be good at everything.

All the women spoke of coming from traditional families where fathers were the providers and mothers were responsible for raising the children and taking care of the home. Many followed in this tradition, whereas others felt strongly about sharing parenting responsibilities with husbands.

Ellen was the clearest example of a young adult stage mother who expected to co-parent with her husband. Ellen always worked several part-time jobs from her children's infancy to the present. She clearly viewed her husband as a partner in caring and raising their two daughters, despite the traditional family upbringing she had. She discussed what her husband did in caring for the children in contrast to herself:

> He [her husband] was always the better one to be around if they were going to do a batch of cookies because he wouldn't mind if things got spilled along the way and they'd take care of it later. He spent a lot of, ever since they were newborns, a lot of time with them alone, which is different from my childhood. My mother was at home all the time and my father had a seven-day workweek and my mother devoted herself to being home. So we have closer to a sharing. What are the things he did? Well, as they were infants, he did all their material needs, as well as being there as the other parent.

Later she adds in the interview:

> I've always said that he could be the parent who would take care of them full time and I could work and it would probably be better for their overall health. Now, I don't think that's quite true and I don't think he would agree, but there were certainly times when they were littler when he would have been.

Ellen, age 46, was at the younger end of this mothering stage. Perhaps her younger age accounts for her viewing her husband as a co-parent. Ellen's view of fathering was similar to the other young adult stage mothers in their early 40's. These mothers may have been influenced by the 1970s women's movement to strive for equality in the home, whereas the older mothers in this group may have been less affected by the women's movement and more established in their attitude toward parenting roles. Thus they were more comfortable with the traditional gendered parenting paradigm.

Jane's view illustrated the older mothers' attitudes regarding parenting. At age 59, she was over a decade older than Ellen. Brought up in a traditional family structure, Jane thought it was important to raise her two sons in the same manner. She took care of the house and children while her husband worked until the children were school age. Then she worked part time so that she could be home in the mornings and after school. She clearly felt this was the right way to raise children and noted a "trend" in more women staying home:

> A lot of young mothers again now are trying to stay home with their children. Not that you have to, but I decided that I wanted to when they were young. I see the trend coming back...it depends where they're living; what lifestyle they are used to. Sometimes they have to have two salaries to keep up with what they want to do, so they feel they have to do this. The younger friends that I have, there are three of them. One is at home with her children and the other one told me at Christmastime when they have their children she's going to quit her job and stay home. And the other one said the same thing. So I think the trend is coming back to try to be there to care for your children when they are young; be there when they're at home.

Jane's older son was recently divorced and returned home to live for 6 months. His young daughter also stayed with them part of the time. It was interesting to hear Jane discuss her son's fatherhood role. I asked Jane about her definition of fatherhood:

> I think they're [fatherhood and motherhood] very similar. We're seeing it probably more and more now with our son going through the divorce. The father tends to do all the care and meet all the needs of the children as the mother can, especially if the mother is working also. But they both have to provide for the day care. They both can provide for all the needs. It's more difficult for one person to do it than two. But the father can provide equally as well.

The mothers' convictions around work and fatherhood were linked and were based on their choosing to work outside of the home or not. As one would expect, the women who worked outside the home believed in more equitable sharing of childcare and household tasks with their husbands. The women who stayed at home saw themselves as the primary caretaker of the house and children and their husbands as the financial provider.

The Perfect Mother Image

Throughout my research I have used a social constructionist approach to examine experiences of motherhood. The basic assumption of social construction is that people view the world differently based on personal history, individual characteristics, social experiences, and environmental contexts (Coltrane, 1998). Social construction is the process by which people develop an understanding of the world and themselves. This approach provides a basis to explore the multiple realities of motherhood for the women in my research. As I noted earlier, images of mothers are so present in literature, art, and political discourse. To what extent do women try to achieve a certain motherhood image? How does this affect their mothering? I asked all the mothers in my studies how they would define the perfect mother, one woman answered, "A god." "Someone who is incredibly encouraging," noted another. These are obviously unattainable and unrealistic goals that have become culturally ingrained for many women.

Yerxa (1993) described occupations as daily pursuits that are self initiated, goal directed and socially sanctioned. The occupation of mothering certainly fulfills those criteria. However, the socially sanctioned aspect of mothering is confusing to women because of the many mixed messages and cultural images of motherhood in our society. The concept of what constitutes a good mother is viewed through the lens of culture and time. For example, middle-class American mothers in the 1950s and 1960s were expected to stay at home and be full-time mothers and supportive wives. Today most American mothers work outside the home. Thus, the expectation of what is acceptable for being a good mother has shifted from staying at home to working outside the home. However, women, especially mothers of young children, still feel acutely the tension between work and mothering.

To further illustrate the point that the occupation of mothering is embedded in a cultural context, LeVine (1994), an anthropologist, showed videotapes of middle-class American women tending to their babies to a group of mothers in southwestern Kenya. The Kenyan women were shocked at the lack of attention the American mothers paid to their fussy babies. They surmised that the American women must be incompetent mothers. The

way we mother is learned from the culture we live in, and thereby our image of what constitutes a good mother is culturally derived. How does this cultural image affect mothering practice?

Many of the women in my study made reference to an image of a perfect mother, as if there is an elusive ideal "out there." Often these references were in regretful or self-derogatory contexts. Patricia, the 78-year-old mother of successful 40-something, twin daughters, remarked,

> I remember telling my kids; "I'm doing the best I can." I would tell them that and "I know that I'm not doing everything, but I am trying to do what I can." They kind of grew up with that. So I thought, well, it's true, I'm not a perfect mom and I don't pretend to be. So I am just going to do what I can and hope that it ends up right.[1]

Soon after this comment, Patricia became tearful and noted, "They've had...you know, they've not had the best life. I mean they had things that are rough in this life." Patricia was divorced and had to work full time, which was less common during the late 1950s and early 1960s, when she was raising her daughters. She felt guilty that she could not be at home for them and could not adequately provide financially for them. Rebecca, a 38-year-old mother of three daughters, also voiced her feelings of not being the ideal mother:

> If I knew then what I know now, I'm not sure it [motherhood] would have been one I would have taken on because of the endlessness, it's constant. I'm glad I chose it for all the reward it's had. Sometimes I don't think I'm the best mom there is, although that was my goal when I started out.[1]

Rebecca's ambivalence about mothering is evident, and she is not alone in her feelings. There appeared to be much guilt among the mothers in my study of not always saying or doing the right thing with their children. Where does this sense of needing to be a "perfect" mother come from? In many of our other adult roles, perfection is not the model. Certainly there is an expectation for competence and consistency, but perfection is not expected, except for mothers. Mothers feel guilty for not being perfect.

Thurer (1994) comments on the image of the good mother as portrayed by the noted American baby expert, Dr. Benjamin Spock. She writes, "He constructs a 'good' mother who is ever-present, all-providing, inexhaustibly patient and tactful, and who anticipates her child's every need. Mother has become baby's servant" (p.258). Is there such a mother, I wondered? "No," was the resounding answer. However, the women in this study were constantly comparing themselves to some ideal. Where does the ideal come from? I suspect there is a connection between this image of the ideal or perfect mother and learning to mother. Women, especially newer mothers, feel that somewhere out there are the answers on how to be the perfect mother, but the information is elusive. Many of the older women in my study noted the lack of information available on parenting while they were young mothers. In contrast, several of the mothers in one of the focus groups had recently become grandmothers and were discussing the amount of literature and technology available to their daughters. Cara observed:

My daughter-in-law, oh you name it. She has all these subscriptions and videos, and she goes to all these sessions and she is just so up on child-rearing. They had tapes that they played in bed at night on her abdomen; played music for this infant.[1]

Another mother, Susan, continued this line of thinking:

Staci keeps three books right there handy and when Hillary is doing something we are concerned about, while she is nursing, she'll flip to the appropriate chapter and she's learned quite a bit.[1]

Mothers seem to be on a quest for the right answer. It is as though if a mother searches long enough, she will find the answers on how to be a perfect mother and thus will ensure the outcome of having a successful child. No matter that many of the popular parenting primers give mixed advice to mothers.

Perhaps this search to be a perfect mother stems, in part, from the influence of Freudian psychology, which makes mothers responsible for the outcome of their children. Chodorow and Contratto (1982) noted the recurrent theme of the perfect mother in psychological and feminist literature as being all powerful. They argue that this image allows for mother blaming, when a child has problems, whether they are biological, academic, or psychological in nature. Karen sums this idea up nicely:

I do think people look at what your children do, who they become, the way they live their lives, and whether you want to believe it or not, and whether you think it is valid or not, it does reflect back to you…But I do think that whether that's valid or not, other people do. They'll say, 'Well, what does your son do? Or what do your kids do?' So I do think there is something like that in it, even though we don't want to say we can take credit for the good or the bad they do, it does somehow seem like we do get judged against that or by that.[1]

Hays (1996), also using social construction theory, describes a model of "intensive mothering" that is centered solely on children's needs (p. 21). This intensive mothering model grew out of the industrial revolution when the dichotomy between home and work began and continued into the 1950s with the ideal family images portrayed in popular television sitcoms like *Father Knows Best*. Research (Thurer, 1994; Hays, 1996) indicates that a mothering ideal is present and fluid throughout history. Thus it is no surprise that the participants in my research were cognizant of a perfect mother image despite the implicit cultural contradictions.

Conclusion

Arendell (2000), in her review of a decade's scholarship of mothering, calls for a greater understanding of what mothers do and how mothering activities change as children grow and mature. It is my hope that this chapter has provided some insights into how mothering evolves and changes as both women and their children age. It is evident, from the participants in my studies, that women viewed mothering as a lifetime occupation. Certainly, the tasks and activities involved in this occupation evolved and changed throughout the stages of motherhood, but nevertheless these women viewed themselves as lifelong mothers. As healthcare practitioners, we need to be cognizant of this important role for many of our clients and not assume that when children become adults, mothering is no longer important.

Mothers of adult children remain invested in their children's lives, often providing both emotional and financial support. They give advice when asked and find it difficult to remain silent at times. They are active participants in their children's lives and find this an incredibly enjoyable mothering time despite the angst of watching adult children make unwise decisions at times. The women in my studies also struggled with wanting to be the best mother they could be and felt guilty that, at times, they did not live up to some ideal image of motherhood.

Mothers of adult children were able to use a wide-angle lens to view their mothering experiences. They reflected on both the joy and pain of mothering and were confident in their mothering skills. This confidence comes from both the children's and the mother's maturation. Mothers have launched their children into adulthood, and the children are now orbiting around their mother planet (Gross, 1985).

I feel that the theme of taboo talk warrants further exploration and is noteworthy for healthcare practitioners. Why is it that mothers of young adult children seemingly become more competitive with each other instead of supporting one another as mothers? Perhaps it is more painful to watch an adult child trip than it is a younger child. Having a child do poorly on a second-grade spelling test has fewer lifelong consequences than failing at a job. When children fail as adults (or appear to do so in the eyes of others), it is very painful for parents.

Consistent with lifecourse theory (Elder, 1987; Setterson, 1999), which argues that attitudes and beliefs are shaped by social, cultural, and historical influences, the participants' view of the father's role was influenced by the historical time period in which they were born and in which they became mothers. The younger mothers wanted more equitable parenting with their husbands, whereas the older mothers were comfortable with the traditional gendered parenting roles. Clearly, the father's voice is missing from my research and could be a source for future researchers to examine.

Last, a lesson for healthcare professionals that I found from these interviews is the importance of truly listening to someone's story. It is only from truly listening that we may have a glimpse of understanding what mothering experiences are like for other women.

Discussion Questions 🐦

- How does motherhood evolve and change over time? What are the tasks and activities of mothering adult children? How are these tasks and activities different from those of mothering young children?

- Describe motherhood as a social-construct. How does context influence women's perception and experience of motherhood?

- What would be your image of a perfect mother? How does this image influence your views of motherhood? What do you think is the prominent cultural image of motherhood? Is this similar to or different from your own image of mothering?

References

Arendell, T. (2000). Conceiving and investigating motherhood: The decade's scholarship. *Journal of Marriage and the Family, 62.* 1192–1207.

Apple, R. D., & Golden, J. (1997). *Mothers and motherhood: Readings in American history.* Columbus, OH: Ohio State University Press.

Berscheid, E., Snyder, M., & Omoto, A. M. (1989). Issues in studying close relationships: Conceptualizing and measuring closeness. In C. Hendrick (Ed.). *Close Relationships* (pp. 63–91). Newbury Park, CA: Sage Publications.

Chodorow, N. (1978). *The reproduction of mothering.* Berkeley, CA: University of California Press.

Chodorow, N., & Contratto, S. (1982). The fantasy of the perfect mother. In B. Thorne, & M. Yalom (Eds.). *Rethinking the family* (pp. 54–75). New York: Longman.

Coll, C.G., Surrey, J. L., & Weingarten, K. (1998). *Mothering against the odds: Diverse voices of contemporary mothers.* New York: Guilford Press.

Coltrane, S (1998). *Gender and Families.* Thousand Oaks, CA: Pine Forge Press.

Elder, G. H. (1987). Family and lives: Some development in lifecourse studies. *Journal of Family History, 12,* 179–199.

Etaugh, C. (1993). Women in the middle years. In F. L. Donmark, & M. A. Paludi (Eds.). *Psychology of women: A handbook of issues and themes.* Westport, CT: Greenwood Press.

Friedan, B. (1963). *The feminine mystique.* New York: Dell.

Francis-Connolly, E. (1998). It never ends: Mothering as a lifetime occupation. *Scandinavian Journal of Occupational Therapy, 5(3),* 149–155.

Francis-Connolly, E. (1999). *A comparison of two motherhood stages: Experience, practice and meaning.* Unpublished doctoral dissertation, The University of Michigan, Ann Arbor.

Francis-Connolly, E. (2000). Toward an understanding of mothering: A comparison of two motherhood stages. *American Journal of Occupational Therapy, 54(3),* 281–289.

Glenn, E.N. (1994). Social constructions of mothering: A thematic overview. In E. N. Glenn, G. Chang, & L. R. Forcey (Eds.). *Mothering: Ideology, experience and agency* (pp. 1–29). New York: Routledge.

Gross, Z. H. (1985). *And you thought it was all over: Mothers and their adult children.* New York: St. Martin's.

Hays, S. (1996). The cultural contradictions of motherhood. New Haven: Yale University Press.

Hochschild, A. (1989). *The second shift.* New York: Avon.

Hofferth, S. L. (1998). Health environments, healthy children: Children in families. (A report on the 1997 Panel Study of Income Dynamics). Ann Arbor, MI: Institute for Social Research, University of Michigan.

Howard, J. A., & Hollander, J. (1997). *Gendered situations, gendered selves.* Thousand Oaks, CA: Sage.

Kaufman, G., & Uhlenberg, P. (1998). Effects of life-course transitions on the quality of relationships between adult children and their parents. *Journal of Marriage and the Family, 60,* 924–938.

Knowles, J. P., & Cole, E. (1990). *Woman-defined motherhood.* New York: Harrington Park Press.

LeVine, R. (1994). *Childcare and culture: Lessons from Africa.* Cambridge: Cambridge University Press.

Lupton, D., & Barclay, L. (1997). *Constructing fatherhood: Discourses and experiences.* Thousand Oaks, CA: Sage.

McMahon, M. (1995). *Engendering motherhood: Identity and self-transformation in women's lives.* New York: The Guilford Press.

Oakley, A. (1974). *The sociology of housework.* New York: Pantheon.

Phoenix, A., Woollett, A., & Lloyd, E. (1991). *Motherhood: Meanings, practices and ideologies.* Thousand Oaks, CA: Sage.

Polakow, V. (1993). *Lives on the edge: Single mothers and their children in the other America.* Chicago: The University of Chicago Press.

Rich, A. (1976). *Of women born: Motherhood as experience and institution.* New York: W. W. Norton & Co., Inc.

Rossi, A. S., & Rossi, P.H. (1990). *Of human bonding: Parent-child relations across the lifecourse.* Hawthorne, NY: Aldine de Gruyter.

Ruddick, S. (1980). Maternal thinking. *Feminist Studies, 6,* 342–367.

Ruddick, S. (1989). *Maternal thinking: Toward a politics of peace.* Boston: Beacon Press.

Salwen, L. V. (1990). The myth of the wicked stepmother. In J. P. Knowles & E. Cole (Eds.). *Woman-defined motherhood* (pp.117–125). New York: Harrington Park Press.

Setterson, R. A. (1999). *Lives in time and place: The problems and promises of developmental science.* Amityville, NY: Baywood Publishing Company.

Sommerfeld, D. P. (1989). The origins of mother blaming: Historical perspectives on childhood and motherhood. *Infant Mental Health Journal, 10,* 14–24.

Thurer, S. L. (1994). *The myths of motherhood.* Boston: Houghton Mifflin Co.

U.S. Bureau of the Census (1997). *Statistical abstract of the United States: 1997* (117th edition). Washington, DC: Author.

Wasserfall, R. (1993). *Reflexivity, feminism and difference.* Human Services Press.

Weiss, R. (1994). *Learning from strangers: The art and method of qualitative interview studies.* New York: The Free Press.

White, L. K. (1994). Coresidence and leaving home: Young adults and their parents. *Annual Review of Sociology, 20,* 81–102.

White, L. K., & Rogers, S. J. (1997). Strong support but uneasy relationships: Coresidence and adult children's relationships with their parents. *Journal of Marriage and the Family, 59,* 62–76.

Yerxa, E. (1993). Occupational Science: A source of power for participants in occupational therapy. *Journal of Occupational Science: Australia, 1,* 3–10.

Zarit, S. H., & Eggebeen, D. J. (1995). Parent-child relationships in adulthood and old age. In M. H. Bornstein, *Handbook of parenting, volume 1: Children and parenting* (pp.119–128). Mahwah, NJ: Lawrence Erlbaum Associates, Publishers.

Source Credits

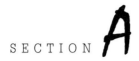

MAKING BEDS OF POETRY
(AND LYING IN THE WORDS)

Renee Norman

I'm just going upstairs to write poetry and make beds.

I don't know how to
make beds
out of fabric springboard stuffing
or write poetry
out of gossamer webbed lace

The sheets are wrinkled
in the stanzas
blood-stained with dots of fearfulness
I don't want to change them
but I can't see to pull them up over
images of uselessness

I don't mind picking up the nighclothes
and tossing them into the dirty laundry
but
it's hard to display them
between the rhythm of the words
everyone is always annoyed
when I return
the special toys and tempo
to the wrong person

Does everyone smooth the bed covers
like this
wondering where the lines came from
staring
at the quilt
on the page
pleased with restored order
which lasts and stays static
for about two minutes

Am I just fooling myself
into believing that I
need to make the beds of words
or could

I think I should have washed the sheets
and written letters home

Reprinted with permission from R. Norman (2002), Making Beds of Poetry (and Lying in the Words), Journal of the Association for Research on Mothering, Volume 4, No. 2, pp. 17–18.

SECTION B
Mothering Occupations in the Context of Special Challenges : Mothers

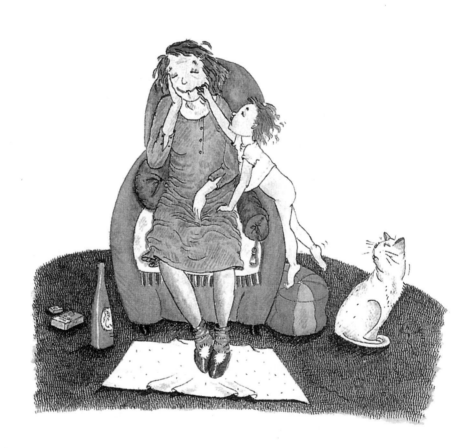

Drawing by Mary Leunig, reprinted with permission.

CHAPTER 9

Mothering Capacity and Social Milieu

Gwynnyth Llewellyn, PhD

David McConnell, PhD, BAppSc(OT)

Anticipated Outcomes

We anticipate that, after reading this chapter, readers will:

- Consider whether, or how, the transient caring behavior of others constitutes mothering

- Consider our argument that mothering is a learned occupation

- Have an increased understanding about mothers with intellectual disability

- Gain a deeper understanding of mothering as a social process dependent on opportunities for learning

- Consider that mothering is a learned occupation and that mothering capacity is a quality of the mother's social milieu

- Reflect on who may be part of a mother's life and the contributions they make to mothering occupations

Introduction

This chapter critiques the commonly accepted notion that mothering capacity can be understood as an individual trait. Instead we argue that mothering capacity is a function of the social milieu in which it occurs. Mothering, therefore, far from being an inherent virtue, is a learned occupation. We further argue that success or lack of success in learning mothering is dependent in a large part on opportunities for learning, which in turn are a function of the mother's social environment, relationships, and social network—in other words, her social milieu. Taking the case of mothers with intellectual disability, condemned in child protection practice as inadequate mothers based on their lower intelligence quotients, we demonstrate the false assumptions that underpin the notion of mothering as an individual trait. We propose that, to further develop an understanding of mothering occupations, the task for researchers is to incorporate explicit examination of the social milieu in which these occupations are embedded. We conclude by offering some beginning questions to advance this new research agenda.

The focus of this chapter is on mothering capacity, specifically, how it is viewed and what the ramifications are for vulnerable mothers. We dispute the dominant view that mothering capacity is somehow locked up within the individual and the myth that mothers are more or less solely responsible for the health, development, and socialization of their offspring. We question this traditional rendering of mothering as an individual trait. Instead, we argue in this chapter for a different conceptualization of mothering capacity—that is, as a quality of mothers' social milieu. Understanding that mothering capacity is a function of embedded social processes is critical to any examination of mothering occupations. In brief, we will argue that mothering occupations can be understood only in relation to the social milieu in which they occur.

Our interest in this topic stems from over a decade of research with mothers with intellectual disability. We began by talking to mothers about who was "there for them" to assist them in their mothering occupations. From a series of studies with mothers with young children, we developed an interview guide to help practitioners and researchers discover, from the mother's perspective, the help available to her. In doing so, our attention was increasingly drawn to exploring how, in industrialized countries, the construct of mothering and the associated notion of mothering capacity are conceptualized. This led us to critique the commonly accepted view of mothering

capacity as an individual trait and to explore alternative explanations for this construct. This chapter represents the current state of our thinking on this topic. In this chapter we limit our discussion to a perspective that begins with the mother, widens out to consideration of her social milieu, and returns to raising questions about how we might examine mothering capacity as a function of this social milieu. We are also acutely aware that our conceptualization is developed primarily within "western" notions of mothering, neglecting for the most part traditions about mothering in other communities and cultures. Notwithstanding, we offer our current conceptualization to encourage debate and discussion among researchers, practitioners, and educators on the complex concepts of mothering, mothering capacity, and mothering occupations. In doing so, we also hope that vulnerable mothers will no longer be subject to judgment and intervention based only on perceptions of their individual capacity to engage in mothering occupations.

To explore and explain our conceptualization, we take as our example mothers with intellectual disability. Mothering and intellectual disability are terms that do not come together easily. The mythic image of the "perfect mother" and the stereotype of people with intellectual disability as eternal children are pervasive and irreconcilable. Intellectually disabled women are therefore rarely considered even in works that include other disabled mothers (e.g., Morris, 1996). In contrast, we have been continually struck by the extraordinary "grit" and "craft" that mothers with intellectual disability display under extraordinary circumstances, not the least of which is the pessimism that prevails about their capacity to engage in mothering occupations.

We draw on our empirical work with mothers with intellectual disability in this chapter for three reasons. Following Goodnow and Collins (1990), we propose that examining mothering in the extreme affords unique insights. It provides the opportunity to critically examine taken-for-granted assumptions about mothering. Because, as we will argue, these assumptions are deeply embedded in tacit knowledge (Polanyi, 1966) about what constitutes mothering, it requires an unusual situation to force critical examination. The second reason is that mothers with intellectual disability are possibly the most marginalized in our community. It is doubtful whether any mothers experience closer or more constant scrutiny than they do (Booth & Booth, 1994; McConnell & Llewellyn, 1998; Tymchuk, Llewellyn, & Feldman, 1999). The intrusion of the state in their lives makes nonsense of the public-private divide normally respected in the mothering occupation. Mothers with intellectual disability are only too aware of this scrutiny, and many are plagued by fears of "the welfare" coming to take their children away. Our research and that of our colleagues in Europe and North America suggests that their fears are well grounded; as many as one in every two children born to mothers with intellectual disability are removed (Bishop et al., 2000; McConnell, Llewellyn, & Ferronato, 2000; Taylor et al., 1991). Our final reason is that their situation demonstrates the more generalized neglect of the highly socialized and social nature of mothering occupations in the literature.

This chapter begins with a story to illustrate our reflections on the social nature of mothering occupations. We follow this with an overview of the traditional view of mothering as an individual trait, institutionalized in societal structures and processes. By way of example, we present the case of child protection practice. We then argue that mothering is not inherent; it is learned in many ways, not the least of which is through practice. To illustrate the learned nature of mothering, we draw on a 2-year ethnographic study with mothers and fathers with intellectual disability. The findings from this study led to further exploring the multiple influences on mothering occupations, including the social milieu in which these occupations are embedded. To discuss this social milieu, we draw on data from several studies in which mothers with intellectual disability identify who is "there for them." For the final section, we turn our attention to the implications of the social milieu for understanding mothering occupations.

A World Full of People

From the moment a child is born, his or her world is full of people. We immediately think of parents, family, friends, and neighbors. However, of course, there are many more people in a child's life. Some are fleeting acquaintances; some are quite intimately involved with the child. There are the people who appear to a greater or lesser extent in the course of everyday activities, such as the person sitting next to mother and child on the bus, the postman, and the mother's best friend. There are the people who hold positions officially sanctioned in the care of children, such as the preschool teacher, after school care supervisor, recreation leader, and so on. And there are many of them. Salzinger (1990) noted that, although the networks of mothers and their young babies are almost identical and quite restricted, the rate at which they accumulate new contacts begins to accelerate around 4 months after the baby's birth. By the end of 7 months, an infant's contacts may number about 100 people.

Before we dismiss these contacts too quickly as being of little consequence to mothering occupations, here is a practical example. A middle-aged man is waiting at a bus stop and a mother with a young child is sitting beside him. The child is around 3 years old and visibly distressed. The conversation initiated by the man might go something like this: "What are all those tears about? Sit quietly now, and I have something to show you." Child stops screaming momentarily. Man seizes the opportunity and slowly and deliberately opens his briefcase and peeks inside. The child, overcome by curiosity leans over and also looks inside. Out comes a photo. The photo (and many others behind it) is of a dog—a border collie. The border collie is swimming. The man continues, "Look at this picture of my puppy. His name is Panda. Can you say that, Panda? It's spelled P-A-N-D-A. See, he's swimming. Do you like swimming?" And the conversation meanders on. The child, fascinated, is now quiet, looks through the photos, tries to copy the dog's name, talks about his own dog, and so on.

In this exchange, not only is the mother relieved that her screaming 3-year-old is now quiet, but someone who until a few minutes ago was a total stranger has "mothered" her child, however momentarily. Employing Ruddick's (1989) three-pronged framework for maternal work, we can understand that during this interlude:

1. The child was drawn from a potentially dangerous situation, throwing himself around at a busy bus stop (preservation).
2. The child was distracted to become quiet and listen (social acceptability).
3. At the same time, the child was given an opportunity to learn a new word, engage in a conversation, and so on (growth).

The picture of young children being mothered by a number of people—both adults and older children, both kin and non-kin—is a familiar image across the world, yet surprisingly neglected in western notions of mothering. Fostering, too, has been commonplace in societies that do not regard mothers and fathers as having "exclusive" rights over the rearing of their children. This may be done to provide additional resources for a child, for a family, or in the face of accident (for example, the death of mother, father, or both), as the only course of action for ongoing childrearing. Fostering may also be done in the face of sociocultural burden. For example, a child who is "different" may be viewed as an economic handicap and sent to live with extended family, as in McNeil's experience of being born an albino in India (McNeil, 2001).

The difficulty in recognizing this strong tradition of mothering as a social occupation appears to be derived, as Dalley (1988) suggests, from being "raised in the normative framework of western culture in which parents cling to their rights of possession over their children, and where they regard the socialization and training of their children as both their exclusive duty and function" (p. 97). Perhaps another reason for the neglect of the shared, social nature of mothering occupations is that, as illustrated by our example of the older man and the child, it is so commonplace, so ordinary, so taken for granted that we,

whether researchers or practitioners, do not even notice its existence. Instead we focus our attention on the individual and micro level of mothering occupations, with only peripheral attention to mothers' social relationships. (Bronfenbrenner, 1979) In so doing, we risk limiting our investigations to mothering as an individual trait and ignore the social milieu in which mothering occupations are embedded. We now turn to critiquing the traditional view that mothering and therefore mothering capacity is embedded within an individual.

Mothering Capacity as Individual Trait

Present day mothers are expected to bear the burden of responsibility for the nurturing of their offspring, and to do so with little communal support or honor accorded to mothers in pre-industrial societies (Doumanis, 1983; Maher, 1987). A romanticized vision of the nuclear family as autonomous and self-sufficient assumes that this structure is both necessary and sufficient for raising children. This view emphasizes the individual responsibility of mothers and downplays the responsibility of the collective. The organization of maternal work, mostly behind the four walls of the family home, further isolates mothers. Their isolation is compounded by societal beliefs about the perfect mother and the implications for children and society should mothers fail these expectations. Thurer (1994) observes that such expectations "cast a long, guilt-inducing shadow over real mothers' lives" (p. xi).

The perfect mother is, *of course,* unerring in love and duty: she is selfless (her child's needs always come first) and self-sufficient (though dependent on a male breadwinner); she is always present (at home) and attentive to her child's every need; she is patient and longsuffering; and, she is diligent in providing instruction, discipline, and stimulation (Hofferth, 1997; Thurer, 1994). If we accept the current western mythology—deeply seated as it is in the collective unconscious—then the well-being of children and thus society's future depend almost entirely on the quality of the mothers (Hofferth, 1997; Thurer, 1994). Nurture holds sway in this debate. *Bad* mothers become the scapegoat for society's ills: unemployment, crime, drug addiction, and mental illness, just to name a few.

Child Protection Practice

Institutionalization of the view that mothering is a quality or trait of individual women is clearly seen in child protection systems across the western world. Yet the cruel and uncaring mother mythologized in the media is, in fact, rarely encountered in child protection practice (Buckley, 1999; Clarke, 1993; Parton, 1995; Pelton, 1989; Thorpe, 1994). Most cases do not feature battered babies. Evidence of willful maltreatment, if present, is rarely clear and compelling. Instead, a body of research suggests that child protection cases typically involve children and families marginalized by poverty, social isolation, addiction, disability, and/or minority status (Fernandez, 1996; Gough et al., 1989; Lindsey, 1994; Morton, 1999; McConnell et al., 2000; Parton, 1995; Pelton, 1989; Thorpe, 1994). These are families who lack the material and social means to offset the impact of situational or personal problems, which, in turn, are often precipitated by adversity and deprivation (Belsky, 1993; Garbarino, 1977; Jack, 1997; Jamrozik & Sweeney, 1996; Pelton, 1982, 1997). Although the language used in child protection practice talks about families and parents, the discursive intent is focused on mothers. We draw attention to this discursive practice in the next paragraph.

Surprisingly, given this evidence, social and environmental stressors play a minor role only in workers' understanding of mothering difficulties or child maltreatment (McGillivray, 1992). Across countries and jurisdictions, child protection authorities view the parent, typically taken to mean the mother, as the problem (Farmer & Owen, 1998; Fernandez, 1996; King & Trowell, 1992; Lindsey, 1994; McConnell et al., 2000; Pelton, 1982; Thorpe, 1994). As Clarke (1993) observes, poverty, isolation and other deprivations are mistakenly conceptualized as predictive risk factors rather than circumstances that help explain child maltreatment.

The individualizing discourses of medicine and psychology lend legitimacy to this view and, in turn, to child protection processes. The diagnostic-prognostic reasoning typical of the clinical sciences focuses on individual traits to explain and anticipate behavior. For example, the diagnostic assessment tools psychologists use to assess parenting, although fathers are rarely assessed, are based on an assumption of individual capacity. Intelligence tests are among those most frequently used (Budd, Poindexter, Felix & Naik-Polan, 2001). The individual's circumstances and environment receive little or no consideration. Attribution of difficulties with parenting to the mother reinforces the assumption that childrearing is the province of one person acting alone. King and Trowell (1992) summarize thus:

> Within these individualizing discourses the social meaning—all those environmental and circumstantial factors that are outside the immediate control of the family—tends to be lost as a cause of harm to children or as a way of alleviating harm (p. 20).

The view that mothering capacity is contained within the individual is well illustrated by the treatment of mothers with intellectual disability in the child protection system—indeed, this is the definitive case. Diagnostic label and intelligence quotient alone are frequently used to determine intellectually disabled mothers as incapable (Haavik & Menninger, 1981; Hayman, 1990; Hertz, 1979; Payne, 1978). Family and disability service workers also work from the assumption that low intelligence is inextricably linked to mothering capacity (Crain & Millor, 1978; Llewellyn, Bye, & McConnell, 1997; McConnell & Llewellyn, 1998).

The dominant view of mothering capacity is evident in the literature on parents with intellectual disability, now spanning a period of more than 60 years. Numerous studies have examined the capacity of parents with intellectual disability to care for their children. Here again, the term parenting is loosely used when, indeed, the literature refers almost exclusively to mothers. As Llewellyn (1990) noted in a review article, up to that time only five fathers had appeared anywhere in the literature. In the intervening decade, fathers have slowly begun to appear (e.g. Llewellyn, McConnell & Honey, 2001), although their appearance is typically limited to articles reporting intervention programs. Authors addressing issues of parental capacity almost exclusively continue to report samples that contain only mothers (e.g., Feldman & Walton-Allen, 1997; Keltner, 1994; Tymchuk & Andron, 1992).

Significant is the consistent finding that there is no obvious relationship between mothering and IQ, and that intellectual (dis)ability *per se* is a poor predictor of an individual mother's competency to care for her offspring (e.g. Booth & Booth, 1993; Borgman, 1969; Budd & Greenspan, 1985; Dowdney & Skuse, 1993; Feldman, 1994; Llewellyn, 1990; Mickelson, 1947; Mira & Roddy, 1980; Tymchuk & Feldman, 1991). Still the myth prevails: researchers, policy makers, and practitioners incorrectly continue to investigate maternal IQ as a predictor of mothering capacity. Although the dominant view of mothering capacity continues to underpin child protection responses, consideration of alternative, less invasive means of securing and promoting the welfare of children are excluded.

Decision Making in Child Protection Processes

Concerned by the mounting evidence of discrimination against mothers with intellectual disability (McConnell & Llewellyn, 2000), we recently undertook a study of the child protection process. The broad aim of this study was to obtain prevalence and outcome data for parents with disabilities (more broadly defined to include intellectual, psychiatric, physical, and sensory disabilities) and their children appearing before the Children's Court in the state of New South Wales (NSW), Australia, and to investigate decision making in the child protection process. The study involved a review of court files of all child protection matters finalized over a 9-month period (May 1, 1998 to February 1, 1999) at two children's courts in Sydney, a city of approximately 4 million people, in Australia. In

all, this amounted to 407 care matters involving 622 children. In addition, 155 child protection officers, 34 lawyers and all 8 specialist children's magistrates (children's court judges) were interviewed, and we spent 35 days in the courtrooms observing court proceedings.

The prevalence and outcomes data from the study are reported elsewhere (McConnell et al., 2000; Llewellyn, McConnell, & Ferronato, 2003). In short, we found that mothers with intellectual disability were involved in almost one in ten cases initiated by the statutory child protection authority. Furthermore, their children were significantly more likely than the children of parents without a disability, or parents with a psychiatric disorder and/or suspected of drug/alcohol use, to be placed out-of-home in foster or residential care.

In line with previous findings (Glaun & Brown, 1999; Lynch & Bakley, 1989; Tymchuk & Andron, 1990), allegations of child abuse were rare, and when these were made, the alleged perpetrator was seldom the mother with an intellectual disability. The typical case was, instead, an allegation of neglect defined as inadequate provision. In 41.2 percent of cases there were concerns about the mother's lack of insight and resistance to statutory intervention. A recurring theme was the mother's incompetence in managing her own affairs: for example, maintaining a tidy and hygienic home environment, managing her finances and choosing appropriate partners. Child protection officers described these cases as "the saddest cases of all," and further:

> In their own mind, in their world, they dearly love the child and they're doing the best they can with what they've got... and that's true...but it's not good enough for that kid.

Evaluation of a mother's capacity to "lift her game" and to do so without ongoing service support was the key factor in determining whether the child was removed and the subsequent decision about where the child should be placed. We found that the authorities usually held little hope that mothers with intellectual disability would be able to provide "good-enough" mothering. Their strong tendency to conflate intellectual disability with perceived mothering deficiency resulted in a generalized assumption that this group of mothers needed 24-hour supervision for an extended period. In the words of one child protection officer, "the disability (and by implication the risk to the child) isn't going away." Or, as one magistrate put it:

> If they've got that disability, you can't fix it. If there's impairment to the brain there's nothing you can do to fix it. They don't know how to cook the child a meal... and they are never going to learn how to cook that meal because they can't.

Set against these pessimistic and outdated beliefs is a substantial body of evidence that demonstrates successful mothering by many mothers with intellectual disability (for example, Booth and Booth, 2000; Keltner, Wise, & Taylor, 1999; Llewellyn, 1995, 1997). There is also abundant evidence that mothers with intellectual disability can and do learn, apply new knowledge, and maintain new skills (Budd & Greenspan, 1985; Feldman, 1994; Tymchuk & Feldman, 1991; Tymchuk, 1990). These skills include basic childcare such as bathing, changing diapers, and cleaning baby bottles (e.g. Feldman, Case, & Sparks, 1992); home safety and emergencies (e.g., Llewellyn, McConnell, & Honey, 2001; Tymchuk, Andron, & Hagelstein, 1992; Tymchuk et al., 1990a & b); parent-child interaction and play (e. g., Feldman et al., 1985; Feldman et al., 1986; Keltner, Finn, & Shearer, 1995); decision making (e.g., Tymchuk et al., 1988); responding to common problematic parenting and social situations (e.g., Fantuzzo et al., 1986), and menu planning and grocery shopping (Sarber et al., 1983).

This mounting evidence negates the stereotyped view that mothering is an individual trait linked to intelligence. If this were the case, all mothers with low intelligence would, *ipso facto*, be incompetent. An alternative view acknowledges the many influences on mothering occupations and mothering practices. From this perspective, mothering capacity is context bound rather than a trait of individuals. To ex-amine mothering in context, we turn to cross-cultural and sociohistorical perspectives to understand the multiple influences on mothering occupations.

↜ Mothering as a Learned Occupation

Women are not born with mothering know-how; mothering is a learned occupation. This learning does not take place in a social vacuum. Rather, and this is the crucial point, it occurs through many and varied social exchanges, which are socially and culturally bound. Consequently, there is cross-cultural variation in childrearing practice: mothering behaviors are not givens (for a review, see Harkness & Super, 1996). Indeed, what comes to be considered mothering in any given society results from complex sociocultural processes.

Mothering know-how and norms are passed on, but each generation modifies, adds to, and subtracts from this socially and culturally shared stock of knowledge. Consequently, mothering occupations not only vary across cultures, but also over time; mothering occupations and practices are historically specific. An illustrative example comes from Smart's work on *Deconstructing Motherhood*. Smart (1996) points out that what we regard as good and bad practices, and for that matter whom we regard as good and bad mothers, is a matter of fashion. These practices become rule laden so that mothers who follow them are seen as good and bad mothers remain deliberately or willfully ignorant of the "right" practices to be followed. She notes, "These (practices) could range from allowing the infant to sleep in the parental bed (bad), to allowing it to sleep in the same room (all right for the first few months only), to failing to provide enough fresh air (bad), to swaddling to not swaddling, and right through to the modern rules on whether to place a baby on its front (bad now although good in the 1970s and 1980s) or its back (good in the 1990s) to sleep" (p. 46).

Mothers, however, do not passively absorb and reproduce this know-how and the norms of their particular society and culture. Mothers actively shape the society and culture in which they are situated. Following the sociological perspective of symbolic interactionism (Blumer, 1969), mothering occupations can be seen as constructed by, and in turn construct, the work that mothers do in their respective societies. As Valsiner and Litvinovic (1996), observe how mothering occupations are regarded comes from:

> … the form of their parallel constructions of conceptions, ideas, and attitudes about parenting and childrearing in general and also in the form of those symbolic constraints on thought and action that are not directly related to parenting but affect the shaping of parental behaviours (p. 63).

Mothering occupations are recognized by practices and behaviors and, in turn, these practices and behaviors inform the work that mothers do. Following Ruddick's (1989) seminal analysis, we understand that maternal work results from the universal demands imposed on those responsible for children. These demands are ensuring the preservation, growth, and social acceptability of the child. Of these, preservation of the vulnerable child is considered pre-eminent. This is supplemented by nurturing the child's emotional and intellectual growth. The final demand is that children's growth is shaped in socially acceptable ways. In essence, what being a mother means for Ruddick is "to be committed to meeting these (three) demands by works of preservative love, nurturance, and training" (Ruddick, 1989, p. 17)

Maternal work captures the everyday responsibilities, tasks and activities inherent in meeting these demands. For Ruddick (1989), those doing maternal work develop distinctive ways of thinking about the world. This view is derived from the philosophy of practicalism, which posits that distinctive ways of knowing arise out of practices. Thus, knowing about mothering (maternal thinking) arises out of practicing mothering. At a deeper level of understanding, practicalism suggests that as a person pursues certain goals associated with a practice and, as that practice is simultaneously defined and refined, so the particular practices make (or come to make) sense. In other words, as we come to understand more fully, our understanding shapes the outcomes we pursue "as the practical pursuit of the end shapes our understanding" (Ruddick, 1989, p. 14).

The mothering occupation is therefore not biologically determined or gendered, despite appearances to the contrary. Mothering is learned by those doing mothering work. Across cultures and within societies, many women and men who are not biological mothers are maternal workers. Maternal thought according to Ruddick (1989) develops from this practice of mothering irrespective of gender or biological or social relationship to the child or children. Engaging in this daily practice of maternal work promotes learning about protecting, nurturing, and training children. We illustrate the learned nature of mothering by way of example from a study of mothers and fathers with intellectual disability.

Mothers and Fathers with Intellectual Disability Learning Mothering

In an ongoing research project spanning several studies, we have explored how mothers and, to a lesser extent, fathers with intellectual disability learn mothering occupations (Llewellyn, 1995, 1997; Llewellyn et al., 1999; Llewellyn & McConnell, 2002; Llewellyn et al., 2002). Their experiences reveal the complex web of social interactions that constitutes the learning experience.

An ethnographic study with six couples with intellectual disability over a 2-year period revealed three primary sources and means of learning for these parents (Llewellyn, 1997). From their own accounts, they relied heavily on the first source, that is, childhood memories and family traditions, for knowledge of what and what not to do. Take Rosalind for example. For her, it was important to follow her family traditions (involving set routines) because, in her words, "my great grandmother, she was a good mother to my grandmother, and she was good to my mother, and my mother was good to me." By contrast, Margaret, fostered with her twin sister as a young child only to be placed (without her sister) in an institution as a young adolescent, began a new family tradition as she learned to use different disciplinary methods in contrast to her foster family's methods of extreme physical force.

A second source was following the example set by other people, especially family members. This strategy was usually employed when the couple's existing knowledge or skills could not meet the demands of a novel situation. For example, help was sought (usually from professionals) when emergencies arose, such as the child swallowing a potentially harmful substance. In less dramatic situations, such as infant teething, most often the couples initially employed "tricks of the trade" learned from someone else. Continuing to use a particular trick depended on whether it was successful or not, for example, in reducing the baby's discomfort.

The third and final source of learning came from, as Ruddick (1989) suggested, the daily practice of "doing parenting." The mothers and the fathers learned by making mistakes, changing routines, and trying alternatives. Although they generally felt positive about being responsible for their own learning, this was not always so, particularly if this type of learning was the only option. For example, Allan strongly asserted a positive value for "learning by yourself" as "it is the only way to learn." In contrast, his wife Ruth recalled bitterly how:

> I did it all from my own learning myself, I didn't learn from anyone else. I didn't get any help from Allan's mum, I didn't get any help from my mum ... I really had no help from Allan's family and I had a sick baby and they never really came around and helped me at all which was a bit upsetting cause they were only around the corner, I didn't have no help.

Learning about the multifaceted responsibilities and tasks of mothering is, of course, not straightforward. The mothers and fathers in this study often talked about the conflicting advice they received. Different strategies were used to deal with this. Some of these mothers and fathers tried out alternative pieces of advice to "see what worked"; others rejected the advice and crafted their own ways of doing things.

Mark and Elizabeth provide an example of how parents learned their "own way" based on ideas from others. This couple frequently sought out and listened to suggestions from hospital nursery staff, from staff at a mother-baby unit, and from friends and family. They based their decisions on these suggestions. For example, when they experienced some difficulty developing a feeding routine with their first child, Samantha, they received advice from both the hospital and the mother-baby unit on a feeding program. Elizabeth recalled this time as follows:

> We had a program (feeding schedule) that we were following from the hospital and when we went to Z. (the mother-baby unit) they gave us this program to follow, so we said, oh well we'll follow this, and then we ended up ... when we got home we didn't like Z.'s way of doing it ... so we said oh well, we'll go back to the hospital's way, because we kind of liked that best, and anytime I get into strife I just ring the nursery up and say look I've got this problem can you help me, they usually do.

As these mothers and fathers demonstrate, those engaged in mothering occupations draw their ideas from multiple sources. Acquiring ideas and learning mothering is not a passive process. Mothering requires lifelong learning. Childrearing presents both familiar and novel challenges, often simultaneously. Circumstances change and life takes unexpected turns. More to the point, children are not predictable or passive recipients of care; meeting their needs demands adaptation or innovation on the run. Engaging in mothering occupations requires, as the mothers and fathers with intellectual disability in this study demonstrate, agency in choosing one idea over another, exercising choice to select who will be regarded as "expert", decoding multiple ideas to encode one's own particular parenting practices, and as Backett (1982) suggests, accepting and at the same time rejecting advice because "it is a good idea but it wouldn't work with my child." We now turn our attention to the social milieu in which this mothering takes place.

🕊 Mothering in a Social Milieu

The starting point is the common-sense observation that relationships with others— partners, family members, friends, and sometimes professionals—hold a place of great significance in our lives. To varying degrees, the paths our lives take, our actions, and how we feel and think about ourselves are influenced by those whose lives intersect with our own.

The literature on mothering occupations already suggests that mothers' relationships are complex and their individual significance varies (Kellegrew, 2000; Primeau, 2000, Segal, 2000). At any point, these relationships may be characterized by unconditional positive regard, conflict ridden, or somewhere in between. Relationships may be a vital resource or a constraint as mothers negotiate life's transitions and unexpected turns (Francis-Connolly, 2000). Mothers are embedded in networks of relationships with friends, family members, and significant others who may support or negate their mothering occupations (e.g., Pierce & Frank, 1992).

We argue that, to understand mothering as a social process, we need first to examine more closely the influence of social relationships on those engaged in mothering occupations. To date, our research has focused on the social networks and relationships of biological mothers of young children. To begin, we present three vignettes to illustrate the diversity of mothers' social environments. Following this, we summarize the findings from several studies that help explain how mothering occupations are strongly influenced by and in turn influence mothers' social milieu.

lic housing. Currently, Elaine has a restraining order against her husband. The support of her mother and sister were vital in persuading Elaine to break from her abusive husband. It was her mother who called the police and her sister who persuaded her that she was "better off without him." Elaine says that she would be lost without their support—knowing that her mother and sister are "behind (her) all the way" is vitally important.

For Elaine, the hardest thing about being a mother is "loneliness." She would desperately like to have a partner—"Do I get to go out with a new man? When is it going to happen? You think, no man is that stupid, who'd want to do that? Who'd want to be with me and my kids?"

Elaine phones her mother and sister almost every day, but lives too far away to see them more than a couple of times each week. With the assistance of a local community worker, Elaine has applied for housing near to her mother. In addition to providing critical moral support, her mother and sister help her budget and manage her money, and "spoil the kids" with gifts. Elaine also knows she can call on them in a crisis.

On a day-to-day basis, Elaine manages all childcare and household management tasks without any support. Don and Pam, two workers from local social service agencies are also important sources of support. Don has been a source of information, explaining to Elaine the meaning of the restraining order. He has also provided practical and emotional support. Elaine talked about the heater, which needed replacing, and purchasing an Easter hamper, both of which Don organized for her. Pam has also been a "great support" to Elaine, organizing early intervention services and attending play groups to help Jacob, who is a little behind in his development, and doing so quickly. Elaine says Pam "sure doesn't muck around!" 🕊

🕊 Vignette: *Elaine*

Elaine, age 32, is separated from her husband, living alone with her two young sons, Shane (age 10 months) and Jacob (age 3 years) in pub-

🕊 Vignette: *Sarah*

Sarah, age 33, is a single mother, who lives in her parent's household with her two children, Katrina (age 5) and Alissa (age 3). Katrina is in kindergarten, attending a regular school. Alissa goes to day care 3 days each week, at which time Sarah earns a small sum working part time in a workshop where she does sewing.

Sarah's parents, Judy and Robert, assume a lot of responsibility for the care of the children. They help get the children up each morning, dress them, prepare their meals, take them to school or day care, and pick them up in the afternoon. Many childcare tasks such as these are done for Sarah, despite her desire to do them herself: "I want to learn all that. Mum and Dad won't be around forever to do that. I don't know why I can't learn!"

Sarah would like a place of her own, "to be my own boss in my own kitchen." Often she feels that her parents thwart her role and responsibility as mother. Sarah says, "When you're with your mum and dad and you have got other people around you, you seem to have more than one boss. I'm like a boss, ... mum and dad is like a boss too. Three of us being the boss of the kids telling them what not to do, and what to do... ."

On weekends, Sarah often takes the children and stays at her brother and sister-in-law's place. Her parents then get a break from the children, and Sarah gets a break from her parents. Sarah says she wouldn't ask her parents to mind the children on weekends anymore, "Dad can get very cranky, I think Dad is getting tired. Mum and Dad's tired, cause Mum and Dad are getting to that age, you know...."

Sarah admits that there are good times and bad times with her parents. "When I'm upset," says Sarah, "it is usually over my parents." For emotional support and advice, Sarah turns mainly to Rebecca, a support person from a local service agency, or to Mrs. Smith, her supervisor at work. Sarah says that sometimes she will try to speak with her parents, but it is hard if they are not going to listen, or say they are too busy.

After having had a series of social workers, Sarah now has a special rapport with Rebecca. The fact that Rebecca has two children of her own is especially important to Sarah. Often they go out to a coffee shop, just to talk. Rebecca assists with the completion of forms for such things as Social Security benefits, and currently

she is helping Sarah to apply for her own place in a nearby public housing estate.[1]   ⌘

⌘ Vignette: **Karina and Paul**

Karina, age 34, and Paul, age 31, have two sons, David (age 7) and Brad (age 3). They live in public housing in a Sydney suburb. Both Karina and Paul are at home full time, relying solely on Social Security benefits for income. Paul would like to get a job, but without the ability to read or write, he has had no good fortune.

Karina, smiling, describes both children as "a real real handful." David has Fragile X syndrome and is hyperactive. He attends a special school, and after hours, goes to respite care. Their younger child Brad is developmentally delayed. Brad is a "real full-time baby," refusing to be cared for by anyone but Karina. Currently, a community social worker is helping to enroll him in a local preschool for the next school year.

With day-to-day childcare and household management tasks, Karina relies on Paul's support. Paul sometimes does the vacuuming, helps Karina with the cooking, and hangs the laundry out. In the mornings he helps David dress and get ready for school, and in the evenings he helps get the children into bed. Karina, however, cannot always rely on Paul's help, "It all depends on how busy he is."

The demands of childrearing have placed Karina and Paul's marriage under a lot of stress. At times, Karina says, "Paul just can't handle the pressure." Karina described a recent incident when she was "nagging" Paul to help her with the children. He responded by leaving her to manage on her own while he took time out with friends. At such times of crisis, Karina turns to Paul's mother, Marie, whom she describes as "the most important (support) person in the whole world."

Marie lives within walking distance of their home. In the past, when the children were younger, Marie gave Karina much practical support, buying necessities such as diapers, babysitting, and helping Karina establish a routine. Now Karina sees Marie only about once a month, and looks to her for advice and emotional support, particularly in relation to her marriage difficulties. Marie, however, "has problems of her own" and advises them to "sort things out for (them)selves."

In addition to Paul and Marie, Karina identified her sister Joanna and her social worker as people in her social environment. Joanna supports Karina by giving her "hand-me-down" clothes for the kids and occasionally talking with her over the phone. Karina rarely sees Joanna because she lives quite a distance away, and Joanna's husband doesn't like to "be involved." Karina, however, had no reservations about the support she has received from a local community social worker. "Whenever I need anything, whenever I want anything, she helps us out." The social worker supports Karina by arranging school and respite placements, filling in forms, and supporting Karina' requests to the Department of Housing. For example, Karina recently decided that she needed a fence around her front yard for her children's safety. Her social worker helped her to obtain it.[1]

✒ Exploring the Mother's Perspective

As these vignettes demonstrate, our approach to understanding the mothers' milieu aims to explore, from the mother's perspective, whom she perceives as being "there for her" and what these people provide (Llewellyn et al., 1999; Llewellyn & McConnell, 2002). We have gathered data over a 4-year period in 3 studies involving 70 mothers with preschool-age children under the age of 6 years. In each case we used a standard method to investigate three aspects of mothers' social networks and relationships. These are:

1. Quantity and composition of their support networks
2. Structural characteristics (e.g., frequency of contact and geographical proximity)
3. Functional characteristics (e.g., type of support provided)

These data were obtained in interviews using a semi-structured protocol, the Support Interview Guide (SIG, Llewellyn & McConnell, 2002). We developed this guide based on social support and personal network theory (House, Umberson & Landis, 1988; Pierce, Sarason & Sarason, 1996; Tracy & Whittaker, 1990; Tracy & Abell, 1994). A copy of the SIG is available from the first author.

The SIG uses simplified language, colored response cards, and graphics to illustrate support dimensions such as closeness. In the first part, mothers are asked to identify those people "who help/support you, and people who you can turn to for help when you need it." The names of people identified are written in the relevant sections of a social network map, viz. people in the household, family members who do not live with the mother, friends, neighbors, and paid service providers. Based on this exercise, support network size and composition are computed. The people whom mothers regard as helpful or supportive are designated as their supportive ties. As reported previously (Llewellyn et al., 1999), we define a supportive tie as the "helping unit" nominated by the mother. Thus, a supportive tie may be one individual, for example, the mother's mother, or it may be more than one, for example, the mother's sister and her husband. The relevant criterion is how the mother identifies the helping unit.

In the second part of the SIG, the mother is asked to indicate the relative closeness of each supportive tie by writing the name of each person in one of three concentric circles. For example, in the inner circle the mothers write (or the interviewer records) the names of people to whom they feel so close that "it would be hard to imagine life without them." The names of people who are "not all that close" are written in the outer circle. The next part of the interview uses response cards to explore other structural characteristics of the mother's personal network, including frequency and type of contact with each supportive tie, duration of the relationship, geographical proximity, and how comfortable the mother feels in asking for/receiving support from each supportive tie.

The final section of the SIG uses graphic representations to explore the functional characteristics of the mothers' support networks. Mothers indicate what type of help is offered: practical support, information or advice, emotional support, and/or social companionship. Examples are given for each type of support, and the mother is asked to give a different example to ensure that she understands each support type. This functional characteristic data is used to determine the sources of each type of support and compute multiplexity, which is defined as the number of different types of support available from each supportive tie.

Through the course of these studies, we have come to understand that the people whom mothers describe as "there for them" can be thought of as the mother's self-identified social milieu, or in other words, the environment in which they carry out their mothering occupations. *One key finding of these studies is the centrality of family members in their lives regardless of their living situation.* Overall, mothers feel closest to, and most comfortable with, family members. Family members provide more types of support than formal ties and friends and neighbors and are also the primary source of practical/tangible and emotional support. However, this close involvement of family members in mothers' lives conceals the fact that many mothers are estranged from their own parents, siblings, and other relatives. Quite a few of the mothers nominate their partner's parents and siblings and not their own as family members. Closeness to family members does not assume, however, that their advice is always supportive. As Tucker and Johnson (1989) have shown, *family members can be either competence promoting or competence inhibiting.*

The second key finding relates to the place of formal ties in the mothers' lives. Service providers are the second largest group of supportive ties and the primary source of information and advice. Mothers' relationships with these service providers are, however, relatively short term and characterized by relatively infrequent contact. *In general, mothers do not feel close to their service providers or comfortable in asking for or receiving support.* These views about service providers may be potential obstacles to mothers gaining support services. Mothers may be fearful of too close a contact with service providers, a fear stemming from their awareness of close scrutiny from "the welfare," as we noted earlier. This is congruent with reports of others (e.g., Taylor, 1995).

The third key finding is that *mothers identify few supportive ties with friends and neighbors.* One in four mothers have no such ties. When mentioned, friends and neighbors are mainly a source of social companionship—people to be with and do things with such as going shopping, to the movies, and to the local club. This absence of friends is of grave concern given their importance as an indicator of quality of life and social integration for other adults with intellectual disability (Newton et al., 1994; House et al., 1988).

Most significantly, variation in mothers' social environments is caused by their living arrangements. In other words, the mothers' social milieu is a function of the households in which they reside. We have identified three distinct household types: mothers living alone with their child/children; mothers living in a parent/parent figure household; and, mothers living with partners. Typical support network features for each group are shown in Table 9–1.

Mothers with Intellectual Disability Who Live Alone with Their Child or Children in the Community

The social milieu for mothers such as Elaine, in the first vignette, is service centered. These mothers rely more on formal ties that tend to provide more varieties of support. They tend to have relatively small support networks, and their relationships are relatively short term. Moreover, these mothers perceive their relationship to service providers to be significantly closer than that of mothers in both other household groups, and they feel significantly more comfortable in asking for and receiving support from them in comparison to mothers living in a parent/parent figure's household. This group of mothers living alone appears to be the most socially isolated. In this they are also probably the most vulnerable because they have such a heavy reliance on service providers, who are less likely to remain constant than family members.

Table 9–1 Support network typology		
Service centered	Local family centered	Dispersed family centered
• Typical of mothers living alone with their children, in either the community or supported accommodation	• Typical of mothers living in a parent/parent figure's household or with significant others.	• Typical of mothers living with partners in the community.
• Relatively small network size • Mothers have a relatively high proportion of formal ties providing multiple kinds of support	• Supportive ties live relatively nearby, with whom they have frequent in-person, but infrequent phone contact.	• Relatively large support networks
• Mothers feel relatively close to formal ties • Relatively infrequent contact with family ties who tend to be widely dispersed	• Mother's supportive ties are stable (i.e., the mother has known them for relatively long period of time.)	• A high proportion of family ties
• Mothers have known supportive ties for a relatively short period of time (less stable social relationships)	• Mothers have a relatively high proportion of formal ties, but these provide a narrow range of support types and are not perceived as being close.	• A relatively low proportion of formal ties, friends, and neighbors. • Family ties are relatively dispersed, living further away. Frequency of phone contact is therefore high.
• These mothers feel quite comfortable asking for/receiving support from supportive ties.	• These mothers do not feel all that comfortable asking for support—perhaps suggesting a desire for greater independence.	• Relatively stable networks • Mothers feel relatively "close" to their supportive ties and comfortable asking for and receiving support.

Source: Llewellyn & McConnell (2002).

Mothers Living in a Parent/Parent Figure's Household

Sarah, in the second vignette, is one such mother. Although the social milieu of these mothers is family centered, with frequent contact in geographically close surroundings, they feel least comfortable asking for and receiving support. This discomfort may be indicative of a desire by these mothers to be more independent from their families and more a part of local community life (Llewellyn et al., 1999). This suggests a role for service providers to engage mothers in activities outside their family home and to, again, work to increase mothers' opportunities to develop relationships with friends or neighbors.

Mothers Living with Partners

The social milieu of Karina, in the third vignette, is also family centered. However, in contrast to mothers living in a parent/parent figure household, there is much less frequent in-person contact because their family members are quite dispersed geographically. The high proportion of family ties in their social environment is at least partly because of two sets of families, their own and their partner's. These mothers view their supportive ties as significantly closer than do mothers in both other household groups. Their relationships are more enduring, and they are more comfortable asking for support.

The varying characteristics of the three social environments suggest that *mothers' living arrangements have differential effects on their opportunities for advice and learning and thus their mothering occupations.* This suggests the critical importance of systematically exploring a mother's social environment if we are to understand the ways in which she carries out her mothering occupations. So, in our example, the mother living in a parent/parent figure's household, by definition, will be subject to more parental advice and less professional advice. The opposite holds true for single mothers living alone. Mothers living with partners can turn to the partner or to their family members or those of their partner.

The conclusion we draw is that *mothers with intellectual disability and their mothering occupations cannot be extracted from their social environment.* From this, we suggest that the capacity to engage in mothering occupations is a function of mothers' social milieu; in this case, those persons whom mothers identify as being there for them, the roles they play, and the tasks and activities they undertake. There are other aspects of mothers' social milieu yet to be explored. Our studies to date have focused attention only on those people identified by the mothers as significant to them. For example, we have yet to explore the contribution to mothering capacity of the many other people with whom mothers come in contact in their everyday mothering lives.

ᴥ Conclusion

In this chapter we have argued that mothering is best understood as a deeply embedded social occupation and mothering capacity as a quality of mothers' social milieu. Three observations were offered to support our argument. The first is that there are many social influences on children and their development. The second observation is that mothering is a learned occupation; this learning takes place within a particular social, cultural, and historical context, through interactions with others, and over a lifetime. The third observation is that people other than mothers engage to a greater or lesser degree in maternal work.

How we conceptualize mothering is not a trivial academic exercise. We have demonstrated, using the case of mothers with intellectual disability, that the taken-for-granted view of mothering capacity as a trait or quality of individual women has potentially devastating consequences for vulnerable families. It is no coincidence that the vast majority of children who are removed by statutory child protection authorities come from poor and marginalized families. Yet, mothers are easily scapegoated. It seems that the effects of

poverty, social isolation, and so on are harder to deal with and easier to ignore.

How we view mothering and mothering capacity is therefore political. If we accept the view that mothering capacity is somehow locked up inside individual women, then we accept the status quo in determining mothering capacity. The conceptualization presented here demands a different response. Mothering occupations are learned and carried out in a social context. To determine mothering capacity, therefore, we need to investigate the quality of the mothers' social milieu. To do so requires researchers and practitioners to explore mothers' social environments, their relationships and support networks, and the assistance or lack thereof that these offer to the mother from her point of view.

We have presented our conceptualization in this chapter to encourage discussion and debate in the emerging literature focused on occupational engagement. As researchers, we are keen to expand the research agenda to incorporate explicit examination of the social milieu in which mothering occupations are embedded. There are many questions to be explored. We offer to researchers, practitioners, and educators only a few as a starting point. Acknowledging that many people can engage in maternal work, we need to ask: How do other people besides the child's mother become engaged in this work, is their work the same or different, and how is it maintained over time? Given that multiple people may be involved, how do mothers negotiate with others the tasks of mothering and also the responsibilities? And finally, for practitioners working with vulnerable families, how can practice be expanded to take account of mothers' social environments? A useful beginning will be reducing attribution of mothering difficulties to individual mothers—being slower to judge and more intent on understanding the social milieu in which the mother is carrying out her mothering occupations.

Discussion Questions ᴊᴥ

- We argue in this chapter that mothering capacity is a quality of the mother's social milieu, drawing on work with mothers with intellectual disability. Is this argument context bound, that is, pertaining only to this particular group? One way to answer this question is to examine our arguments using as the example another group of mothers with whom you are familiar.

- Views of mothering are deeply embedded in sociocultural-historical experience. Critiquing these views offers considerable challenge. Particularly confronting is the notion that transient or short-term interactions between adults and children may constitute mothering. Attempt to formulate an argument that short-term or transient engagement in maternal work (Ruddick, 1989) does not constitute mothering.

- We observe that the taken-for-granted view of mothering capacity as a trait or quality of individual women has potentially devastating consequences for vulnerable families—mothers are easily *scapegoated*. Consider the relationship between how mothering capacity is viewed and how family and community services are delivered. What are the potential implications for vulnerable families of a welfare system, premised on the view that mothering capacity is a quality of the mother's social milieu?

References

Backett, K. C. (1982). *Mothers and fathers. The development and negotiation of parental behaviour.* London (UK): Macmillan.

Belsky, J. (1993). Etiology of child maltreatment: A developmental-ecological analysis. *Psychological Bulletin, 114*(3), 413–434.

Bishop, S. J., Murphy, J. M., Hicks, R., Quinn, D., Lewis, P. J., Grace, M., & Jellinek, M. S. (2000). What progress has been made in meeting the needs of seriously maltreated children? The course of 200 cases through the Boston Juvenile Court. *Child Abuse & Neglect, 24*(5), 599–610.

Blumer, H. (1969). *Symbolic interactionism. Perspective and method.* Englewood Cliffs, CA: Prentice-Hall, Inc.

Booth, T., & Booth, W. (2000). Against the odds: Growing up with parents who have learning difficulties. *Mental Retardation, 38*(1), 1–14.

Booth, T., & Booth, W. (1994). *Parenting under pressure. Mothers and fathers with learning difficulties.* Buckingham (UK): Open University Press.

Booth, T., & Booth, W. (1993). Parenting with learning difficulties: Lessons for practitioners. *British Journal of Social Work, 23,* 459–480.

Borgman, R.D. (1969). Intelligence and maternal inadequacy. Child Welfare, XL VIII (5), 301–304.

Bronfenbrenner, U. (1979). *The ecology of human development.* Cambridge, MA: Harvard University Press.

Buckley, H. (1999). Child protection practice: An ungovernable enterprise? *The Economic and Social Review, 30*(1), 21–40.

Budd, K., & Greenspan, S. (1985). Parameters of successful and unsuccessful interventions with parents who are mentally retarded. *Mental Retardation, 23,* 269–273.

Budd, K. S., Poindexter L. M., Felix, E. D., & Naik-Polan, A. T. (2001). Clinical assessment of parents in child protection cases: An empirical analysis. *Law and Human Behavior, 25*(1), 93–108.

Clarke, R. (1993). Discrimination in child protection services. The need for change. In L. Waterhouse (Ed.). *Child abuse and child abusers. Protection and prevention* (pp. 178–190). London (UK): Kingsley.

Crain, L. S., & Millor, G. K. (1978). Forgotten children: Maltreated children of mentally retarded parents. *Pediatrics, 6*(1), 130–131.

Dalley, G. (1988). *Ideologies of caring. Rethinking community and collectivism.* London (UK): Macmillan.

Doumanis, M. (1983). *Mothering in Greece: From collectivism to individualism.* New York: Academic Press.

Dowdney, L., & Skuse, D. (1993). Parenting provided by adults with mental retardation. *Journal of Child Psychology & Child Psychiatry, 34*(1), 25–47.

Fantuzzo, J. W., Wray, L., Hall, R., Goins, C., and Azar, S. (1986). Parent and social skills training for mentally retarded mothers identified as child maltreaters. *American Journal of Mental Deficiency, 91*(2), 135–140.

Farmer, E., & Owen, M. (1998). Gender and the child protection process. *British Journal of Social Work, 28,* 545–564.

Feldman, M. A. (1994). Parenting education for parents with intellectual disabilities: A review of the literature. *Research in Developmental Disabilities, 15,* 229–332.

Feldman, M. A., Case, L., Towns, F., & Betel, J. (1985). Parent education project 1: The development and nurturance of children of mentally retarded parents. *American Journal of Mental Deficiency, 90,* 253–258.

Feldman, M. A., Case, L., & Sparks, B. (1992). Effectiveness of a child care training program for parents at-risk for child neglect. *Canadian Journal of Behavioural Science, 24*(1), 14–28.

Feldman, M. A., Towns, F., Betel, J., Case, L., Rincover, A., & Rubino, C. A. (1986). Parent education project II: Increasing stimulating interactions of developmentally handicapped mothers. *Journal of Applied Behavior Analysis, 19,* 23–37.

Feldman, M. A., & Walton-Allen, N. (1997). Effects of maternal mental retardation and poverty on intellectual, academic, and behavioural status of school-age children. *American Journal on Mental Retardation, 101*(4), 352–364.

Fernandez, E. (1996). *Significant harm. Unravelling child protection decisions and substitute care careers of children.* Aldershot: Avebury.

Francis-Connolly, E. (2000). Toward understanding of mothering: A comparison of two motherhood stages.

American Journal of Occupational Therapy, 54(3), 281–289.

Garbarino, J. (1977). The human ecology of child maltreatment: A conceptual model for research. *Journal of Marriage and the Family, 39,* 721–735.

Glaun, D. E., & Brown, P. F. (1999). Motherhood, intellectual disability and child protection: Characteristics of a court sample. *Journal of Intellectual and Developmental Disability, 24*(1), 95–105.

Goodnow, J. J., & Collins, W. A. (1990). *Development according to parents. The nature, sources, and consequences of parents' ideas.* Hove and London: Lawrence Erlbaum Associates, Publishers.

Gough, D. A., Boddy, F. A., Dunning, N., & Stone, F. H. (1989). *The management of child abuse: A longitudinal study of child abuse in Glasgow.* Glasgow, Scotland: University of Glasgow, Social Paediatric and Obstetric Research Unit.

Haavik, S. F., & Menninger, K. A. (1981). The retarded parent and child neglect laws. In S. F. Haavik & K. A. Menninger (Eds.). *Sexuality, law and the developmentally disabled* (pp. 87–104). Baltimore: Paul H Brookes.

Harkness, S., & Super, C. M. (Eds.) (1996). *Parents' cultural belief systems. Their origins, expressions, and consequences.* New York: The Guildford Press.

Hayman, R. L. (1990). Presumptions of justice: Law, politics, and the mentally retarded parent. *Harvard Law Review, 103,* 1201–1271.

Hertz, R. A. (1979). Retarded parents in neglect proceedings: The erroneous assumption of parental inadequacy. *Stanford Law Review, 31,* 785–805.

Hofferth, S. L. (1997). Book review. Hays, S. (1996). *The cultural contradictions of motherhood.* New Haven, Connecticut: Yale University Press, *The American Journal of Sociology, 103*(1), 243.

House, J. S., Umberson, D., & Landis, K. R. (1988). Structures and processes of social support. *Annual Review of Sociology, 14,* 293–318.

Jack, G. (1997). Discourses of child protection and child welfare. *British Journal of Social Work, 27,* 659–678.

Jamrozik, A., & Sweeney, T. (1996). *Children and society: The family, the state and social parenthood.* Melbourne: MacMillan.

Kellegrew, D.H. (2000). Constructing daily routines: A qualitative examination of mothers with young children with disabilities. *American Journal of Occupational Therapy, 54*(3), 252–259.

Keltner, B. (1994). Home environments of mothers with mental retardation. *Mental Retardation, 32*(2), 123-127.

Keltner, B., Finn, D., & Shearer, D. (1995). Effects of family intervention on maternal-child interactions for mothers with developmental disabilities. *Family and Community Health, 17*(4), 35–49.

Keltner, B., Wise, L. A., & Taylor, G. (1999). Mothers with intellectual limitations and their 2-year-old children's developmental outcomes. *Journal of Intellectual & Developmental Disability, 24*(1), 45–57.

King, M., & Trowell, J. (1992). *Children's welfare and the law: The limits of legal intervention.* London (UK): Sage.

Lindsey, D. (1994). *The welfare of children.* New York: Oxford University Press.

Llewellyn, G. (1997). Parents with intellectual disability learning to parent: The role of informal learning and experience. *International Journal of Disability, Development and Education, 44*(3), 243–261.

Llewellyn, G. (1995). Relationships and social support: Views of parents with mental retardation. *Mental Retardation, 33*(6), 349–363.

Llewellyn, G. (1990). People with intellectual disability as parents: Perspectives from the professional literature. *Australia and New Zealand Journal of Developmental Disabilities, 16*(4), 369–380.

Llewellyn, G., Bye, R., & McConnell, D. (1997). Parents with intellectual disability and mainstream family agencies. *International Journal of Practical Approaches to Disability, 21*(3), 9–13.

Llewellyn, G., & McConnell, D. (2002). Mothers with learning difficulties and their support networks. *Journal of Intellectual Disability Research, 46*(1), 17–34.

Llewellyn, G., McConnell, D., Cant, R., & Westbrook, M. (1999). Support networks of mothers with an intellectual disability: An exploratory study. *Journal of Intellectual and Developmental Disabilities, 24*(1), 7–26.

Llewellyn, G., McConnell, D., & Ferronato, L. (2003). Prevalence and outcomes for parents with disabilities and their children in an Australian court sample. *Child Abuse and Neglect, 27,* 235–251.

Llewellyn, G., McConnell, D., & Honey, A. (2001). Healthy and safe: NSW Parent-child health and well-being research and development project. Report to the NSW Ageing and Disability Department. University of Sydney.

Llewellyn, G., McConnell, D., Russo, D., Mayes, R., & Honey, A. (2002). Home based programs for parents with learning difficulties: Lessons from practice. *Journal of Applied Research in Intellectual Disabilities, 15*(4), 341–353.

Lynch, E. W., & Bakley, S. (1989). Serving young children whose parents are mentally retarded. *Infants and Young Children, 1*(3), 26–38.

McConnell, D., & Llewellyn, G. (2000). Disability and discrimination in statutory child protection proceedings. *Disability & Society, 15*(6), 883–895.

McConnell, D., & Llewellyn, G. (1998). Parental disability and the threat of child removal. *Family Matters, 51,* 33–36.

McConnell, D., Llewellyn, G., & Ferronato, L. (2000). *Parents with a disability and the NSW Children's Court.* Lidcombe, NSW: University of Sydney, Family Support and Services Project.

McGillivray, A. (1992). Reconstructing child abuse: Western definition and non-western experience. In M. Freeman & P. Veerman (Eds.). *The ideologies of children's rights* (pp. 213–236). Amsterdam: Kluwer Academic Publishers.

McNeil, S. (2001). A journey of discovery. In M. Priestley (Ed.). *Disability and the life course. Global perspectives* (pp. 79–88). Cambridge (UK): Cambridge University Press.

Maher, T.F. (1987). The loneliness of parenthood. *Social Service Review, 61*(1), 91–101.

Mickelson, P. (1947). The feeble-minded parent: A study of 90 family cases. *American Journal of Mental Deficiency, 51*, 644–653.

Mira, M., & Roddy, J. (1980). *Parenting competencies of retarded persons: A critical review.* Unpublished manuscript, University of Kansas Medical Center, Kansas City, KS.

Morris, J. (Ed.)(1996). *Encounters with strangers: Feminism and disability.* London (UK): Women's Press.

Morton, T.D. (1999). The increasing colorization of America's child welfare system: The overrepresentation of African-American children. *Policy & Practice of Public Human Service, 57*(4), 23–33.

Newton, J. S., Horner, R. H., Ard, W. R., LeBaron, N., & Sappington, G. (1994). A conceptual model for improving the social life of individuals with mental retardation. *Mental Retardation, 32*, 393–402.

Parton, N. (1995). Neglect as child protection: the political context and the practical outcomes. *Children & Society, 9*(1), 67–89.

Payne, A. T. (1978). The law and the problem parent: Custody and parental rights of homosexual, mentally retarded, mentally ill and incarcerated parents. *Journal of Family Law, 16*, 797–818.

Pelton, L. H. (1997). Child welfare policy and practice: The myth of family preservation. *American Journal of Orthopsychiatry, 67*(4), 545–553.

Pelton, L.H. (1989). *For reasons of poverty: A critical analysis of the public child welfare system in the United States.* New York: Praeger.

Pelton, L.H. (1982). Personalistic attributions and client perspectives in child welfare cases: Implications for service delivery. In T. A. Wills (Ed.). *Basic processes in helping relationships* (pp.81-101). New York: Academic Press.

Pierce, D., & Frank, G. (1992). A mother's work: Two levels of feminist analysis of family centered care. *American Journal of Occupational Therapy, 46*(11), 972–980.

Pierce, G. R., Sarason, B. R., & Sarason, I. G. (Eds.). (1996). *Handbook of social support and the family.* New York: Plenum Press.

Polanyi, M. (1966). *The tacit dimension.* Garden City, NY: Doubleday Anchor.

Primeau, L. (2000). Divisions of household work, routines, and child care occupations in families. *Journal of Occupational Science, 7*(1), 19–28.

Ruddick, S. (1989). *Maternal thinking. Toward a politics of peace.* New York: Ballantine Books.

Salzinger, S. (1990). Social networks in child rearing and child development. In S. M. Pfafflin, J A. Sechzer, J. M. Fish, & R. L. Thompson (Eds.). *Annals of the Academy of the New York Academy of Sciences, 602:* 171–188.

Sarber, R. E., Halasz, M. M., Messmer, M. C., Bickett, A. D., & Lutzker, J. R. (1983). Teaching menu planning and grocery shopping skills to a mentally retarded mother. *Mental Retardation, 21*(3), 101–106.

Segal, R. (2000). Adaptive strategies of mothers with children with attention deficit hyperactivity disorder: Enfolding and unfolding occupations. *American Journal of Occupational Therapy, 54*(3), 300–306.

Smart, C. (1996). Deconstructing motherhood. In E. B. Silva (Ed.). *Good enough mothering* (pp. 37–57). London (UK): Routledge.

Taylor, S. J. (1995). "Children's division is coming to take pictures." Family life and parenting in a family with disabilities. In S. J. Taylor, R. Bogdan and Z. M. Lutfiyya (Eds.). *The variety of community experiences: Qualitative studies of family and community life* (pp. 23–45). Baltimore: Paul H Brookes.

Taylor, C. G., Norman, D. K., Murphy, J. M., Jellinek, M., Quinn, D., Poitrast, F. G., & Goshko, M. (1991). Diagnosed intellectual and emotional impairment among parents who seriously mistreat their children: Prevalence, type, and outcome in a court sample. *Child Abuse & Neglect, 15*, 389–401.

Thorpe, D. (1994). *Evaluating child protection.* Buckingham: Open University Press.

Thurer, S.L. (1994). *The myths of motherhood: how culture reinvents the good mother.* New York: Penguin.

Tracy, E. M., & Abell, N. (1994). Social network map: Some further refinements on administration. *Social Work Research, 18*, 56–60.

Tracy, E. M., & Whittaker, J. K. (1990). The social network map: Assessing social support in clinical practice. *Families in Society: The Journal of Contemporary Human Services, October*, 461–470.

Tucker, M. B., & Johnson, O. (1989). Competence promoting vs. Competence inhibiting social support for mentally retarded mothers. *Human Organisation, 48*, 95–107.

Tymchuk, A. J. (1990). Parents with mental retardation: A national strategy. *Journal of Disability Policy Studies, 1* (4), 43–56.

Tymchuk, A. J., & Andron, L. (1990). Mothers with mental retardation who do or do not abuse or neglect their children. *Child Abuse and Neglect, 14*, 313–323.

Tymchuk, A.J., & Andron, L. (1992). Project parenting: Child interactional training with mothers who are mentally handicapped. *Mental Handicap Research, 5*(1), 4–32.

Tymchuk, A. J., Andron, L., & Hagelstein, M. (1992). Training mothers with mental retardation to discuss home safety and emergencies with their children. *Journal of Developmental and Physical Disabilities, 4*(2), 151–165.

Tymchuk, A. J., Andron, L., & Rahbar, B. (1988). Effective decision-making/problem solving training with mothers who have mental retardation. *American Journal on Mental Retardation, 92*, 510–516.

Tymchuk, A. J., & Feldman, M. A. (1991). Parents with mental retardation and their children: Review of research relevant to professional practice. *Canadian Psychology, 32*(3), 486–494.

Tymchuk, A. J., Hamada, D., Andron, L., and Anderson, S. (1990a). Home safety training with mothers who are mentally retarded, *Education and Training in Mental Retardation, 25,* 142–149.

Tymchuk, A. J., Hamada, D., Andron, L., and Anderson, S. (1990b). Emergency training for mothers with mental retardation, *Child and Family Behavior Therapy, 12,* 31–47.

Tymchuk, A. J., Llewellyn, G., & Feldman, M. A. (1999). Parenting by persons with intellectual disabilities: A

timely international perspective. *Journal of Intellectual and Developmental Disability, 24*(1), 3–6.

Valsiner, J. J., & Litvinovic, G. (1996). Process of generalization in parental reasoning. In S. Harkness and C. M. Super (Eds.), *Parents' cultural belief systems. Their origins, expressions, and consequences* (pp. 56–82). New York: The Guildford Press.

Source Credits

1. The vignettes "Sarah" and "Karina and Paul" are reprinted with permission from the *Journal of Intellectual and Developmental Disability,* previously published in Llewellyn, G., McConnell, D., Cant, R., &

Westbrooke, M. (1999). Support networks of mothers with intellectual disability: An exploratory study. *Journal of Intellectual and Developmental Disability, 24*(1), 16–18.

CHAPTER 10

Experience of Mothers with Disabilities: Learning from Their Voice

Ruth S. Farber, PhD, MSW, OTR

Anticipated Outcomes

I anticipate that, after reading this chapter, readers will:

- Understand range and individual differences of experiences

- Understand the influence of their child's developmental issues

- Understand the meaning of participation in maternal occupations

- Understand the importance of adaptation in occupations

- Understand the importance of social supports

- Understand the potential interaction of participation, well-being, social support, and health

℀ Introduction

A chance event inspired my interest in studying mothering with a disability. A delightful woman arrived at the family-centered care class I teach to substitute as a guest speaker on disability issues. She had cerebral palsy with substantial motor involvement and functional limitations. At the break we discovered that we were both mothers with adolescent children and with similar parental challenges. She showed me a picture of her daughter as well as a picture of herself pregnant in a wheelchair. The image of a happy pregnant woman in a wheelchair seemed incongruous to me. I could not recall images of mothers in wheelchairs from popular culture. My puzzlement about this cultural blind spot stimulated my desire to learn more about this area.

The same guest speaker told me about the thoughtful and creative way in which she psychologically bonded with her daughter and directed and assisted in her care, although she had substantial physical limitations in her ability to give direct hands-on care. It made me think: What is the essence of motherhood? This question reminded me of a similar one that women I studied grappled with when they chose to combine careers and family and had to fulfill the role of mother in a nontraditional way (Farber, 1988).

I began speaking with other women with disabilities who were actively mothering. I learned of the special challenges these mothers with disabilities experienced. It was incredible to me how much bias, stigma, and invisibility they had to contend with. They also told me of the unfounded assumption of incompetence they experienced. These mothers were resourceful women who had to be especially steadfast to not internalize this stigma and to establish their own unique model of mothering (Farber, 2000). All of these experiences stimulated and prepared me to begin my study of mothers with disabilities.

℀ Background

In the past decade there has been a rapidly expanding body of scholarship about mothering and motherhood. Arendell (2000) described the shift in focus from examining the quality of the mothering and its effect on the children to including the mother's subjective experience. In contrast, research on mothers with disabilities or chronic illness has continued to be understudied (Cohen 1998; Radtke & Van Mens-Verhulst, 2001), and the voice and perspective of mothers with disabilities or chronic illness is relatively absent (Farber, 2000; Morris, 1995). Mothering is a central human experience, which has both universal and culturally specific aspects. That is, mothers are both similar and unique. Mothering is a deeply personal, subjective experience, and it involves participating in culturally common "maternal practices" (Arendell, 2000, p. 1194). In addition to mothers having continual dynamic social interaction with their children, they are expected to participate in and orchestrate many diverse maternal activities, ranging from the provision of their child's concrete needs for nurturance, shelter, and safety to the provision of a stimulating psychosocial environment for their child's overall development and socialization (Maccoby & Martin, 1983). Motherhood has been considered a normative aspect of adult development (Erikson, 1980), a central component of many women's adult identity (Wollett & Marshall, 2001) and personality organization (Gutmann, 1975), and a source of self-worth (Tardy, 2000). Being a mother can influence well-being both positively and negatively (Oberman & Josselson, 1996). For many people, it gives life meaning (Umberson, 1989). Although being a mother is an experience that many individuals assume will be accessible to them (if they choose it), this has not been true for women with disabilities.

The number of parents with disabilities is growing (National Resource Center for Parents with Disabilities, Fall 1998). As a result of technological and biomechanical advances in medicine, individuals born with disabilities are leading longer and fuller lives that could include conceiving, bearing, and nurturing children. Professionals work with women who have congenital or acquired disabilities and choose to become a parent, and with mothers who acquire a disability or chronic illness after they have had children. The Independent Living and the Disability Movements (Morris, 1995; Thomas, 1997), with their expectation for full participation in chosen life experiences, including motherhood, make exploring this issue particularly salient at this time.

Historically, women with disabilities were not viewed as people who could conceive and nurture future generations (Collins, 1999; Sprill, 1987; Morris, 1995). Because of discriminatory attitudes (and negative stereotypes) entrenched in our societal, governmental, and health-care system, it has been suggested that women with disabilities may not be able to easily actualize their true choice to become a mother (Collins; Cohen, 1998). According to Collins (1999), for women with a disability, the "right to express sexual needs" and the choice to become a mother "are often restrained or denied" (p. 300). Thomas (1997) also describes the health-care prejudices that women with disabilities face with their decision to have children, including the medical/health-care professionals' perception of medical risk, concerns about the fairness to the child, and capability to respond to a child. In a qualitative study of women with disabilities, Thomas found that almost all experienced some degree of "fear to be judged inadequate as a mother" (p. 633), with consequences that could lead to loss of custody of their child.

Legal Issues

The unfounded belief that individuals with disabilities will be unfit parents that exists in our culture also exists in our legal system (Asch & Fine, 1988; Gilhool & Gran, 1985; Morris, 1995) and is reinforced by legal precedents. Laws prohibiting individuals with disabilities (epilepsy, retardation, or psychiatric illness) to marry or have children existed in many states (Asch & Fine). Although there have been social and civil rights trends toward full life involvement for persons with disabilities, there are still "only a handful of progressive states that refused to treat disability as prima facie evidence of parental unfitness and possible detriment to the child" (Gilhool & Gran, 1985, p. 30). Individuals with physical disabilities continue to have their right to child custody legally

challenged. In an interview conducted by Greenspan, a researcher in child custody and disability issues, he found that "because a parent has a disability the system throws all kinds of roadblocks in the way" (De Angelis, 1995, p. 39). This bias also occurs in the psychological assessment of parents that courts use. A fair assessment would include examining the parent and total family environment and support, not relying exclusively on scores of a psychological test. This is not always carried out.

✒ Professional Literature

There has been evidence of a pathological or biased lens used with examination of parenting with a disability in the literature as well. Meadow-Orlans (1995) observed that studies of individuals with disabilities tend to be driven by a deficit, rather than a coping perspective, "ignoring the natural adjustments made by the human organism to biological risk and disability" (p. 64). Earlier writing on the effects of parenting with a disability generally concluded that having a disabled parent in the home adversely affected the child's development in areas such as sex-role identity, interpersonal relationships, physical health, and so forth (Buck & Hohmann, 1981, 1983). Many of these initial findings may have been based on speculation rather than on empirical evidence. In a seminal paper, Buck and Hohmann (1983) described the methodological flaws in previous research, including the absence of control groups, the combining of dissimilar parent groups (such as those with psychiatric and physical disabilities) and less reliable instrumentation, which may have confounded the results. In contrast, Buck and Hohmann (1981) used a more sophisticated research design and found that children with fathers who had spinal cord injuries were not (as previous research had suggested) adversely affected on a number of psychological variables.

Cohen (1998) found shortcomings similar to those found by Buck and Hohmann (1983) in her more recent review of the literature on parenting with a disability. Her findings also challenged the common assumption that there is a role reversal in caregiving with parents with disabilities and their children. She found that the opposite is true. The parents in her study took extra care not to assign their parenting tasks to children. There are many mediating factors about the parenting experience with individuals with disabilities. Coates, Vietz, and Gray (1985), from their review of the literature, underscored the importance of including family process variables as either a predisposing or mediating factor on how the disability will affect the child. Criticism concerning the lack of voice of the person with a disability in the literature has also come from the Disability Movement (Thomas, 1997; Morris, 1995, 1993).

Because of this historical lack of voice of mothers with disabilities and prevalence of negative stereotyping in the literature, the purpose of this chapter is to describe the variation in the normative experiences of mothers with disabilities. Extra care was given to be neutral and open to positive aspects of these mothers' adaptation to achieve balance. I believe that this perspective will add another dimension of knowledge to inform clinical reasoning, allow a more realistic response to mothers with disabilities, and promote collaborative planning for more relevant goals.

An additional purpose of this chapter is to explore the interrelationship between maternal self-description, participation in chosen maternal practices, and perception of social support across the family life cycle. This concept showing the interrelationships between phenomenology, or subjective experience, participation, what mothers do, and social interactions within a community, is illustrated in Figure 10–1. This systemic schema suggests the importance of developing interventions to foster positive self-perception, maximizing participation in chosen maternal practices, promoting social support, and facilitating both attitudinal and physical accessibility to community resources.

ℒ❦ Mothers' Self-perception, Participation, and Well-being

In this section of my chapter, I will describe aspects of mothering relevant to the understanding of mothering with a disability. The major features are maternal self-perception and the subjective experience of being a mother, as well as the doing or participating in culturally valued maternal practices (Arendell, 2000). For mothers with disabilities, this can be especially complex and inextricably connected. What one experiences and believes about one's self affects what one does, and what one does affects self and identity. For people with disabilities, "doing" can be limited by internal and external constraints.

Women's maternal self-perception and experience can be influenced by many factors. Francis-Connolly (2000) studied the occupation of mothering and found that the women (without disabilities) had an "illusive ideal" of the perfect mother. She describes this ideal as socially constructed. Francis-Connolly found that the women in her study were constantly comparing themselves to this ideal and at the same time feeling guilty for not being perfect. Other researchers describe this idealized and selfless maternal myth (Falk, 2000). This myth affects women's experience of self. According to McMahon (as cited by Falk, 2000), women judge their worth as a person through motherhood. Falk also found that women felt "pressure" to conform to "cultural representations and social expectations associated with motherhood" (p. v). Images of ideal mothers in early television, like Donna Reed, may have also contributed to this phenomenon.

Like other women, mothers with disabilities can also compare themselves to an idealized version of a mother, and they share similar struggles with the discrepancy between the actual mother and the myth. However, this may be further compounded by the complexity of their disability or chronic illness and societal reactions to it (Farber, 2000). Grant (2001) found that the mothers with disabilities struggled with their "preconceived notions of motherhood" and found themselves not being able to be the mother they wanted to be (p.327).

This comparison to the "ideal mother" may affect their subjective experience of mothering, quality of relationships, and beliefs about what they should be doing as mothers. My previous research (Farber, 2000) suggested that mothers with disabilities seemed to have intuited culturally common activities that they

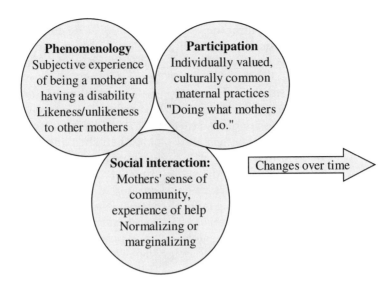

Figure 10–1 *Mothers with disabilities: Phenomenology, participation, and social interaction.*

believed that other mothers did, and valued doing them. The importance of this feeling of universality, of being like other mothers, may be connected to a need to feel part of a larger community of mothers, which is important to all mothers (Tardy, 2000; Oberman & Josselson, 1996). In the next section I will discuss this process of doing, or participating in the maternal or social role.

🐾 Participation

In general, participation in life situations, life roles, and life tasks has been shown to be vital to the quality of human experience and functioning (Cantor & Sanderson, 1999; Law, 2002). The concept of participation is addressed from several health-related sources. One source is the World Health Organization (WHO) and its development of the International Classification of Functioning, Disability and Health (ICF), a system that was designed to provide a unified and standard language and framework for the description of health and health related issues (WHO, 2001). ICF includes activity and participation together as central domains of health. Participation is defined as " participation in a life situation," while activity "is the execution

of a task or action" (WHO, p. 10). Disability is seen as an "umbrella term for impairments, activity limitations, or participation restrictions" (WHO, p. 1).

Quality of life has been also been linked to participation in the social role (Ware, 2001; Johnston, 2001). In the presentation on quality of life issues and traumatic brain injury, Johnston stated the importance of activity in relation to quality of life. He stated his belief that a person's activities are connected with the person's feeling and thoughts about them (Johnston). Ware, on the other hand, described role participation as the most important factor in health-related quality of life. He presented preliminary evidence from a new structural model in which physical and mental health components interacted with participation to create a health-related quality of life concept cross-culturally.

Cantor and Sanderson (1999) have written that "sustained participation in personally and culturally valued tasks enhances well-being" (p. 230) by providing meaning and a sense of personal agency. Social well-being, a by-product of participation in life tasks, occurs through having a strong connection to others and gaining access to instrumental resources. According to Cantor and Sanderson, when activities are autonomously chosen, intrinsically motivating, and occur in the context of the individuals' daily life, enhancement in the well-being of the individual is optimal.

The importance of women participating in maternal and domestic role activities cannot be underestimated for many women (McDonough, 1996). According to Walmsley (1993) "For some women who are denied the opportunity to be caregivers, caring becomes a valued activity to be sought, rather than an oppressive burden to be shifted" (p.131). Bowlby, Gregory, and McKie (1997) described the doing housework and safeguarding family life as "doing gender" or the enactment of normative gender role, establishing a membership in that gender (p. 346).

This interaction of being and doing is especially poignant for women with disabilities, when "doing" may be more challenged by physical limitations, psychosocial factors, and/or environmental obstacles. According to Morris (1995), "disabled women are often prevented from participation in such [caregiving] relationships because they do not receive appropriate help and or live in an appropriate physical environment" (p. 90). In an earlier study, Morris (1989) found that women with new paralysis valued their lives by the degree to which they were able to participate in their roles as mothers and wives. Therefore, in the next section, I discuss the role of *participation* in the lives of mothers with disabilities who participated in my research studies during the past 5 years (Farber, 2000).

🐚 My Current Research

Because in my studies I found that the child's age and developmental differences appeared to affect the mothering experience differentially, I interviewed more mothers with adolescent children and reanalyzed the previous data for this age group for the study presented in this chapter. Also, because earlier data suggested the importance of the women's occupational engagement in parenting, I conducted a secondary analysis of the overall findings to explore the role of maternal participation.

In preparation for this study, I consulted a panel of experts in the disability community who were also mothers. Their input was invaluable in developing the interview questions. Additional interview questions were added for the interviews of mothers of adolescent children. I conducted in-depth interviews to uncover the nature of their mothering experience. The interviews, lasting 1 to 2 hours, were audiotaped and then transcribed. Member checking was done by telephone. Data were coded and analyzed for themes using the constant comparison approach of grounded theory (Strauss & Corbin, 1990). Also, data were compared to narratives of mothers from the disability community, which were published in anthologies of women's stories (Finger, 1985; Hyler, 1985; Matthews 1983).

Participants

The sample (n=10) was composed of mothers with diverse disabilities, including physical or sensory disability and/or chronic illness (Table 10–1). The snowball sampling technique utilized contacts in the nondisabled and disabled communities (within a large urban university and a university hospital) to recommend mothers for the study who had a physical or sensory disability and were currently parenting and living in the community. The mothers interviewed were also asked if they knew other women who were eligible for this study.

The majority (8 out of 10) of the women described in this chapter chose to have children or continued their pregnancy after they acquired their disability. As one mother said, it felt like her "destiny" to have a child. Two of the women were diagnosed within close proximity to the pregnancy and birth (one of these women went on to have a second child after the diagnosis). One mother acquired her disease when her children were in their teens. Some mothers continued pregnancies in spite of potential risk to their own health.

Names and identifying information were changed to protect the anonymity of the participants. Four of the key informants are described in the following vignettes. Other participants in my study will be described throughout the text with their narratives. They are all described in Table 10–1.

Name (fictitious)	Age of mother	Age of youngest child	Number of children	Race	Diagnosis
					Table 10–1. Demographic information about mothers with disabilities (n = 10)
Jean	39	9 months	2	Caucasian	Fibromyalgia
Sue Ann	31	4 years	2	Caucasian	Multiple sclerosis
May	35	4 years	1	Caucasian	Multiple sclerosis and diabetes
Rachel	43	7 years	1	Caucasian	Multiple sclerosis
Judy	44	9 years	1	African-American	Cerebral palsy
Crystal	36	10 years	2	African-American	Scoliosis and kidney disease
Gerry	55	11 years	4	Caucasian	Retinitis pigmentosa
Sally	47	12 years	1	Caucasian	Parkinsonism
Katrina	51	14 years	1	Caucasian	Spinal cord injury
Arielle	55	16 years	2	Caucasian	Parkinsonism

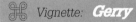

Vignette: *Gerry*

Gerry is a 55-year-old educated, resourceful, and articulate woman who has had a rare degenerative eye disease since the age of 7 and is now legally blind. Although she describes motherhood as a major "dream of my childhood," she works full time in a professional capacity as well. Gerry has four children ranging in age from 11 to 31, the youngest being from her second marriage. She described her second husband as dramatically different from the first in his support and empowering attitude toward her and sharing of parenting responsibilities.

Gerry had few worries when she became pregnant with her first child, and she had confidence about figuring out necessary adaptations. Her first baby had some medical problems, and Gerry was caught off guard when an in-law assumed that these problems were related to her blindness. Gerry's previous "nondisabled" view of herself was shaken when she was made very aware of her "inabilities" and "burden" for the first time in her life. Her experience in having her second child has been substantially different from that with her first child. Not only does she have more life experience; her second husband, the father of her second child, has been described as supportive and empowering toward her. At this point in her life, she described her

resourcefulness and the obstacles that she had to overcome with pride as a mother.

Vignette: *May*

May is a 35-year-old articulate and thoughtful married woman with a 4-year-old son. She worked in a management capacity until she was laid off, around 6 months before the interview. At the time of the interview she had been diagnosed with multiple sclerosis for around 10 years.

May and her husband "knew" they wanted children when they married. Within the first 2 years of marriage, May was diagnosed with insulin-dependent diabetes and multiple sclerosis. The couple was very concerned that it would prevent them from having a child. They dealt thoughtfully with the uncertainty of the disease and found an absence of "documentation" about negative results (except that some people have exacerbations at about 6 months) with multiple sclerosis. They realized that May could be either okay or "bedridden" in 6 months. Their extended families were "pretty devastated" and fearful when they were told of the pregnancy after 6 years of a childless marriage. In spite of this, the couple was very determined to have a baby and planned for all possible contingencies.

⌘ *Vignette:* **Sally**

Sally is a 47-year-old married mother with a 12-year-old son. When she received her master's degree, she felt that her life was "perfect." Then she moved to live with her boyfriend in another city, with plans to marry if the relationship worked out. The day after she became officially engaged, she was scheduled for medical tests because of previous ambiguous symptoms. The test results were not conclusive at that time. Once they were married, Sally became pregnant sooner than she had planned, which she described as "a calendar mistake." Although Sally didn't feel "ready to have a baby," she and her husband knew they eventually wanted a child. She also described herself as being "in denial" about how much was wrong. During her pregnancy, she had trouble distinguishing symptoms of Parkinsonism from symptoms of pregnancy. After months of this ambiguous, unfolding dual experience, she was finally diagnosed with Parkinsonism when her son was 4 months old.

⌘

⌘ *Vignette:* **Rachel**

Rachel, a 43-year-old married woman who retired as a teacher because of having multiple sclerosis, had a 7-year-old son. She was diagnosed at age 31, and as soon as she told her neighbor, she was given the advice, "Please don't get pregnant" (based on negative anecdotal evidence). She and her husband first considered adoption, but found out that she could only adopt in one state in the United States because of the multiple sclerosis. Eventually she and her husband told a doctor that she wanted to get pregnant. He made her aware of more recent research and supported their decision for her to try to get pregnant, which she describes as "the best decision we ever made." During the pregnancy she had some problems with sensation in the vaginal area, so she wore a baby monitor.

Although at the time of the interview Rachel was unable to walk independently and had some difficulty with hand function, she said that she was grateful that she had her intellectual functioning. Because of safety concerns when her baby was young, she and her husband decided to have help at home (such as an au pair) while he worked.

⌘

✒ Findings and Discussion

From my analysis of the research data, four major themes emerged. These were:

■ Maternal self-description that included feelings of being *just like other mothers, unlike other mothers,* or *unlike other mothers and it is okay to be different)*

■ Participation that included *nonparticipation to adaptive participation*

■ Perception of interpersonal environment that included experiences *fostering normalization and adequacy*

■ Experiences *stimulating feelings of marginalization or inadequacy*

■ Developmental changes

These themes will be more fully described in the following section of this chapter.

Maternal Self-description

Maternal self-descriptions reflected one of these three categories: *just like other mothers, unlike other mothers,* and *unlike other mothers and it is okay to be different.* I noted that with some participants there were fluctuations in the maternal self-description between categories, over the course of the interview and follow-up call. However, for most participants, their self-description demonstrated either a primacy of having a disability and being different or seeing the disability at the margins of their life. This later capacity to minimize the disability has been described as a way to help the person carry on with usual activities of everyday life (McDonough, 1996; Charmaz, 1991)

This phenomenon could also be seen as the degree of acceptance or nonacceptance of self with a disability. Self-acceptance is considered a beneficial psychological characteristic of an individual with a disability, as well as an important factor in parenting (Hanna & Edwards, 1988). "Disabled parents who view themselves positively are better equipped to cope with disability and establish healthy personalities" (Hanna & Edwards, p. 42).

Corbin and Strauss (1987) also described variation in the way individuals come to terms with their disability or illness experience. People experience falls on a continuum from nonacceptance to acceptance, with some going beyond to "transcendence," which they define as being able to "find real joy in living . . . even though their performance may now be severely limited" (Corbin & Strauss, p. 271). The way the participants in the Corbin and Strauss study described themselves as mothers, similarly, varied from a source of pride and comfort to a painful longing, or both.

Just Like Other Mothers

On one end of the continuum, some participants in this study defined themselves as *just like other mothers*. Judy, a 44-year-old mother with cerebral palsy, who had a 9-year-old daughter, had been working full time as an administrative assistant for over 20 years. She was able to walk with crutches when her child was born, but at the time of the interview, she depended on a wheelchair for mobility. Italics will be used for emphasis given by the mothers in their narratives. In discussing her reaction to finding out she was pregnant, Judy said, "There's no difference between me and Joe Blow over there, except for *I have a little disability*. But the disability does not stop me from being the parent that I am—*the good parent that I am*."

Another mother, Katrina, a businesswoman who was a paraplegic for 13 years before she had her daughter (14 years old at the time of the interview), emphasized, "The only thing I can't do is walk." She frequently described herself as being *like other mothers*. Katrina spoke of the commitment she made to herself when she found out she was pregnant with her daughter:

> I made a decision … that I would do everything within my power to have her have as normal a childhood as possible. Obviously, being in a wheelchair … going to a playground is a little bit difficult. You know, swings … wheelchair in sand—you spin your wheels … we would go to playgrounds and I would just see a mother

and say, hey, I can't push her, will you? And of course—I mean, always people would be more than glad to help you out. So in that respect, [my daughter] always had *the most normal upbringing….*[1]

Unlike Other Mothers

In the above section, participants emphasized how they were *like other mothers*, and how their offsprings' childhoods were like those of other children. In contrast, other participants emphasized how they were *unlike other mothers*. This was based primarily on the activities they could not do. The following quotes illustrate this difference, emphasizing the painful loss experienced by one mother. Sally, who had developed Parkinson's disease simultaneously with her pregnancy, spoke about her son, who was 11 years old at the time of the interview, and how she felt:

> I was a good skater. I can't skate now… I would love to skate with him. But I can't … when he was younger, I was always afraid that something was going to happen to him … I wouldn't be able to rescue him. So I avoided doing a lot of activities … *I really missed being able to do what other mothers were able to do with their kids* (Farber, 2000, p.264).[1]

Another mother, Sue Ann (with multiple sclerosis), who had an assertive 6-year-old daughter, observed:

> She sees her friends at school, they're doing this and that. But one day specifically—she asked me to put her hair in pony tails and then she was really yelling at me…that she guesses that the only time she's going to be able to have pony tails is if her Aunt, or Grandmom puts them in for her because *I can't do it. Well, that made me feel like crap.*(Farber, 2000, p. 264).[1]

Several of the mothers who repeatedly spoke about being *unlike other mothers* had chronic progressive illnesses like Parkinson's disease, multiple sclerosis, or fibromyalgia, with fatigue challenges. In contrast, two women with these same chronic illnesses did not describe the primacy of being *unlike other mothers*. This fatigue involvement may contribute to less participation because of not having the energy to overcome obstacles or make adaptations. But it may not be sufficient to explain withdrawal from participation completely.

Unlike Other Mothers and It Is Okay to be Different

The third description found in this theme was mothers feeling *unlike other mothers and it is okay to be different.* Several mothers described ways they had made adaptations that satisfied their parental role. For May, the mother with multiple sclerosis, which affected her balance and caused periods of extreme fatigue, the following themes of loss and sadness were repeated periodically in her description of mothering her 4-year-old son during the interview:

> I'd say the biggest sadness in it is that I can't do things with him, like go to the park. I see mothers throwing Frisbee, having kick ball, soccer, whatever—and I can't do that... I don't shop. You know, so that's sad ... But I can't be the parent that's playing ball or kicking around with him and stuff like that. That's the sad part (Farber, 2000, p. 264).[1]

However, when the same mother was asked what she thought was important for parents with a disability to know, she responded:

> Not everybody's the same... My son could have a wonderful time learning. ... I could teach him a lot of things regarding the zoo, for example. Doesn't mean we have to go. There's videos. There's story books. We read a lot of books. So we talk about it ... That's doing it differently is what I mean. ...*So we can get the same thing accomplished. It's the same end, different means* (Farber, 2000. p. 264).[1]

This acceptance of adaptation, *"same end, different means,"* was echoed by other mothers. A mother who ran with her daughter as a co-athlete was transformed into an avid fan of her sports events. However, mothers varied in their choices to make or not make adaptations in order to participate in maternal practices. The mother's unique adaptation in maternal activities will be discussed in the following section describing the type of participation.

Maternal Participation

The women in this study were involved in many activities that ranged from *normal participation* to *adapted participation* to *nonparticipation,* that is, role withdrawal or loss. Maternal activities occurred within the home or community. The mothers who appeared to come to terms with their disability (Corbin & Strauss, 1987), seeing themselves as *like other mothers,* or *unlike other mothers and it is okay to be different,* seemed to offer more spontaneous descriptions about their normative or adapted participation in their children's lives. Some of these included their use of activity adaptation/reconfiguration, or selective participation in which they used energy conservation, reprioritization of activities, or environmental adaptation such as household reorganization, to make maternal practices more accessible and safe. In the interviews, these mothers conveyed a sense of pride and determination to make their maternal participation as full as possible and their children's lives as normal as possible. As an involved observer, I was often impressed by the creativity and resourcefulness in adaptations to make their involvement in their child's life as normal as possible. Gerry, the mother with a progressive visual impairment, described the way in which she adapted her reading to her daughter when she was younger:

> I wanted to be like a really good parent. I wanted to give them whatever I thought a fully sighted parent could do. It was hard for me to read to them and do some puzzles and things. You know, I had to select toys and books that I could manage. And when they got older I had a lot of books memorized. I bought a lot of Dr. Seuss books because I can memorize them and I mean, you know, I could read them close up and after—a—well, I had like photographic memory until I was 35 so it was easy. And ah, so I would do things like that. I knew that reading was very important and I wanted them to have all the visual skills that children should have.[1]

May, the mother with multiple sclerosis and a large baby as a result of diabetes, had balance problems after the baby was 6 months old. She described her physical symptoms: "I can walk but not properly. Sometimes my fatigue is a very big factor. I get very tired. I can't stand for any real length of time …" She both readjusted the place where she gave care to her baby and completely reorganized her home to make it more accessible:

> When he was so young at that time that it—you can easily like play on the floor, sit on the floor with him, you know, as he crawls around or get his clothes and change him on the floor. [Adapted participation: Activity reconfiguration]
>
> I never usually use the cane in the house. I do a lot of wall walking when necessary. We don't use stairs. Our bedroom is downstairs. His bedroom is downstairs. We deliberately didn't use upstairs. Originally we were upstairs. I needed to be close to the kitchen, to the bathroom, to the baby's room. [Adapted participation: Household reorganization]
>
> I adjust as I do throughout this whole life. When I'm tired I just don't do what I was planning to do that day. I do sitting. I sit all the time when I'm cutting food or whatever, I have to sit. I balance out things that I have to go out and do. We go out and do it in the morning when I have the most energy type of thing. If it's something I can take him with me, I bring him with me as much as possible. [Adapted, selective participation: Energy conservation][1]

On her own, this mother considered the baby's needs, her physical condition and limitation, and adapted the activity and environment to maximize her participation. Rachel, another mother with multiple sclerosis, spoke about her frustration at not being able to "jump" in the car and drive her 7-year-old son places because she had not yet obtained her adapted van. However, she effortlessly added, "So we sort of prioritize the things that we can do together. It's a little bit more restricted. We work on the computer together. We do a lot of reading together. We do some artwork" (Farber, 2000, p. 265).

In contrast, Jean, a 39-year-old mother with fibromyalgia and two daughters under 6, viewed her situation through the lens of loss, that is, role withdrawal, and felt "out of sync" with other mothers:

> I struggle with taking care of them [the children] … I really do. In fact, that's where all my energy goes. I have no energy left over for any—for anybody, including myself or my husband.[1]

She continued to describe how it was with her first child, and then described the difference with her second:

> I was able to get out of the house, able to get the car carrier into the car, you know, get the baby and the carrier into a shopping cart, that kind of thing. Now I can't do that … I've got two kids' schedules now to try to accommodate to and I don't rest when I can rest…when I need to rest cause *I don't get time to rest* and then I also feel very trapped now because I, I can't—it's really hard for me to get out of the house with [second child].[1]

These mothers' participation in their home and/or community also seemed related to the perception of their interpersonal environment. In the following section I will describe their perception of interpersonal environment and social support.

Perception of Interpersonal Environment

Different experiences were described by the participants in this study in regard to role sharing, accepting help, and sense of community. In the literature there are many subtleties to consider in helping people with disabilities. This section will address the complexities of offering support to mothers with disabilities. Thomas (1997) described how there is an internal pressure to be seen as a good enough mother and present as managing normally. Thomas discussed assistance that is described as not helpful. This is when the mother feels a loss of control, the activity is taken over, or there is a lack of specific enough information to help her. This may inhibit her in asking for help. Also, mothers in Thomas' study did not want it to be assumed that they needed help. They wanted to be asked about what assistance they really wanted, and if they wanted help, and asked how they wanted it given. Morris (1995) believes that the "provision of accessible housing and equipment, and of personal

assistance over which they have control, enables disabled women to participate in the
kind of relationships—with all their dilemmas, joys and sorrows—that nondisabled people take for granted" (p. 90).

In this study (Morris, 1995), two main categories of perception of the interpersonal
environments were identified: experiences
fostering participation, normalization, and
adequacy and experiences stimulating feelings
of marginalization or inadequacy. Experiences
that fostered normalization and adequacy
included:

- Being willing to provide or providing
complementary or supplementary parental activities (i.e., role sharing)
- Giving support
- Having a facilitative attitude

In contrast, some participants described
ambivalence to the assistance or role-sharing,
especially when it was perceived as highlighting their inadequacy or feelings of being left
out. The participants' perception of role sharing or receiving assistance from the spouse,
children, and professional caregivers and
their sense of community is described in the
following paragraphs.

The Spouse

The mothers reported a variation in
arrangements made and reactions to the way
spouses shared childrearing and provided
support. May, one of the mothers with multiple sclerosis, which has an uncertain course,
described a powerful discussion with her
spouse regarding future role sharing before
making the decision to have a child, which included a contingency plan:

> If I was going to do this [have a child] . .
> we needed to prepare for whatever was
> going to happen. My husband was willing
> to be full time… he would do everything
> … He knew that if necessary, he would do
> whatever he had to do to take care of the
> child… So if mother and father are both
> together, then the child gets 100%
> (Farber, 2000, p. 265).[1]

This is an example of a couple being proactive in preparing for the unknown contingencies that may occur with this woman's illness.

This couple was explicit about what may be
necessary, and what they are willing or not willing to give if needed, in anticipation of having
a child. Their contracting process is similar to
the one recommended for dual-career couples
in planning the extent of parenting and role
sharing needed to combine career and parenthood in an equitable way (Farber, 1988).
This is empowering to both marital partners
because they are consciously entering this
arrangement. The ability to make an effective
contract is dependent on the individual's self-
awareness, ability to face the disease possibilities squarely, and the quality of individual and
collective communication. With chronic illness and disability, the importance of effective
communication may be even more "vital to the
family' than usual (Rolland, 1994, p. 71).

Gerry, the mother with a visual impairment,
described the positive importance of role sharing and support to her comfort as a mother:

> My first husband would never read to me.
> My second husband would, so we read
> things together when we had a baby, so I
> was kind of a little better prepared (for
> delivery) …My second husband was more
> comfortable with me as a visually im-
> paired person and I was more comfort-
> able (Farber, 2000, p. 265).[1]

More conflicted feelings emerged from several other participants regarding role sharing
with a spouse. Sue Ann, the mother with multiple sclerosis and two children (4 and 6 years
old) described the following mixed feelings:

> Their dad has filled that gap… I don't
> know if he had a conception … on what a
> father was supposed to do or be, but
> based on my performance as a mom, it's
> been wonderful. *Almost even too
> wonderful…* Last year, he insisted on tak-
> ing the kids canoeing… I opted to stay
> home. The kids wouldn't let me forget
> that…Why didn't you come canoeing?
> (Farber, 2000, p. 265).[1]

While reflecting on these words, this participant added later that, although she was both
truly grateful for her husband's help, at the
same time his ability to do things reminded
her of what she could not do and brought up
feelings of loss and envy.

The Child

The mothers' perception of their interaction with their children varied between mothers and was influenced by the personality, temperament, gender, and age of the child. There is a de facto assumption of the existence of role reversal in care between parents with disabilities and their children that was not found by Cohen (1998), who instead found that parents used "vigorous caution when assigning tasks to their children" (p.1). However, normatively, children progressively take on more self-care and family or household responsibilities as they get older. When a parent has a disability and needs specialized help, one may occasionally find "breaches" in the traditional, hierarchical parent-child helping relationship boundaries (Rolland, 1994). Sometimes breaches can be necessary for family functioning, and only become dysfunctional if role expectations are age inappropriate and rigid. Rachel, the mother with multiple sclerosis, described her 8-year-old:

> He's a big help. *He has dubbed himself my royal footman* ... when I need help with things ... like getting into bed ... When he was about 3 and a half ... I couldn't get into his room and sit down on the rocking chair to read to him anymore. Since then we, we've been reading at night in my bedroom and so he helps me get into bed (Farber, 2000, p. 265–266).[1]

Two mothers describe their adolescent daughter(s) as coaches or facilitators. Arielle, who has Parkinson's disease, described her relationship with her adolescent daughters:

> Both girls really showed a lot of caring and concern. They kind of were watching and if they ever could help out with something. One daughter would grab my arm if we were walking in the mall you know, if she saw I was having trouble... The other noticed how I would be holding my right leg back, [and said] just "do this."[1]

Katrina, the mother with paraplegia, described her teenage daughter in the following way:

> You know, she never, never took no for an answer. I mean, unless, unless there was ten stairs to climb and she knew at that point, that, okay, wheelchair and stairs don't mix. She knew that much. But if it were just like a little step, she'd look at me and go, *you can do that.* Just do it. You know, I mean. *So she pushed me.*[1]

Three of the participants described their children's response to the parental request for assistance as one of ambivalence. This ambivalence may be especially accentuated by gender and age, with the accompanying need for individuation, as illustrated by Sally, the mother with Parkinson's disease, and her preadolescent son:

> He has two phases. When he's in a sweet phase... he's just wonderful. He helps me. He does things for me... On the other hand, he's got this other phase where he resents having to do everything for me ... This little boy has had to take on responsibility... for taking care of me (Farber, 2000, p. 266).[1]

Professional Caregivers

According to Rolland (1994), in families that have a member with a disability or chronic illness, professional caregivers can become part of the "health related family unit" (p. 71). In describing mothers with disabilities, Morris (1995) suggests that it is important for the woman to have control over and direct the way personal assistants help with giving care. An example she gives is of a mother who requested that if her child fell, her assistant should pick the child up and bring him or her to the mother for a kiss. Although there was another caregiver, the mother wanted it to be clear to her child that she herself "was her mother" (Morris, p. 88). Some participants described the auxiliary parental support from caregivers very positively, particularly when they felt supported in their role. Gerry stated:

> I had a baby nurse who was very helpful cause she showed me a lot of things that you need to learn when you're a new mom. And she was aware that ... I had a vision problem... She was very supportive

and said, you'll be fine... You're experiencing being a new mom pretty much like any other new mom (Farber, 2000, p. 266).[1]

Rachel, the mother with multiple sclerosis and a 7 year-old son, had full-time child help since her son was 6 months old. She said:

> I don't know that it was shared parenting but perhaps akin to the role of a mother that's working who has her child in childcare for a long period of time during the day. And as the years progressed—somebody had said to me once, God that must be so difficult on him to get a new au pair every year or whatever, but *he realizes that Mommy and Daddy are constants.*[1]

Sally, the mother with a movement disorder from Parkinson's disease, described this poignant scenario in which she felt grateful but envious. This was bittersweet, like the mother whose husband's involvement reminded her of her inability to be involved:

> Sylvia (childcare provider) was so important... she was able to give him what I couldn't. It really meant a lot to me ... Sometimes I'd see her ... carrying him on her hip and *I was kind of envious...* That was something I couldn't do. But ... *it made me happy* to see him getting it from somebody (Farber, 2000, p.266).[1]

There were reported instances when individuals received unsolicited help or help "beyond what was asked for" from paid caregivers or family. This was described as an "invasion of boundaries" by some participants, similar to the findings of Thomas (1997) mentioned earlier. The net effect of this unnecessary help is the disempowerment of the individual with the disability (Thomas, 1997; Morris, 1995).

Community

Oberman and Josselson (1996) described the importance of mothers becoming part of a "maternal community" to mitigate the isolation that can occur with the central parenting responsibilities in nuclear families (without the support of extended family). Being part of a larger community of mothers can help mothers cope with the potential frustration and loneliness of their situations. Tardy (2000) described both the need of mothers to be "known and understood" (p. 455) as well as for tangible assistance. Accessibility to maternal communities and other communities may be more complicated for mothers with disabilities.

Participants in this study described a continuum of feeling related to their perceptions of their communities and their subsequent involvement in their communities, either for themselves or for their children. Social support and social integration, a component of community integration, have been associated with life satisfaction and health-related quality of life in individuals with disabilities and chronic conditions (Burleigh, Farber, & Gillard, 1998). Four participants who depicted a positive sense of community described intact groups as providing opportunities for shared individual or family activity. Some of the community groups were traditional community resources like play groups and schools. Others provided a context in which people like themselves, who were mothers, artists, or people with disabilities, could interact and participate in shared individual or family activities such as the multiple sclerosis walk. A mother who previously described poignant loss at not being similar to or doing childcare activities like other mothers, mentioned the participation in this last resource with positive affect and pride. She proudly shared a news clipping with me about her and her family's participation in the multiple sclerosis walk. Rachel, who was an artist, mentioned her excitement at the newly found physical accessibility to a community resource:

> I've been at the art center since I was 11 years old. It's my 2nd home and it got to the point where I can't do the steps any more. My father raised money to—to purchase for the art center mechanisms that—you put the wheelchair into it, it climbs the steps. It's really neat.[1]

Katrina, the mother with paraplegia who was a wheelchair user, described a situation in which there was a flight of stairs to her daughter's classroom or the nurse's office. However, the spirit of the administration made her so comfortable that she described her access to school in a seamless and effortless way. For instance, if her child was sick and she was called to pick her daughter up, the principal would say, "No problem" and walk the child to her car, or for parent conferences, the teacher would easily meet her on the first floor. It felt natural for her to be a frequent visitor to the school, doing things mothers do, like bringing her child lunch, participating in school book sales, and so forth. Also, she offered the observation that she was proud to model the naturalness of a woman with a disability being involved in the everyday life of her child.

Three participants described aspects of communities as nonsupportive or potentially hostile, especially in families in which children had preadolescent or adolescent peers. To prevent their children from being stigmatized regarding the mother's disability, because, as one mother said, "kids can be cruel," some mothers used humor or taught avoidance techniques to their children to circumvent or deal with teasing. Crystal, who had visible scoliosis and restricted height, described a verbal confrontation with a stranger regarding her disability and an incident in which her 8-year-old son and another child had a physical altercation. Another informant, Judy, the mother with cerebral palsy, felt marginalized by her community of fellow workers. She emphatically expressed her experience as living in "two separate worlds," "one [of persons] with disabilities and one without."

Three mothers who had invisible disabilities in which unpredictability of energy was an issue, described feelings of being out of sync. One participant, Jean, a mother with fibromyalgia who had two daughters aged 9 months and 5 years, described how she would longingly watch other mothers walk by her house with their strollers, going to the playground, and not have the energy to join them. As a group, these mothers with fatigue issues felt badly for not being able to participate in a cooperative nursery school or car pool in a regular way, or at a certain time of the day. When their requests for more flexibility or ac-

commodations were not responded to affirmatively, this added to their feeling of being *unlike other mothers.* The importance and type of community involvement varies with the age of the child. The next section will describe some highlights of children's developmental changes and the ways mothers experienced them.

Developmental Change

The primary focus of this chapter has been on the experience of the mothers with disabilities. However, there are inevitable changes in the parent-child relationship as the child grows up that affect the mother's experience. This process can be accounted for from a family developmental psychology perspective (L'Abate, 1994), which allows the examination of each individual family member's growth within the relational development of the family. Using this approach, Cusinato (1994) suggests that there is a continual adaptation process inherent in parenthood, in which the parent changes simultaneously with the growth and development of the child. However, when there is a disability, not only is there the complexity of a mutually interacting family system, but there is also the nature of the disease itself, with its onset and progression (or constancy), to integrate into the totality of the couple and family's experience (Rolland, 1994).

Initially children need intensive physical, hands-on care, which may be complicated for parents with physical and sensory disabilities to a varying degree, depending on their disability and the adaptations or resources they have available. Cohen (1998) found that a "preponderance of disability related problems mothers had parenting their children occurred in physical care-taking tasks that mothers perform for their children through the ages five " (p. 2). In my current study, Sally, who had Parkinson's disease, reported great difficulty trying to get socks on her moving baby because of periods of muscular rigidity and tremor. This compounded her feeling that she couldn't be or do things like other mothers.

Gerry, who had visual losses, found many adaptive ways to feed her child, find his mouth, and change his diaper without visual clues. She mostly described herself as being *just like other mothers*, acknowledged the difficulty, but proudly described the many resourceful adaptations she developed with her firstborn and subsequent children.

Because of the rapid growth in early years, continual resourcefulness and problem solving for new situations are necessary. For mothers with infants or small children, innovative equipment has been developed to assist parents with caregiving tasks: for example, accessible cribs, infant care seats attached to wheelchairs, baby bathtubs at the level of the wheelchair (De Moss, Rodgers, Tuleja, & Kirshbum, 1995). However, the mother has to freely want and be willing to seek and accept adaptive methods of mothering. According to Culler, Jasch, and Scanlan (1994), when the parent is empowered to make the decision, the utilization of adaptive equipment can help them conserve energy and improve task performance and safety for the baby.

The dependent infant soon becomes the exploring toddler, and the parent has to figure out how to allow this to unfold, yet provide safety during the exploration. This was not without anxiety for some. Mothers in this study found ways to respond to this developmental period by specially childproofing areas in their home that they could manage with their disability. Also, in the community, the mother with a visual problem had her child wear bright colors, which she could see, and one mother, in a wheelchair, had rules that her daughter stayed near her chair in open places and visited playgrounds that had enclosed areas.

As the child becomes school age, more interaction with the community occurs. This is where the school faculty's attitude and physical accessibility to classrooms, as well as participation in extracurricular or community activities, become an issue. Cohen (1998) also found that attitudinal and architectural barriers were described as more "numerous and deleterious to the mother's ability to parent their children" (p. 2) as the children matured.

In the limited literature on mothers with disabilities, there is even less written on par-

ents with a disability who have adolescent children. There were a few areas that were especially noteworthy in the descriptions of the experiences of women with children who were either preadolescent or adolescent. These included separation-individuation issues, driving, and monitoring behavior and discipline.

Separation/Individuation

The parental reaction to the adolescent and accompanying separation-individuation can be profound. Like other mothers, mothers with disabilities expressed the normal developmental bittersweet experience of parenting adolescents. Sometimes a child was described as a typically "obnoxious" or "demanding" teenager. Mothers described their own experience of falling off the pedestal, the mothers being perceived as "dumb" or "uncool" and being needed less. Their reactions were similar to those described by Steinberg and Steinberg (1994) in their study of nondisabled parents, which included feelings of abandonment, rejection, jealousy, loss, and powerlessness. However, some mothers embraced the burgeoning autonomy and tolerated the normal dethroning, whereas others took it more personally or fluctuated between these two states. This personalization became disability related for a few. Some particularly poignant narratives described the mother who felt more incompetent because of her disability (mentioned later), or two mothers whose visual difficulties were associated with their feeling of rejection or stigma for their children.

This bittersweet feeling of a child growing up was described by Arielle, the mother with Parkinson's disease, who noticed a change in her relationship with her adolescent daughter. She noticed that recently her husband was more involved in her daughter's life, helping her with decision making regarding going out into the world. Arielle was experiencing more cognitive difficulties, particularly when she was in affectively charged situations. She consciously felt that it was important for her husband and daughter, and did not want to "interfere." However, when asked if she thought this was the normal bittersweet feeling about a child growing up, she responded: "This is more painful, I didn't feel as if I had as much choice.... I feel embarrassed I have this weakness. I can't function as competently [about helping her with decision-making]."

Driving

Not being able to drive was an issue for a number of the mothers. Mothers' feelings about this varied with the degree of internalization of this as an accepted maternal practice and their subsequent interpretation as being "*not like other mothers*" when they could not fulfill this role. Sally reported:

> Now, when I'm dyskinetic I really shouldn't be driving... It's very hard on him. It's hard for him. He feels trapped in this house with me and can't go anywhere. I realize that most parents of kids that age are—most mothers from what I've been able—spend their lives carpooling their kids.[1]

In contrast is the discussion of this same issue by Gerry, the mom with a visual impairment (*unlike other mothers and it is okay to be different*):

> Not being able to drive was a major issue. My kids had to learn to take public transit. They had to walk... , it wasn't so horrible but [sometimes] they couldn't participate...*I had to let them go... further afield on public transit than other parents would have.* They sometimes complained ...They got wet. They got cold ... But at least [they] will be able to drive someday ... it's not forever (Farber, 2000, p. 265).[1]

Monitoring Behavior or Discipline

Most of the mothers (4 out of 5) who had preadolescent and adolescent children felt that the disability made it "a little harder" to monitor their children's behavior or discipline them. However, the following two conveyed a sense of personal agency in their attitude about establishing authority. The following mother, Crystal, had significant scoliosis and related restricted height, along with kidney disease, and describes her relationship to her son, who is one of a set of twins:

> Discipline is a challenge. He [my son] is a little bit taller than I am so you know the challenge comes a lot I think because we're like the same height or eye level... they think that you know well. I'm taller than mommy, and...but *I always tell them, you might be taller but I'm bigger when it comes* to discipline (They were her height since age 7).[1]

Gerry described the following:

> So discipline, monitoring their behavior *was a little harder*, but I have to admit that when they were young I pulled some mean things on them *like magical things like Mommy will find out somehow* so that they wouldn't pull that on me. *I'd tell them I knew what they were doing even though I didn't.*[1]

She also described how she would connect with her daughter's friends, using self-effacing humor to help them be more comfortable. This, in turn, helped her to know how her child coped in group settings.

The two mothers who had Parkinson's disease and energy concerns seemed to attribute making previously weak areas more labored and problematic to the disease:

> I mean I had trouble with being a good planner and organizer anyway in terms of my consistency as a parent—like following through you know, rules or limits or whatever. And I wasn't good at it anyway to begin with so the Parkinson's definitely affected that it you know—it got at one of my weak spots...
>
> My son knows how to manipulate me. I have always been a lousy disciplinarian. But I think having a disability enhances that. I mean if it weren't such a physical effort for me to get up and do something to reinforce something, I'd be more likely to do it, and it would be easier.[1]

All mothers have to continually adapt to the changing needs of their children and balance nurturance with setting limits. Some mothers in this study had resourcefully adapted to the age-related changes of the child, but for others their disability interfered with their satisfaction and the self-perceived effectiveness of their own parenting.

✒ Implications

Research Implications

Mothering is an intense, complex, and profound human experience. This chapter described the experience of motherhood from a subjective (being) and a participation (doing) perspective. It also described the impact of the mothers' interpersonal world and developmental challenges with the growth of their children. The purpose of this chapter was to describe the variation in the normative experiences of mothers with disabilities while secondarily describing the potential interrelationship between maternal self-description, participation in chosen maternal practices, and perception of social support across the family life cycle, as illustrated in Figure 10–1.

As a whole, the women in this study were educated and resourceful. Although at times these women shared painful experiences and losses, they also showed great pride in meeting the challenges of being mothers. As with any qualitative study, the results may not be generalizable to all mothers with disabilities, but perhaps the description of their rich stories can inform future research, theory, and practice in working with these mothers.

On the whole, this was a group of women who were very motivated to be mothers. This was demonstrated by the fact that 8 out of 10 chose to pursue or continue a pregnancy after their disability was clearly diagnosed, in spite of potential health risks for themselves. Subsequently, they were very invested in the role. Because disability can frequently restrict choices (Cardol, 2000), making a choice such as becoming a mother can be viewed as an "exercise of agency" (McDonough, 1996, p. 17). Fulfilling caregiving roles and taking on family responsibility can also be viewed as a component of the construct of social participation (Noreau, Fougeyrollas, & Tremblay, 2001). An important quality of social participation is autonomy in the choice of meaningful activities (Law, 2002; Cardol, 2000). Becoming a mother is very meaningful to many women.

The first theme, maternal self-description, appeared to reflect the continuum of acceptance of self with disability, as well as the degree to which their disability was either central or peripheral to the experience of self as mother. For mothers who primarily felt *just like other mothers*, their adaptation and participation in the maternal role appeared effortless and seamless. Their disability seemed to be on the periphery of their mothering. They minimized differences between themselves and other mothers and described trying to make their child's life "as normal as possible." In the current study, mothers who felt *just like other mothers* seemed to reach a state of "coming to terms' with their disability and even "transcendence," which occurs when individuals "overcome their bodies in such a way that they are able to find real joy in living" (Corbin and Strauss, 1987, p. 271).

Corbin and Strauss (1987) also found chronic illness (with resultant disability) was, for the most part, "something to be managed and taken into consideration, but certainly not the only aspect of life" (p. 251), although they describe this as more difficult to do with more severe and frequent symptoms. Most of the mothers (across diagnoses) in this study either saw themselves as *just like other mothers* or *unlike other mothers and it is okay to be different*. However, the three mothers who felt most *unlike other mothers*, with accompanying sadness or feelings of frustration, had either a different psychosocial adjustment to their disability or a chronic illness with more severe symptoms that made it less possible to put the disability in the background. For example, Sally, the woman with Parkinson's, had very visible difficulties with tremors and movement during the interview. In contrast, the 3 out of the 5 mothers who felt *like other mothers* and demonstrated less distress about mothering with a disability had serious but relatively stable disabilities. Further research is needed to explore the effect of the seriousness and frequency of symptoms, perception of health, and type of disability on women's acceptance of self as an adequate mother.

It is also possible that mothers with disabilities may truly be like other mothers in their unfair comparison to a culturally idealized myth of the perfect selfless mother (Francis-

Connolly, 2000; Farber, 2000). The quest for this socially constructed perfect mother is hard enough for mothers without disabilities, but it may make mothering even more challenging for women who are simultaneously grappling with the disability experience. This can be further compounded by the "fear of being judged" as an inadequate mother found in the literature (Thomas, 1997, p. 633), with even higher external stakes such as potential legal consequences and loss of custody.

In terms of maternal participation, the women in this study did what mothers do. Their involvement in activities ranged from *normal participation* to *adapted participation* to *nonparticipation*, role withdrawal or loss. Mothers who felt *like other mothers* or *unlike other mothers and it is okay to be different* spoke of the normalcy of their participation and adaptations they made. In addition to autonomy and choice being important to participation, a supportive and facilitating environment is important as well. Recent disability consumer-oriented research is not examining independent functioning per se, but the quality and choice in type of participation (Cardol, 2000), the level of participation with or without environmental adaptation, technical or human assistance, and the person's satisfaction with this participation (Noreau, Fougeyrollas, & Tremblay, 2001). The mothers who felt *just like other mothers*, and *unlike other mothers and it is okay to be different* reported their participation or adapted participation with comfort and sometimes pride. The mothers who withdrew from either personally or culturally valued maternal activities (without substitution or adaptation) expressed this as a painful loss. More research is needed to clarify the complexities of level of participation, type of assistance, and use of technology and satisfaction level of mothers with disabilities.

Participation is always "influenced by the environment in which activities are to be performed " (Noreau, Fougeyrollas, & Tremblay, 2001, p. 8). Mothers in this study reported interpersonal environments that either fostered participation, normalization, and adequacy or stimulated feelings of marginalization or inad-

equacy. They reported experiences of their spouses, children, and professional caregivers, and sense of community. Experiences that fostered normalization and adequacy included:

- Being willing to provide or providing complementary or supplementary parental activities, for example, role sharing
- Giving support
- Having a facilitative attitude

In contrast, some participants described ambivalence toward assistance or role sharing, especially when it was perceived as highlighting their inadequacy or feelings of being left out.

It is beyond the scope of this study to examine the effect of the external physical environment in terms of facilitating or inhibiting conditions, as well as access to technical assistance, or the new adaptive parenting equipment available to facilitate their parental functioning. However, further research is needed to examine the effect of both external and interpersonal environmental supports on mothers' participation and well-being. Figure 10–2 postulates a model that includes the elements illustrated in Figure 10–1, with the addition of health, as perceived by the individual and as discernible through the severity and frequency of symptoms.

The findings regarding the developmental changes in childhood are complex. Initially, children need intensive physical, hands-on care, which was found to be complicated for some mothers in this study. Also, protecting them in the larger environment was problematic for some. Cohen also (1998) found that a "preponderance of disability related problems mothers had parenting their children occurred in physical care-taking tasks that mothers perform for their children through the ages five "(p. 2). However, their psychosocial adjustment and their narrative script of being *just like other mothers* or *unlike other mothers and it is okay to be different* seemed related to their perception of the difficulty of the adjustment needed. The severity of symptoms, or more advanced disease states, may also affect self-perception; however, further research is needed to clarify this issue.

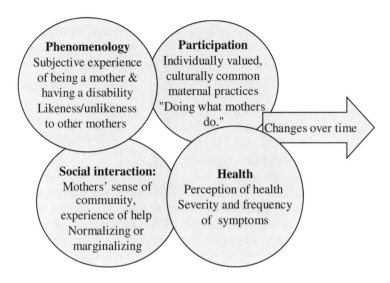

Figure 10–2 *Mothers with disabilities: Phenomenology, participation, social interaction, and health.*

In addition, some limitations seemed to be more problematic with adolescents. Both mothers who had Parkinson's disease reported greater distress regarding their difficulties with teenagers. One mother attributed this to difficulty with consistency, slowness, and difficulty with cognitive functioning under emotionally intense situations. However, it is relevant to note that mothers without disabilities who have adolescents also report experiencing emotionally intense situations. One mother had difficulty related to the fact that she was not able to physically follow through and reinforce discipline. In contrast, other mothers with more predictability of movement, and without possible cognitive sensitivities, described their handling of these issues with more ease.

Again, more information from larger samples is needed about the self-perception and well-being of mothers with disabilities, normative maternal participation, and perception of support over the family life cycle. This evidence would be helpful for developing a consumer-oriented model to explain the interrelationship of the developmental needs of the mother and family, the continual developmental needs of the child, and the effects of the changes in health status related to disability or chronic disease. Based on this normative mode, a comprehensive plan for health promotion/health enhancement and relevant outcomes for rehabilitation for mothers with disabilities could be developed.

Practice Implications

The primacy of being a mother cannot be underestimated for many women, with or without a disability. Numerous women with disabilities have experienced either invisibility or a deficit lens in regard to their being a mother. Therefore, it is essential that professionals working with mothers who have disabilities be self aware and genuinely sure of their ability to appreciate the unique ways of mothering that they will see, and be strongly committed to support the strengths and resourcefulness of these mothers. Based on the findings of this study, there are a number of issues that professionals need to be sensitive to:

- The mother's unique maternal self-description
- Her choice, preferred level, and satisfaction with maternal participation
- Her perception of personal and community support
- Changes in the developmental needs of the child

Professionals need to be aware of the normal variation in the mothers' self-acceptance or nonacceptance of self with a disability. In general research with disability groups, impairment severity is not correlated to quality of life (Johnston, 2001). Therefore, coming to terms with one's self with a disability (Corbin & Strauss, 1987) theoretically could contribute more to functioning and quality of life than the disability itself. For the health practitioner, it is important to explore how each woman perceives herself as a mother with a disability, and how central or marginal the disability is to her identification as a mother. Is the mother comparing herself to other mothers and feeling like or unlike them? Or is she comparing herself to the unattainable, illusive ideal of the perfect mother that mothers without disabilities have been found to compare themselves to (Francis-Connolly, 2000)? Helping a mother identify her internal dialogue through active listening or observation may be useful. Mothers with disabilities can be helped to be aware of these counterproductive comparisons, and helped to value what they can do (Grant, 2001) and to accept and appreciate their uniqueness as a person and as a mother.

"Being" and "doing" were found to be interrelated for mothers with disabilities. Therefore, in addition to working toward helping mothers accept themselves (being), ways of maximizing maternal participation should be encouraged. The mothers in my study appeared to value participating in culturally traditional maternal practices, which in turn made them feel *like other mothers*, even when they used adaptation. The degree of perceived similarity in participation seemed to be related to the sense of well-being and personal agency they projected. The degree of perceived dissimilarity in participation seemed to be related to distress.

Mothers may have unique preferences for specific maternal involvement in traditional or nontraditional ways. These preferences need to be explored with each mother. What maternal activities are most important to this mother? This is especially important for mothers who have problems with physical activity or fatigue as a consequence of their disability. It may be valuable to explore ways of helping mothers to foster psychological connectedness to their child through talk, play, or the sharing of community activities, either in person or through new technology, when physical activity or energy is severely limited. Prioritization or reprioritization may be particularly important for energy conservation. Also, because many mothering activities have several subactivities "enfolded" within another activity. For example, giving a bath may be a chance for socialization or for helping one's child relax before bedtime, as well as for hygiene (Griffin, 2002), and the specific qualities of the desired activity should be clarified.

Another factor that should be considered is the mother's need for human or technical assistance to participate as fully as she wishes to in her choice of maternal activities or assistance needed for adequate childcare. Sometimes this is a straightforward process with professionals such as occupational therapists evaluating the impairment and matching assistance or adapted equipment to the mothers' needs. However, complications in this process could occur when a mother sees herself through a deficit lens as *unlike other mothers* and sees the adaptation or assistance as further proof of this deficit. Also, if a mother is fearful of being judged incompetent because of her disability, it may be more difficult for her to ask for, or trust, assistance. A sense of safety and trustworthiness needs to be cultivated in the helping relationship to allow some mothers to ask for help from family or professionals. Asking for help or adaptation may also need to be reframed as a strength. Requiring additional human assistance needs to be normalized as role sharing, which working mothers who do not have a disability often have to do. Asking for help should not be perceived as a weakness or deficit.

Professionals need to be aware of the possible symbolic meaning of participation for mothers with disabilities. Homemaking activities, which can appear mundane, cannot be taken for granted and "relinquishing them may engender feelings of incompetence" (McDonough, 1996, p. 19). The importance of participation was further described by McDonough regarding women's striving to perform homemaking activities: "The women's attempts to meet expectations associated with normative social role can be seen as the exercise of agency in a context in which choices are not always evident" (p. 17). In my study, women who felt more *like other mothers* (or same ends, different means) reported participation more frequently and effortlessly in both adapted and nonadapted ways.

Participation can be influenced by the environment (Noreau, Fougeyrollas, & Tremblay, 2001). In my study, mothers felt bolstered when the interpersonal environment facilitated normalcy and adequacy, or were able to make necessary accommodations. Being treated like other mothers and being able to participate like other mothers can be a product of good social support. Group membership in the community was also found to be essential both emotionally and instrumentally for mothers without disabilities, and to prevent isolation (Oberman & Josselson, 1996; Tardy, 2000). Opportunities to foster participation in natural maternal communities or cyber-support groups should be encouraged. Community participation is important; therefore, health professionals could take a proactive role in facilitating both attitudinal and physical accessibility in the community for their clients whenever possible. It also may be important to educate significant others regarding the importance of offering help in ways that respect the autonomy and centrality of the mother's role.

Last, the development of the child and accompanying psychosocial stages bring unique stage-related challenges to being a parent. Mothers with a disability need similar and unique support, depending on the age-related needs of the child. When the child is young, adapting to and involvement with direct care is a primary concern. Professionals need to be aware of the unique adaptation, as well as adaptive childcare equipment and technology now available for parents with disabilities. As the child ages, more complex psychosocial needs emerge. Mothers with disabilities, like other mothers, may need support to function during the emotional intensity of adolescence. Improving access to normative community supports and contact with other mothers may be especially important at certain developmental periods.

Conclusion

Being a mother is a profound human experience, which many women, with or without disabilities, want to have a chance to actualize. Professionals can make a significant difference in the lives of mothers with disabilities by increasing self-acceptance and maximizing meaningful participation in the mothering role, helping mothers obtain useful social support, and making connections to important communities and resources, as well as helping mothers with the transitions necessary for stage-related changes in their child.

Discussion Questions

- How would you explore the issue of adaptive childcare equipment for a mother who does not feel "like other mothers" and may see it as a sign of her limitation?

- A mother had a comfortable relationship with her school-age child and felt competent with her mothering involvement. Now her child is turning 13, and she senses that the child is embarrassed by her and doesn't want to do as much with her. With what issues might they be struggling? Can you identify how normative or unique to the disability each of these issues may be?

- What would you do if a mother who was experiencing extreme fatigue wanted more maternal involvement? How would you help her?

References

Arendell, T. (2000). Conceiving and investigating motherhood: The decade's scholarship. *Journal of Marriage and the Family, 62*(4), 1192–1207.

Asch, A., & Fine, M. (1988). Introduction: Beyond pedestals. In M. Fine & A. Asch (Eds.). *Women with disabilities: Essays in psychology, culture and politics* (pp. 1–38). Philadelphia: Temple University Press.

Buck, F. M., & Hohmann, G. W. (1981). Personality, behavior, values and family relations of children of fathers with spinal cord injury. *Archives of Physical Medicine and Rehabilitation, 62,* 432–439.

Buck, F. M., & Hohmann, G. W. (1983). Parental disability and children's adjustment. *Annual Review of Rehabilitation,* pp. 203–239. New York: Springer.

Bowlby, S., Gregory, S., & McKie, L. (1997). "Doing home": Patriarchy, caring and space. *Women's Studies International Forum, 20,* 343–350.

Burleigh, S. B., Farber, R. S., & Gillard, M. (1998). Community integration and life satisfaction after traumatic brain injury: Long-term findings. *American Journal of Occupational Therapy, 52*(1), 45–52.

Cantor, N., & Sanderson, C. A. (1999). Life task participation and well-being : The importance of taking part in daily life. In D. Kahneman, E. Diener, & N. Schwarz (Eds.). *Well-being: The foundations of hedonic psychology* (pp.230–243). New York: Russell Sage Foundation.

Cardol, M. (2000). Beyond disability: Assessing participation and autonomy in medical rehabilitation. Published master's thesis, Department of the Academic Medical Centre in Amsterdam, the Netherlands.

Charmaz, K. (1991) *Good days, bad days: The self in chronic illness and time.* New Brunswick, NJ: Rutgers University Press

Coates, D. L., Vietze, P. M., & Gray, D. B. (1985). Methodological issues in studying children of disabled parents. In S. K. Thurman (Ed.). *Children of handicapped parents: Research and clinical perspectives* (pp.155–180). New York: Academic Press.

Cohen, L. (1998). Mothers' perceptions of the influence of their physical disabilities on the developmental tasks of children. *Dissertation Abstracts International, 59,* 3090.

Collins, C. (1999). Reproductive technologies for women with physical disabilities. *Sexuality and Disability, 17*(4), 299–307.

Corbin, J., & Strauss, A. L. (1987). Accompaniments of chronic illness: Changes in body, self, biography and biological time. *Research in the Sociology of Health Care, 6,* 249–281.

Culler, K. H., Jasch, C., & Scanlan, C. (1994). Child care and parenting for the young stroke survivor. Topics in Stroke Rehabilitation: *Child Care and Parenting Issues. Spring* (1), 48–64.

Cusinato, M. (1994). Parenting over the family life cycle. In L. L'Abate (Ed.). *Handbook of developmental family psychology and psychopathology* (pp. 3–23). New York: Wiley.

De Angelis, T. (1995, January). Custody battles challenging for parents with disabilities. *APA Monitor,* p. 39.

De Moss, A., Rodgers, J., Tuleja, C., & Kirshbum, M. (1995). *Adaptive parenting equipment: Idea Book 1.* Berkeley, CA: Through the Looking Glass: National Resource Center for Parents with Disabilities.

Erikson, E. H. (1980). *Identity and the life cycle.* New York: W. W. Norton & Co.

Farber, R. S. (1988). Integrated treatment of the dual-career couple. *The American Journal of Family Therapy, 16*(1), 46–57.

Farber, R. S. (2000). Mothers with disabilities: In their own voice. *American Journal of Occupational Therapy, 54*(3), 260–268.

Falk, M. (2000). The real and ideal mother: The experience of motherhood in light of the ideal. *Dissertation Abstracts International,* AAT 9992447.

Finger, A. (1985). Claiming all of our bodies' reproductive rights and disability. In S. Browne, D. Connors & N. Stern (Eds.). *With the power of each breath* (pp. 292–307). Pittsburgh: A Women's Publishing Company.

Francis-Connolly, E. (2000). Toward an understanding of mothering: A comparison of two motherhood stages. *American Journal of Occupational Therapy, 54*(3), 281–289.

Gilhool, T. K., & Gran, J. A. (1985). Legal rights of disabled parents. In S. K. Thurman (Ed.). *Children of handicapped parents: Research and clinical perspectives* (pp. 11–33). New York: Academic Press (Harcourt Brace Jovanovich, Publishers).

Grant, M. (2001). Mothers with arthritis, child care and occupational therapy: Insight through case studies. *British Journal of Occupational Therapy, 64*(7), 322–329.

Griffin, S. D. (2002, June). A bath to get clean or get settled for sleep: The meaning of everyday mothering activities for mothers. Poster presented at the 13th World Congress of Occupational Therapist, Stockholm, Sweden.

Gutmann, D. (1975). Parenthood: A key to the comparative study of the life cycle. In N. Datan & L. E. Ginsberg (Eds.). *Life-span developmental psychology* (pp. 167–184). New York: Academic Press.

Hanna, D. V., & Edwards, P. A. (1988). Physically disabled parents and their normal children: Assessment, diagnosis, and intervention. *Holistic Nurse Practitioner, 2*(2), 38–47.

Hyler, D. (1985). To choose a child. In S. Browne, D. Connors & N. Stern (Eds.). *With the power of each breath* (pp. 292–307). Pittsburgh: A Women's Publishing Company.

Johnston, M. (2001, November). *Quality of life issues in traumatic brain injury.* Paper presented at Quality of Life Measurement, Building an Agenda for the Future, Kessler Medical Rehabilitation, Research and Education Corporation, Parsippany, NJ.

L'Abate, L. (1994). (Ed.). *Handbook of developmental family psychology and psychopathology.* New York: Wiley.

Law, M. (2002). Participation in the occupations of everyday life. *American Journal of Occupational Therapy, 56*(6), 640–649.

Maccoby, E. E., & Martin, J. A. (1983). Socialization in the context of the family: Parent-Child interaction. In P. H. Mussens (Ed.). *Handbook of Child Psychology.* Volume 4 (4th ed., pp. 1–101). New York: John Wiley & Sons.

Matthews, G. F. (1983). *Voices from the shadows: Women with disabilities speak out.* Ontario, Canada: Women's Educational Press.

Meadow-Orlans, K. P. (1995). Parenting with a sensory or physical disability. In M. H. Bornstein (Ed.). *National Institute of Child Health and Human Development. Handbook of parenting: Vol. 4. Applied and practical parenting* (pp. 57–84) Mahwah, NJ: Erlbaum.

McDonough, P. (1996). The social production of housework disability. *Women & Health, 24,* 1–25.

Morris, J. (1995). Creating a space for absent voices: Disabled women's experience of receiving assistance with daily living activities. *Feminist Review, 51,* 68–93.

Morris, J. (1993). Feminism and disability. *Feminist Review, 43,* 57–70.

Morris, J. (1989). *Able lives: Women's experience of paralysis.* London (UK): The Woman's Press.

National Resource Center for Parents with Disabilities (Fall 1998): *Parenting with a disability.* Volume 6 (1). Berkeley, California: Through the Looking Glass.

Noreau, L., Fougeyrollas, P., & Tremblay, J. (2001). Measure of life habits: *Life-H, User's Manual.* Quebec, Canada: International Network on the Disability Creation Process.

Oberman, Y., & Josselson, R. (1996). Matrix of tension: A model of mothering. *Psychology of Women Quarterly, 20,* 341–359.

Radtke, H. L., & Van Mens-Verhulst, J. (2001). Being a mother and living with asthma: An exploratory analysis of discourse. *Journal of Health Psychology, 6*(4), 379–391.

Rolland, J. S. (1994). *Families, illness and disability: An integrated model.* New York: Basic Books.

Sprill, L. C. (1987, April). *Sexuality, childbearing, and family planning for physically challenged women.* Paper presented at Public Health Social Work Institute, University of Pittsburgh, Graduate School of Public Health, Pittsburgh, PA.

Steinberg, L., & Steinberg, W. (1994). *Crossing paths: How your child's adolescence triggers your own crisis.* New York: Simon & Schuster.

Strauss, A., & Corbin, J. (1990). *Basics of qualitative research: Grounded theory procedures and techniques.* London (UK): Sage Publications.

Tardy, R. W. (2000). But I am a good mom: The social construction of motherhood through health-care conversations. *Journal of Contemporary Ethnography, 28*(4), 433–473.

Thomas, C. (1997). The baby and the bath water: Disabled women and motherhood in a social context. *Sociology of Health & Disease, 19*(5), 632–643.

Umberson, D. (1989). Parenting and well-being. *Journal of Family Issues, 10*(4), 427–439.

Van Loon, R. A. (2000). Redefining motherhood: Adaptation to role change for women with AIDS. *Families in Society, 81*(2), 152–161.

Walmsley, J. (1993). Contradictions in caring reciprocity and interdependence. *Disability, Handicap & Society, 8*(2), 129–142.

Ware, J. (2001, November). *Quality of life measurement: The evolution of the field.* Paper presented at Quality of Life Measurement, Building an Agenda for the Future, Kessler Medical Rehabilitation, Research and Education Corporation, Parsippany, NJ.

Woollett, A., & Marshall, H. (2001). Motherhood and mothering. In R.K. Unger (Ed.). *Handbook of the psychology of women and gender* (pp. 170–182). New York: Wiley.

World Health Organization (2001). *International Classification of Functioning Disability and Health.* Geneva, Switzerland: Classification, Assessment and Surveys and Terminology Team.

Source Credits

CHAPTER 11

Mothers with Chronic Illness: Reconstructing Occupation

Karin Opacich, PhD, MHPE, OTR/L, FAOTA

Teresa A. Savage, PhD, RN

 Anticipated Outcomes

We anticipate that, after reading this chapter, readers will:

- Acknowledge the internal and external characteristics that shape the experiences of women with chronic illnesses

- Recognize the factors that may enhance or diminish quality of life for women with chronic illnesses

- Appreciate the occupational complexities of mothering for women living with chronic illnesses

- Understand the importance of developing strategies that empower women to meet the challenges of mothering for women who have chronic illnesses

✍ Introduction

About the Authors

Over many years of providing health-related services to children, we came to understand and appreciate the critical influence that women can exert in family and community life. When women who are mothers face the added challenge of addressing personal chronic illness, quality of life for the entire family can be either enhanced or diminished. We (Karin Opacich and Teresa Savage) have collaborated over the years in ethics deliberations and in teaching. Some of the issues addressed in this chapter first emerged in a course we taught entitled *Women, Feminism, and the Health-Care Professions*.

In addition to academic roles, one of us (Karin Opacich) has spent many years providing occupational therapy in both home and hospital settings. In these settings the illness experience is defined by personal attributes, family relationships, culture, economic resources, and the environment. Her recent research is about women with HIV/AIDS and exploring the way that women rearrange their occupations to accommodate their illness, their perceived quality of life, and the relevance of health-related services available to them. Even healthy mothers were observed to experience role overload, and mothers coping with their own illnesses adapt their roles in a variety of ways.

One of us (Teresa Savage) is a nurse ethicist who has worked in pediatrics throughout her entire career. Having worked as a staff nurse in neonatal intensive care and as a clinical nurse specialist in pediatric neurology, she has witnessed the evolution of chronic health problems and their effect on the family. Her ethics education and experience, along with her clinical background, permitted her to counsel families and facilitate decision-making. Although contact with mothers focused on their children's health issues, the interactions gave her insights into how mothers cope and adapt. It was not unusual for the mother of a child with a health problem to develop health problems of her own. She learned that women, as mothers, often have a different perspective of their own illness than women who are not mothers.

✍ Overview

Using examples of chronic illness characterized by trajectories reflecting both physiological and social consequences, we have attempted to frame illness from a feminist point of view (Dan, 1994; Krieger, 1994). We have also considered cultural attitudes toward illness and a cultural perspective of caregiving and receiving. Relationships, the significance of life partners, disruption of intimacy, and support systems are acknowledged to shape the illness experience for women. It is recognized that, for women, the mothering role, however that is expressed, extends over a woman's lifetime regardless of personal status. In some cases, role reversal, parentification of children, or dependence on aging parents occurs among women with chronic illnesses. This can raise issues about parental competency and decisional authority. Women with chronic illnesses, struggling with such issues as self-reliance and interdependence, might understandably manifest ambivalence about compliance with regimes or recommendations. To fully appreciate women's experience of chronic illness, it is necessary to examine the resources available to them, the negotiation entailed, the routes of access, and the demands of managing those resources. Although some might associate these concerns with public health, all those committed to improving health and quality of life, including occupational therapy practitioners, must understand principles of social justice and must address inequity in order to achieve those ends (Townsend, 1993, 1996; Whiteford, Townsend, & Hocking, 2000). Understandably, women experiencing chronic illness interact with the medical establishment; thus they may form a "guarded alliance" with agencies and health-care practitioners.

Only by understanding the full biopsychosocial picture of chronic illness can health-care practitioners plan and offer relevant and potentially effective interventions to women. If one of the primary goals of care is to preserve occupational competence and occupational coherence (Christiansen, 1999) in the interest of quality living, health-care practitioners must commit to the preservation of *meaningful doing* as that is constructed by women. This chapter endeavors to raise consciousness about the phenomena, challenges, and opportunities encountered by women living with chronic illnesses.

ᖶ Occupational Challenges and Interventions

Women with chronic illnesses are faced with tremendous challenges and choices in attending to their own health needs while preserving the integrity of their families, however these are defined. Chronic illness, no matter how slow, rapid, or intermittent the progression of symptoms along the trajectory, necessitates reconstruction of occupations. Sometimes, as in the example of HIV given later in this chapter, this reconstruction leads to improved quality of life. More commonly, chronic illness threatens meaningful doing.

Quality of life seems to be levied according to the extent to which individuals can fulfill their life plans, however trivial or elaborate those plans might be (Christiansen, Little, & Backman, 1998). In response to any threats or alterations to well-being, the overarching goal of occupational therapy is to promote *quality living* as expressed through *meaningful doing* (Wilcock, 1998; Zemke & Clark, 1996; Christiansen, 1999). The primary goals of occupational therapy in the treatment of women with chronic illness are to preserve or engender *occupational competencies* and to promote *occupational coherence*. (Christiansen, 1999; Opacich, 2002). *Occupational competencies,* simply stated, are the repertoire of skills, strategies, and experiences we bring to the mundane and extraordinary challenges we encounter in doing the things we deem meaningful. *Occupational coherence* is the result of implementing our competencies to construct lives that make sense, that flow logically, that are satisfying, and that represent our life plans. Guidance for assessing occupational performance and establishing specific

occupational problems can be found in the Framework for Practice (American Occupational Therapy Association [AOTA], Commission on Practice, 2002). With the ultimate agenda of promoting performance in areas of occupation, the occupational therapist, in conjunction with other health professionals treating women with chronic illness, may need to address performance skills, performance patterns, context, activity demands, and client factors as these change in response to the illness. The Matrix of Occupational Status (Fig. 11–1) was generated by one of us (Opacich) when sifting through narrative data of her research. We think that this might be a useful tool for organizing data and representing the extent to which a chronic illness has affected a variety of women's occupations, regardless of the narrative tool or template used.

It should be remembered that women's occupations tend to represent "enfolded" activities, a term used by Bateson (1996) when she likened women's occupations to the construction or composition of artistic work. She noted, "Holistically, the composing of a life, the combination of elements, and the balancing and harmonizing of them is in itself an art form" (pp. 10, 11). It becomes increasingly apparent that if only the substrates, or prerequisite skills and tasks entailed in occupations, are addressed, without attending to their integrity and complement, it is unlikely that occupational coherence will be enhanced. Additionally, intervention must be relevant to the real life of each woman receiving treatment. To ascertain what is relevant, collaborative reasoning is most likely to yield positive outcomes. Ethical health practitioners must recognize and attend to the underlying social issues that determine the options available to each woman; doing this may entail empowering others or advocating on behalf of others.

ᖶ The Sociopolitical Context

To understand the impact of chronic illness on women, it is necessary to appreciate the sociopolitical context in which illness occurs. The World Health Organization has long acknowledged that the health of any society is

Occupational Domain	Associated Occupational Roles	Occupational Status				
		Discontinuation	Disruption	No Change	Adaptation	Augmentation
Work	parent/caregiver					
	homemaker (IADL)					
	employee (remunerated)					
	entrepreneur					
	vocational trainee					
	student					
Play Leisure	spectator					
	participant/observer					
	hobbyist					
	athlete					
Self-Care	spiritual/devotional life					
	personal care (ADL)					
	health-related care					
	personal advocacy					
	intimacy/sexual expression					
Occupational Context	home environment					
	family support					
	network of friends					
	financial support					
	neighborhood/community setting					
	health-care facility					
	social agencies					
	church/temple/mosque					
	place of employment					
	other					

Figure 11–1 *Matrix of Occupational Status*

inextricably related to the health of its women (WHO, 1995). Because women manifest "enfolded occupations," they exert influence well beyond childbearing and childrearing in family systems. Whether by personal choice or economic necessity, the role of mothering is rarely the only role assumed by modern women, and it is not uncommon for women to engage in the activities and tasks of multiple roles, sometimes simultaneously, both within and outside the home.

Although such roles may be expressed differently in each society, women assume roles as household managers, caregivers of elderly parents or other relatives, entrepreneurs, members of the workforce, community activists, and more. Research in neuropsychology has suggested a tendency of women to process information diffusely rather than linearly, a characteristic that probably contributes to the skill of "multitasking." The capacity for attending to multiple agendas is clearly an asset when it comes to mothering

(Speck et al., 2000; Weekes, 1994). When women are challenged by chronic illness, they must first reckon with their own health needs in order to preserve the integrity of their families and fulfill their chosen roles. For women who are unaccustomed to attending to their own needs before those of others, attending to a chronic illness may seem self-indulgent.

Evolving Paradigms in Identifying Health Needs of Women

Medicine as an organized and regulated profession is relatively young, and the explosion of medical wisdom reflects the evolution of microbiology and epidemiology in the last century. As more rigorous science and systematic research advanced insight into disease processes, women were largely considered unsuitable subjects in investigations until the 1980s because of their menstrual cycles and childbearing potential, functions over which they had little social or political voice. Historically, women have been undiagnosed or misdiagnosed, stereotyped or stigmatized, and even excluded from the benefits of scientific investigation that yielded effective interventions (Sherwin, 1992; Lawrence & Wernhouse, 1994). Exclusion of women in research has resulted in gaps in understanding about gender-specific presentations and manifestations of some chronic illnesses. The epidemiological history of HIV/AIDS in the United States can serve as a case in point. Because the proportion of women infected with HIV in the United States was so small in the early years of the epidemic, their unique symptoms and experiences were misunderstood. When HIV/AIDS definitions were amended in 1993 to include disease expressions unique to women, statistics reveal a dramatic increase in HIV/AIDS incidence in women. According to surveillance data from the Centers for Disease Control (CDC), the proportion of women infected with HIV rose from 7 percent in 1985 to 25 percent in 1999, and that figure is expected to increase (CDC, 2002). Today it is well established that women manifest HIV differently, and that valuable information leads to earlier detection and more effective management of the disease.

If gender has been considered at all in the treatment of ailments, women have been characterized as vessels and either sexualized or defined in terms of childbearing. Although some might disagree, modern women clearly have more options than their historical sisters. Wife and mother were socially acceptable and socially expected roles for women living at the turn of the 20th century, particularly women born into families with social currency. Access to education and career opportunities were somewhat restricted, even for women of means, and only those willing and able to defy social convention dared to aspire to autonomous roles within and beyond the home. Women's pursuits were often diminished and their maladies paternalistically regarded as characteristics of the "weaker sex."

Coinciding with the early development of modern medicine, classic literature such as Charlotte Perkins Gilman's short story, *The Yellow Wallpaper* (Gilman, 1973, 1899) and Kate Chopin's novel, *The Awakening* (Chopin, 1976), poignantly depict women whose lives

and illnesses were mistakenly described in terms of feminine propensities or fragility as those were defined largely by men. Both of the women portrayed in these famous stories were prohibited from pursuing personally meaningful occupation. Edna Pontellier, the central character in *The Awakening*, unfulfilled by the roles of wife and mother, becomes so despondent that she drowns herself. In *The Yellow Wallpaper,* a young woman, whose husband is a physician, narrates her own descent into psychosis after the birth of her first child. A medically prescribed intervention called the *Weir Mitchell Rest Cure* and described in Gilman's short story (Olfson, 1988) was most often imposed on women from the wealthier strata of society for a variety of misinterpreted symptoms, including postpartum depression. The rest cure entailed enforced idleness and avoidance of mental and physical exertion, which more likely exacerbated the condition. Motherhood was regarded as a source of stress, and the rest cure required that women be relieved of their mothering responsibilities altogether. Over the past few years, there were tragic deaths of children in the infamous cases of Susan Smith from Maryland, who locked her two children in a car and rolled them down a boat ramp; Marilyn Lemak, an Illinois nurse estranged from her husband, who tranquilized and smothered her three children; and Andrea Yaeger from Texas, whose fundamentalist husband opposed her taking antipsychotic medications, and who drowned her children one by one in the bathtub. All three women have been convicted and incarcerated. These women appear to have had serious chronic mental health issues that affected their ability to mother. Their cases suggest that recognizing mental illness continues to be confounding. Continuous care and adequate support for mothering women, especially for those with chronic illnesses, would seem an essential ingredient for positive outcomes. The potential consequences of minimizing an array of chronic illnesses of women who are mothers have received much public attention, which must be translated into more caring vigilance and aggressive intervention in the future.

With regard to both sex and conception,

women were traditionally expected to comply with the wishes of men, certainly within and sometimes outside the bonds of marriage. There are still many cultures and circumstances in which women are subjugated to the will of men (Rodriguez-Trias, 1992). Women have suffered and even died from folkloric remedies and clandestine abortions for unwanted pregnancies. Distribution of information and the means for preventing pregnancy were legally prohibited in the United States until such laws were repealed in 1972. Until that time, women were not empowered to advocate for a broader and deeper understanding of even their reproductive health. From 1969 until 1973, when the court case of *Roe v. Wade* decriminalized abortion in the United States, an underground group known as The Abortion Counseling Service of Women's Liberation, *aka Jane*, operated in Chicago and provided both information and access to skilled abortionists for thousands of women (Kaplan, 1995). Since the expiration of the statute of limitations, activists in *Jane* have been revealing the stories of women who, in many cases, were married working-class women desperate to prevent bringing another child into their families. Access to abortion as a birth control strategy, however, continues to be contentious and debated on both moral and political grounds, and measures for terminating pregnancy cannot be taken for granted in the future. Even in societies where personal freedom is assured, women may not be empowered to exercise freedoms such as reproductive choice within their relationships. Whether before or after conception, when women do not have the opportunity to choose motherhood as an occupation, they may be less able to manage when personally faced with a chronic illness.

In the 1980s, the women's movement yielded a number of *feminine standpoint* theories. Carol Gilligan's book *In a different voice: Psychological theory and women's development* (1982) made a major contribution, along with other seminal works of the feminist movement that contributed to increased awareness of the unique health needs of women (Aptheker, 1989; Belenky, et al., 1986; Eisler 1987; Smith, 1987). Women's health issues extend beyond reproductive health. Krieger and Fee (1994) contend that the dearth of information addressing women's health impedes our ability to address inequality in meeting the health needs of women and places women in a position of socioeconomic disadvantage. At long last, there are contemporary initiatives in research and education (e.g., the Women's Health Initiative) that focus on women's health and are appropriately multidimensional and sensitive to the ways that women find meaning in their lives (Dan, 1994). As another example, the United States Department of Health and Human Services (2000) tacitly integrates the interests of women in its goals and objectives. This important document includes a template for gathering comprehensive population information that more clearly establishes the context in which health and chronic illness occur. Accumulation of these data, including data about women, is intended to render a more accurate picture of the risk and prevalence of disease. The projections can be used in health policy and planning to more efficiently and effectively develop relevant health related services conceived and designed to meet the needs of women.

ᘓ Recurring Themes in Chronic Illness

Cultural Perspectives of Chronic Conditions

Everyone is rooted in a culture of origin, even though the premises and practices associated with that culture might be challenged as one experiences a broader multicultural world. Regardless of gender, it is important to ascertain the *meaning* of illness (and particularly chronic illness) within the cultural context of the individual. Although western medicine looks to science for explanation of disease, many other cultural perspectives linger. For example, Arviso-Alvord, herself a Navajo and a surgeon (Arviso-Alvord & Cohen van Pelt, 1999), describes being challenged by the work of translating illness into the Navajo belief structure necessary to establish trust among her people. In another cultural context, fiction written by African-American authors is frequently replete with mysticism and spiritual explanations for an array of maladies (Bambera, 1980; Marshall, 1983; Naylor, 1988). Customs and taboos reflected in Chinese culture might prohibit direct discussion of illness, necessitating a more tangential approach (Becker et al., 1998; Ma, 2000). Some years ago, one of us (Karin Opacich) suggested to a young Chinese woman who suffered an idiopathic cerebrovascular accident (CVA) that walking through her familiar neighborhood would be a good next step in her recovery. The young woman indeed complied by walking through the neighborhood— before dawn, to hide the shame of her condition. Among religious Hispanic families, the scientific approach to the treatment of chronic illness might be superficially accepted, but much energy is devoted to appealing for divine intervention. Along with the physician, nurse, and therapist, a family from Mexico might be consulting a "curandera" or other folk healer or spiritualist (Colucciello & Woelfel 1998; Trotter, 2001). Although it is never advisable to stereotype, it is critically important to explore the cultural infrastructure in which a woman's experience of chronic illness unfolds.

Cultural Perspectives of Caregiving and Care Receiving

Just as culture influences interpretations of illness, it also shapes the way in which care is administered and received in a society. Those who minister to women with chronic illness must be culturally competent and sensitive to issues that arise in a specific cultural context (Wells & Black, 2000). Almost universally, women assume caregiving roles and responsibilities. In a study exploring the motivation of women who were primary caregivers for a family member, 14 distinct factors were identified (Guberman, Maheu, & Maille, 1992). Most of these factors were related to the attitudes and values of the caregiver. Although the caregiving role seems a natural outgrowth of feminine expression, women tend to be less comfortable soliciting and receiving care, even when they are affected by chronic illness. Not surprisingly, when women experience chronic illness, they are reluctant to abdicate caregiving roles. Particularly in cultures that emphasize or limit women to caregiving roles, loss of these roles may result in loss of self-worth or social status (Schaefer, 1995; Thomas, 1997). Even healthy women are subject to role strain (Spurlock, 1995), but women fulfilling the demands of their usual roles while coping with their own compromised health may be even more vulnerable.

Lifetime Mothering

According to Thomas (1997), "A mother is expected to be selfless, ever-nurturing, and indefatigable, and she feels tremendous guilt if unable to achieve this ideal" (p. 546). Implications for women whose illnesses interfere with their roles and routines are even greater. The demands and activities associated with mothering change as children grow, develop independence, and leave their families of origin, but mothering continues even though it may be expressed differently (Francis-Connolly, 2000). Both Thomas and Francis-Connolly established that women take on the burdens and concerns of others, including those of their grown children and grandchildren. At different stages, motherhood is expressed in different forms, and according to Francis-Connolly, some women perceive that relating to grown children is the most gratifying experience of motherhood. In some cultures, women commonly assume responsibility for raising grandchildren, extending the mothering period well beyond their own childbearing years. The following vignette illustrates this point.

> ⌘ *Vignette:* **Irene's Story—Lifetime Mothering with Chronic Pain Syndrome**

Irene, now almost 70 years old, married her lifetime partner at 18 years of age. She had been married a little over a year when she slipped on the stairs and injured her cervical spine. Her treatment and protracted rehabilitation entailed hospitalization, traction, pain medications, and thermal modalities. This was the first incident in what was to become a lifetime of joint pain, traumatic injuries, and surgeries. Luckily, Irene's young husband provided loving support during this and subsequent episodes throughout their marriage.

Because they really wanted children, Irene willingly accepted the prospect of difficult pregnancies. After one miscarriage, Irene carried her first child to term when she was 21, spending much of her pregnancy on bed rest. Five years later, she delivered her second child after a similar course. Irene refers to her children as her greatest joy in life. After the birth of her children, Irene became a full-time homemaker, and she very much enjoyed, cooking, baking, antiquing, and home decorating. During her marriage, the family moved several times to accommodate Irene's husband's job, so those skills were put to good use. Irene states that whenever they moved, she placed a high priority on establishing a home to ease the transition for her children.

For the most part, Irene was able to fulfill her roles with assistance from her husband, her own mother, and an occasional housekeeper. Her symptoms seemed to increase in her 30s when her children were in grade school. She reports a period of tremendous headaches, fatigue, and fever that resulted in a 6-week hospitalization. Although she experienced bouts of illness, she recalls having been an active participant in the lives of her children, who would grow up to be highly successful professionals. Sporting activities were the only ones in which she remembers she could not participate. Irene does not recall her children showing that they were upset by her illness, and feels that they took things in stride. She recalls only one incident when her young son included in a school essay, "My mom has a lot of headaches, but she's better now."

Today Irene is preparing for shoulder reconstruction, a prospect that she perceives as exhausting. To date she has had five total knee replacements, along with many other medical interventions for pain and discomfort. Nevertheless, Irene still very much enjoys her adult children and her three grandchildren, whom she sees often. She flies out of state to visit intermittently and requires some assistance for mobility in airports and planes. Her endurance and tolerance for driving has recently diminished, and she reluctantly depends on others more frequently for transportation. When asked what positive things come from being a mother with a chronic illness, Irene unhesitatingly states, "If you have a chronic illness, you can be so much more compassionate to family and friends." Since her husband's death, Irene has spent more time with friends and tries to help others who are having a hard time.

In retrospect, Irene says that she probably didn't rest enough while mothering her young children, and she tries to respect her need for rest periods now. She encourages the use of psychological support services, stating that she should have used these more frequently. Irene and her family always belonged to a church, and she valued visits and conversations with her pastor. When asked what advice she would give those who provide health care to women with chronic illnesses, she noted that professionals need to be more patient and to demonstrate caring, particularly trying to understand the experience of women raising children. She specifically noted that a gentle touch or a reassuring pat on the shoulder would be appreciated.

Commentary: Irene's Story

To begin, the Matrix of Occupational Status (Fig. 11–2) quickly illustrates the occupational nature of Irene's life at the time of her interview.

The matrix illustrates that most occupational features of Irene's life are currently stable and perceived as sufficiently intact to fulfill her immediate life plans. In some areas, her narrative indicates that satisfactory adaptations have been made contributing to the overall quality of her life. The matrix can also help practitioners to decide where further assessment might be warranted. For instance, knowing that Irene is about to undergo a major joint replacement surgery, one would anticipate disruption in some areas of occupation and increased reliance on family, friends, and health-care providers.

The social and economic resources available to Irene have clearly enhanced her quality of life and ability to live independently. Because the cumulative effects of her illness seem to become more debilitating as she ages, one might expect to see more disruption of

Occupational Domain	Associated Occupational Roles	Occupational Status				
		Discontinuation	Disruption	No Change	Adaptation	Augmentation
Work	parent/caregiver				X	
	homemaker (IADL)				X	
	employee (remunerated)			X		
	entrepreneur			X		
	vocational trainee			X		
	student			X		
Play Leisure	spectator			X		
	participant/observer		X			
	hobbyist				X	
	athlete		X			
Self-Care	spiritual/devotional life			X		
	personal care (ADL)				X	
	health-related care				X	
	personal advocacy			X		
	intimacy/sexual expression	X				
Occupational Context	home environment				X	
	family support				X	
	network of friends					X
	financial support			X		
	neighborhood/community setting			X		
	health-care facility			X		
	social agencies			X		
	church/temple/mosque			X		
	place of employment			X		
	other					

Figure 11–2 *Matrix of Occupational Status—2*

occupations over time, requiring new forms of adaptation to preserve coherence. Mothering has been the single most important occupational role in Irene's history, and health-care practitioners may need to help her express that role in different ways as her dependency needs increase. For example, even though she is still physically able, Irene prefers not to drive and increasingly depends on her daughter to provide her transportation, resulting in some friction because of busy schedules. Identifying alternative forms of transportation might enhance Irene's independence and reduce the burden on other family members. Given the illness trajectory and prognosis, Irene is likely to need some form of assisted living in the near future, and health-care providers can provide anticipatory guidance that will facilitate planning and transitioning.

⚘ Relational Shifts

Support structures for women with chronic illnesses coincide with social and economic status. Women with means plot a different social trajectory than do women who are unmarried, unemployed, and/or uninsured. As women with chronic or progressive illnesses deplete their respective resources, they are often forced to rely on family members for emotional, economic, and mechanical support. As illness progresses and abilities decline, women frequently find themselves once again dependent on their aging parents. When children are involved, family constellations may be reconfigured and decisional authority transferred to grandparents or other family designees. These dramatic shifts in family structure can lead to conflict, manifested in depression or expressed as behavioral problems (Quinn-Beers, 2001; Kahle & Jones, 1998; Lange, 1996). Involvement with children can be a source of joy and self-esteem for a mother with a chronic illness. However, during the course of chronic illness, women may find themselves depending on their children to assume adult responsibilities, a phenomenon known as *parentification* (Valleau, Bergner, & Horton, 1995). Some children respond to these expectations with precocious maturity, whereas others become resentful and oppositional. In either case, placing extra demands on children engenders guilt among mothers who are more accustomed to meeting dependency needs than indulging them.

As family structures change, shifts in decisional authority are likely. Some women succeed in exercising parental authority in spite of chronic illness (Elmberger, 2000). When a disease process affects cognitive function, the best interests of children must take priority. Women facing deteriorating health may elect to appoint a guardian as a way of participating in the future of their children. In some jurisdictions, there is no mechanism for ensuring this transition without relinquishing legal custody. Particularly in terminal phases of illnesses (e.g., AIDS), women may become increasingly concerned about the placement of their children after their deaths (Dumaret et al., 1996; Andrews, Williams & Neil, 1993). Planning for the welfare of children may be a critical and highly stressful occupation for women in the end stages of chronic illnesses.

Self-Reliance, Interdependency, and Support

Women first diagnosed with a chronic illness typically experience a period of disbelief characterized by feelings of loss and fear (Schaefer, 1995; Rosenfeld & Gilkeson, 2000). Until symptoms occur, a woman may have little awareness of the illness and lack incentive to gather information pertaining to it. When the illness begins to demand attention, Schaefer (1995) contends that women enter a period of "discovery." This may entail consulting health professionals and learning to recognize and manage symptoms. Initially, women experiencing illness may resist medication or other medical regimes.

The value of shared experience is evident in the literature describing an array of chronic illnesses (Wyatt & Friedman, 1996; Williams, et al., 1997). Women tend to place high value on caring, and groups constituted around caring as a primary purpose seem to be useful for women coping with chronic illness. Feminist ethics postulates that women express caring and valuing through relationships (Guberman, Maheu, & Maille, 1992; Sherwin, 1992). Connectedness, as that is expressed in meaningful relationships, appears to be an important part of responding to protracted illness. Many women report inadequate support from spouses or life partners in addressing their health issues, reinforcing the importance of building supportive relationships and friendships (Andrews, Williams, & Neil, 1993; Schaefer, 1995; Thomas, 1997; Kenney, 2000). Role conflict and role overload are common among modern women. Many healthy women find themselves juggling priorities and being overwhelmed, and women with chronic illnesses may feel unable to manage the additional burdens that compromised health or healthcare regimens add to their lives.

When caring for others competes with caring for self, women with compromised health tend to defer to the needs of others, sometimes at the expense of their own well-being. When illness is part of the scenario, Farber (2000) contends that successful adaptation is contingent on both individual and family resilience. Interviews with mothers with disabilities revealed the desire to be as much like other mothers as possible. Mothers with health challenges commonly needed to enlist support from family members and health-care providers or "auxiliary caregivers" to achieve a state of family equilibrium. Farber suggests that the role of health-care professionals is to assist women to make unique adaptations to their circumstances rather than aspire to an idealized notion of perfect mothering.

Many women lack the resources necessary to care for themselves effectively. "Resources" encompass information, finances, access to relevant health services, housing, adequate nutrition, and transportation. It has been noted that women forego resources allocated for their own health care to increase the resources available to their families (Lea, 1994). Angus (1994) remarks that "…in comparison to men, women's basic needs are poorly met in all societies" (p. 26). The various resources necessary for achieving and maintaining health are cited repeatedly in the literature as directly related to positive outcomes, but women, particularly poor women, have had fewer opportunities to garner these resources (Angus, 1994).

As illness progresses, some women enjoy

deeper friendships, seek spiritual revelation, and discover unknown personal strengths. Bayer (1993) speaks directly to the importance that women with chronic and terminal illnesses place on expressing and adhering to their values. He contends that women express their values through personally meaningful choices and actions, notions that are very familiar to occupational therapy practitioners. Even when women are coping with declining abilities, the presence of children seems to afford women opportunities to connect and contribute. Andrews, Williams, and Neil (1993) noted that children can minimize isolation, engender a sense of purpose, provide a source of self-esteem, and deter engagement in high risk behaviors.

⚓ The Biopsychosocial Nature of Chronic Illness

Although chronic illness affects older women more than younger women, it can occur at any point in the life span. Where it occurs in the lifespan will have a profound effect on the woman's life. Chronic illness may begin in childhood and persist throughout adult life. Disorders such as sickle cell disease, diabetes, juvenile rheumatoid arthritis, or systemic lupus erythematosus can all begin in childhood. Chronic illness contributes to the shaping of the child's personality. The family's response to the chronic illness; the interactions among the family, the child, and the health-care system; and the society's attitudes toward the disorder all converge to integrate the chronic condition within the identity of the child. Defining and managing the chronic condition is the work of the child and family, and ideally, positive strategies are practiced and learned by the child. The socially acceptable approach to chronic illness is to triumph over it, persevere despite it, and conceal its presence. The struggle between wanting to conceal it and wanting external validation creates a paradox for women (Schaefer, 1995). Alterations in appearance, through either changes in the body or the need for equipment or assistive devices, tend to be a source of embarrassment instead of an enhancement to the corporeal self. How

the chronic illness is managed, both physically and psychologically, will affect how the child manages it in adulthood. In turn, the child who becomes the woman with a chronic illness has the illness as an integral part of her identity.

Certain disorders can affect the woman's decision to become a mother. Some conditions affect a woman's fertility or her likelihood of carrying a fetus to term. The treatment regimen of some conditions (e.g., anticonvulsant therapy for seizure disorder, chemotherapy for cancer) may be teratogenic. Therefore a woman may choose to risk health problems by foregoing treatment that may be damaging to the pregnancy or fetus. The decision to become a mother, whether through pregnancy or adoption, rests on the woman's assessment of her ability to raise a child. Chronic illness often poses limitations in a woman's energy level. The woman may also be concerned that her illness may shorten her life expectancy. Weighing all the risks and benefits of the particulars of her situation, the woman decides whether or not she will become a mother.

Society may view some women, those with chronic illness or disability, as unfit to be mothers. Thomson (1997) maintains that society infantilizes women with disabilities and sees these women as "objects of other people's virtue" (p. 26). The same is true for women with chronic illness, especially when that illness is apparent to others, by the use of equipment such as a wheelchair, oxygen tank, or insulin pump. However, women managing their illness have three types of work: illness related work, biographical work, and everyday-life work (Corbin & Strauss, 1988, p. 90). Having children may be part of the biographical work of the woman with a chronic illness. Participating in this normal cycle of human existence may be one of the woman's efforts in not surrendering to her illness. Rearing a child will also be part of her biographical work and everyday-life work. Bowden (1997) says, "the mothering connection provides a privileged example of the possibilities of human connectedness.. . . Seen as the functionally necessary and natural realm of affection and love, enduring and unconditional openness, and responsiveness to the particular material, emotional and social needs of another person, mothering frequently carries the full weight of ideological constructions of caring" (p. 21). Mothering permits, even demands, that attention be focused on the child. The illness no longer becomes the focus of her existence; her child is that. Managing the chronic illness involves prioritizing needs and available resources, balancing workload, negotiating the division of labor, facing disruptions in the management plan, and maintaining hope and commitment (Corbin & Strauss, 1988). The most difficult aspect of motherhood may be fighting societal prejudice.

A later midrange theory of chronic illness in women suggests that women move from an initial phase of "extraordinariness" to "ordinariness" (Kralik, 2002). The initial shock and accommodations are "extraordinary" in the lives of women who are diagnosed with chronic illness, but they often incorporate the changes in their everyday lives and strive for returning to an ordinariness of life and continuing to meet the needs of others. Feminist principles support this transition, although the transition is usually not linear but cyclical. Paterson (2001) identifies this transition as the "shifting perspectives model."

Although a chronic illness may be acquired and cannot be inherited, such as renal failure related to antibiotic treatment of an infection, there may be a societal perception that a woman with a chronic condition should not reproduce. However, there are some disorders that are known to be hereditary, such as polycystic kidneys, in which the kidneys contain many cysts that interfere with normal renal function. With the availability of abortion, there may be the expectation that any woman who is aware of the possibility of bearing a child with a chronic, life-threatening condition would choose to avoid pregnancy or abort if she becomes pregnant. Mairs (1996) sees this attitude as delivering a message to people who are sick and/or disabled. *We're doing everything we can to exterminate your kind*, the social message would read, *and we'd get rid of you too if only we knew how* (p. 112). Mairs was 29 and the mother of two children when she learned she had multiple sclerosis (MS). She describes be-

ing "wracked by guilt" (p. 34) that she was not "normal" for her children. Yet her children, as adults, told her that the transition of being cared for and then caring for her was gradual and seemed natural. As Mairs required more assistance and her husband died, her physician asked her if her children would provide this assistance; Mairs rejected the notion. She did not want to be the sick person in her children's lives. Yet she later considered that they may have wished to provide this assistance, even though she initially did not give them the opportunity. The assumption is that any adult who cannot be independent is a burden to society. This assumption translates into a "subtle pressure" (p. 121) to reject life-sustaining treatment, or accept assistance in dying. American culture, in its individualism, sees a dependent life as intolerable, especially when one's children are expected to provide assistance to the dependent parent. Yet the purported "suffering" of the person with the chronic illness or disability may not be caused by the disorder but by society. Mairs does not dismiss the suffering caused by the disorder:

> Everybody, well or ill, disabled or not, imagines a boundary of suffering and loss beyond which, she or he is certain, life will no longer be worth living. When I reach the wall, I think I'll know. Meanwhile, I go on being, now more than ever, the woman I once thought I could never bear to be (pp. 121–2).

She does not condemn the women with MS who seek assistance in dying. Rather, she suggests that one may underestimate the conditions one is willing to endure. Her message is instructive in light of the popularity of advance directives.

Self-Determination

The Patient Self-Determination Act of 1991 (PSDA) had its beginnings in the case of Nancy Cruzan. Nancy was a young woman, in her 20s, who was found pulseless and unresponsive in a field after crashing her car on an icy road. She was diagnosed as being in a persistent vegetative state after a period of time, and her parents petitioned the court to permit the withdrawal of her feeding tube. The State of Missouri refused their request because the parents did not meet the court's standard of evidence (clear and convincing evidence) that Nancy would refuse tube feedings. Her case was argued before the United States Supreme Court, who agreed that Missouri could hold the petitioners to the state's high standard of evidence. Not until more people who knew Nancy came forward to testify that Nancy would not want to live in her present condition, did the court permit her feeding tube to be withdrawn, which allowed her to die of dehydration. To avoid having similar cases decided by the courts, Congress drafted and passed the PSDA. All health-care facilities, agencies, clinics, and insurers were required to ask if the patient/client had an advance directive or if they wanted assistance in completing one. The law did not require a person to have an advance directive, but it required that the person be asked about having or creating one.

Advance directives are documents that indicate a person's health-care preferences regarding life-sustaining treatment should that person become incapacitated and unable to communicate preferences. Governed by state laws, advance directives vary from state to state. In general, there are two kinds of advance directives: living wills and durable powers of attorney for health care. The following vignette illustrates this point.

⌘ Vignette: *Linda's Story—A Living Will*

Living wills are activated if a person who has a terminal illness becomes incapacitated and there is a decision to be made regarding further life-sustaining treatment. For example, Linda is a 52-year-old woman with a 10-year history of breast cancer. She was aggressively treated 10 years ago when she was first diagnosed and, until 3 years ago, believed the cancer was in remission. While her cancer was actually in remission, she drafted a living will stating that she would not want to be kept alive by use of machines if there was no hope of her surviving without the machines. She has three children, and believes that she is obligated to accept all treatment to stay alive for as long as she can, unless it is clear that she is dying and machines will only prolong the dying process. ⌘

Commentary: Linda's Story

In order for her living will to be activated, Linda must be incapacitated and must be considered to be dying. She can stipulate those treatments that she does not want except for food and fluid. Living wills do not permit foregoing nutrition and hydration. In Nancy Cruzan's case, a living will would not have been useful. She did not have a terminal illness and could not request discontinuation of tube feedings through a living will.

Suppose that Linda had drafted a durable power of attorney for health care. This document authorizes a surrogate decision maker, someone who Linda believes will make decisions as she would, whenever Linda is incapacitated and a decision needs to be made. If Linda is incapacitated because she is under anesthesia during a procedure, and a decision regarding life-sustaining treatment must be made, Linda's surrogate decision maker can make that decision. If Linda lapses into a coma and needs life-sustaining treatment to stay alive, the surrogate decision maker would authorize or refuse the treatment, based on what he or she believes Linda would want. Should Linda recover from the coma and is no longer incapacitated, decision-making authority reverts back to Linda.

Advance directives are predicated on people's ability to look into the future and project how they will feel about a future situation. As Mairs (1996) observed, the point at which she thought she could not bear to live kept moving. Keeping a written document up to date as one's perspective changes is very important. Advance directives are most useful as a communication tool in articulating one's wishes about life-sustaining treatment to one's family and health-care providers.

Assistance in dying is different from advance directives. If Linda had written in her living will that she wanted to be given a lethal overdose of medication if she lapsed into a coma from which she was not expected to recover, her wishes could not be honored. Even in Oregon, the only state that legally permits assistance in dying, one must be capable of ingesting a lethal overdose orally, without assistance from another person. An injection cannot be given, nor can anyone place the pills in the person's mouth or crush them and give them by tube. If Linda lived in Oregon, repeatedly asked her physician to give her a prescription for a lethal overdose, and was considered competent by her physician, she would be able to fill the prescription, take the pills by mouth, and end her life. No other state permits physician-assisted suicide.

Although cancer is often viewed as a terminal illness, people can be cured, or can live with cancer in remission. Breast cancer, initially treated and in remission, can be considered a chronic illness, especially if the woman continues oral chemotherapy for several years. Life decisions are made considering the chronic illness. Table 11–1 illustrates a matrix displaying chronic illness, potentially life-threatening complications of those illnesses, and life-threatening illnesses or conditions.

The first column in Table 11–1 represents a number of common chronic illnesses. These conditions can occur in childhood and persist throughout a woman's life, or can present in adulthood. Although the conditions are chronic, there may be episodic crises that are typical, such as sickle cell crisis with sickle cell disease, an asthma attack, or breakthrough seizures in a long-standing seizure disorder. Life-threatening complications are found in the second column of Table 11–1. Life-threatening complications can be caused by progression of the disorder or complications of treatment for the disorder. The third column lists conditions that are life threatening but not necessarily stemming from a chronic condition. The onset of these conditions is usually sudden versus the static or slow progression of a chronic illness. Having time to become knowledgeable about the condition, live with it, and consider the future with it provides a better foundation for the woman to make decisions.

A mother with a chronic illness can incorporate the illness into her everyday life, or the illness can become more prominent. How the mother views her chronic illness is based on her premorbid personality, her family's response to the illness, and her psychological and social resources. The illness can be used for secondary gain, as a way to garner sympathy or to manipulate others. This is illustrated in the following story.

⌘ *Vignette* : Mrs. Allen's Story—Seeking Sympathy

Mrs. Allen was in her 30s and her children were school age when she was diagnosed with "an enlarged heart and elevated blood pressure." She was given a number of medications (digoxin, a diuretic, and an antihypertensive) and continued to take the medication over the years. Her physician did not limit her activities, but her excess weight caused limits in her endurance and stamina. She attended community activities (church, bridge, lunches with friends) but insisted, because of her "heart condition," that her children and spouse perform all the household chores (cleaning, cooking, laundry, grocery shopping, errands). Her illness became a source of resentment on the part of her family, who thought she was capable of more physical exertion than she displayed. Mrs. Allen would declare that she was having a "spell" and had to "take to her bed" whenever her children would talk of moving out, getting married, or moving away. As a result, the children, especially her daughters, proceeded with their plans on their mother's timetable for fear their actions would precipitate a worsening of their mother's condition, or even her demise.

⌘

Commentary: Mrs. Allen's story

As this story is written, it suggests that Mrs. Allen used her chronic condition as a way of manipulating her family. Although she may have had legitimate limitations requiring assistance with her activities of daily living, the timing of her *spells* raised suspicion that her *relapses* were within her control. In her family's view, Mrs. Allen assumed a *sick* role because there were benefits to her. In a different story, which follows, a woman rejects the sick role.

Table 11–1 Potential manifestations of chronic illnesses

Chronic illness	Life-threatening complications	Life-threatening illnesses
Alzheimer's disease	DP: Inability to swallow	Accidents
Amyotropic lateral sclerosis	DP: Inability to swallow or breathe	Asphyxia, profound
Arthritis	Complications of anti-inflammatory treatment	Burns, extensive
Asthma	Acute "attack"—inability to breathe	Head injury, internal injuries, massive
Cancer	Complications of treatment	Cancer unresponsive to treatment
Cardiac disease	Complications of treatment, DP	Cardiac arrhythmia, acute, untreated
Cerebrovascular accident (CVA)	Complications of treatment	CVA, massive
Chronic fatigue		
Chronic obstructive pulmonary disease	DP	Hydrocephalus, acute, untreated
Crohn's disease	Infection, failure to thrive	Liver failure, transplant rejection
End-stage renal disease	Infection, failure to thrive	Poisoning, acute
Fibromyalgia		
Gastroesophageal reflux disease	Complications of treatment	
Insulin-dependent diabetes mellitus	DP: renal, cardiac, PVS effects	
Irritable bowel disease	Complications of treatment	
Multiple sclerosis	DP: Inability to swallow	
Osteoporosis	DP: Fractures near spinal cord	
Parkinson's disease	DP: Inability to swallow	
Post-polio syndrome	DP: Inability to breathe or swallow	
Rheumatoid arthritis	Complications of treatment	
Seizure disorder (epilepsy)	Status epilepticus, medication side effects	
Sickle cell disease	Ischemia to vital organs, stroke	
Stroke	Same as CVA	
Traumatic brain injury	Inability to protect airway	
Tuberculosis	Inability to protect airway	

DP = disease progression; PVS = peripheral vascular system

Vignette: *Mrs. Bates' Story— Managing Illness as Part of Life*

Mrs. Bates, on the other hand, was diagnosed with insulin-dependent diabetes in her late teens. At age 28, she and her husband carefully weighed the potential risks of a pregnancy, as well as the stress of parenting, and decided to become parents. Mrs. Bates managed her illness as a routine part of the family life—her diet,

exercise, blood glucose testing, and insulin injections were as routine and unobtrusive as brushing her teeth and feeding the dog. Having children posed a challenge in managing her diabetes, but she worked to keep the disease "in its place." She did not want her life to revolve around her diabetes, although all of the decisions she made considered the effect on her health. Despite careful management of her condition, she developed diabetic retinopathy and nephropathy. Her vision was impaired to the point where she could no longer drive, and her nephropathy eventually progressed to renal failure, requiring dialysis. She planned how she would get transportation to and from the dialysis center and began learning Braille. Her family insisted on driving her to appointments and urged her to participate in research to improve her vision. They worried at times that Mrs. Bates' acceptance seemed like resignation to the inevitable, and they wished she would "fight" against her deterioration. She felt greatly supported by her family but also in control of her life and her decisions.   ⌘

Commentary: Mrs. Bates' Story

Mrs. Bates rejected the *sick* role, even as her health deteriorated. She was determined not to *burden* her family with the care needs. Although the case descriptions are thin and somewhat stereotypical, they are meant to illustrate differences in how mothers and their families adapt to chronic illness. The illness can become the focal point from which all other issues emanate and are measured, or it can be one of many considerations in the family's life plans.

Corbin and Strauss (1988) identified the "Domino effect" as a "downward spiral of loss of control" (p. 117) when resources are inadequate, the workload becomes overwhelming, the routine becomes disrupted, such as through exacerbation or progression of the disorder, and the motivation to continue the struggle is lost. To maintain equilibrium, they advise "planning for resource consumption, keeping negotiations open for division of labor, managing the total workload, and finding emotional support" (p. 124). Thomas (1997) would add that psychotherapy may help the woman discover what she really wants and needs.

✒ HIV/AIDS as a Metaphor for Chronic Illness

To illustrate the many dimensions of chronic illness and its concomitant effects on occupation, HIV/AIDS can serve as a metaphor for chronic illness because it insinuates itself into virtually every aspect of life. Along the illness trajectory, HIV/AIDS requires tremendous resources to maintain health, alleviate symptoms, and address the end-stage disease (Hall, 1994; Cowles & Rodgers, 1997). The majority of women who have contracted HIV emanate from marginalized populations reflecting a plethora of social justice issues (Schneider, 1992; Sowell, Moneyham, Aranda-Naranjo, 1999). Based on surveillance data accumulated by the CDC through 1999, African-American and Hispanic women represent 78 percent of the women identified as having HIV in the United States, even though they represent less than a fourth of the total population (CDC, 2002a). Thirty-eight percent of the women with HIV were infected through sex with an injecting drug user, and another 25 percent were directly infected through drug use. Examining the sociopolitical context in which HIV/AIDS is experienced by women renders a fairly comprehensive picture of what it is like to overcome social disadvantages, parlay limited resources, access relevant health-care services, and muster the psychic and material resources that enable quality living. Because of scientific advances, people with HIV/AIDS are able to live increasingly longer and healthier lives as long as the appropriate resources are available (CDC, 2002b).

From an occupational performance perspective, women with HIV/AIDS are particularly interesting and instructive. Given the demographics of HIV-positive women in the United States, many of those infected have developed few occupational competencies, and their histories often reveal disempowerment, poor role development, unhealthy behaviors, and chaotic existence (Driscoll et al., 1994; Stevens, 1996). The diagnosis of HIV is, for some, a pivotal event that leads to healthier, more cohesive lives. The ensuing story of Cleo not only reveals the themes of chronic illness addressed in this chapter but also attests to the process of *reconstructing occupation* after HIV infection (Opacich, 2002). Using the *Occupational Performance History Interview* (OPHI-II: Kielhofner et al., 1998, 2001) and another semi-structured interview focusing on health and health-related experiences, the narrative revealed the before- and after-illness events and occupations that shaped a unique life.

⌘ Vignette: *Cleo's Story—Reconstructing Occupations*

Cleo, a 48-year-old African-American woman, looks 10 years older than her age. She speaks frankly and quietly about her life without apology, punctuating her story with gratitude for her rather *miraculous remission*. Despite her diagnosis of full blown AIDS, she is responding to a multiple drug protocol. Cleo was released from the hospital 7 months before the interview, having been found lying comatose on the floor. She emerged from a state of virtual oblivion after 3 months in the hospital, a period of time she refers to as one when she "died." Since that experience, Cleo has virtually been delivered from the destructive life that she was leading and is slowly recovering her health. When asked about life before HIV, she began with the story of her family.

When Cleo was 15 years old, her older sister's boyfriend met her at school one day on the pretense of treating her to lunch. He raped her. Confused and terrified, she told no one until her pregnancy became evident, and she refused to reveal the father of her baby. Having no other options, she withdrew from school, resided with her grandmother, and took a job with a local merchant. Shortly after her child was born, Cleo ventured to use her talent for singing to procure employment as a lounge singer, a career that supported her into her 20s. In that environment, she was introduced to alcohol and began to drink heavily. In the ensuing years, she had relationships with other men, two of which resulted in children. At some point, her sister introduced her to heroin, and she began using it intravenously, occasionally *turning a trick* (selling sex for money) to support her drug habit.

Although Cleo learned in 1996 that she was HIV positive, she made no attempt to learn about her illness or to change her lifestyle, believing herself to be doomed. She describes herself as "mad at the world" during that period. When, finally, her body could no longer withstand the abuse, she collapsed. Medically, her

HIV had progressed to AIDS, and she had contracted pneumonia and tuberculosis. She was not expected to survive, but she clung tenaciously to life, and she seemed to awaken to an entirely different life at that. Cleo attributes this to the intercession of God, and she reports that the urge to use drugs vanished.

Today Cleo has established a different routine. She resides with her youngest daughter, whom she characterizes as her *love child* and who is also HIV positive, and assists with the care of her three grandchildren, one of whom is HIV positive. Cleo rises early and dutifully starts each day with prayer and meditation. She sings every day, but now she "sings for God." When she is feeling well enough, she works in her eldest daughter's store. Knowing that her medication regimen is critical to her survival, she diligently swallows pills at intervals throughout the day. Her daily routine includes "eating right" and reading the Bible. She attends church regularly and attends support meetings. Cleo says that her "whole world turned around," and she relays contentedly that "I got people who love me." ⌘

Commentary: Cleo's Story

Even though she has a life-threatening, chronic illness that can be plotted far along the illness trajectory, Cleo has been restored to reasonable health and perceives herself to be enjoying a life that, while not perfect, is of acceptable quality. The Matrix of Occupational Status (Fig. 11–3) illustrates the general nature of Cleo's occupational life at this point in time.

In light of her history, Cleo's profile conveys a good deal of adaptation and enhancement of occupation despite her disease status (AIDS). Imbedded in Cleo's story are allusions to aforementioned themes. Social stigma and ignorance about HIV/AIDS deterred her from seeking treatment at the point of diagnosis. Culturally, her life story is characterized by social inequities: poverty, disrupted education, violence, lack of access to care, and limited options in relation to her health and life choices even though she expresses no surprise or bitterness about those constraints. Although she had developed some occupa-

Occupational Domain	Associated Occupational Roles	Occupational Status				
		Discontinuation	Disruption	No Change	Adaptation	Augmentation
Work	parent/caregiver					X
	homemaker (IADL)				X	
	employee (remunerated)				X	
	entrepreneur			X		
	vocational trainee			X		
	student			X		
Play/ Leisure	spectator			X		
	participant/observer				X	
	hobbyist				X	
	athlete			X		
Self-Care	spiritual/devotional life					X
	personal care (ADL)				X	
	health-related care					X
	personal advocacy					X
	intimacy/sexual expression	X				
Occupational Context	home environment				X	
	family support					X
	network of friends					X
	financial support				X	
	neighborhood/community setting			X		
	health-care facility					X
	social agencies					X
	church/temple/mosque					X
	place of employment					X
	other					

Figure 11–3 *Matrix of Occupational Status—3*

tional roles and competencies, these were not exercised while chemical dependency dictated her behavior. One of the themes emerging from the research and exemplified by Cleo's story is *the desire to be perceived as a good mother*. During her recovery, Cleo has begun to repair fractured relationships, especially with her children, and she expresses joy in caring for her grandchildren. She seems to have resumed her mothering role, especially in supporting her youngest daughter, who is newly diagnosed with HIV. She has assumed a major caretaking role for her grandchildren and even shares a room with them. Reflecting her newfound spirituality, Cleo believes that God saved her life to help this adult daughter, who is struggling with her own recovery.

It is quite evident that Cleo's mothering role is a major element of her recovery, a role that greatly enhances her self-reported quality of life. As Cleo's illness progresses, she will be challenged to make additional adaptations and to explore ways to preserve those occupations and roles from which she derives the greatest meaning. Because she is now well connected with family, friends, and a team of health-care providers, it is likely that she can avail herself of services and support to make that happen.

Recommendations for Use and Generation of Research

Although there is a relatively small body of literature specific to women with chronic illness, it is important for health-care providers to use accumulated wisdom in making clinical decisions. Moreover, health and social care professionals can contribute to the accumulation of knowledge and evidence by designing, collaborating, and/or implementing studies that enlighten health-care providers and policy makers about the unique experiences, responses, and needs of women with chronic illnesses. Neither quantitative nor qualitative studies alone will reveal the whole rich story, and one approach can inform the other. Practitioners who consume and apply research to benefit women should discretely select credible evidence that protects the interests of women. For those who venture to design original research, particular attention ought to be paid to select methodologies that are sensitive to the nature and needs of women (Guerrero, 1999).

ᨀ **Conclusion**

Chronic illnesses are, by nature, multidimensional. In addition to impacting the physiological health of a woman, chronic illness is superimposed on personal and social circumstances that render the experience of the illness unique to each individual. Mothering occupations are inevitably shaped by the illness and the concomitant adaptations and disruptions that may ensue for a woman and her family. Although numerous internal and external factors contribute to both the physiological and social trajectories of chronic illness, resources, relationships, and relevant health related services are major determinants of occupational coherence and quality of life. Women with chronic illnesses are best served when their health-care providers grasp and address not only their medical needs but also the contextual and performance issues that support meaningful doing and especially mothering.

Discussion Questions ᨀ

- What factors, aside from disease symptoms, might you need to examine in order to provide relevant health-related services for women with chronic illnesses?

- Given the same chronic illness, how might the occupations of a woman with ample resources differ from the experience of a woman with few resources?

- What occupational challenges might you anticipate for a young woman with three

children under 10 who is suffering from cardiomyopathy?

- Looking at a particular chronic illness, how might culture influence mothering occupations differently?

- How might a given chronic illness shape mothering occupations across the life span, and what anticipatory guidance might you reasonably provide at points along the illness trajectory?

References

American Occupational Therapy Association, Inc. (2002). *Occupational therapy practice framework domain and process.* Bethesda, MD: American Occupational Therapy Association, Commission on Practice.

Andrews, S., Williams, A. B., & Neil, K. (1993). The mother-child relationship in the HIV-1 positive family. *Image: Journal of Nursing Scholarship, 25*(3), 193–198.

Angus, J. (1994). Women's paid/unpaid work and health: Exploring the social context of everyday life. *Canadian Journal of Nursing Research, 26*(4), 23–42.

Aptheker, B. (1989). *Tapestries of life: Women's work, women's consciousness, and the meaning of daily experience.* Amherst, MA: University of Massachusetts.

Arviso-Alvord, L., & Cohen van Pelt, E. (1999). *The scalpel and the silver bear.* New York: Bantam Books.

Bambara, T. C. (1980). *The salt eaters.* New York: Vintage Books.

Bateson, M. C. (1996). Enfolded activity and the concept of occupation. In R. Zemke & F. Clark (Eds.). *Occupational science: The evolving discipline* (pp. 5–12). Philadelphia: F. A. Davis.

Bayer, D. L. (1993). Women approaching death. *The American Journal of Hospice and Palliative Care,* May/June, 28–32.

Becker, G., Beyene, Y., Newsom., E. M., and Rodgers, D. V. (1998). Knowledge and care of chronic illness in three ethnic minority groups. *Family Medicine, 30*(3), 173–178.

Belenky, M. F., Clinchy, B. M., Goldberger, N. R., & Tarule, J. M. (1986). *Women's Ways of Knowing.* Basic Books.

Bowden, P. (1997). *Caring: Gender-sensitive ethics.* New York: Rutledge.

Centers for Disease Control, National Center for HIV, STD and TB Prevention, Divisions of HIV/AIDS Prevention. (2002, November). *HIV/AIDS among US women: Minority and young women at continuing risk.* Retrieved November 1, 2002, from *CDC: http://www.cdc.gov/hiv/pubs/facts/women.htm*

Centers for Disease Control, National Center for HIV, STD, and TB Prevention, Divisions of HIV/AIDS Prevention. (2002, November). HIV/AIDS Update: *A glance at the HIV epidemic.* Retrieved November 2, 2002 from *CDC: http://www.cdc.gov/nchstp/od/news/At-a-glance*

Chopin, K. (1976). *The awakening.* (Ed. 1). New York: Norton.

Christiansen, C. H. (1999). Defining lives: occupation as identity: An essay on competence, coherence, and the creation of meaning. *The American Journal of Occupational Therapy, 53*(6), 547–558.

Christiansen, C. H., Little, B. R., & Backman, C. (1998). Personal projects: A useful approach to the study of occupation. *The American Journal of Occupational Therapy, 52*(6), 439–446.

Colucciello, M. L., & Woelfel, V. (1998, Fall). Child care beliefs and practices of Hispanic mother. *Nursing Connections, 11*(3), 33–40.

Commission on Practice of the AOTA. (2002). Framework for Practice. Bethesda, MD: AOTA Publications.

Corbin, J. M., & Strauss, A. (1988). *Unending work and care: Managing chronic illness at home.* San Francisco: Jossey-Bass.

Cowles, K. V., & Rodgers, B. L. (1997). Struggling to keep on top: Meeting the everyday challenges of AIDS. *Qualitative Health Research, 7*(1), 98–120.

Dan, A. (1994). (Ed.) *Reframing women's health: multidisciplinary research and practice.* Thousand Oaks, CA: Sage Publications.

Driscoll, M., Cohen, M., Kelly, P., Taylor, D., Williamson, M., & Nicks, G. (1994). Women and HIV. In A. J. Dan (Ed.), *Reframing women's health: Multidisciplinary research and practice* (pp. 175-186). Thousand Oaks, CA: Sage Publications.

Dumaret, A. C., Boucher, N., Torossian, V., & Donati, P. (1995). *Early Childhood Development & Care, 1123,* 65–76.

Eisler, R. (1987). *The chalice & the blade: Our history, our future.* San Francisco: Harper.

Farber, R. S. (2000). Mothers with disabilities: In their own voice. *American Journal of Occupational Therapy, 54*(8), 260–268.

Francis-Connolly, E. (2000). Toward an understanding of mothering: A comparison of two motherhood stages. *American Journal of Occupational Therapy, 54*(3), 281–289.

Gilligan, C. (1982). *In a different voice: Psychological theory and women's development.* Cambridge, MA: Harvard University Press.

Gilman, C. P. (1973, 1899). The yellow wallpaper. (Ed. 1). New York: Feminist Press.

Guberman, N., Maheu, P., & Maille, C. (1992). Women as family caregivers: Why do they care? *The Gerontologist, 32*(5), 607–617.

Guerrero, S. H. (Ed.). (1999). *Gender-sensitive & feminist methodologies: A handbook for health and social researchers.* Quezon City: University of the Philippines Center for Women's Studies.

Hall, B. A. (1994.). Ways of maintaining hope in HIV disease. *Research in Nursing & Health, 17,* 283–293.

Health and Human Services (2001). *Healthy People 2010, November 2000.* McClean, VA: International Medical Publishing, Inc.

Kahle, A., & Jones, G. (1998). Adaptation to parental chronic illness. In A. J. Goreczny & M. Hersen (Eds.). *Handbook of pediatric and adolescent health psychology*

(pp. 387–399). Needham Heights, MA: Allyn & Bacon, Inc.

Kaplan, L. (1995). *The story of Jane: the legendary underground feminist abortion service.* New York: Pantheon Books.

Kenney, J. W. (2000). Women's 'inner-balance': A comparison of stressors, personality traits and health problems by age groups. *Journal of Advanced Nursing, 31*(3), 639–650.

Kielhofner, G., Mallinson, T., Crawford, C., Nowak, M., Rigby, M., Henry, A. D., & Walens, D. (1998). *The user's manual for the Occupational Performance History Interview (Version 2.), OPHI-II.* Chicago, IL: University of Illinois at Chicago.

Kielhofner, G., Mallinson, T., Forsyth, K., & Lai, J. (2001). Psychometric properties of the second version of the occupational performance history interview (OPHI-II). *The American Journal of Occupational Therapy, 55*(3), 260–276.

Kralik, D. (2002). The quest for ordinariness: Transition experienced by midlife women living with chronic illness. *Journal of Advanced Nursing, 39*(2), 146–152.

Krieger, N., & Fee, E. (1994). Man-made medicine and women's health: The biopolitics of sex/gender and race/ethnicity. *International Journal of Health Services, 24*(2), 265–283.

Lange, S. M. (1996). Evaluating the impact of chronic illness on children. *Dissertation Abstracts International, 57*(5-B), November 1996, 3433.

Lawrence, L., & Weinhouse, B. (1994). *Outrageous practices: The alarming truth about how medicine mistreats women.* New York: Fawcett Columbine.

Lea, A. (1994). Women with HIV and their burden of caring. *Health Care for Women International, 15,* 489–501.

Ma, G.X. (2000). Barriers to the use of health services by Chinese Americans. *Journal of Allied Health, 29*(2), 64–70.

Mairs, N. (1996). *Waist-high in the world: A life among the nondisabled.* Boston: Beacon Press.

Marshall, P. (1983). *Praisesong for the widow.* New York: Penguin Books.

Naylor, G. (1988). *Mama Day.* New York: Tinccnor & Fields.

Nyborg, H. (1994). The neuropsychology of sex-related differences in brain and specific abilities: Hormones, developmental dynamics, and new paradigm. In Vernon, P. A. (Ed.). *The neuropsychology of individual differences* (pp. 59–113). San Diego: Academic Press.

Olfson, M. (1988). The Weir Mitchell rest cure. *Pharos Alpha Omega Alpha Honor Med Soc,* Summer, *51*(3), 30–32.

Opacich, K. J. (2002). *Reconstructing occupation after HIV infection: Lessons from the lived experience of women.* Unpublished doctoral dissertation, University of Illinois, Chicago.

Paterson, B. (2001). The shifting perspectives model of chronic illness. *Image, Journal of Nursing Scholarship, 33,* 21–26.

Quinn-Beers, J. (2001). Attachment needs of adolescent

daughters of women with cancer. *Journal of Psychosocial Oncology, 19*(1), 35–48.

Rodriguez-Trias, H. (1992). Women's health, women's lives, women's right. (editorial) *American Journal of Public Health, 82*(5), 663–664.

Rosenfeld, A. G., & Gilkeson, J. (2000). Meaning of illness for women with coronary heart disease. *Heart & Lung: Journal of Acute & Critical Care, 29*(2), 105–112.

Schaefer, K. M. (1995). Women living in paradox: Loss and discovery in chronic illness. *Holistic Nursing Practice, 9*(3), 63–74.

Schneider, B.E. (1992). AIDS and class, gender, and race relations. In J. Huber & B. E. Schneider (Eds.). *The social context of AIDS* (pp. 19–43). Newbury Park: Sage.

Sherwin, S. (1992). *No longer patient: Feminist ethics & health care.* Philadelphia:Temple University Press.

Smith, D. E. (1987). *The everyday world as problematic: A feminist sociology.* Boston: Northeastern University.

Sowell, R. L., Moneyham, L, & Aranda-Naranjo, B. (1999). The care of women with AIDS: special needs and considerations. *Nursing Clinics of North America, 34*(1), 179–99.

Speck, O., Ernst, T., Braun, J., Koch, C., Miller, E., & Chang, L. (2000). Gender differences in the functional organization of the brain for working memory. *NeuroReport, 11*(11), 2581–2585.

Spurlock, J. (1995). Multiple roles of women and role strains. *Health Care for Women International, 16,* 501–508.

Stevens, P.E. (1996). Struggles with symptoms: Women's narratives of managing HIV illness. *Journal of Holistic Nursing, 14*(2), 142–61.

Thomas, S. P. (1997). Distressing aspects of women's roles, vicarious stress, and health consequences. *Issues in Mental Health Nursing, 18,* 539–557.

Thomson, R. G. (1997). *Extraordinary bodies: Figuring physical disability in American culture and literature.* New York: Columbia University Press.

Townsend, E. (1993). 1993 Muriel Driver Lecture:

Occupational therapy's social vision. *Canadian Journal of Occupational Therapy, 60*(4), 174–84.

Townsend, E. (1996). Institutional ethnography: A method for showing how the context shapes practice. *Occupational Therapy Journal of Research, 16*(3), 179–199.

Trotter, R. T. 2$^{nd.}$ (2001). Curanderismo: A picture of Mexican-American folk healing. *Journal of Alternative & Complementary Medicine, 7*(2), 129–131.

United States Department of Health and Human Services (2000). *Healthy People 2010 (Volume I).* McLean, VA: International Medical Publishing, Inc.

Valleau, M. P., Bergner, R. M., & Horton, C. B. (1995). Parentification and caretaker syndrome: an empirical investigation. *Family Therapy, 22*(3), 157–164.

Weekes. N. Y. (1994). Sex differences in the brain. In Zaidel, D. W. (Ed.). *Neuropsychology:* Handbook of perception and cognition (2nd ed.) (pp 293–315). New York: Academic Press.

Wells, S., & Black, R. M. (2000). *Cultural competency for health professionals.* Bethesda, MD: American Occupational Therapy Association.

Whiteford, G., Townsend, E., & Hocking, C. (2000). Reflections on a renaissance of occupation. *Canadian Journal of Occupational Therapy, 67*(1), 61–69.

World Health Organization (1995). *Women's health and human rights.* Platform for Action presented at the Fourth World Conference on Women, Beijing, 1995. Document retrieved Oct. 27, 2002, from *http://www.who. int./hhr/information*

Wilcock, A. (1998). *An occupational perspective of health.* Thorofare, NJ: Slack, Inc.

Williams, A. B., Shahryarinejad, A., Andrews, S., & Alcabes, P. (1997). Social support for HIV-infected mothers: Relation to HIV care seeking. *Journal of the Association of Nurses in AIDS Care, 8*(1), 91–98.

Wyatt, G., & Friedman, L. L.(1996). Long-term female cancer survivors: Quality of life issues and clinical implications. *Cancer Nursing, 19*(1), 1–7.

Zemke, R., & Clark, F. (1996). *Occupational science: The evolving discipline.* Philadelphia, PA: F. A. Davis.

CHAPTER **12**

Mothers with Mental Illness: An Occupation Interrupted

Elizabeth Anne McKay, PhD, MSc, DipCOT, SROT

Anticipated Outcomes

I anticipate that, after reading this chapter, readers will:

- Explore the impact of severe mental illness on the occupation of mothering
- Share the women's diverse and difficult experiences of mothering
- Identify implications for practice and future research

 Introduction

> If motherhood is an occupation
> which is critically important to society
> the way we say it is, then there should
> be a Mothers' Bill of Rights.
> Mickulsci (1936)

The above call for a Mothers' Bill of Rights, first suggested many years ago, may indeed be a way for the occupation of mothering to be recognized and supported by society today. If it is needed for mothers generally, it is certainly required for women who experience mothering with a mental illness; they have

to meet the challenge of fulfilling a complex but commonplace occupation in extraordinary circumstances. This chapter will present the reality of this experience from the perspectives of four Scottish women who recounted their unique experiences of mothering as they shared their life histories.

The development of my interest in women with severe mental illness originates from my experience, initially as an occupational therapist and later as a university lecturer with responsibility for the provision of mental health education for undergraduate and postgraduate occupational therapists. This interest stemmed from my first post as an occupational therapist, in which I worked in the long-stay psychiatric wards of the Royal Edinburgh Hospital, Scotland. Here there were women who had been admitted to the psychiatric service for not adhering to society's norms, for example, having an illegitimate child. The result was a lifetime spent in an institution. I often wondered about these women, their experiences, and the child from whom they had been separated. Similarly, within acute psychiatric wards, I found that the multidisciplinary team inadequately considered women's roles as main carers of children and others. The focus was on stabilizing the woman's mental status and discharging her back to her community, with no or very limited follow-up that had implications for supporting her role and responsibilities as a mother.

My continuing interest in women's mental health issues resulted in my doctoral study, which explored the lived experience of women with severe mental illness (McKay, 2002). In my study, mothering emerged as a significant theme from the findings. Mothering from the women's perspective was a multidimensional occupation involving many diverse tasks that changed over time. The women in my study seemed to have experienced mothering as an interrupted occupation. The interruptions took two main forms: a cessation of the mother's direct involvement in mothering for differing periods of time or the mother's mental health status interfering with her perceived capacity to mother.

Mothering is considered a co-occupation, with both the mother and her child being active participants in this shared occupation (Primeau, 1996). Ruddick (1989) identified the concept that mothering involves sustaining the child's health and promoting the child's development to facilitate progress to adulthood, so that the child is able to contribute to society. However, mothering has been taken for granted (Larson, 2000). The literature reflects the concept that mothering is important to society. Therefore occupational therapists and other health professionals need to be involved, along with others, in working with mothers to facilitate and support their mothering role.

For occupational therapists, supporting the occupation of mothering is a significant part to play if we are to maintain a mother's ability to respond to the needs and well-being of her children (Oates, 1997). This role is essential to support mothers with mental illness who find themselves trying to deal with the occupation of mothering in less than ideal circumstances. Such involvement would be beneficial to both mothers and children by preventing or reducing the stress or isolation experienced by mothers and, importantly, lessening the possible adverse effects that may arise because of a mother's mental illness. The effects of maternal mental illness on children may include lack of stimulation, neglect, and isolation resulting in developmental delay. It may increase the risk of emotional and physical harm to the children and, at the extreme end, risk of fatal abuse (Gopfert, Harrison and Mahoney, 1999). This chapter will provide insights, using the women's own words, into how their valued occupation of mothering was interrupted by mental illness.

I conducted the work for this chapter in Scotland for my doctoral study. I explored the lives of women with enduring mental illness, using qualitative methodology, specifically life history, to understand how they viewed their past, their present, and their possible future. I analyzed the resultant data using the constant comparative method. In the process of this work, the women's narratives brought to the fore their unique experiences of being a mother, bringing up children, and dealing with their own mental illness.

The participants described mothering as an occupation that was extremely meaningful to them, although they experienced many difficult problems. The women highlighted their early mothering experiences, although for all the participants this was some time ago. They reported that they received little understanding of their situations or, indeed, practical support to help them to continue with this significant role.

What emerged from the findings was a continuum of mothering from pregnancy to being a grandmother. This continuum portrayed the different aspects that affected their capacity to mother as their children developed. An important aspect from the women's perspective was their roles as grandmothers. For all, this was a highly valued role that offered them opportunities to have a more positive mothering experience. The chapter highlights implications for practice and research and challenges us to recognize the importance of mothering for all our clients.

✎➤ Historical Overview of Women with Severe Mental Illness

The following literature presents an overview by first emphasizing the lack of relevant sources. Second, the review charts chronologically the growth of awareness and the need for research and change. Figures would indicate that women and men are equally represented within the severely mentally ill population, each forming around 50 percent of that population. Yet women with severe mental illness are little studied. Wahl (1992) concluded that this situation left a gap in knowledge. This is partly explained by Payne (1995), who discusses the difficulties of seeing this particular population. He argued that the specific needs of individuals and subgroups become organized around the most dominant group. In the case of people with severe mental illness, the most dominant group is perceived to be men who suffer from schizophrenia; thus women's invisibility is increased as a result of being overshadowed by this group.

That said, women hold a particular place in the story of psychiatry. From the earliest time, women who were considered different in their culture have been labelled as many things, from witches to being possessed by evil spirits to insane (Roffe & Roffe, 1995; Chesler, 1996). As the 18th century started, the formalization of psychiatric care within the United Kingdom was beginning. Women quickly became the main recipients of this budding specialism, often not at their own choice, and it could be argued they have been over-represented as patients ever since. Generally, women outnumber men in mental health services as a whole (Office for Population Censuses and Surveys (OPCS), 1994). One of the explanations of this figure includes the idea that women, by their nature, seek help more than men. An alternative view, especially through the 19th and 20th centuries, was that women were oppressed by men in male-dominated institutions within a similarly male-dominated society. This patriarchal view of psychiatry is well documented (Chesler, 1972; Showalter, 1985; Ussher, 1991).

A third perspective is the notion of gender bias in the diagnosis and care of women with mental illness. Busfield (1996) maintains that the official psychiatric classifications, namely International Classification of Diseases (ICD10) and the Diagnostic and Statistical Manual (DSM-1V) were developed to be gender neutral. However, she argues that the "formal, surface, gendered-neutrality does not mean that the categories themselves are constructed independently of gender" (p. 103). She highlights the fact that occasionally gender-specific symptoms are included as well as statements that flag up the likely gender balance of the disorder. For example, in ICD10 anorexia nervosa is highlighted as a disorder more likely found in women.

One group of women who are included in the general female population, but whose experiences are rarely reflected in the literature, are women with severe mental illness (Repper, Owen, Perkins, Deighton & Robinson, 1996, Harlene & Bernhard, 1994). As a specific group, women with severe mental illness have been little covered in the literature over the last 30 years. It was not until the early 1980s that the group began to receive attention, and not until the 1990s that some attempt at addressing the lack of research was evidenced. The literature falls into two main categories. First, there is the literature that highlights the evidence that women have been discriminated against within mental health services (Test & Berlin, 1981; Carmen, Russo, & Miller, 1981; Repper, Perkins, & Owen, 1998; Ritsher, Coursey & Farrell, 1997). Second, there is the body of literature that offers different perspectives or proposes alternatives for working with women (Harlene & Bernhard, 1994; Nahmias & Froelich, 1993; Cowan, 1996).

In 1981, two articles were published that reinforced the need for more research. These works were not research, but reviews of relevant literature drawn from a variety of areas including women's studies, mental health, roles, and social contexts. The first paper, by Test and Berlin (1981), argued that women with severe mental illness were still considered almost genderless by clinicians and researchers. It highlighted that, even when these groups considered gender, their responses often followed the stereotypic route that placed women in traditional roles and contexts. Women were offered treatment options that did not meet their needs but were seen as being socially appropriate. They also proposed that women's longevity might mean that their care over time is the most disadvantaged and neglected. They hypothesized that the homemaker role may provide flexibility because it offers a high tolerance for unusual behavior. But it is accompanied by a low profile in the community that can lead to isolation and possible social exclusion. Furthermore, there are other disadvantages attached to the homemaker role, such as increased stress and economic pressures with little reward, resulting in low self-esteem and status.

Test and Berlin (1981) also identified that women with severe mental illness may incur serious limitations across a spectrum of areas, including social, living, and work contexts. They argued that little was known of this group in relation to their lives and their experiences as women, mothers, wives, lovers, and carers. Little was known about them also as a client group, and some areas were rarely discussed, including sexuality, sexual health, exploitation, and abuse. These authors called for "responsible" research to explore the many facets of these women's lives, to advance the understanding of their experiences, and to create appropriate services.

The same year saw the second of the review articles. Carmen, Miller, and Russo (1981) clearly discuss inequality and women's mental health. Although this review is not specifically geared to women with severe mental illness, many of the issues discussed are relevant. The authors strongly present the case that mental health workers need to address the societal institutions that affect women with mental health problems. The paper presents some of the inequalities that women face, such as social inequality increased by women's participation in work, pay issues, types of occupations, and financial concerns, to name but a few. These authors reiterate Test and Berlin's (1981) call for more research in relation to women with severe mental illness.

In another review article, the position of women with severe mental illness is explored against the background of an increasing interest in women's physical and mental health (Bachrach, 1985). The author states that these women need special attention and that in the past they have been reduced to general statements and therefore "desexed" or perceived as genderless. She states,

> Heightened awareness of—and responsiveness to—women's gender specific treatment needs require more than knowledge of objective circumstances; it requires social endorsement as well (p. 1064).

Bachrach acknowledges that some of the endorsement has to come from the women's movement. She further identifies the areas that should be included when planning for this specific group, namely, homelessness, skills training, family planning, and social networks. She, too, supports Test and Berlin's (1981) view that gender stereotyping results in lower expectations for women than men, and therefore reduced opportunities for women. Later, Bachrach & Nadelson (1988) reiterate this point, describing how services for women are based on lower performance expectations. The above literature is from an American perspective. It is not until 1991 that the UK literature begins to discuss some of these issues in another special edition, this time from the *British Journal of Psychiatry* looking at "Women and Psychiatry." One article in this special supplement highlights issues for women in the development of mental health services (Subotsky, 1991). It describes how in Camberwell, London, services have developed that follow a woman's cycle approach. Subotsky discusses the need to listen to the patient's experience and the importance of the role of the consumer as both a patient and carer. She adds a note of caution: "These women-orientated services may not automatically follow, unless specifically fostered" (p. 21).

The question of women and mental health begins to surface in other professions other than psychiatry and psychology throughout the 1990s. From a UK nursing perspective, Faugier (1992) discusses that, although it is not fashionable and service providers and developers may not wish to hear it, there is a substantial body of evidence that points to the many differences in the mental health of men and women. She identifies that the majority of mental health problems, excluding schizophrenia and addictions, are more commonly diagnosed in women. She also criticizes psychiatry for ignoring the differences in the rates of mental illness between the sexes and for tending to adhere to a gender-neutral view of mental illness. Faugier further argues that we need to make attempts to understand and analyze the nature of such differences. She is critical of nursing as a profession for not doing enough to address gender issues. She highlights the need for the education of health professionals, not only nurses, and for this education to place gender issues centrally in our work and our curricula. The Health Department of the Commonwealth Secretariat has recently endorsed this view of incorporating gender and health issues into health professional education (Harding & Sills, 1999).

It is not until 1993, in another review article, that occupational therapy addresses the question of women and mental health generally. Nahmias and Froelich (1993), American occupational therapists, focus on gender role stereotypes and the implications of these for occupational therapists. They highlight how essential it is that occupational therapists fully understand social cultural contexts and the theories specific to women's psychological development. They draw heavily on some of the articles mentioned previously, acknowledging that "gender-related issues are virtually absent in the occupational therapy literature" (p. 40). The authors advocate an essentially feminist approach to be used with women to enhance interventions. They purport that occupational therapy, as a profession, has been slow to respond to the changing climate.

Insofar as this is the case, they call for occupational therapists to explore their attitudes and beliefs and how these translate into ways of knowing and ways of working with women.

An article from an American nursing viewpoint offers a feminist perspective of the literature regarding women with severe mental illness (Harlene & Bernhard, 1994). The authors initially reinforce the silence of these women, stating that the limited information available narrows our thinking and that, as a result, there is not only missing knowledge, but also a range of distortions. They assert that three factors dominate the situation. First, women are "other" in a male-norm society. Second, severe mental illness is viewed differently from physical illness and, last, healthcare personnel are educated in the dichotomy of mind/body split. They propose that these factors affect both the health care of women with severe mental illness and their status as a population at risk. They reviewed the existing literature and concluded that feminist literature on health and mental health has avoided severe mental illness. They further suggest that the literature concentrated on mostly white, educated, middle-class women's issues, such as career, relationships, and topics that have previously received little attention, such as cancer. A third aspect of this literature is the need to address abuse of women, including battering, rape, and the overprescribing of drugs. They highlight that schizophrenia and bipolar disorders are not mentioned, whereas depression is consistently identified.

Harlene and Bernhard (1994) assert that this group of women's "invisibility enhances [their] vulnerability" (p. 83). The invisibility of these women is increased by the gap in the research literature, which has failed to include the standpoint of women with severe mental illness. They advocate that the valuing and validating of personal experience is an aspect of quality feminist work: "Women's lived experience should be the starting point for all health efforts" (p. 85).

Another view of the field of women's mental health issues is presented from a Canadian perspective (Cowan, 1996). Cowan argues that it is only over the past 2 decades that women's mental health has been brought into the wider societal context. She proposes that there is a need for a woman-centered therapeutic approach, but adds that deep-seated bias and oppressive ways of working have to be acknowledged and changed. She, too, supports Faugier in calling for staff to address these issues in both their practice and their educational courses.

The call for these issues to be addressed in both practice and education has been supported by various campaigns from the early 1990s on. In the UK, the mental health charity MIND (1992) published a policy paper stating that "women's experience in society, from birth until old age, generally exposes them to greater stress than men" (p. 7). They too advocated that the way forward lies in providing women with the service options they wish, including choice of woman-only space, women workers, adequate childcare, and the chance to explore the causes of their distress. This policy document also emphasized the need for training in gender and race issues. These calls have been supported by other organizations and professions, including *Good Practices in Mental Health* (1994) and the *Royal College of Nursing* (RCN) (1994).

It has been shown that the literature highlights several major themes in relation to women and mental illness. These include the reliability of diagnostic criteria, the lack of gender recognition, limited and stereotypic treatment opportunities, raising awareness of the needs of women with mental illness, increased sensitivity to meet women's needs, and the application of feminist thinking in practitioners' ways of working. However, all acknowledge the lack of relevant research.

ᴥ Women with Severe Mental Illness: The Research Perspective

A large body of work records the rate of mental illness in mothers (Cleaver et al, 1999). However, as has been highlighted above, little research has explored the experiences of women with severe mental illness generally, or specifically examined their roles as mothers. Three recent studies have dealt specifically

with women and severe mental illness. In each of these, mothering is considered, but not as a central issue.

From a North American perspective, Ritsher, Coursey, and Farrell (1997) aimed to explore the issues related to living with severe mental illness by use of a questionnaire. The questionnaire was developed using focus groups to identify the topics. Two groups of women with severe mental illness and a third of mental health practitioners were studied. The resultant questionnaire was then distributed to a range of urban, suburban and rural psychiatric rehabilitation centers in Maryland, USA. The sample population consisted of 107 women and 59 men. It is not clear whether all attendees at these centers were asked to be included or how, if any, attempts were made to refine the sample.

The study set out to address three main areas: issues in living with severe mental illness, interpersonal relationships, and relationships with healthcare providers. In addressing living with severe mental illness, the researchers wished to explore whether men and women gave different explanations for their symptoms. They also explored how living with severe mental illness affected women's sense of themselves and their satisfaction with their life. A third aspect focused on their formative experiences and their current goals. Under the heading of "Interpersonal relationships," four main areas were included: friendships and social supports, abuse, romantic and sexual relationships, and parenting.

The results demonstrated that more women were diagnosed as having affective disorders, whereas men were more likely to have schizophrenia. There was a significant difference in the distribution of these two types of illness as has been noted before. The women in the sample were, on the whole, slightly older, and similarly, their onset of illness was later than for men. When asked about the causes of their problems, women more than men cited "bad things in the past" or "the result of the way I was raised." The results from the first two areas that relate to being a mother will be highlighted below.

The first area addressed issues in "living with severe mental illness" (Ritsher, Coursey,

& Farrell, 1997). When considering the impact of mental illness on their lives, most women reported being moderately affected. Just less than half (47 percent) of women felt that the mental illness had forced them to give up or to change their life goals, such as jobs, attending college, or, importantly for women, having children. Clearly, these women had lost completely or had to significantly modify the course of their life in relation to their personal ambitions.

The second area to be considered encompassed the women's interpersonal relationships; mothering is included within this section (Ritsher, Coursey & Farrell, 1997). With regard to mothering, 62 percent of the women were likely to have had at least one child, with only 17 percent of the men having one child. Eighty-two percent of the mothers reported that they were able to raise or help raise at least one of their children. It is clear that more women than men had children and the majority were involved to some degree in caring for their children. Twenty-nine percent of the women identified that the illness had made it harder for them to be "good" parents.

An interesting aspect that arose was the place of medication in relation to pregnancy. More than half of the women reported that if they became pregnant they would stop taking medication, even though this might lead to a relapse of their mental illness. Similarly, the women were worried that continuing to take their medication might affect the child before birth or during breast-feeding (Ritsher, Coursey & Farrell, 1997). There is a need here for more information and education for women around this particular subject.

A frustration from this study is the lack of detail or examples of the ways in which mothers were able to help raise their children or, indeed, what made it harder for them to be good parents. The questionnaire method, although useful in accessing large numbers of subjects, loses the opportunity to collect rich data or the individual's unique perspective. Nonetheless, this study concluded that, for women with severe mental illness, "the illness is not the center of these women's identities" (Ritsher, Coursey & Farrell, 1997; p. 1280). Most women felt that the illness had had some

adverse impact on their lives. However, the survey did not explore whether the adversity the women experienced was a result of the illness or the secondary consequences of the illness, or as is likely, both. The study does illustrate that severe mental illness can be seen as complex with many effects on the lives of women.

A British study placed women with severe mental illness at its core (Repper, Perkins, Owen, Deighton & Robinson, 1996). This research used feminist methodology to explore the experiences of women. The study aimed to investigate the acceptability and adequacy of services for women with serious mental health problems. The study, conducted in Nottingham, UK, used a variety of research methods to ascertain the women's experiences. These included in-depth interviews, questionnaires, and focus groups. Two research papers that report the results of this work have been published.

The first to be considered is the work of Owen, Repper, Perkins, and Robinson (1998). They evaluated the adequacy, accessibility, and responsiveness of the services provided for women. Fourteen women's views were collected through focus groups to gain an understanding of the impact of severe mental illness on their lives. The results indicated that women were more likely to be divorced or widowed and to have children. It found that the women were more often living with a spouse or a cohabitee or lived alone with children. Analysis of the data revealed two main themes, namely, loss and hope.

The findings of Owen et al. (1998) revealed that the women in their study had an overwhelming sense of loss throughout their lives, which had been exacerbated since the onset of their mental illness. Their losses were considered under three main headings. Under the heading "Loss in present lives," women reported experiencing loss of past relationships including partners and children, as well as loss of independence and work. Secondly, the women described "loss as a result of symptoms," which included an inability to cope. For example, they experienced reduced energy, as well as having little control over their symptoms and the negative side effects of medication. The final loss concerned "opportunities in the mental health services." In this section, the women reported that they had lost opportunities for meaningful activity in their lives. They also had lost contact with other women, for example, past friends or relatives. Finally, the women highlighted the loss they felt with regard to having little input to decisions that affected their lives. The other major finding was that these women continued to have hopes. These were "very ordinary aspirations: they wanted to get married, have friends, a job, a house, and something to do with their time" (Owen et al., 1998; p. 287). However, they needed help and support for these hopes to be realized. An important finding was the emergence of "powerlessness of the women" across all aspects of their lives. The authors advocated that women should be empowered to make choices and be supported in their choices. This is particularly important if these decisions involve children. Women need accurate information, time, and support to make informed choices. They stress that services must work to reduce women's sense of loss and to support their future aspirations.

The Owen et al. (1998) study provided valuable information from the focus groups about the experiences of women using mental health services. It is unclear if the women were consulted about the findings. A relatively small number of women participated in the 5 focus groups, 14 in all, so results cannot be generalized, but the study provides a useful baseline for further investigation.

The second paper arising from the original 1996 study was by Repper, Perkins, and Owen (1998). The authors utilized the same data but treated it differently. They decided that in analyzing the data according to themes as in the previous study, the women's actual experiences were not reflected. This article sought to present the women's perspectives more completely. They reconstructed the focus group transcripts to discover that 8 of the 14 participants had told their "life story" in the course of the groups. Their findings told of social disadvantages predating the women's mental health problems. These included poverty, divorce, and for some of the women, sexual abuse. The participants identified other issues

such as loss of children, relationships, home, and work; and a lack of understanding about what had happened to them. The women's hopes and aspirations, as highlighted in the previous work, were tempered by staff attitudes, which did not support them or deemed their wishes unrealistic. The researchers concluded that the effects of such negativity on women with reduced self-confidence could only be detrimental to their well being in the long term. The range of women's experiences reflected loss across personal, social, and material spheres, with the women importantly reporting experiences that predated their mental health problems.

To conclude this section, these three studies (Ritsher et al., 1997; Owen et al., 1998; Repper et al., 1998) illustrated that women with severe mental illness experience "losses" across social, personal and material spheres, including a loss or reduction of their roles as mothers. The presence of mental illness may affect a mother's capacity to care for her child in a range of different ways, including parenting skills, their perceptions of being a parent, control of their emotions, neglect of physical needs, and attachment and separation issues.

These areas were found to some degree in my own work (McKay, 2002). My study explored the lived experiences of women with severe mental illness, not only their illness narratives, but also their whole life story, with an emphasis on their occupational functioning.

This phase of the work took place over a 2-year period, 1999 to 2001, and is presented in the following paragraphs.

✍ Narrative Inquiry: Exploring the Lived Experience of Women with Severe Mental Illness

Mattingly (1999) regards narratives as being event and experience-centered, which creates experiences for the listener or audience. She considers the narrative form as being particularly appropriate for addressing illness and healing experiences. In narrative terms, the "illness or disability" is considered as an episode within the larger context of the individual's life history. Williams (1984) posits that during certain times of crisis, of which illness could be considered an example, the life story is lost. The routine narrative can become confused, resulting in some reworking of the narrative to account for the disruption. The reconstruction is necessary "both in order to understand the illness in terms of past social experience and to reaffirm that life has a course and the self a purpose" (p. 179). Such narratives hold our experiences together in some order, allowing links to the past, present, and most importantly, the future.

Narrative enables people to make sense of their own lives. Kielhofner and Mallinson (1995) state: "Stories are interpretive vehicles through which one's life is made coherent and takes on meaning" (p. 63). Narratives have been used in occupational therapy to explore a range of issues. This body of literature encompasses work illuminating clients' narratives (Clark, 1993; Price-Lackey & Cashman, 1996; Fanchiang, 1996; Mostert et al., 1996) highlighting student and educational issues (McKay & Ryan, 1995; Ryan & McKay, 1999; Fortune, 1999). Other work considers the therapeutic potential of narrative (Polkinghorne, 1996; Hughes, 2002) and narrative as a research method (Mallinson et al., 1996; Frank, 1996; Frank, 2000).

Research Approach

For my study, narrative inquiry using life history was used to explore the lived experience of women with severe mental illness. Frank (1996) defined life history as "a narrative approach in which empirical methods are used to reconstruct and interpret the lives of an ordinary person " (p. 252). Life history can be considered a form of biographical research drawn from anthropological and social science research (Creswell, 1998). The use of life history as a research method has increased as attention has turned to exploring the meaning of lives. Therefore, life history can be used to enhance our understanding of how particular people experience and adapt to major life events. As Schempp (1995) states: "The life is seen as being lived in a time, and place under particular circumstances rather than a simple collection of events" (p. 115). The life history

method was chosen to gain insight into and to comprehend the lives of women with severe mental illness. This allowed for a detailed exploration of each woman's lived experience, enabling the unique diversity of her life to be described and represented.

Gaining Access to the Women

Because I wished to gain access to women with severe mental illness who were living in the community, I approached a Mental Health Resource facility in Glasgow, Scotland. Possible participants were made aware of the study through two methods, either meeting with myself over a number of sessions at the facility or responding to an advertisement I placed in the center's newsletter. Once I had made contact with possible participants, further information was given and I sought their informed written consent. This study adhered to the ethical procedures of my university.

Interviewing the Women

Five women agreed to take part in the study. Each had two in-depth interviews, approximately 18 months apart. On both occasions, the participants were interviewed in their own homes, at their convenience. The interviews were tape recorded. The first interview focused on their life history and asked what Spradley (1979) described as the "grand tour" question. I asked an open-ended descriptive question: "Tell me your life history." This was used to encourage the participants to tell their stories as freely as possible. Atkinson (1998) stated that "the less structure a life story interview has the more effective it will be in achieving the goal of getting the person's own story in the way, form and style that the individual wants to tell it" (p. 41). Following verbatim transcription, a biographical framework of key dates and events identified by each of the women was constructed. In addition, concept maps of their major life themes were also developed at this time.

The second interview consisted of three distinct aspects building on the first interview. These were a review of the participant's biographical details, presentation of the initial themes via the concept map, and last, questions of a retrospective nature and questions with a future orientation.

An overview of the participants is found in Table 12–1. All but one of the participants were mothers. Vignettes of the four mothers are presented below.

Vignette: *Marguerite*

Marguerite had one daughter, age 30 at the start of this study. Marguerite had recently become a grandmother; her new granddaughter was only 6 months old. Marguerite had several interests, including church activities, singing in the choir, and taking part in educational classes. Although she took early retirement from her employment, she was keen to find a part time job. Marguerite has had contact with psychiatric services from her teens. She was one of five children; three of her siblings, also suffer from mental illness. Marguerite lived with her parents and cared for them till their deaths.

Vignette: *Helen*

Helen, the oldest woman in the study, had one daughter, age 52. She had two grandsons who at the time of the study were in their 20s. Helen was becoming increasingly frail. She lived in a small apartment that she had organized to maximize her independence. Helen felt that she was becoming more isolated from her friends because of her lack of mobility; she was unable to use public transport. She had recently stopped attending the mental health day center and she missed this contact with others very much.

Throughout her life, Helen has been an activist for improved mental health services and facilities.

Vignette: *Pat*

Pat had three children, two sons and a daughter, ages from 27 to 31 years. She too was a grandmother, although she had contact with her daughter's son, only. She became ill when she was bringing up the children on her own. At the time of the interview, she lived in an apartment with her youngest son, who was 27 years old. She too had several interests; she attended the mental health day center and enjoyed creative writing. She was very pleased when some of her work was published. She enjoyed writing about her early experiences of the Scottish countryside. She had a twin sister.

Vignette: *Pam*

Pam had one son, age 27. Pam grew up on a working farm. From an early age she wished to be a teacher and worked towards this goal. She worked for many years with children ages 5 to 12 years old. Recently she left teaching because of her recurrent mental illness. She appreciated the countryside and enjoyed walking and travel. She too had become involved at a local level in trying to improve both inpatient and community facilities for mental health users. She met her current partner while in the hospital.

Table 12–1	Characteristics of the women				
	Age at the beginning of the study	Year of birth	Marital status	Living with	Diagnosis
Helen	74	1924	Widowed	Alone	Depression
Pat	60	1938	Divorced	Son	Depression
Marguerite	53	1945	Divorced	Alone	Bipolar disorder
Pam	49	1950	Divorced	Partner	Bipolar disorder
Sarah	48	1952	Single	Alone	Post-traumatic stress

✎ Narrative Analysis

Polkinghorne (1995) discussed two different approaches to analysis of narrative. The first "analysis of narratives" is useful to discover commonalties across subjects and is the most often used analytical method. The second "narrative analysis" is better for discovering unique and diverse perspectives. In this latter approach the data were actions, events, and happenings, which through analysis and the use of emplotment, produced stories. Emplotment is the organization of events into an order. It is through reordering that meaning is derived from the narrative. I therefore selected narrative analysis because of its focus on the individual in her context and culture. In my work, five unique narratives were created through this process.

In addition, the data were analyzed using the constant comparative method to identify common shared experiences (Maykut & Morehouse, 1994). From this analysis process six themes emerged. Within the theme of life roles, mothering emerged as an important and separate subtheme for the four women who were mothers. This subtheme will form the remainder of this chapter.

✎ The Findings: Who's Minding the Mothers?

This study took place at a time in the women's lives that was long after their early mothering experiences. Francis-Connolly (2000) highlighted that the occupations of mothering are different across the life span. She emphasized that with preschool children the focus for the mother is on caretaking activities and meeting the basic needs of the child, whereas with "young adults the focus of motherhood is emotional and supportive activities" (p. 281). For the women in this study, their children at the time of the first interview were all adults, with the youngest being 27.

This distance in time offered the women a retrospective view of their mothering experiences from their current life stage. Several of the women, reflecting on their involvement in the study, stated that at an earlier stage in their lives they would have felt unable to take part in this type of research. Table 12–1 shows that the women in this group were similar to the participants in the Owen et al. (1998) work, with three of them being divorced and one widowed.

These four mothers identified motherhood as a significant and meaningful life role. Different aspects of their unique experiences as mothers are presented here and supported by extracts from their individual narratives to portray their experience. In this study, mothering emerged as a multidimensional occupation. It was considered an occupation that was longitudinal, with mothering roles and issues changing over time. Three of the four women were grandmothers, and the meaning of this specific role will also be explored. This continuum of motherhood, from being pregnant to being a grandmother, was represented in this group of women's narratives (Fig. 12–1). Although at first glance this continuum may seem self-evident, it raises key areas that may have implications for service providers.

Pregnancy, the beginning of the journey, will be considered first. For both Pam and Helen, the pregnancies were unexpected. For Pam, the pregnancy was unplanned, and as it continued, she began to take medication for depression to help her cope with her situation.

Helen was unaware that she was pregnant, and when it was confirmed early in her marriage, her reaction was one of fear. Helen stated: "I didn't want the baby I was carrying...I knew I had to have it." She was unprepared for motherhood. The baby was not something she had planned for at such an early stage in her married life. As a result, she felt frightened and that she had no control over what was happening to her. These initial feelings continued after the birth of her daughter and may have affected her ability to form a positive attachment with her.

Attachment was to be a major issue for Marguerite also. She had had several past episodes of bipolar disorder that resulted in admissions to psychiatric hospitals. Her difficulties came to a head when Marguerite experienced postpartum psychotic illness following her daughter Linda's birth in 1968. At this time there were few mental health special-

- Pregnancy
  Fear
  Adjusting
  Coping

- Childbirth and infancy
  Attachment
  Separation
  Developing caring

- Early childhood
  Children's needs first
  Sustaining contact
  Providing for their needs

- Adolescence
  Resentment
  Changing dynamics

- Adulthood
  Support: Practical and financial
  Guidance

- Grandmother
  Revisiting motherhood
  Experience and practice
  Positive identity

Figure 12–1 *The mothering continuum: Issues for mothers with a mental illness.*

ist services available to her. For example, *Mother and Baby Units* were not generally found in psychiatric hospitals in the UK, although they had been suggested as early as 1948 to avoid the twin dangers of separating mother and child (Main, 1948). This absence of service and the potential risk of child neglect and infanticide related to postpartum psychosis resulted in Marguerite spending nearly 2 years in the hospital (Kohen, 2000). Therefore her opportunities to develop a relationship with her baby were severely interrupted. Marguerite recalled that even breast-feeding was for

her problematic: "The poor child never got fed because there was not enough milk for her."

While in the hospital, Marguerite recalls, she was involved with occupational therapy. As a new mother, she was encouraged to make a teddy bear for her daughter, an appropriate and hugely meaningful task for her, at that time. Her engagement in this occupation provided both process and a finished product. Her involvement in constructing the bear enabled her to attend and concentrate on this purposeful task, building her confidence with tools and materials, and it also offered a focus and structure to her hospital stay. The finished product was, needless to say, very important to her because it was a gift for her daughter. She recalled that being engaged in this task was very important to her.

> I remember I made a red teddy for my
> baby; it was in Ted Heath's time [Prime
> Minister of the UK] so this was Red Ted. I
> just remember that bit.

As her admission continued, her daughter went home to be cared for by her husband and her mother-in-law. Marguerite's time with the baby was interrupted and restricted to short ward visits, and later weekend home visits when these were feasible. She believed that she did not have the opportunity to bond or to form a positive attachment with her daughter over this crucial period. As attachment had been problematic, separation would also become an issue for Marguerite.

As her admission continued, Marguerite was frightened that she was "going to end up permanently in the hospital." Therefore she decided to leave the hospital and return to live with her parents. She chose to leave her daughter in the care of her husband and his family. She then had to make another decision concerning custody of Linda because her husband wanted a divorce. Marguerite was advised that she should not seek custody.

> The lawyer said because of my history
> there would be very little chance of me
> getting custody and it would be very trau-
> matic to go up there and be asked all
> those questions and all this to come out
> in court.

As a result, Marguerite found herself in a situation in which she was unable to be involved in caring for her young daughter in anything but a peripheral role. This separation was very difficult and continued to affect her relationship with Linda over the intervening years. Her experiences support the findings of Stein et al. (1991), who identified that separation can affect the mother's relationship with the infant and may set up long-term worrying influences. In Marguerite's experience, her relationship with her daughter was always strained. When her daughter was in her teens, she completely rejected her mother, wanting nothing to do with her. Marguerite was aware that she was always on the periphery of her daughter's life and had no real influence with her. This poor relationship may have hindered her daughter's understanding of Marguerite's situation and her understanding of mental illness.

Similarly, Helen and Pam felt unable to cope with their roles as mothers after the birth of their children. At different stages, both felt unable to look after their children. However, each took a different approach to her dilemma to compensate for the perceived inability to cope. Helen's daughter, Julie, was born in 1946, and at this time the family was living in postwar London. Helen had suffered from depression for a number of years. She recalled:

> When I had that breakdown in London, I spoke to a doctor. She asked me if I had any problems. I'd never had a house. I'd had to live with Tom, Dick and Harry. There was a war on. I had to live that way, I had to plan my life their way: don't make a noise, keep the baby quiet. It was tense and worrying.

As Helen's depression continued, she felt increasingly unable to care for her 6-year-old daughter. She felt that her extended family would be able to help her. So, in 1952, the family returned to Helen's home, Glasgow. Once there, Helen seemed to hand over the care of Julie to her husband. She felt that Julie was fine; her father loved her and was there for her, and as an only child she had material luxuries that others did not. This action by Helen,

although done for the best of reasons, may have reinforced her less-than-positive relationship with her daughter. This concurs with the findings of Kohen (2000), who stated that "insecure attachments are more frequent in children who have mothers with a history of depression" (p. 169).

Pam, who also had a depressive illness, managed things differently. In 1971, she had her son, Craig. After his birth, she returned to college to finish her degree. This proved to be a difficult time. Nevertheless, she achieved her degree, though a year later than planned.

Pam, her husband and son were now living in an apartment. She recalled her feelings from that time:

> I was going to be the perfect mother. God, it drove me round the bend. I couldn't stand it being stuck in this apartment with this child crying and too young to tell me what was wrong.

Pam soon started back on medication. Following a chance meeting with the head teacher of the school where she had her final teaching placement, she was offered a job. She jumped at this chance. She hired a caregiver for Craig and took up the post. She worked part time in the school from January to June.

This job proved to be a turning point for Pam. She described her feelings of relief: "It was great for me, it meant I was using the brain, I was getting some exercise." Craig, too, benefited from his mother's job. Pam believed that the time she spent with him improved qualitatively. "I had a great time in the afternoons with Craig. I always spoke a lot to him and spent a lot of time with him." However, the job finished and, as the summer went on, Pam was soon back to feeling unable to cope. She just could not stand being at home. She felt trapped. "You know, the four walls [were] clawing in." She actively sought another teaching job. Craig went back to his caregiver. She did worry for Craig because he was the only child at the caregiver's home. Nevertheless, she took the job, which lasted a year. She then began full-time employment in a local school and Craig went to nursery school full time, this time with other children.

Pam's return to work enabled her to cope better with her role as mother. Her role as a teacher provided a counterbalance to the demands of mothering that she found so difficult. Her actions may have also been beneficial for Craig in the long-term; research shows that depressed mothers may have a range of negative influences on their child. Stein et al. (1991) studied 19-month-old babies of depressed mothers. They found that these children were less responsive, less interactive, and showed less positive affect than those in the control group. Craig may have doubly benefited from having time away from his mum with the caregiver and experiencing better quality time with mum when she returned from work. These different compensatory strategies adopted by Helen and Pam seemed to help both of them to cope emotionally and practically with their roles as mothers, although the impact of those strategies on the children is not known.

Pat's experiences offer a different perspective of motherhood. In 1970, she had two children, a son and a daughter. However, Pat's marital relationship was deteriorating rapidly, with her husband being abusive and violent. "I had to in the end get away and make a life for the children and myself…He had started turning on them as well as me." So she took the two children and set up a new home in Glasgow. She remembered, "It was really quite bad. You just kind of plodded on from bit to bit. Sometimes it felt like from hour to hour." At this time, she was pregnant with her third child. Her second son was born in 1971. Pat was 33 years old and had sole responsibility for three children. Importantly, she had no relatives locally to offer much-needed support.

Life for Pat over the next few years was arduous; she had financial problems, but her main concern was the children's welfare. She explained:

> You've got to pay the rent…All that is in your mind is you've got to pay the rent. You've got to pay the bills, you've got to put food in your children's stomachs and you've got to feed and clothe them and you've got to give them heat and light…That was the main thing on my mind…You dreamt about it.

Pat's life revolved around caring for the children, but the lack of money was a constant source of worry. Weich and Lewis (1998) emphasised that continued financial strain is strongly associated with the onset and maintenance of mental disorders. In addition, she had little time for herself to meet her own needs. She explained, "You've got to try and survive and make sure that they get all they need… I was never out. I couldn't afford to go out." On one occasion, a friend convinced her to go out for the evening. Pat hired a caregiver for the children. However, on her return home, the children were misbehaving. The following day, her eldest son announced "that it wasn't fair that mum had gone out." Pat explained: "He thought I had no right to be going out to do something I wanted to do…I said to myself, I'll never go out again until they are grown up."

Pat continued to hold the family together. The children were now all at school. However, Pat was worried, anxious, and tearful. She felt unable to care for her children and was concerned for their safety, both from the perspective of not being able to meet their needs and from worrying about who would care for them if anything happened to her. Furthermore, Phillip and Hugman (as cited in Göpfert, Harrison & Mahoney, 1999) identify that parents fear their children will be removed from the family by the authorities. She became increasingly depressed. Her experiences were reflected in the work of Popay and Jones (1990), who identified that mothers who bring up children alone have consistently worse health than those in two-parent homes. As Pat's health deteriorated, she sought admission to a local psychiatric hospital and placed her children in local authority care. Pat had continued anxiety about her children being in care. For example, how were they being cared for by others? Gopfert, Harrison and Mahoney (1999) identified that anxiety concerning their children's care can negatively affect the mother's mental health. This was echoed in Pat's story; at this time, her family were all separated, and they would never live together again as a family. Separation was to be a common issue for Pat and Marguerite.

Both experienced motherhood from a distance, and clearly their occupation as mothers was interrupted. With Marguerite it was almost immediately after her child was born and with Pat sometime later. They both worked hard to maintain contact with their children, although this was often in difficult and extreme circumstances.

Marguerite's situation in regard to maintaining contact with her daughter was exacerbated by an incident that occurred not long after she returned to her parents' apartment. This incident had serious repercussions for herself and on her ability to mother Linda. She recalled:

> I had stood on the window-sill, I remember thinking do I want to do this? But, I looked down and I lost my balance and I came down [the building] all on one side…I had serious problems at that time… I've no husband, I've no daughter, and I've nothing what is there?

Today Marguerite believes that the fall was not a suicide attempt, she said that had she meant to kill herself, she would have. Nonetheless, the resultant injuries from the fall were very serious, and Marguerite had a long period of hospitalization and a range of operations over a number of years. However, as she slowly recovered, she did not allow her physical difficulties to interfere with her contact with her daughter. "I went down [to visit her] with two [walking] sticks, I went down with one [walking] stick."

Pat, too, showed similar determination; when in the hospital and much later, when she lived in a community mental health house, she fought to maintain contact throughout with her children. This was made more difficult as the children were not kept together. The two boys were in the same local care home and her daughter was placed elsewhere. Pat had to assert herself and her status as a voluntary patient to be allowed to leave the hospital and attend her children's reviews. Pat's experience highlighted that when women were patients in a hospital, the multidisciplinary team did not recognize the importance of her mothering role. As a result, they hindered rather than supported the maintenance of her maternal role. For example, Pat was not included in decisions regarding her children's care. She felt excluded and perceived that her status as a capable and caring mother was under question. This increased her anxiety and may have reduced her ability to ask for support. Professionals involved with mothers at this time should be sensitive to the mothers' roles and responsibilities, facilitating the provision of necessary frameworks to reassure and support the mother.

However, both Pat and Marguerite demonstrated courage, strength, and resolve to continue their relationships with their children against this backdrop of physical and institutional barriers. After several years, Pat left the hospital to live in a group home. Her eldest children, now young adults, had set up home elsewhere. Her youngest son, Mark, now 17, was living in an independent living apartment, and he decided that he would move into the group-home to be with his mother. The mental health or social services did not sanction his action. Meanwhile, Pat had been trying to find alternative accommodation, and in March 1991, she and Mark moved into their new family home.

Following the idea of a motherhood continuum, three of the women in the study became grandmothers: a pivotal role for each of them. Doyal (1995) reminds us that the role of grandmother is much valued, "offering women greater autonomy than at any other point in their lives" (p. 40). The beneficial role of grandmothers in supporting mothers and children has been little researched. However, a study by Fergusson and Taylor (1998) showed that grandmothers could provide reassurance for families with young children, thus reducing inappropriate attendance at accident and emergency departments for nonserious injury or illness. They suggested that the absence of an involved grandmother in a child's care is one marker of family vulnerability.

In my study, involvement as a grandmother was highly valued by the women, often proving to be a turning point, although their experiences as grandmothers were very different. This role has proved to be very important for the women and their grandchildren in a variety of ways, as we shall see. Helen, as a grandmother, became the legal guardian for her two grandsons because of her daughter's and her son-in-law's alcohol addiction. This resulted in Helen's active involvement with her grandsons' upbringing. She said:

> I may not have been the best mother to Julie, but I was her mother when she needed me…I was the one who looked after her kids…she's never put a nappy on.

Helen offered Julie's children both practical and emotional support. Today, she still maintains contact with her grandsons, although she is more involved with her youngest grandson. Helen feels he was most adversely affected by his parents' addiction problems. She continues to worry about him. She regularly contacts him by phone and, whenever possible, offers financial help and respite from his social circumstances.

Pat's role as grandmother is marred by her poor relationship with her eldest son. As a result, she rarely sees these grandchildren. However, she is actively involved with her daughter and her daughter's son. She has been able to support them. "I'm always there for them and I always will be no matter what." Francis-Connolly (2000) considered mothers as "invested participants … they provided emotional support to [their children] and gave them advice on everything from car loans to parenting" (p. 287). All the women were actively involved, to some degree, in their children's and grand children's lives.

For Marguerite, although she had maintained contact with her daughter over the years, the relationship at times had been very difficult, with Linda rejecting Marguerite for a time. However, her continued presence in her daughter's life finally came to fruition with the birth of her granddaughter, Hannah, in 1998. Marguerite's growing involvement with her granddaughter was an opportunity for her and Linda to develop their relationship further. Her grandchild, in some way, bridged the gap and provided a focus for both Marguerite and Linda. Importantly, her involvement with her granddaughter enabled her to experience many of the milestones she had missed previously. She explained, "I'm reliving what I missed out on with Linda through my grand-

daughter. It's like a second chance." Similarly, as a grandmother she has felt and experienced common situations to those of her peers and is able to contribute and identify herself as a grandmother, something she missed out on as a mother. Significantly for her, she is able to have a role that is sanctioned by society and one that she loves. Overall, it was clear that being grandmothers offered a way for the women to remain active participants in their children's lives, offering emotional and practical support.

On reflecting on their roles as mothers, their perceptions of themselves as parents emerged from the findings. Specifically, they discussed how they felt guilty about being inadequate mothers and the effect this had on their children. For example, Pat felt guilt at placing the children in care. This guilt was further intensified when she discovered much later that both boys were sexually abused while in care. Guilt was evident in all the women's accounts. Tanner (2000) adds that as "motherhood is such a central component of women's identifies that [any] perceived 'failures' in this area hit at their very core" (p. 292).

Another perception evident in the women's narratives is "blame;" they perceived that they were somehow at fault. Here, the women blamed themselves for things that occurred in their families. For example, Helen continues to ponder on her daughter's long-standing alcohol problem: was her own depressive illness a factor? For all the mothers, the idea of not making the grade or falling short of being "a proper mother, a good mother, or a perfect mother" recurs throughout the women's narratives. It was unclear whether the expectation of being a perfect mother was a personal or a societal expectation or both. Nonetheless, it was evident that they believed they fell far from the ideal in their relationships with their children. This feeling agrees with Ritsher et al. (1997) in whose study 29 percent of the mothers felt that their mental illness had made it harder for them to be "good mothers." This also corresponds to recent findings in an UK study of mothers with arthritis (Grant, 2001). Similarly, Farber (2000) cites Francis-Connolly (1997, who found that:

The women held an "illusive ideal" of the perfect mother that was socially constructed. Her participants were constantly comparing themselves to this ideal and, at the same time, "feeling guilty for not being perfect" (p. 267).

It seems that the women in my study were similar to other groups of mothers. They were seeking maternal perfection that may be an unattainable goal for all mothers. However, perhaps for mothers with disabilities, both seen and, in the case of mental illness, unseen, this is an added factor that they have to contend with and be supported through. Furthermore, people involved in professional interventions must be careful not to compound mothers' feelings of inadequacies or further reinforce the ideal of the perfect mother.

For all the participants, being seen as a good mother and a good grandmother were powerful motivators. Today, according to the participants, most of them have stable relationships with their children, although these relationships may be either positive or negative. Their situations probably reflect the varied relationships experienced by all parents and their children.

Overall, being a mother, for these women, seemed to encompass being there for the children, supporting them, protecting them, giving advice, and moving them safely to adulthood. The participants believed that they failed to some degree to achieve this goal. There is, for each of them, a sense of loss in relation to being a mother. Some perceived their experiences to be diminished or narrowed in comparison to other mothers as a result of their mental illness. It is clear from their narratives that the women in my work experienced lack of support and feelings of powerlessness and were often socially isolated. It is useful to remember that these are identifiable factors linked to increased vulnerability to mental distress.

To conclude, all the women whom I had interviewed experienced mothering to some degree as an interrupted occupation as a result of their mental illness. For those who are now grandmothers, this role offers and affords a more positive experience of mothering. They clearly value this opportunity to be engaged with their grandchildren and benefited from developing a different relationship with their own children. The implications of these findings will be considered.

⤷ Messages from Mothers—Implications for Practice and Future Research

This final section will discuss the implications for practice and research. It contains messages for a range of practitioners as well as academics. For the women in this study, whose experiences spanned several decades of mental health care, the message is clear: mothers with mental illness need support. As individuals, they each experienced little support or indeed little recognition of their unique and complex roles as mothers. Not all mothers with mental illness will require support with the occupation of mothering, but some will, and all should be asked if they have unmet needs in respect of their capacity to mother. Assessment procedures concerned with maternal capacity should be supportive rather than punitive. In addition, such assessments should acknowledge their strengths and not undermine the mother's identity or confidence.

Mothers must be partners in the process because they may have a range of strategies or developed solutions that will work for them if they are provided with the necessary information or support. There is a need for the development and provision of services across inpatient and community services: importantly, not just supporting new mothers, but also supporting mothers who have recurrent episodes of mental illness and who therefore face a range of different issues as their children grew up and their caring demands change. There is also a need to work with mothers and families to include their insider perspective to change or design services.

It is important, too, that children and young people have access to explanations and support when their mother becomes ill or is hospitalized. How different such an approach may have been for Helen's and Pat's children we will never know. Explanations and age-appropriate education on what was happening to their mothers may have helped their children to understand they were not to blame or how they could best help. That said, children's contact with services should be welcoming and informative. Appropriate resources should be available for children when they accompany their mothers or visit hospital or mental health facilities. The provision of suitable environments and staff members who are able to interact appropriately with children is essential.

It is also important that the family be placed at the center of the decision-making process. Health professionals, including occupational therapists, have a part to play in working with women to support their roles as mothers. This may include coordinating practical support or developing effective coping strategies to deal with the pressures of mothering. The use of occupation to develop positive infant-mother relationships is well documented. Occupational therapists can be involved with mothers in structuring their day, maximizing their abilities to encourage appropriate play and create environments that facilitate their child's development. We have a responsibility to provide information and advice on local community supports and possible networks. These may not be necessarily linked to mental illness organizations. For example, local mothers' and children's groups can be found in churches and community centers. Being aware of local groups that can offer support and reduce the isolation often experienced by mothers is essential. We may need to help mothers engage with such groups. In working with mothers, we must remain sensitive to their needs, and therefore our interventions need to complement their needs and not burden them further. We should work in partnership with mothers, identifying suitable times and places for interventions to take place, with childcare available if necessary.

Children should also be included in the occupational therapist's reasoning because there is increasing recognition of the needs of children with mentally ill parents (Hetherington, 2000). Such children require a range of support mechanisms, including education

on mental illness and opportunities to discuss their own experiences and develop coping skills. Professionals must understand the mental health issues and be aware of the effects of mental illness. However, they must also be aware of child protection issues.

The research cited in this chapter has included a range of methodologies; all the work has contributed to the field. However, there are implications for future research. Francis-Connelly (2000) previously identified the need for research across the continuum of motherhood. My own work did not set out to examine mothering explicitly, although its importance to the participants emerged as a strong finding. The occupation of mothering for women with mental illness is clearly an area of study that warrants further action and research. The work presented here could be replicated with a larger cohort, or in other cultures and countries. Similarly, specific research aimed at further exploring the occupation of mothering could be undertaken; different research methods may offer valuable insights. Furthermore, research is needed to examine and understand the occupation of mothering from a range of perspectives and differences over time. Opportunities exist for multidisciplinary research. Importantly, this requires involving mothers who are both current and past consumers of services to play an important role in the design of research and the implementation and dissemination of the findings.

♪ Conclusion

This chapter has presented an overview of women with severe mental illness. It has highlighted that, until recently, this group of women had received little attention and that little was known of their lives and their experiences of mothering. My work has added, in a small way, to the existing knowledge base. What clearly emerged from the study was that mothering was a significant and meaningful occupation for these women and that they had received little or no support in this role from either mental health or social services. If we are to create better services for future mothers and their children, we need to be proactive to ensure that, in whatever area of practice we find ourselves, we do not negate that mothering is the core role and the most meaningful occupation for many of our clients. By giving women the opportunity to highlight their needs and issues, we may be in a position to offer practical, educational, and emotional support. Such support may make a difference in the lives of women with mental illness. It may enable them to experience mothering as a positive occupation that they can jointly share with their children, with few or no interruptions.

Discussion Questions 🐾

- How can mothers be placed at the center of assessment in a way that values their skills and contributions?

- What staff training is required to support mothers with mental illness?

- If society values mothering, what role can health and social care professionals play in addressing the inequalities that increase women's vulnerability to mental distress?

- In what ways, methodologically, can we further address the occupation of mothering?

References

Atkinson, R. (1998). *The life story interview* (Vol. 44). London (UK): Sage Publications.

Bachrach, L. L. (1985). Chronic mentally ill women: Emergence and legitimation of program issues. *Hospital and Community Psychiatry, 36*(10), 1063–1069.

Bachrach, L. L., & Nadelson, C. C. (Eds.) (1988). *Treating chronically mentally ill women*. Washington: American Psychiatric Press Inc.

Busfield, J. (1996). *Men, women and madness: Understanding gender and mental disorder*. London (UK): Macmillan Press.

Carmen, E. H., Russo, N. F., & Miller, J. B. (1981). Inequality and women's mental illness: An overview. *American Journal of Psychiatry, 138*, 1319–1330.

Clark, F. (1993). Occupation embedded in a real life: Interweaving occupational science and occupational therapy. *American Journal of Occupational Therapy, 47*(12), 1067–1078.

Chesler, P. (1972). *Women and madness*. New York: Doubleday and Co.

Chesler, P. (1996). Women and madness: The mental asylum. In T. Heller, G. Reynolds, R. Gomrn, R.

Muston, & S. Pattison (Eds.). *Mental Health Matters: A Reader* (pp. 46–53). London (UK): MacMillan Press Ltd.

Cleaver, H., Unell, I., and Aldgate, J. (1999). *Children's needs—Parenting capacity. The impact of parental mental illness, problem alcohol and drug abuse, and domestic violence on children's development*. London (UK): The Stationery Office.

Cowan, P. J. (1996). Women's mental health issues: Reflections on past attitudes and present practices. *Journal of Psychosocial Nursing, 34*(4), 20–24.

Creswell, J. W. (1998). *Qualitative inquiry and research design: Choosing amongst The five traditions*. London (UK): Sage.

Doyal, L. (1995). *What makes women sick: Gender and the political economy of health*. London (UK): Macmillan Press Ltd.

Fanchiang, S. P. C. (1996). The other side of the coin: Growing up with a learning disability. *American Journal of Occupational Therapy, 50*(4), 277–285.

Farber, R. S. (2000). Mothers with disabilities: In their own voice. *American Journal of Occupational Therapy, 54*(3), 260–268.

Faugier, J. (1992). Taking women seriously. *Nursing Times, 88*(26), 62–63.

Fergusson, E., & Taylor, B. (1998). Grandmothers' role in preventing unnecessary accident and emergency attendances: Cohort study. *British Medical Journal, 717*, 1685.

Fortune, T. (1999). Students' fieldwork stories: Reflecting on supervision. In S. E. Ryan & E. A. Mckay (Eds.). *Thinking and reasoning in therapy: Narratives from practice*. Cheltenham (UK): Stanley Thornes.

Francis-Connolly, E. (2000). Toward an understanding of mothering: A comparison of two motherhood stages. *American Journal of Occupational Therapy, 54*(3), 281–289.

Frank, G. (1996). Life histories in occupational therapy clinical practice. *American Journal of Occupational Therapy, 50*(4), 251–264.

Frank, G. (2000). Venus on wheels: Two decades of dialogue, on disability, biography, and being female in America. Berkeley, CA: University of California Press.

Good Practices in Mental Health (1994). *Women and mental health: An information pack of mental health services for women in the UK*. London (UK): Good Practices for Mental Health.

Göpfert, M., Harrison, P., & Mahoney, C. (1999). *Keeping the family in mind. Participative research into mental ill health and how it affects the whole family*. Liverpool (UK): University of Liverpool.

Grant, M. (2001). Mothers with arthritis, childcare and occupational therapy: Insight through case studies. *British Journal of Occupational Therapy, 64*(7), 322–329.

Harding, F., & Sills, M. (1999). *Gender and health: Curriculum outlines*. London (UK): Commonwealth Secretariat.

Harlene, A. C., & Bernhard, L. A. (1994). Health care dilemmas for women with serious mental illness. *Advances in Nursing Science, 16*(3), 78–88.

Hetherington, R. (2000). *The Icarus Project. Professional interventions for mentally ill parents and their children: Building a European model. Executive Summary of the Final Report to the European commission.* London (UK): Centre for Comparative Social Work Studies, Brunel University.

Hughes, J. L. (2002). Illness narrative and chronic fatigue syndrome/myalgic encephalomyelitis: A review. *British Journal of Occupational Therapy, 65*(1), 9-14.

Kielhofner, G., & Mallinson, T. (1995). Gathering narrative data through interviews: Empirical observation and suggested guidelines. *Scandinavian Journal of Occupational Therapy, 2,* 63–68.

Kohen, D. (Ed.). (2000). *Women and mental health.* London (UK): Routledge.

Larson, E. A. (2000). Mothering: Letting go of the past ideal and valuing the real. *American Journal of Occupational Therapy, 54*(3), 249–251.

Main, T. (1948). Mothers and children in psychiatric hospital. *Lancet, 11,* 845.

Mallinson, T., Kielhofner, G., & Mattingly, C. (1996). Metaphor and meaning in a clinical interview. *American Journal of Occupational Therapy, 50*(5), 338–346.

Mattingly, C. (1999). *Healing dramas and clinical plots: The narrative structure of experience.* Cambridge: Cambridge University Press.

Maykut, P., & Morehouse, R. (1994). *Beginning qualitative research. A philosophic and practical guide.* London (UK): Falmer Press.

McKay, E. A. (2002). *"Rip that whole book up—I've changed": Life and work narratives of mental illness.* Unpublished doctoral dissertation, University of Strathclyde, Glasgow.

McKay, E. A., & Ryan, S. E. (1995). Clinical reasoning through storytelling: Examining a student's case-story on a fieldwork placement. *British Journal of Occupational Therapy, 58*(6), 234–238.

Mickulsci, B. A. (1936). Motherhood: A gift of love (1991). Philadelphia: Running Press.

MIND (1992). *Stress on women: Policy paper on women and mental health.* London (UK): National Association for Mental Health.

Mostert, E., Zacharkiewicz, A., & Fossey, E. (1996). Claiming the illness experience: Using narrative to enhance theoretical understanding. *Australian Occupational Therapy Journal, 43,* 125–132.

Nahmias, R., & Froelich, J. (1993). Women's mental health: Implications for occupational therapy. *American Journal of Occupational Therapy, 47*(1), 35–41.

Oates, M. (1997). Patients as parents: The risk to children. *British Journal of Psychiatry, 170* (supp. 32), 22–27.

Office for Population Censuses and Surveys (1994). *Surveys of psychiatric morbidity in Great Britain bulletin No. l: The Prevalence of psychiatric morbidity among adults aged 16–64 living in private households in Great Britain.* London (UK): OPCS.

Owen, S., Repper, J., Perkins, R., & Robinson, J. (1998). An evaluation of services for women with long-term mental health problems. *Journal of Psychiatric and Mental Health Nursing, 5,* 281–290.

Payne, S. (1995). The rationing of psychiatric beds: Changing trends in sex-ratios in admission to psychiatric hospitals. *Health and Social Care in the Community, 3,* 289–300.

Polkinghorne, D. E. (1995). Narrative configuration in qualitative analysis. *Qualitative Studies in Education, 8*(1), 5–23.

Polkinghorne, D. E. (1996). Transformative narratives: From victimic to agentic life plots. *American Journal of Occupational Therapy, 50*(4), 299–305.

Popay, J. & Jones, G. (1990). Patterns of wealth and illness among lone parents. *Journal of Social Policy, 19,* 499–534

Price-Lackey, P., & Cashman, J. (1996). Jenny's story: Reinventing oneself through occupation and narrative configuration. *American Journal of Occupational Therapy, 50*(4), 306–314.

Primeau, L. A. (1996). Work versus non-work. The case of household work. In R. Zemke & F. Clark (Eds.). *Occupational Science: The evolving discipline* (pp 57–70), Philadelphia: F. A. Davis.

Repper, J., Perkins, R., Owen, S., Deighton, D., & Robinson, J. (1996). Evaluating services for women with serious and ongoing mental health problems: Developing an appropriate research method. *Journal of Psychiatric and Mental Health Nursing, 3*(1), 39–46.

Repper, J., Perkins, R., & Owen, S. (1998). 'I wanted to be a nurse...but I didn't get that far': women with serious ongoing mental health problems speak about their lives. *Journal of Psychiatric and Mental Health Nursing, 5,* 505–513.

Ritsher, J. E. B., Coursey, R. D., & Farrell, E. W. (1997). A survey on issues in the lives of women with severe mental illness. *Psychiatric Service, 48*(10), 1273–1282.

Roffe, D., & Roffe, C. (1995). Madness and community care: A medieval perspective. *British Medical Journal, 311,* 1708–1713.

Royal College of Nursing (1994). *RCN Guidelines,* Number 30. London (UK): Royal College of Nursing.

Ruddick, S. (1989). *Maternal thinking: Towards a politics of peace.* Boston: Beacon Press.

Ryan, S., & McKay, E.A. (Eds.) (1999). *Thinking and reasoning in therapy: Narratives from practice.* Cheltenham(UK): Stanley Thornes.

Schempp, P. (1995). Life history and narrative: questions, issues, and exemplary work. In J. A. Hatch & R. Wisniewski (Eds.). *Life history and narrative.* London (UK): The Falmer Press.

Showalter, E. (1985). *The female malady: women, madness and English culture 1830–1980.* London (UK): Virago.

Spradley, J. (1979). *The ethnographic interview.* New York: Rinehart & Winston.

Stein, A., Gath, D., Bucher, J., Day, A., & Cooper, P. (1991) The relationship between postnatal depression and mother child interaction. *British Journal of Psychiatry,* 158: 393–397.

Subotsky, F. (1991). Issues for women in the development of mental health Services. *British Journal of Psychiatry, 158* (suppl. 10), 17–21.

Tanner, D. (2000). Crossing bridges over troubled waters?: Working with children of parents experiencing mental distress. *Social Work Education, 9*(3), 287–297.

Test, M. A., & Berlin, S. B. (1981). Issues of special concern to chronically mentally ill women. *Professional Psychology, 12*(1), 136–145.

Ussher, J. (1991). *Women's madness: Misogyny or mental illness.* London (UK): Harvester Wheatsheaf.

Wahl, O. F., & Hunter, J. (1992). Are gender effects being neglected in schizophrenia research? *Journal of Abnormal Psychology, 86,* 195–198.

Weich, S. & Lewis, G. (1998). Poverty, unemployment and common mental disorders: Population based cohort study. *British Medical Journal, 317,* 15-119.

William, G. (1984). The genesis of chronic illness: Narrative reconstruction. *Sociology of Health and Illness, 6*(2), 175–200.

CHAPTER *13*

Mothering from Prison: It Can Be Done!

Cristina Jose-Kampfner, PhD

Introduction
The Problem
Factors Leading to Incarceration
Nonviolent Crimes: Drugs and Property Offenses
Poverty
Unemployment
Mothers' Histories of Abuse
The Arrest Experience: The Beginning of Occupational Deprivation
The Children Suffer
Voices of Mothers and Their Children
Pregnancy and Giving Birth
A Ghost Mother: Mothering from Prison
Visitation
Phone Calls and Letters
Mothering and the State
How the Children's Visitation Program Supports Mothering
Conclusion

 Anticipated Outcomes

I anticipate that, after reading this chapter, readers will:

- Understand the occupational deprivation that occurs when women who are mothers are incarcerated and are unable to perform many of their mothering occupations

- Have an increased understanding of the lives of mothers in prison and of the lives of their children from their mothers' firsthand stories

- Understand how mothering can continue even in the difficult context of prison and that social justice demands that this basic human right—to important human relationships like mothering—be supported

- Be better equipped to respond to the unique needs of women who are mothering from prison in the spirit of social justice

- Consider the unique needs of women who are mothering from prison within the context of their own personal and professional lives

ℒ✦ Introduction

I think of myself, my identity, as a mother first, then as a Latina, then as a woman with a profession. I am a college professor. I have a doctoral degree in clinical psychology. I am a community organizer and I have many other roles. These roles are complementary. However, when it comes to being a mother, that is the role that defines who I am, what has always been central in my life. My children are at the core of my identity. As a counselor in a prison, I was often moved by the pain and constant worry that these women had concerning their children. While working in a prison, I was often overcome by the painful thought, "What would I do if I were in prison and could not touch or see my children whenever I wanted?" It seemed that worrying about their children was often the only mothering occupation available for the women in prison. These women prisoners and I share love for our children. When these women talked about their children, the expressions on their faces changed, and they seemed to be different people. Like all mothers, they showed photographs of their children and commented on their qualities. When I finished my doctorate, I asked the women prisoners who had generously helped me to make the study possible what I could do for them (Jose, 1985). Their unanimous answer was, "We want regular visits with our children." All these women wanted was to visit with their children, to touch and hold them. The love these mothers had for their children was the force that made it imperative for me to keep struggling with a prison administration that was not interested in having a visitation program for incarcerated women, which I was struggling to create. Often the struggle to get this program created seemed impossible, but the women's love for their children would not let me quit. It took 4 years of bureaucratic efforts to get a program approved.

With the help of women doing life sentences in prison, I founded the Children's Visitation Program (CVP) in southeast Michigan in 1988. This program is the social action that resulted from my doctoral research. The CVP has taken place one Saturday each month for the past 15 years. It is held in the women's prison visiting room that is converted just for the afternoon into a playroom where mothers can play, read stories, do their children's hair, and talk and listen to their children who have been brought to the prison to visit their mother. In short, for 4 hours, women who are in prison can do intensive mothering (Jose-Kampfner, 1991). The CVP relies on volunteers who provide transportation to the children for their visits. I also coordinate this volunteer component, in which a particular child (or children) from a family is assigned a transportation volunteer. Volunteers pick up the children and later return them to their current homes. I provide support and guidance to these volunteers as they form important relationships with the children. When the first meeting of the CVP happened, the sight of these mothers and their children holding each other with faces of joy and contentment was worth all the years of effort. The intense mothering that is done in 4 hours that must hold these children until the next visit keeps me working with these women and their children. I also continue to do research related to this program (Jose-Kampfner, 1991, 1995).

In this chapter I will present the stories of some women who are mothering from prison. I have given them pseudonyms to protect their confidentiality. I will highlight the meaningfulness of mothering for women that creates the possibility of mothering from prison, a place of occupational deprivation.

ℒ✦ The Problem

It is estimated that more than 1.3 million minor children in the United States have mothers under correctional sanction (Greenfield & Snell, 1999). A majority of women who are incarcerated are mothers of children under the age of 18 (Mumola, 2000). The actual numbers can vary, depending on the agency that reports them. This is likely because women who are sentenced to prison tend to hide information about their children. They fear that the state will take their children away from them. From my experience working with mothers in prison, 80 percent is a reasonable estimate of women who are mothering. In Table 13–1, some other relevant statistics about parents in general, and mothers in particular, are presented. These statistics were based on a 1997 Survey of Inmates in State and Federal Correctional Facilities as reported by Mumola, a policy analyst for the Bureau of Justice. Because this chapter focuses on women who are mothering from prison, the most relevant information for this discussion includes the percentage of mothers in prison reporting living with their children before admission (64 percent), the variety of placements for children during their mother's incarceration—the largest percentage living with grandparents (52.9 percent), and the degree and type of contact reported by mothers with their children during incarceration. These statistics are helpful in defining the scope of the problem of mothering from prison.

♨ Factors Leading to Incarceration

Nonviolent Crimes: Drug and Property Offenses

Women are in prison because they have committed, in a large majority, nonviolent crimes. Women are considerably more likely than men to be incarcerated for nonviolent offenses such as drug or property offenses (Mauer, Potler, & Wolf, 1999). However, many people who commit the same crimes are not "doing time" in prison. Minorities, especially African-Americans and Hispanics from low socioeconomic backgrounds, are more likely to be incarcerated. Drugs are a case in point. There are millions of illegal drug users who are not in prison. Women doing time in prison for drug-related crimes have increased tremendously since 1981, and they account for the large increase in women prisoners. The inception of the war on drugs in the 1980s has had a much more profound impact on poor minor-

Table 13–1 Selection of relevant facts about parents in prison and their children in the United States*		
The issue	**Parents involved**	**Percentage**
Number of state and federal prisoners with children under age 18	721,500 prisoners were parents to 1,498,800 children	
Mothers in state prisons who reported having more than one child	Actual number of mothers was not provided in the report	45
Parents' living arrangements before incarceration	Number of mothers and fathers who reported living with their children	Mothers 64 Fathers 44
Living arrangements for children after their mothers' incarceration	Child(ren) living with other parent who is not in prison Child(ren) living with grandparent Child(ren) living with another relative Child(ren) living in foster home/agency placement Child(ren) living with other relatives, friends, or others	28 52.9 25.7 9.6 10.4
Mothers reporting weekly contact with their children	Mothers in the state prisons who reported weekly contact Mothers in the state prisons who reported phone contact Mothers in the state prisons who reported contact via mail	60 40 45
Maintaining personal contact with children from prison	Mothers who reported not having a personal visit with their children since admission to prison	54
Parental ethnicity and incarceration	Likelihood of African-American children having a parent in prison Likelihood of Hispanic children having a parent in prison Likelihood of Caucasian children having a parent in prison	7 2.6 0.8

*Derived from Mumola, 2000 analysis of United States Bureau of Justice statistics

ity women. In 1986 one of every eight women in prison (12 percent) was convicted of drug felonies. In 1996, this rose to one in three (37 percent) (Mauer, Potler, & Wolf, 1999).

When women are incarcerated for a violent offense, they are twice as likely as men to have committed their offense against someone close to them, such as an abusive spouse (Mumola, 2000). The circumstances of violent crimes for which women are convicted often involve a woman acting in self-defense against an abusive male partner or as an accomplice to a male partner who is the one who actually commits the violence involved in the crime.

Poverty

What appears to be a determinant of the incarceration of women is poverty. The majority of incarcerated women are poor. Additionally, their poverty works against them in sentencing. This issue is illustrated in the following vignette.

⌘ *Vignette:* **Lola**

Lola was 24 years old when she was sentenced for attempted murder, which occurred while she was being beaten by her abusive boyfriend during an argument about his abandonment of her and their children. Excerpts from her pre-sentence report, the report prepared by a probation officer upon which a judge relies in deciding what sentence to impose, state:

> Lola does have four illegitimate daughters fathered by three different men. About the only thing the fathers seemed to share in common is that none of them support their children. ... They are presently in the custody of their maternal grandmother ... and are supported by ADC.
>
> Lola's employment record is practically non-existent. For short periods of time in the past, she has worked as a cook. For the most part, Lola appears to have been content to live off Welfare. At the present time, she has no income, savings, assets, or large debts.
>
> To be realistic, it is felt that sentencing in this matter should be envisioned as strictly punitive. To date, respondent has led a remarkably parasitic and useless lifestyle. Although opportunities for rehabilitation exist in prison, we are less than optimistic with prospects that Lola will avail herself of them. Respondent has never been a contributing member of society in the past and we fear she will continue to live off the public in the future whether she is incarcerated or on the street.

Based on this pre-sentence report, Lola was sentenced to life in prison, although she could have received a much shorter sentence if she had been a woman of means who could pay a lawyer to uncover evidence and build a case using expert witnesses.   ⌘

Unemployment

Another factor to consider is women's employment status. In many cases, before a mother's arrest, her family typically survived on less than $600 per month. Sixty percent of women in state prison were unemployed before their incarceration, and nearly 30 percent of women prisoners were receiving welfare assistance immediately before their arrest. Thus, women are more likely than men to be serving sentences for drug offenses (39 vs. 29 percent respectively) and other nonviolent crimes (44 vs. 40 percent) that have a base in economic motives (Greenfield and Snell, 1999).

Poverty imposes stress on mothers struggling to support a family—stress that is often expressed in frustration, despair, and depression. Poverty also functions as a precursor to abuse. McLoyd (1990) argues that poor mothers experience higher levels of stress and are more punitive toward their children than mothers who are financially secure, making poor children more likely to be physically abused. Thus, addressing the structural variable of poverty is critical, not only because it is an important risk factor in its own right, but also because of its connection to other criminogenic influences such as child maltreatment, delinquency, and substance abuse. Although these factors are generally examined individually, multiple factors may accumulate and interact to create a destructive pathway that leads from poverty to prison.

Mothers' Histories of Abuse

Most women prisoners (57 percent of state prisoners and almost 40 percent of federal prisoners) have histories of being physically and/or sexually abused before incarceration. More than a third of women in state prisons (36.7 percent) and almost a quarter of women in federal prisons (23.0 percent) suffered physical and/or sexual abuse as children. Significant numbers of women (28 percent of state prisoners and 15 percent of federal prisoners) suffered both physical and sexual abuse at some time in their lives. Similarly, almost 37 percent of state prisoners and 23 percent of federal prisoners were abused as children age 17 or younger; 45 percent of state prisoners and 31 percent of federal prisoners were abused at age 18 or older, and almost 25 percent of state prisoners and 14 percent of federal prisoners were abused as both children and adults. Additionally, 37 percent of state prisoners and 21 percent of federal prisoners suffered rape or attempted rape before admission to prison. Not surprisingly, 80 percent of abused women had used illegal drugs regularly and 69 percent of abused women reported drinking regularly at some point in their lives (Harlow, 1999).

These figures were compiled on the basis of surveys conducted between 1995 and 1997. These numbers are probably lower than the actual reality because of the many reasons why women do not report abuse in general, and specifically because of the distrust most women prisoners have of authority. The distrust of authority itself is rooted in their experiences of abuse: almost 91 percent of women in state prison and 95 percent of women in federal prisons who disclosed their abuse in these surveys knew their abusers, and the overwhelming majority of their abusers were family members and spouses/ex-spouses or boyfriends/girlfriends (Harlow, 1999). Neither do these figures reflect the reality of the repeated and virtually inescapable abuse these women suffered at the hands of abusers who lived in their own homes and the constant feelings of fear, dread, and anxiety suffered in anticipation of the next incident between incidents of abuse.

It is important to note here that women who are mothering from prison are, in many respects, not that different from women who are not in prison and are mothering. In both groups there are good mothers and not-so-good mothers. In both groups there are histories of abuse, poverty, and unemployment. In both groups there are women who strongly desire to be good mothers and others who do not. But there is one major difference between women who are mothering from prison and women who are not, and that is the multiple marginalizations that are experienced by the women in prison.

This discussion raises the question of whether a woman who has committed a crime can still be a good mother (Schram, 1999). Are these circumstances—being a woman in prison and being a good mother—mutually exclusive? That question is problematic because it implies a definition of a good mother. I contend that there is no one universal definition of a good mother because such a definition depends on multiple factors, such as culture, age of the child, etc. Therefore, I believe that no one circumstance, specifically that of having committed a crime, can negate the desire and need that a woman has to be a good mother.

☙ The Arrest Experience: The Beginning of Occupational Deprivation

For most women prisoners, the occupational deprivation that begins with the separation from their children at the time of their arrest is dramatic and frightening (Whiteford, 2000). These mothers are not given time to make arrangements for their children, but try to arrange for them to go with someone as soon as possible after they arrive at the police station. For women arrested on a murder charge, it probably means that this is the last time, if ever, they will see their children in the "free world." The term "free world" is used by most of the women to refer to the world outside the prison. For the children, it marks the beginning of a long, bitter journey of separation. Some children will not see their mothers for a year or two. Some will never see their mothers again. This issue is illustrated in the experience of three mothers, Jean, Sarah, and Lynn, who are quoted in the following paragraphs.

Jean was 17 years old when she was arrested. Because she was married, although not living with her husband, she was treated as an adult.

> My son was two years old when I got here. He did not really understand what was going on when the police took me to be questioned. That was the last day I saw him.

Sarah had left her daughter at a friend's house on the day of the arrest.

> When I was arrested, my daughter was with my friend. She did not see me any more until much later. When I was in the county jail before I was sentenced, the hardest thoughts to live with, for me, were that I may never see my daughter again. My aunt was very angry with me for what happened. I could not see my daughter, and my aunt would not come and see me so I could know what was going on with my daughter.

Lynn tells about her arrest:

> The day I was arrested is so painful that it has been erased from my mind. I cannot even think about it. I remember faces, the faces of my children, the room where I was when the police came to arrest me—that is all I can remember. The first memory I have is when I was at the county jail. I used to think of my children and ask myself why? Why? Why did you do that? I would think of my children being mocked at by their friends about me. I could not see them. I wanted to know what they were thinking, but I was ashamed to see them too. Now I always get into big depressions when the facts sink in. If I ever come out of here, my kids will be grown-people and I will have missed all these years with them. That can never change. You lose your children, and when you come out of here, you find strangers that you have to get to know as grown-ups.

The children may or may not be present at the arrest. When children are not present in the home at the time of the arrest, many of the arresting officers do not even ask the women if they have any children. If they do ask, no attention is paid to critical arrangements for childcare. Historically, police conduct has been appalling in their disregard for the children's needs.

When the children are present at the time of the parent's arrest, at best, police tend to overlook them, giving them no explanations, much less reassurances. Stanton's study (1980) of children with mothers in jail reports that 80 percent of the children had been present at the time of arrest. Usually the children are taken away in a police car, often separated from their mothers, and are taken to the police station, where they wait separated from their mothers until someone, either a relative, friend, or social services agent, arrives to take them.

Alice, a prisoner and mother of three children who, at the time of the arrest, were 8, 6, and 4 years old, commented:

> The day the police came to get me, I was getting ready to send the kids to school. The children were at the store with me. They could not understand what was going on, neither did I. I have never been in trouble with the police. I asked the policeman what was going on, and he said I was charged with conspiracy to kill my husband. The two younger kids were clutching (sic) into my legs crying. The older one started to cry, and the only thing that she wanted to know was if I was coming back soon. I told them not to worry, that this was a mistake. I told them I was coming back soon. So the kids stayed until their father came. How little I knew of the nightmare that was to follow.

Nancy, another mother who was in prison, talks about her feelings about the occupational deprivation:

> Every day when my children are spread apart from each other, someone is preparing their daily meal at dinner time. About 400 miles away, their mother is sitting on a bunk bed, listening to music, crocheting, reading, writing a letter or

just relaxing … something is terribly wrong with this picture. There are other alternatives to this situation; solutions that would benefit the welfare of the children.

At worst, police treat children the same way they treat their mothers, pointing guns at them and ordering them away from their mothers, up against walls or onto the floor. The children also suffer by having their personal and special belongings searched by the police. "The police got my teddy bear and tore it up with a knife," said one 6-year-old.

Another mother who was a prisoner, Carla, tells us:

> The day I was arrested my two-year-old and my four-year-old were home. The police burst into my house and cut open the heads of my four-year-old daughter's dolls to search for drugs as my child looked on in tears. They handcuffed me and led me away without giving me an opportunity to comfort my children.

Cindy has two children, ages 11 and 5 years. When she came to prison, her youngest was 3 months old. Cindy tells us:

> The day I was arrested…I remember it so well. The children were scared and so was I. Elsa (the oldest daughter) did not want to let me go. The policeman said to her that I will be back soon but that I must go now. She believed him and let go. It took almost nine months before I saw her again. You know, Elsa, my oldest child, was just seven when I left her.

Some children will go to relatives. Children have told me that they were sent in a taxi to a grandmother's house at 3 AM when the police came to the house. Even relatives, however, are not an adequate substitute for a child's mother. Many women just want to give custody to a family member so that the state will not become involved, even when they realize that sending the child to an unstable relative or chaotic family situation is not an optimal placement for the child.

Another mother, Barbara, recalls:

> I have been in prison for eleven years. The day I was arrested is still very vivid in my mind. The day I got picked up to go to jail I did not want to leave my child with my mother. The thought of my child having to go through all I went through living with my mother…it hurt to think of him feeling what I used to feel as a child. Would she beat him up the same way I was? Would she call him "liar" like she used to do with me? Would he feel lonely and helpless like I felt? All these questions came to my mind. The pain was unbearable. I had no choice. The choices were my mother, where at least I would know what kind of home that was, or someone else whom I would not know.

Some of the children will be placed in foster care homes and will be separated from their brothers and sisters in addition to their mothers. Jodie's four children are separated in different homes and towns. Jodie's mother told me:

> They have made orphans of the children. They cry and miss their parents whom they love and were good to them.

For women convicted of a crime and sentenced to incarceration, entering prison was the transition between their role as mothers and being relegated to sitting on the sidelines of their children's lives or losing them altogether. Parenting from prison is very difficult because in most states the incarceration of mothers is considered neglect of the children, and if the sentence is longer than 2 years, mothers can lose their parental rights (Beckerman, 1991).

The Children Suffer

> My children are the ones that are suffering the most. My son, Stanley, always asked me, "Mama, when are you coming home?" I replied, "Soon." After six years he said, "Mama, soon sure takes a long, long time."—Lovetta

Women with children are arrested daily in the United States. In spite of this reality, the consequences for their children have not been addressed (Baunach, 1985; Dressel, Porterfield, & Sandra, 1998; Greene, Haney, & Hurtado, 2000; Henriques, 1982). Judges do not take into account the number of children the women have before giving them their sentences. If the judge considers the children at all before sentencing the women, it is usually negatively. If it is decided that a woman has not performed her maternal role according to middle-class social values, this fact will count against her in her sentencing.

The conspiracy of silence that surrounds parental incarceration is ubiquitous and leaves the children severely isolated, forcing them to cope as best they can alone with their overwhelming feelings of trauma, loss, grief, depression, anger, and guilt. Even if the children are present at the arrest, the conspiracy of silence about their mother's location is common. Most children are misinformed. A 5-year-old told me one day while we were leaving the prison: "Cristina, can I tell you a secret? My grandmother thinks that this is a hospital but this is a prison. Please don't tell her anything." The wall of silence is erected from the time of arrest. Children are told little or nothing about what is happening or why, and the adults involved show little or no inclination to listen to the children's feelings and concerns. This process of withholding from the children information about what is happening to their mothers and to them, and of effectively silencing the children from expressing their feelings and concerns, continues throughout the children's experience of their mothers' incarceration.

The children did not commit a crime, but they are often stigmatized at school, church, and among peers and their peers' mothers. Children of imprisoned mothers are frequently rejected or taunted by friends, relatives, and teachers. Children then react through aggressive or withdrawn behavior or with regression, nightmares, enuresis, insomnia, truancy, poor achievement, deep depression, and even suicide.

To the children, even in the most ideal home setting, it feels as if they are isolated, alone, bearing the experience of their mothers' incarceration as if it were a secret only they know about. It seems as if their feelings do not matter and even that they should not have feelings about losing their mother to incarceration. This is the one consistent message that children receive from every venue of society with which they have contact during their mothers' incarceration.

On the outside, the children suffer without their mothers. When a mother is incarcerated, children generally move to a different household. The majority begin living with a relative, especially a grandparent, but others go somewhere else, such as foster care. New rules of conduct in possibly unfamiliar settings await them. Relatives may resent taking on a new parenting role or may possess insufficient health, finances, or other resources to do so. Unlike the case with foster parents, who are paid adequately for caring for children and who have access to paid support services, financial aid and support services available to relatives are minimal to nonexistent. On the average, children with mothers in prison move three to four times. Jamul, one of the children who participated in the Children's Visitation Program, had moved seven times during 2 years. Some of the children in the study had been moved to different homes of family members as many as nine times. This carries with it the problem of changing schools and friends.

In a study that I conducted (Jose-Kampfner, 1995), I found that some of the children with mothers in prison suffered post-traumatic stress disorder or depression. Often the children felt homeless because they could be moved if the family member or foster parent is upset with their behavior or if the health or economic situation of the family member or foster parent changes. For the children in my study, there had been no evidence of these conditions before their witnessing their mother's arrest and the subsequent forced separation from their mother. After these events, they were exhibiting hyperactivity, attention deficit, delinquency (for example, stealing or fighting), teenage pregnancy, withdrawal from social relationships, and/or retreat into denial and fantasy. About 75 percent of the children studied reported symptoms including depression, difficulty in sleeping, concentration problems, and flashbacks about their mother's crimes and arrests (Jose-Kampfner, 1995). Four of the seven children interviewed reported hearing their mother's voices sometimes. Other children reported difficulty in concentrating. The caretakers interviewed agreed with the symptoms that the children reported, but did not know what to do and did not think that it was because of their mother's incarceration, but rather a "problem of the child."

Other research on incarcerated mothers and their children has often focused on how children's lives are affected by their mothers' incarceration. Studies have examined and evaluated visits and contact between mothers and children (Baunach, 1985; Bloom & Steinhart, 1993; Johnston, 1995c; Stanton, 1980), care and placement of the children (Baunach, 1985; Beckerman, 1994; Johnston, 1995a; Sametz, 1980), legal issues with regard to custody and care (Barry, Ginchild, & Lee, 1995; Bloom & Steinhart, 1993; Smith, 1995; Stanton, 1980), and interventions and social services (Hairston & Lockett, 1987; Johnston, 1995b; Weilerstein, 1995).

It is usual for children to suffer from the effects of poverty and other marginalizations before their mothers go to prison. Their mothers' incarceration adds one more marginalization. Research on the topic of children of prisoners has linked parental incarceration with social, emotional, and cognitive delays among the children as well as behavioral problems at home and at school (Fritsch & Burkhead, 1982). Having a parent in prison is particularly hard on those children who had a positive relationship with the offender. They mourn the loss of their parent and tend to exhibit reactions like denial, guilt, anger, low self-esteem, lack of motivation, depression, and sadness.

ɛ♥ Voices of Mothers and Their Children

Children and their mothers suffer deeply when mothers are taken away to be imprisoned. The vast majority of these women were the primary caregivers for their children, who spent most of their time with their mothers and looked first to their mothers for support. Even when this was not the case and the mothers were often absent from the children's home or were "neglectful" by the standard of the middle class, mothers were still of integral importance to the lives of their children.

⌘ Vignette: *Sarah*

The story of Sarah illustrates the pain that the mothers suffer.

> I was 19 when the crime happened. I did not know that he had a gun when he went into the gas station. He came out running and told me to drive. He told me the attendant was hurt. The police came to the house and arrested me. When I was arrested, the only person that offered to take care of my two-year-old daughter was my aunt. I had mixed feelings, because I was so unhappy growing up with her, but I had no choice. It was either her or foster care. I did not want my child in foster care. I did not want my child in a situation where the family would be mistreating her, like so many of them do. People do it for money, not out of the goodness of their hearts; you never know what kind of family your kid will end up with. With my aunt, at least, I knew what to expect. I don't have any other family but her. My mother was still alive then, but I really did not know her, and, besides, that would have meant my child will be out of state. My aunt does not bring her to see me. I do not get to see her but once a year. She always has an excuse of not having any money to come from where we live to here. I guess when you live on so little money, you can't ask for much. When you do a long sentence, you are grateful if you at least can keep in contact with your kids. There are so many women that just do not know what happens with her kids. It is so sad when you are doing a long sentence; you lose your parental rights. They do not have to tell you what happened to the kids. It is not your business anymore. When I think of her, my stomach hurts. I cry so often and send her my love and blessing many times during the day. What else can I do? ⌘

Two other mothers, Venesa and Martina, echo the experience of Sarah in the vignette. Venesa, who is serving a life sentence for murdering an abusive husband, shares her experience. During one of our conversations, Venesa said:

> I can hardly remember what happened at the county jail, that is how upset I was. The only thing I recall is that I had a meal with them. As I am saying this to you, my stomach hurts, even after so many years. It is still an open wound.

Martina, a mother of two children, explained, "I never knew how badly my children have been hurt by my incarceration until I sat down and had a serious talk with them after my release."She has two sons. They were 6 and 8 years old when she entered prison. I have known Martina's children for the past 18 years. Their story is a clear example of how the incarceration of their mother has a profound impact on the lives of children. Martina tells us:

> My children grew up feeling grief and abandonment; anger, guilt and shame grew with them. They were called names at schools and the children would say "your mom is in prison." That hurt them. The pain they had was expressed in different ways. My youngest son learned at an early age to detach himself from people who would hurt him. My oldest son's feelings were often displayed through acts of aggression and delinquency behavior. The older he got, the angrier he became.

Martina's younger son finished college and, although he had some serious struggles emotionally, as well as health related, he was able to finish school. Her oldest son is presently doing a life sentence. When I visited him in the prison, he talked about the issues he had living with his grandmother. Although he dearly loved his grandmother, his childhood years spent with her were very painful. I remember him as a child, running on the streets playing. When I visited his grandmother, he would ask me when his mother was coming home. I have to say, with a sinking heart, that we have failed him as a society by ignoring his pain. He was very attached to his mother when the arrest happened, and no consideration was given to his situation.

The effect of a mother's incarceration on her children is a continuing source of concern for many mothers. For example, Maria tells us:

> My older son is having problems in school, and I think, from what I hear, that he is probably involved in drugs too. I have called him, but my mother did not accept the calls. I wrote to him, but I got no answer. He is very angry with me. He thinks I have deserted him. I asked the social worker over here to help me to find out what was happening to him. I wanted to know if he is really involved in drugs. She did not want to. She did not consider this an emergency and, besides, she felt that finding out what was going on with him would be of no use to me. She said I would just be upset, and there was nothing I could do. Every time you ask about your children, they think it is not an emergency. It is not for them, but it is for me.
>
> Ever since I found out about him taking drugs, I cannot sleep at night. I want to help him, but I'm cut off from him. If I was home, it would be different. You cannot be a parent long distance. You hear what other people tell you about them, but you do not know. It hurts to think that I have been eleven years away from them. (Her eyes filled with tears.) You know, your children pay for your crime too.

🐾 Pregnancy and Giving Birth

For some children, the separation starts at the beginning of their lives and birth is marked by sadness and deprivation of attachment with their mothers. I (Jose-Kampfner, 1995) found that 9 percent of women in prisons and jails surveyed revealed having given birth to a child while incarcerated. In Bloom and Steinhart's book (1993), they emphasized the importance of the first year of life for the creation of child-mother bonds. However, with the exception of some correctional facilities in the states of New York, Nebraska, Ohio, and Washington, United States prisons do not allow newborns and young infants to remain with their incarcerated mothers. Some states, such as North Carolina, have enacted legislation that allows a judge to defer incarceration of a pregnant woman convicted of a nonviolent crime until 6 weeks after the birth of her child. This provision allows the mother to experience some bonding with her child and provides her with an opportunity to establish adequate placement for the child (Bloom & Steinhart, 1993).

Except for these few programs, however, women who deliver their babies while in prison must leave their babies in the hospital and return to the prison (Modie, 1997). In most instances, when a woman gives birth during incarceration, she is allowed to spend only a few days at most with her newborn baby after delivery. Essential bonding of mother to infant cannot occur in such a short period of time, and this has serious implications for the future mother-child relationship. This is the most heartbreaking experience I had to endure while working at the prison. The mothers hold on to their babies and do not want to leave. Some mothers try to hurt themselves so they can stay with their baby a little bit longer. These children do not have the option to be breast-fed because their mothers return to the prison without their babies.

Another concern for high-risk pregnant prisoners is the use of shackles and restraints in the delivery room, transportation methods, and the management of perinatal drug addiction. The problem of pregnant, substance-dependent prisoners is complex and has critical implications for both the mother and her unborn child, particularly in relation to detoxification procedures and prenatal and postpartum care. Pregnant prisoners may also suffer emotional problems associated with denial of the right to choose between carrying the fetus to term or terminating the pregnancy (Catan, 1992).

🐾 A Ghost Mother: Mothering from Prison

Most of the mothers in prison will be reunited with their children. However, the children will be motherless for several years. As a child used to say to me, "My mother is like a ghost mother. I know she is there, but I cannot see her when I want to."

Visitation

I have facilitated the visits between children and their mothers through the Children's Visitation Program for many years, and I have seen the importance of these visits. Mothers who visit regularly with their children spend more time discussing important issues with their children. Just like outside mothers, these mothers have the same concrescence about their children, and the visits make it possible for them to mother their children even if the visits are restricted. It has not been unusual to see children in the visitation program sitting in their mother's lap and not moving for 3 hours. All they wanted was to fill themselves with the love of their mothers, hoping it could last them until the next visit.

Children who do not visit with their mothers regularly cannot benefit from this mothering and often are more emotionally affected. Often when I pick up children to bring them to see their mothers during the Children's Visitation Program, I find close to their beds a picture of them and their mothers that we take in the visiting room for them to take home.

Visitation is more difficult for incarcerated mothers and their families than for men. Koban (1983) concluded that female offenders have closer relationships with their children before incarceration than do men and that women's relationships with their children are more affected by incarceration. Koban also found that the women prisoners in her study experienced a significant disadvantage compared to male prisoners in attempting to maintain consistent contact with their children and the caregivers of these children. This is a factor that was associated with problems during reunification with their children. One of the reasons for infrequent visitation or nonvisitation by children of mothers in prison is the distance between the child's residence and the correctional facility (Bloom & Steinhart, 1993). Over 60 percent of the children lived more than 100 miles from the mother's place of incarceration (Mumola, 2000). Trips to the prison require a reliable car and gasoline money, and sometimes food and motel costs that many families do not have.

Another reason for the paucity of visits is that caretakers feel that they have to take care of the children, which takes their time, and visiting becomes one more burden for them. Gender issues also play an important role in visitation between women and their children. It is estimated that 80 percent of the women doing time in prison or jail are single mothers (Stanton, 1980) who were the primary caretakers of their children. Women are economically disadvantaged, and when they go to prison, the support of their children becomes one of their main stresses.

Even when children visit with their mothers in prison on a regular basis, contact may be quite limited. For example, some prisons offer minimal visiting opportunities or have stringent rules regarding legal guardianship, which make it difficult for the children's caregivers to bring them to see their mothers. From 1995 to 2002, the state of Michigan required that the only person who could bring a child to visit be a custodial parent or a legal guardian. For most of the women and children, caretakers other than the father have custody of the children under a legally binding power of attorney allowed under Michigan law. This gives the caretaker the ability to make decisions on behalf of the children, but leaves control of the child's placement with the mother. Legal guardianship in Michigan requires going to court, a task beyond the abilities of many caretakers and incarcerated mothers, in which case the mothers and children are not allowed to see each other for the duration of the mother's incarceration. Legal guardianship also takes away from the mothers all control over the children and places the control with the court and the guardian. After legal guardianship is granted, the guardian can petition the court for permanent custody of the children, and often the courts grant such petitions. Thus, this requirement puts the mother and children at risk of being permanently separated. Consequently, even when caretakers and mothers have the resources to access the courts to acquire legal guardianship status for the caretaker, mothers are forced to choose between risking the permanent loss of their children and seeing them while they remain incarcerated.

This is cruel and unusual punishment that makes mothering impossible. Fortunately, after a trial in Federal Court on the issue in 2000, the Court agreed that this provision violates Constitutional rights and struck down this rule. The Sixth Circuit Court of Appeals affirmed the lower court decision in 2002. So this rule no longer applies to Michigan prisoners and their children, and children who could not see their mothers because of the rule are now allowed to visit them. The State of Michigan, however, has appealed to the United States Supreme Court, and if the Supreme Court reverses the lower courts' decisions, the rules will revert to the conditions that were implemented in 1995.

Many states, including Michigan, continue to set up needless roadblocks to visitation between mothers and their children, both passively (e.g., by locating women's prisons in a place very distant from the place where the children reside) and aggressively (e.g., by imposing rules such as the one described). Motherhood is used inside the prison to punish women. The Children's Visitation Program, although a 100 percent volunteer-run program, is also used to punish women. The institution can pull the privilege of these special visits away at any time.

We must remember that most of these mothers will be reunited with their children some day. Prolonged occupational deprivation very probably diminishes the likelihood of appropriate adaptive responses when these women leave the prison (Whiteford, 2000). Lack of visitation is damaging for the mother/child relationship. In Michigan, the only visits that some of the mothers can have regularly with their children is through the Children's Visitation Program. Unfortunately, only a few women can participate because of the capacity of the visiting room and the large number of women and children. The institution gives priority to the women who have short sentences.

Phone Calls and Letters

Prison rules and regulations intentionally make meaningful contact between mothers, children and caretakers difficult to impossible. Telephoning from the prison is very expensive, and many families have a block on their phones. The cost of an average 15-minute call from prison can be as high as 10 to 15 dollars. As discussed earlier, a great majority of the women come from poor families and the families cannot absorb the expense of phone calls.

Letters are the mothers' main form of contact with their families, followed by telephone calls. These methods of communication are inadequate for a number of reasons. Letters to young children must be read to them and have little meaning to very young children. Information that the children or mothers consider to be strictly confidential between them may not be relayed either in writing or on the phone because the caretaker may read the letter or listen in on the phone conversation. Other mothers send their children little presents that they can afford, such as pieces of gum or candy. Mothers draw cards for their children and send them poems saying how much they love them. The delay between sending letters and receiving a response makes it difficult for mothers to provide comfort and advice about children's difficulties in a timely manner. It is also difficult to provide comfort and advice in a phone call that is repeatedly interrupted by announcements that the call is from a prison and that automatically cuts off at 15 minutes.

Mothering and the State

Women in prison must deal with many issues to keep their parental rights. More than 25 states have laws providing for the termination of parental rights or adoption statutes that explicitly pertain to incarcerated parents (Genty, 1995). Cooperation by the various state departments of corrections has been mixed, with few fully and actively supporting programs to minimize the problem and some failing to provide any programming to address the problem.

The programs for children of women who are incarcerated are often limited to what people are able to do outside the prison with little cooperation from the departments of corrections. Such programs include providing transportation and overnight lodging for regular prison visits, providing legal and other advocacy programs for mothers and children, providing supportive services to children and their caregivers, providing special activities such as camping, and gifts for the children for Christmas and sometimes other important occasions, providing counseling programs for the children and/or the caregivers, and providing family reunification programs and support services when mothers are released from prison.

Some departments of corrections have offered minimal assistance to incarcerated mothers and their children. Many have incorporated parenting classes into their programs for prisoners, although these classes are not aimed at the needs of mothers in prison (Harm & Thompson, 1997). These classes are provided by the departments of corrections or by allowing an outside agency to provide them. Some have allowed outside agencies to facilitate mothers making audio recordings of books and providing the recordings and books to the children. In at least one prison system, young children are allowed to bring in with them one toy that must be constructed in one piece with no moving parts, such as a teddy bear. In 2000, the Bureau of Milwaukee Child Welfare started a program to identify foster children who had incarcerated mothers and to arrange regular visits for them. In addition, prisoners in Wisconsin were given a 1-800 number and a code to call their children at the homes of foster mothers, whose phone numbers remain confidential (Abdul-Alim, 2000).

Some prison facilities have allowed "children's centers" to be instituted. Such centers usually consist of an area in the visiting room where children's toys and books, purchased either through the prisoner benefit fund and/or outside donor(s), are available during visitation, so that prisoners may have more meaningful interaction with their children. Sometimes these children's centers are in a room separate from the visiting room. When the centers are located in the visiting room, the mothers and children are allowed to play with the toys, but usually must still abide by regular visit rules, including that the prisoner may not leave her seat. When the children's center is located in another room, sometimes the mothers are allowed to join their children there and have relatively normal interactions with them. But sometimes access to the children's center is limited to only the children, and volunteer caregivers tend them while their mothers remain in the visiting room with adult visitors (U.S. Department of Justice, 2002).

A few states have cooperated in the institution of halfway houses or community corrections centers where prisoners may be sentenced as an alternative to prison or where prisoners may be transferred when they near the end of their sentences. Such halfway houses allow prisoners and their children to live together and provide supportive services to them. Usually there is an age limit for the children, generally ranging from birth to a few weeks or months thereafter up to a maximum of 6 years old. Consequently, children over the age limit are still deprived of continuous caregiving by their mothers, and when there are multiple children straddling the age limit, the older children still have to live with other caregivers separated from their younger siblings (U. S. Department of Justice, 2002).

At the Nebraska Correctional Center for Women, which houses an average of 273 women, a parenting program started in 1974 and was the first of its kind in the United States (Clement, 1993). From 1974 to the present, opportunities have been provided for overnight visits for children between 1 and 6 years of age. Children in this age group may spend up to 5 nights per month with their mothers. Newborns and children through the age of 16 may have on-grounds day visits in the program area. In 1994, the parenting program expanded to include a second nursery program modeled after the nursery in the Bedford Hills Correctional Center in New York. Pregnant women who meet all of the criteria required by Nebraska are admitted to the program and are allowed to have their infants on facility grounds. The goal is to have the mother and baby leave the prison together by the time the baby is 18 months old. The parenting program includes many classes and workshops on parenting skills, prenatal care, child development, child health and safety, and improving relationships.

The Children's Center at Bedford Hills Correctional Facility in New York was estab-

lished in 1980 (Ryan, 2002). This program provides transportation, overnight lodging, a children's center and playroom in the visiting area, parent education, information, referrals, gifts for children, a nursery, family reunification support, and public education and advocacy. The summer visiting program hosts children of prisoners in nearby homes so that they can take part in extensive visits and special activities with their mothers. The overnight program hosts children one weekend per month during the school year.

The Children's Center provides mothers with training in foster care issues, child custody, and family law. The nursery program allows mother and child to stay together for 12 to 18 months and provides child development training, prenatal workshops, family literacy education, and transitional support for children leaving the program.

North Carolina provides a special visiting area for eligible women who complete an 8-week parenting class. The area provides a homelike atmosphere with a kitchen where a mother can prepare meals, including cookies and birthday cakes, for her children; a living room; a nursery; and toys and books. The visits last from 1 to 3 hours once a month (U.S. Department of Justice, 2002).

The Ohio Reformatory for Women (ORW) established a nursery in June, 2001, where women serving short sentences are allowed to live with their infants. Eligibility criteria ensure that the women and their children leave together. The nursery program provides hands-on parenting instruction and endeavors to address the factors that brought the mother to prison. ORW also offers a once-a-year Merit Family Day when eligible prisoners plan and pay for a full day of activities with their families. Volleyball, music, and prisoner-produced skits are examples of the types of activities offered (U. S. Department of Justice, 2002).

The Tennessee Prison for Women has a weekend child visitation program in which an eligible mother is allowed to spend the entire weekend with one of her children between the ages of 3 months and 6 years in separate quarters away from the general prison population. The unit has single-cell space for 16 women and their children (Glick & Neto, 1977).

The Washington Corrections Center for Women offers a Residential Parenting Program that includes an Early Head Start Program for the children and an enriched environment, as well as parenting skills for minimum security women prisoners who give birth while incarcerated. A "Girl Scout Behind Bars" program is also offered for women prisoners and their daughters. The program meets once a month and the mothers act as leaders to provide craft and educational projects for their daughters (Moses, 1993; 1995).

In addition to Michigan, Missouri, New Jersey, New Mexico, North Carolina, Pennsylvania, Texas, Vermont, Washington, and Wisconsin offer enhanced visiting programs for mothers and their children. The CVP in Michigan's women's prisons was born of the love and care that these mothers have for their children. The Department of Corrections does not pay for it. This program gives the mothers the opportunity to mother their children and be involved in their lives. It took 4 years of hard work and trying to convince the administration to let the program happen, but finally we were allowed to start a "pilot program" that has lasted for 15 years. The institution was not interested in facilitating mothering for the women prisoners, but rather saw the women as prisoners and not in the role of mothers.

How the Children's Visitation Program Supports Mothering

My years of experience with the Children's Visitation Program in southeast Michigan have reinforced my firm belief in the importance of visitation to allow mothering to continue for women in prison. During their visits, children hold on to their mothers and often want just to be hugged during the entire visit. It is almost as if they want to feel all the love they can get to last until the next visit. Although I have conducted this program in the prison and in the jail for many years, I am continually moved by the love and caring that the children and the mothers share during those 4 hours. In addition to holding, the

mothers also give their children advice about school and the importance of getting good grades and other such matters of importance. Teens have a hard time listening to the advice from their mothers, just as they would if their mothers were at home.

Also during the visits, teaching moments occur for these mothers, and they are asked to consider alternative parenting skills and to receive guidance in implementing those skills. At times, however, the clash of class and cultural and socioeconomic bias becomes starkly apparent. For example, I remember one time when a little boy in the program tripped and fell and began crying. His mother walked over to him and said, "Boy, get your black ass up and stop that crying now!" I was surprised by her behavior. So I pulled her aside and told her that I did not think that her response was appropriate because her son comes to visit needing all of the love and comfort he can get from her. I told her I thought she should have picked him up and comforted him. In response, she told me quite frankly that where she and her son lived, if he behaved like that, it could get him killed, and that, if he was to survive, he had to learn to pick himself up when he got knocked down without crying. After thinking about what she said, I realized that her response to her son had been appropriate parenting in the context of the situation in which they actually live. The lesson she was teaching her child was as important as the lessons that middle-class people typically teach their children not to run into the street.

For the reasons I have presented, mothering from prison is difficult because of the enormous barriers to maintaining effective and regular contact with children. Mothers in prison often go to extraordinary lengths to care for their children, including finding appropriate caretakers, interceding between children and their caretakers when necessary, finding new caretakers when necessary, and providing material and emotional support for their children. I was always moved by the many phone calls I received asking me to please check on their children, talk to their teachers, and find out what was going on in their homes. The following vignette illustrates how the women do mothering from prison.

✤ *Vignette:* **Rose**

When Rose was sentenced to 25 years in prison, she had four daughters, the oldest of whom was 6 years old. Her second daughter, who was then 3 years old, had cerebral palsy. At first, the children were placed with her mother. When her mother was no longer able to care for them, Rose convinced her father and stepmother to take them. When her father died, Rose convinced a friend to take all four girls. When the friend found the task too difficult, she called in social services, which decided that the children should be split up and placed in separate foster homes.

Rose then convinced her brother and sister-in-law to step in and take them before the court had a chance to rule on the social services petition. When that arrangement didn't work out, the children were returned to Rose's ailing mother. When Rose's oldest daughter turned 17, she assumed responsibility for her three younger sisters.

The situation for the children was undoubtedly difficult, and definitely left them psychologically scarred. But at least they remained together and had each other throughout their lives. All are adults now with children of their own, but remain close to each other. Rose tells us in her own words what the worry about her children was like:

> I lost ten pounds worrying. Are they allowed to see each other? My children had never been apart. Are they scared? Lonely? Do they worry about me? I was going crazy. There is nothing you can do from jail, except cry and pray that your children will be OK.

For Rose, visitation with her children was sporadic. As each caretaker assumed responsibility for the children, they promised regular visits and tried to fulfill that promise for a while. Then the time, energy, and financial burdens of caring for four children and having to travel so far to visit would set in and the visits would become less and less frequent until the next caregiver took over and the cycle would repeat itself.

Contact by phone and correspondence substituted for visits to the degree possible. In this way, the children could tell Rose what was happening with them. She could give them guidance and help them work through their feelings about everything in their lives, including the fact that Rose was in prison and how hard it was for them to be without her. Letters and phone calls were still inadequate. Often the cost of phone calls was prohibitive for the caretaker. Frequently, attempts were made to prearrange times for phone calls so that the children could be available rather than either having them wait around for a call or risk missing them. But lack of timely access to the phones in the prison often occurred, leaving the children devastated when the call they expected did not come. The children were unable to communicate freely because of the caretaker's presence. Seldom were they able to give Rose a complete understanding of what was going on, even when they could communicate freely. Communication by letter was similarly limited by the child's ability to express herself in writing, by both the child's and Rose's ability to obtain stamps, by the caretaker's willingness to allow uncensored written communication, and by the time lag between the sending and receiving of letters. Nevertheless, Rose remained the one constant force in her children's lives just like any mother.

Her daughters depended on her to help with problems, and she found ways to come through for them. Money was difficult to come by in prison, but Rose managed to work the highest paying prison jobs she could and supplemented her income by making and selling crafts to other prisoners and staff. Nevertheless, this was hardly enough to cover the needs of four children. But Rose made many friends among prisoners serving shorter sentences than she, among volunteers, teachers, lawyers, and others who came to the prison to provide services to prisoners, and among pen-pals she developed on the outside. Thus, when her children were in need of something, Rose called people on the outside until she found someone who could either help directly or who could put her in contact with someone who could help. This is how Rose mothered her children from prison.   ✤

✒ Conclusion

As discussed in this chapter, the majority of the women in prison are poor and the children share this poverty with their mothers. Poverty is a powerful determinant in the cognitive and behavioral development of children (Duncan, Brooks-Gunn, & Klebanov, 1994). This problem needs to be addressed. As a community, we need to understand that sexual abuse, poverty, poor education, and the lack of resources, education, and opportunity must be changed if we want the children of these women to break the cycle of despair. In addition, it is estimated that as high as 83 percent of the children had been either sexually or physically abused or had witnessed violence at home almost identical to the frequency among the mothers themselves. These cycles of abuse need to be interrupted with specific services aimed at providing children with their basic need for safety (Greene, Haney & Hurtado, 2000).

Indeed, the mothers repeatedly told me that they wanted to be present and to function as effective mothers for their children. They wanted to stay away from drugs and to avoid involvement with the people with whom they associated before their incarceration. Again and again, women told me how much they wanted a better life for their children than the life they had. They vividly described the pain it caused them to be unable to make a better life for their children. One woman declared, "My mother was a drug user, and I hated being taken away from my mother. I don't want to be away from my kids any longer. I don't want to make them suffer like I did." They very much want their children to have healthier, happier childhoods, with more opportunities to escape the dependencies that dictated their own lives. Many mothers reiterated: "I don't want to see my child go through everything I went through." Moreover, because of the serious problems with and shortage of homes in the foster care system, these mothers are the most reliable and effective available resources for interrupting such cycles of poverty, abuse, drugs, and criminality.

Mothers and children need contact on a regular basis. Every effort should be made to facilitate frequent and meaningful visits between them. Mothers should be allowed to phone their children and significant others in their children's lives, such as their caretakers and teachers, on a regular basis without having to pay the very high telephone rates that the prison imposes.

Further, helping women to return to society after incarceration is necessary. It is unreasonable to expect that these women, without help, will just incorporate themselves successfully into society. The reasons why they could not do it before they came to prison will still be there on their release. Additionally, they will have a criminal record that will make it more difficult for them to get a job and to find housing. As a community of mothers, we could advocate for programs that will help women to be with their children while dealing with their addiction or the lack of skills for employment that brings them to commit the crime. The children should be helped to have better and more successful access to education, including tutoring programs. The best program would be to avoid the separation between mothers and children by creating alternatives to incarceration, which include leaving the mothers and children together in their own homes, with the mother under house arrest if deemed necessary. Access to special centers that maintain a supportive environment where the women and their children could go for help need to be provided. Mothers could learn parenting skills through guided practice and obtain assistance in accessing other appropriate support services. Previously incarcerated women who had successfully made the transition to the "outside world" could provide staffing. They could serve as role models of success and could use their unique understanding to assist the women and their children. This could provide an opportunity to stop the cycle of abuse and trauma for these children and their mothers.

It is important to the creation of a humane society that we stop labeling these mothers and children in ways that allow us to ignore and discard them as somehow unworthy of the most basic of human rights, the rights to maintain a family relationship and to develop to their full potential. As long as we persist in seeing them in socially constructed ways that excuse our participation in making them "disposable people," we as a society lose all of the benefits that development of their full potential could add to *our* lives, and we gain only all of the costs of marginalizing them.

Mothering from prison is about understanding the meaning of the African proverb "It takes a village to raise a child." The women need the village, and often they cannot access it from prison. But they certainly advocate for their children with anybody who will listen.

I have presented the problem of mothering in prison to you through the words of mothers and their children and my own experiences with them. To further facilitate your ability to easily access other literature relating to women in prison, I am including a section of Additional Readings.

Discussion Questions 🖎

- What criminal behaviors of a mother should make incarceration of the mother more important than sentencing her to alternatives to incarceration that allow her to remain with her children?

- Can mothers learn parenting skills in the artificial environment of prisons that are transferable to the "free world?" If so or if not, after reading this chapter, what would you suggest?

- Consider what you can do in your community for women in prison who are mothering.

- How can you become an activist for mothers in prison in your personal and professional lives?

- Do you think that a mother who may not be an ideal parent as defined by middle-class, Caucasian parenting because she uses a harsh parenting style, or a mother who has problems with drugs, should be considered an unfit mother?

References

Abdul-Alim, J. (2000). Easing visits to mom in prison. *Milwaukee Journal Sentinel*. Retrieved January 15, 2003, from *http://www.JSOnline.com*

Barry, E., Ginchild, R., & Lee, D. (1995). Legal issues for prisoners with children. In K. Gabel & D. Johnston,

(Eds.). *Children of incarcerated mothers.* (pp 147–166). New York: Lexington Press.

Baunach, P. J. (1985). *Mothers in prison.* New Brunswick, NJ: Transaction Books, Rutgers University Press.

Beckerman, A. (1994). Mothers in prison: Meeting the prerequisite conditions for permanency planning. *Social Work, 39*(1), 9–13.

Beckerman, A. (1991). Women in prison: The conflict between confinement and parental rights. *Social Justice, 18*(3), 171–183.

Bloom, B., & Steinhart, D. (1993). *Why punish the children: A reappraisal of the children of incarcerated mothers in America.* San Francisco: National Council on Crime and Delinquency.

Catan, L. (1992). Infants with mothers in prison. In R. Shaw (Ed.). *Prisoners' children* (pp 13–28). London (UK): Routledge.

Clement, M. J. (1993) Parenting in prison: A national survey of programs for incarcerated women. *Journal of Offender Rehabilitation, 19*, 89–100.

Dressel, P., Porterfield, J. B., & Sandra, K. (1998). Mothers behind bars. *Corrections Today, 60*(7), 90–94.

Duncan, G. J., Brooks-Gunn, J., & Klebanov, P. K., (1994). Economic deprivation and early childhood development. *Child Development Special Issue: Children and Poverty. 65*(2), 296–318.

Fritsch, T. A., & Burkhead, J. D. (1982). Behavioral reactions of children to parental absence due to imprisonment. *Family Relations, 30*, 83–88.

Genty, P. M. (1995). Termination of parental rights among prisoners: A national perspective. In K. Gable & D. Johnston (Eds.). *Children of incarcerated parents* (pp 167–195). New York: Lexington Books.

Glick, R., & Neto, V. (1997). National study of women's correctional programs. Washington, DC: National Institute of Law Enforcement and Criminal Justice.

Greene, S., Haney, C., & Hurtado, A. (2000). Cycles of pain: Risk factors in the lives of incarcerated mothers and their children, *The Prison Journal, 80*(1), 3–23.

Greenfield & Snell (1999). *Women offenders.* (Report No. NCJ 175688). Washington, DC: Bureau of Justice Statistics.

Hairston, C. F., & Lockett, P. W. (1987). Mothers in prison: New directions for social sciences. *Social Work, 32*(2), 162–164.

Harlow, C. W. (1999). *Prior abuse reported by inmates and probationers (Report No. NCJ 172879).* Washington, DC: Bureau of Justice Statistics.

Harm, N. J., & Thompson, P. J., (1997). Evaluating the effectiveness of parent education for incarcerated mothers. *Journal of Offender Rehabilitation, 24*(3–4), 135–152.

Henriques, Z. W. (1982). *Imprisoned mothers and their children.* Washington, DC: University Press of America.

Johnston, D. (1995a). The care and placement of prisoners' children. In K. Gabel & D. Johnston (Eds.). *Children of incarcerated mothers.* (pp 103–123). New York: Lexington Press.

Johnston, D. (1995b). Intervention. In K. Gabel & D. Johnston (Eds.). *Children of incarcerated mothers.* (pp 199–236). New York: Lexington Press.

Johnston, D. (1995c). Parent-child visitation in the jail or prison. In K. Gabel & D. Johnston (Eds.). *Children of incarcerated mothers* (pp 135–146). New York: Lexington Press.

Jose, C. (1985). *Women doing life sentences: A phenomenological study.* Unpublished doctoral dissertation, University of Michigan.

Jose-Kampfner, C. (1991). Mother and child reunion. Two women's programs show that relaxed visitation can improve inmate behavior. *Corrections Today, 53*(7), 130–134.

Jose-Kampfner, C. (1995). Post-traumatic stress reactions in children of imprisoned mothers. In K. Gabel & D. Johnston (Eds.). *Children of Incarcerated Mothers* (pp 89–102). New York: Lexington Press.

Koban, L. (1983). Mothers in prison: A comparative analysis of the effects of incarceration on the families of men and women. *Research in Law, Deviance and Social Control, 5,* 171–183.

Mauer, M., Potler, C., & Wolf, R. (1999). Gender and justice: Women, drugs and sentencing policy. Washington, DC: The Sentencing Project.

McLoyd, V. C., (1990). The impact of economic hardship on Black families and children: Psychological distress, parenting, and socioemotional development. *Child Development Special Issue: Minority Children, 61*(2), 311–346.

Modie, T. (1997). Should babies be kept in prison with their incarcerated mothers? A social work response. *Scandinavian Journal of Development Alternatives and Area Studies, 16*(3–4), 37–55.

Moses, M. C. (1993). Girl Scouts behind bars: New program at women's prison benefits mothers and children. Girl Scout Troop for incarcerated women and their daughters. *Corrections Today, 55,* 132.

Moses, M. C. (1995). "Girl Scouts beyond bars": A synergistic solution for children of incarcerated parents. *Corrections Today, 57,* 24–126.

Mumola, C. (2000). *Incarcerated mothers and their children (Report No. NCJ 182335).* Washington, DC: Bureau of Justice Statistics.

Ryan, R. P. (2002). Mothers behind bars. *Brain, Child, 3*(4), 28–37.

Sametz, L. (1980). Children of incarcerated women. *Social Work, 25*(4), 298–303.

Schram, P. J., (1999). An exploratory study: Stereotypes about mothers in prison. *Journal of Criminal Justice, 27*(5), 411–426.

Smith, G. (1995). Practical considerations regarding termination of incarcerated mothers' rights. In K. Gabel & D. Johnston (Eds.) *Children of Incarcerated Mothers* (pp 183–198). New York: Lexington Press.

Stanton, A. (1980). *When mothers go to jail.* Lexington, MA: Lexington Books.

U. S. Department of Justice. (2002) Serving families of adult offenders: A directory of programs. Retrieved February 8, 2003, from *http://www.nicic.org/pubs/2002/017081.pdf*

Weilerstein, R. (1995). The prison MATCH program. In K. Gabel & D. Johnston (Eds.) *Children of Incarcerated Mothers* (pp 255–264). New York: Lexington Press.

Whiteford, G. (2000). Occupational deprivation: Global challenge in the new millennium. *British Journal of Occupational Therapy, 63*(5), 200–204.

Additional Readings

Adalist-Estrin, A. (1986). Parenting…from behind bars. *Family Resource Coalition Report, 5*(1), 12–13.

American Bar Association (1993). *Children on hold: What happens when their primary caregiver is arrested?* Washington, DC: Author.

Bakker, L. J., Morris, B. A., & Janus, L. M. (1978). Hidden victims of crime. *Social Work, 23,* 143–148.

Balk, D. L. (1983). Adolescent grief reactions and self-concept perceptions following a sibling death: A study of 33 teenagers. *Journal of Youth and Adolescence, 12*(3), 159–170.

Bartlett, R., (2000). Helping inmate moms keep in touch. *Corrections Today, 62*(7), 102–104.

Baunach, P. J.: (1984). *Mothers in Prison.* New Brunswick, NJ: Transaction Books, Rutgers University Press.

Beckerman, A. (1998). Charting a course: Meeting the challenge of permanency planning for children with incarcerated mothers. *Child Welfare, 77*(5), 513–529.

Beckerman, A. (1994). Mothers in prison: Meeting the prerequisite conditions for permanence planning. *Social Work, 39,* 9–14.

Bifulco, A. T., et al. (1987). Childhood loss of parent: Lack of adequate parental care and adult depression. *Journal of Affective Disorders, 12,* 115–128.

Birtchnell, J. (1970). Depression in relationship to early and recent parental death. *British Journal of Psychiatry, 116,* 229–306.

Bistrian, J. (1997). *Incarcerated mothers and the foster care system in Massachusetts: A Literature Review.* Family & Correction Network. Retrieved 6/17/03 from *http://fc-network.org/reading/bistrian/html*

Block, K. J., & Potthast, M. J., (1998). Girl Scouts beyond bars: Facilitating parent-child contact in correctional settings. *Child Welfare, 77*(5), 561–578.

Boudin, K. (1998). Lessons from a mother's program in prison: A psychosocial approach supports women and their children. *Women & Therapy*: Special Issue: Breaking the rules: Women in prison and feminist therapy, II. 21(1), 103–125.

Bowlby, J. (1946). *Forty-four juvenile thieves: Their characters and home-life.* London (UK): Tindall & Cox.

Bowlby, J. (1951). Adverse effects of maternal deprivation. In *Maternal Care and Mental Health.* Geneva: World Health Organization.

Bowlby, J. (1973). *Separation: Anxiety and anger.* New York: Basic Books.

Bowlby, J. (1980). *Attachment and loss.* New York: Basic Books.

Bowlby, J. (1983). *Attachment and loss.* New York: Basic Books.

Breier, A., Kelso, J. R., Kirwin, P. D., Beller, S. A., Wolkowitz, D. M., & Pickar, D. (1988). Early parental loss and development of adult psychology. *Archives of General Psychiatry, 45,* 987–493.

Browne, D. (1989). Incarcerated mothers and parenting. *Journal of Family Violence, 4*(2), 211–221.

Brown, F. (1961). Depression and childhood bereavement. *Journal of Mental Science, 107*, 754–777.

Bush-Baskette, S. (2000). The war on drugs and the incarceration of mothers. *Journal of Drug Issues, 30*(4), 919–928.

Cain, A. C., & Fast, J. D. (1966). Children's disturbed reactions to parent suicide. *American Journal of Orthopsychiatry, 36*, 873–880.

Clark, J. (1995). The impact of the prison environment on mothers. *The Prison Journal, 75*, 306–329.

Cottle, T. J. Angela: A child-woman. *Social Problems, 23*(4), 516–523.

Datesman, S.K., & Cales, G.L. (1983). I'm still the same mommy: Maintaining the mother-child relationship in prison. *Prison Journal, 63*(2), 142–154.

Doyle, J. S., & Bauer, S. K. (1989). Post-traumatic stress disorder in children. *Journal of Traumatic Stress, 2*(3), 275–288.

Eekelaar, J. M. (1973). What are parent rights? *Law Quarterly Review, 89*, 210.

Elizur, E., & Kauffman, M. (1983). Factors influencing the severity of childhood bereavement reactions. *American Journal of Orthopsychiatry, 53*(4), 668–676.

Enos, S. (1997). Managing motherhood in prison: The impact of race and ethnicity on child placements. *Women & Therapy, 20*(4), 57–73.

Fagin, A., & Reid, A. (1991). Moms in jail. *Children Today, 20*, 12–13.

Florida House of Representatives Justice Council Committee on Corrections (1998). *Maintaining Family Contact When a Family Member Goes to Prison: An Examination of State Policies on Mail, Visiting, and Telephone Access.* Tallahassee, FL: Author.

Fuller, L. G. (1993). Visitors to women's prisons in California: An exploratory study. *Federal Probation, 57*, 41–47.

Gabel, K., & Johnson, D. (eds.) (1994). *Children of incarcerated mothers.* Boston, MA: Lexington Books.

Gabel, S. (1992). Behavioral problems in sons of incarcerated or otherwise absent fathers: The issue of separation. *Family Process, 31*, 303–314.

Garfalda, M. E. (1982). Hallucinations in psychiatrically disordered children: Preliminary communication. *Journal of Sociological Medicine, 75*, 181–184.

Gaudin, J. M., Jr. (1984). Social work roles and tasks with incarcerated mothers. *Social Casework: The Journal of Contemporary Social Work, 65*(5), 279–286.

Genty, P. M. (1998). Permanency planning in the context of parental incarceration: Legal issues and recommendations. *Child Welfare, 77*(5) 543–560.

Goldberg, M. E., Lex, B. W., Mello, N. K., Mendelson, J. H., & Bower, T. A. (1996). Impact of maternal alcoholism on separation of children from their mothers: Findings from a sample of incarcerated women. *American Journal of Orthopsychiatry, 66*(2), 228–238.

Hairston, C. F. (1991). Family ties during imprisonment: Important to whom and for what? *Journal of Sociology and Social Welfare 18*(1), 85–102.

Hale, D. C., (1987). The impact of mothers' incarceration on the family system: Research and recommendations. *Marriage and Family Review, 12*(1–2), 143–154.

Hannon, G., Martin, D., & Martin, M. (1984). Incarceration in the family: Adjustments to change. *Family Therapy, 11*, 253–260.

Harm, N. J., Thompson, P. J., & Chambers, H. (1998). The effectiveness of parent education for substance abusing women offenders. *Alcoholism Treatment Quarterly, 16*(3), 63–77.

Huling, T. (1991). *Breaking the silence.* New York: Correctional Association of New York.

Hungerford, G. P. (1996). Caregivers of children whose mothers are incarcerated: A study of the kinship placement system. *Children Today, 24*(1), 23–27.

Johnston, D. (1995). Jailed mothers. In K. Gabel & D. Johnston (Eds.). *Children of Incarcerated Mothers.* New York: Lexington Press, pp 41–58.

Johnston, D. (1995d). Effects of parental incarceration. In K. Gabel & D. Johnston (Eds.). *Children of Incarcerated Mothers.* New York: Lexington Press, pp 59–88.

Jolowicz, A. R. (1981). A foster child needs his own mothers. *Child, 12*(2) 18–21.

Katz, P. C. (1998). Supporting families and children of mothers in jail: An integrated child welfare and criminal justice strategy. *Child Welfare, 77*(5), 495–511.

Korbin, J. E., (1987). Incarcerated mothers' perceptions and interpretations of their fatally maltreated children. *Child Abuse & Neglect Special Issue: Child Abuse and Neglect, 11*(3), 397–407.

LaPoint, V., Picket, M. O., & Harris, S. (1985). Enforced family separation: A descriptive analysis of some experiences of children of black imprisoned mothers. In Spencer, A, *Beginnings: The social and affective development of black children* (3rd. ed.). (pp. 239–255) Hillsdale, NJ: Erlbaum.

Littner, N. (1981). The importance of the natural mothers to the child in placement. In P. A. Sinanoglu & A. N. Maluccio. *Mothers of children in placement* (3rd ed.). New York: Child Welfare League of America.

Lyons, J. (1987). Post-traumatic stress disorder in children and adolescents: A review of the literature. *Developmental and Behavioral Pediatrics, 8*(6), 349–356.

Maeve, M K. (1999). Adjudicated health: Incarcerated women and the social constructions of health. *Crime Law and Social Change, 31*(1) 49–71

Martin, M., (1997). Connected mothers: A follow-up study of incarcerated women and their children. *Women and Criminal Justice, 8*(4), 1–23.

McGowan, B. G., & Blumenthal, K. L. (1978). *Why punish the children? A study of the children of women in prison.* Hackensack, NJ: National Council on Crime and Delinquency.

Moore, A. R., & Clement, M. J. (1998). Effects of parenting training for incarcerated mothers. *Journal of Offender Rehabilitation, 27*(1–2), 57–72.

Morton, J. B. & Williams, D. M. (1998). Mother/child bonding. *Corrections Today, 60*(7), 98–105.

Musk, H. A. (1982). Programs for incarcerated women

and their children: Psychodynamic considerations and implications. *Dissertation Abstracts International, 42*(8-B), 34–60.

Myers, B.J., Smarsh, T. M., & Amlund-Hagen, K., (1999). Children of incarcerated mothers. *Journal of Child and Family Studies, 81*(1), 11–25.

Payton, J. B., & Krocker-Tuskan, M. (1988). Children's reactions to loss of a parent through violence. *Journal of American Academy of Child and Adolescent Psychiatry, 27*(5), 563–566.

Prison Visitation Project. (1993). *Needs assessment of children whose mothers are incarcerated (Grant No. 720-93616D).* Richmond, VA: Department of Mental Health, Mental Retardation, and Substance Abuse Services.

Radosh, P. F., (2002). Reflections on women's crime and mothers in prison: A peacemaking approach. *Crime & Delinquency,* Special Issue: Criminology at the edge: Essays in honor of Richard Quinney, *48*(2) 300–315.

Rosenkrantz, L., & Joshua, V. (1982). Children of incarcerated mothers: A hidden population. *Children Today, 11,* 2–6.

Sach, W. H., Siedler, J., & Thomas, S. (1976). The children of imprisoned parents: A psychological exploration. *American Journal of Orthospsychiatry, 46,* 618–628.

Salm, D. (1993). *Women offenders in the correctional system: Memo no. 7.* Wisconsin State Legislative Council, Madison, Wisconsin; 1993-02-03.

Sanders, J. F., McNeill, K. F., Rienzi, B. M., and DeLouth, T. B. (1997). The incarcerated female felon and substance abuse: Demographics needs assessment, and program planning for a neglected population. *Journal of Addictions and Offender Counseling, 1,* 41–51.

Sandifer, J. L. (2002). *Incarcerated mothers' perceptions and attitudes about parenting.* Association Paper, Southern Sociological Society.

Schafer, N. E., & Dellinger, A. B., (1999). Jailed parents: An assessment. *Women & Criminal Justice, 10*(4), 73–91.

Schoenbauer, L. (1986). Incarcerated mothers and their children: Forgotten families. *Law and Inequality, 4,* 579–582.

Schwartz, I. M., (1989). *The incarcerations of girls: Paternalism or juvenile crime control?* Unpublished manuscript.

Simonds, J. F. (1975). Hallucinations in non-psychotic children. *British Journal of Psychiatry, 129,* 267–276.

Snyder, J., Zoann, K., & Carlo, T. A. (1998). Parenting through prison walls: Incarcerated mothers and children's visitation programs. In Miller, S. L. (Ed.). Crime control and women: Feminist implications of criminal justice policy (pp. 130-150). Thousand Oaks, CA: Sage Publications, Inc.

Sommerfeld, M., (1995). Time well spent: Girl Scouts of America help the daughters of incarcerated women. *Education Week, 14,* 30–31.

Steffensmeier, D. (1995) Trend in female crime: "It's still a man's world." B. Price & N. Sokoloff (Eds.). *The criminal justice system and women* (2nd ed). New York: McGraw-Hill, Inc.

Task Force on the Female Offender. (1990). *The Female Offender: What Does the Future Hold?* Laurel, Maryland: American Correctional Association.

Teather, S., Evans, L., and Sims, M. (1997). Maintenance of the mother-child relationship by incarcerated women. *Early Child Development & Care, 131,* 65–75.

Terr, L. (1983). Forbidden games: Posttraumatic child's play. *Journal of American Academy of Child and Adolescent Psychiatry, 20,* 741–760.

Thompson, P. J., & Harm, N. J. (1995). Parent education for mothers in prison. *Pediatric Nursing, 21,* 552–556.

Wallace, J. J. (1991). Prison and mothering: The hidden punishment. Association paper, Society for the Study of Social Problems.

Ward, D., & Kassebaum, G. (1965). *Women's prison: Sex and social structure.* Chicago: Aldine-Atherton.

Yates, T., and Bannard, J. (1988). The "haunted" child: Grief, hallucinations, and family dynamics. *Journal of American Academy of Child and Adolescent Psychiatry, 27*(5), 573–581.

Young, D. S., and Smith, C. J., (2000). When moms are incarcerated: The needs of children, mothers, and caregivers. *Families in Society, 82*(2), 130–141.

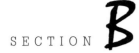

SECTION **B**   *Reflection*

Michael Leunig

God be with the mother. As she carried
her child may she carry her soul. As her
child was born, may she give birth and life
and form to her own, higher truth. As she
nourished and protected her child, may she
nourish and protect her inner life and her
independence. For her soul shall be her
most painful birth, her most difficult child
and the dearest sister to her other children.

Amen

Reprinted with permission from Michael Leunig: Common Prayer Collection, published by Harper-Collins Publishers (Australia) Pty. Ltd. 1993.

SECTION *C*

Mothering Occupations in the Context of Special Challenges: Children with Special Needs

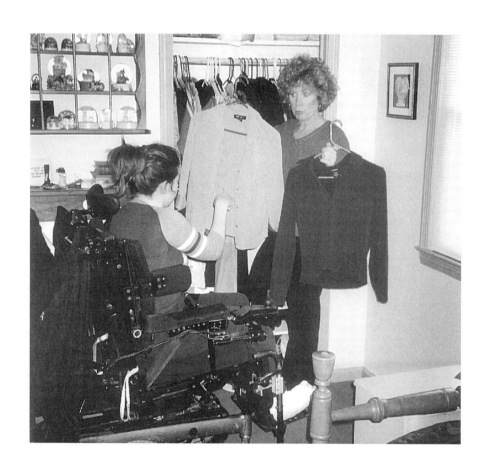

CHAPTER **14**

Activism as a Mothering Occupation

Gwynnyth Llewellyn, PhD
Kirsty Thompson, BAppSc(OT) Hons
Samantha Whybrow, BAppSC(OT) Hons

 Anticipated Outcomes

We anticipate that, after reading this chapter, readers will:

- Have a better understanding of the potential liberating power of mothers' experiences as caregivers

- Identify the occupational activism in the stories of the nine mothers as they negotiated the social systems in which their child and family were embedded

- Consider how activism, as illustrated in this chapter, plays out in three different ways: on behalf of the mother's own child, extending concerns to others, and to make the world a better place

- Explore mothers' activism and develop a deeper understanding of the complex inter-relationships between agency and structure in the lives of mothers of disabled children

✒ Introduction

This chapter introduces the concept of activism as an occupation of mothers of children with disabilities. Our aim is to focus attention on mothers' experiences as caregivers as potentially powerful, liberating, and identity changing, in contrast to the bulk of the literature that focuses on stress, coping, and the burden of care. Drawing on the findings of an interview study with mothers of children aged between 6 and 13 with disabilities and high support needs, we illustrate how mothers proactively and reactively engage with social systems to attain the desired goals for their children. We describe, through the stories of nine mothers, how experiences with social systems shape and frame their lives and the lives of their families. We identify three distinct loci for mothers' occupational activism: on behalf of their own child, extending concerns to others, and to make the world a better place. We conclude the chapter with a discussion of how activism as a mothering occupation highlights the complex inter-relationships between agency and structure in mothers' lives.

We deliberately use the term *activism* to describe the occupational work done by mothers as they struggle to have their children recognized as equally deserving of the opportunities available to other children. Using this term may seem out of place here. Activism is usually reserved for social movements. We typically think of activists as outspoken, even attention grabbing, often in the media, perhaps chained to fences to force radical social change. In the 21st century we think particularly of environmental activists, green parties and policies, and their concerted efforts to provide a "wake-up" call to the destruction that humankind is wreaking upon this planet.

The mothers whose stories grace this chapter do not call themselves activists. Their stories, nevertheless, are rich with activism. Sometimes this activism comes about as a reaction to their child being treated unfairly. At other times it comes about because mothers engage proactively to head off unfair treatment. Some mothers talk about their actions being for their child only. Others act to hold individuals and systems to account when any disabled child is denied his or her rightful place in the world. Mothers in another group talk about their goal to make the world a better place for disabled people. Their purpose is to promote social change more generally. These mothers share a deep commitment to remove the social restrictions, disadvantages, and discrimination leveled against their children. All seek to have the opportunities other children are given—without question—for their own disabled children. They want their children to be welcomed, accepted, and included. None of these mothers are prepared to settle for less, and all are engaged in activism as a mothering occupation.

How did we, the authors of this chapter, "wake up" to mother activism as a mothering occupation? We knew about disability movements. We were, of course, aware that many mothers become leaders in disability-related fields. We had met many of these mothers in disability organizations, in not-for-profit service agencies, on government working parties and committees. We knew and respected the work of these mothers. We marveled at their seemingly endless energy and capacity to engage in "extracurricular" activities while simultaneously maintaining a home and raising children. Many were also engaged in full-time paid employment. How did they do it all, we wondered?

We certainly appreciated their expertise. We valued their insights. We purposefully sought their views on mothering children with disabilities, along with the views of other mothers who appeared less active in promoting opportunities for disabled children. One of us, Gwynnyth Llewellyn, has been engaged in a long-term program of research to understand the rich and complex web of interrelationships between family and disability over the life course. Still, we did not yet recognize activism as an occupation in mothers' lives.

It was not until listening and relistening to over 160 taped interviews with mothers of disabled children that Gwynnyth had the "ah-ha" experience! She had been initially thinking about these data in relation to how mothers develop expertise in caring for their disabled children over time. In the interviews there were many examples of mothering expertise, a topic regrettably underresearched because of the high status accorded professional expertise. Even more pronounced, however, was the wealth of examples in which mothers engaged in pro*active* and re*active* occupational work to get a "fair deal" for their disabled children. Here, it seemed, was activism at work in mothers' everyday lives.

We went on to examine these data more closely. Our analysis revealed patterns in this occupational work of activism. This chapter tells the story of these patterns, drawing on brief vignettes to illustrate the different ways in which mothers engage in activism as a mothering occupation. Our aim is to make clear the purposes behind mothers' activism and the catalysts that propel mothers into action. We also comment on the variety of actions mothers undertake. Although there is an expanding occupational literature on the everyday routines of mothers of disabled children, less is understood about how, why, and in what way mothers "fight" for their disabled children. This chapter begins the process of filling this gap.

The existence of mother activism and its neglect in the professional literature highlight the subtle and not-so-subtle ways in which discrimination against disabled children and their families continues in our societies. We are particularly interested here in the broader societal views of disability and gender and their interrelationship with mothering occupations. Can we imagine a world where mothers of disabled children need not engage in activism as a mothering occupation? Is it not enough for a mother to raise her disabled child without also having to campaign for better social conditions for her child and her family? What responsibility do practitioners bear to join with mothers and work toward making the campaign redundant? We do not provide answers, but rather encourage readers to reflect on these questions as they read mothers' accounts of their occupational work to secure better conditions for their children.

In the next section of this chapter we shall discuss the mothers' accounts of their involvement with school systems. At the time of the interviews, all the mothers had school-age children between 6 and 13 years of age, so much of their lives and those of their families was taken up with schooling. Much of the activism captured in the mothers' stories in this chapter, although not all, therefore addresses educational opportunities and the institutions through which schooling is provided. However, we invite readers to reflect on the issues raised more broadly and to think about how other systems affect the lives of families with disabled children. These could include early intervention, family support, post-school options, employment, leisure programs, or respite care. We also invite readers, if they have not already done so, to become familiar with social activism movements seeking institutional change for people with a disability in many countries around the world. The stories of their successes—and failures—can be read elsewhere (e.g., Driedger, 1987; Kasnitz, 2001). However, our focus in this chapter is on how individual mothers seek social change through activism in their everyday lives.

Before turning to the mothers and their stories, we need to make clear the reasons for our choice of language. We use the term "disabled children" in preference to "children with disabilities." We acknowledge that there are at least two competing traditions in terminology (Corker & French, 1999). On the one hand, there are many who have fought for recognition of people with a disability as people first and having a disability second. This tradition resists the use of the word disabled, which is seen as a stigmatizing label, and instead uses the term people with a disability. On the other, the social model of disability supports the use of the term disabled children (Oliver, 1990). This is based on disability being located within societal structures and cultural beliefs and practices, not within the person. In other words, society disables the person rather than the person suffering a disability. The influence of societal structures provides the context within which activism as a mothering occupation flourishes. Thus, the expression "disabled child" is our term of choice.

The vignettes included in this chapter come from a 3-year research study, *Supporting Families*, funded by the Australian Research Council Strategic Partnerships with Industry Research and Training (SPIRT) Scheme,

Number C79804675. This study, conducted in partnership with the Spastic Centre of NSW, investigated family well-being and out-of-home placement in families with disabled children and high support needs (Llewellyn et al, 2002). The following section briefly outlines the study. This is followed by the mothers' stories.

The Study

Families with children aged from 6 to 13 years having intellectual, physical, or sensory impairment were recruited for the *Supporting Families* study with the help of service agencies in the northern and eastern areas of Sydney, Australia, a state capital city of approximately 4 million residents. The design of the study followed an earlier study with families whose children ranged in age from infancy up to age 6 (Llewellyn et al., 1999). The study set out to investigate the influences on family well-being and the relationship between well-being and families continuing to care for their children at home.

Briefly, the study was based on ecocultural theory (Gallimore, Weisner, Kaufman, & Bernheimer, 1989). Ecocultural theory proposes that the central adaptive problem facing families is the construction of a sustainable, meaningful, and congruent daily routine of family life (Gallimore, Weisner, Bernheimer, Guthrie, & Nihira, 1993). Families go about this in different ways. How they do this depends in part on whether they regard particular environmental factors as resources or constraints. For example, one family may regard support from the extended family as a resource. Another family will determine that help provided by their extended family is a constraint. How families develop a sustainable and meaningful routine also depends on their values, beliefs, and family goals.

Health and social welfare practitioners are familiar with the way in which families in ostensibly similar circumstances construct remarkably varied family settings and make different family decisions. Ecocultural theory explains this in terms of each family's perspective on their resources and constraints interlinked with their beliefs, goals, and values.

Critical to this approach, therefore, is the need to understand each family's perspective on their everyday life from their point of view. A series of instruments were developed to assist this process. Central to these is the Ecocultural Scale Family Interview (Nihira, Weisner, and Bernheimer, 1994). The interview is conducted with whichever family member identifies as the primary caregiver, although typically this is the mother. The interview requires a narrative approach and usually begins with an open-ended question such as "How are things going these days?" During the course of the interview the nine domains of everyday family life identified as consistent across families are addressed (Nihira, Weisner, & Bernheimer, 1994). These domains are:

- Resilience of the family's subsistence base
- Service usage
- Structuring of the home environment
- Family involvement and assistance in childcare and domestic work
- Connectedness of family
- Involvement of child in nondisabled networks
- Involvement of child in disabled networks
- Variety and amount of formal and instrumental help
- Used information from professionals

The 81 families participating in the *Supporting Families* study were interviewed twice over a 12-to-18-month period in 1999 and 2000. These interviews were tape recorded with the interviewees' permission and later transcribed and coded for analysis in response to the study questions about family well-being and out-of-home placement.

Analysis

The analysis conducted for this chapter arose out of Gwynnyth's interest in the development of caregiver expertise over time in families with a disabled family member. Following Smith's (1987) perspective on "doing sociology for women," Gwynnyth listened and re-listened to all taped interviews, coding and subsequently analyzing all instances of activism. Smith's approach requires working upward from women's (in this case, mothers') everyday experiences to understand the relationship between agency and structure in their lives and how the broader social relationships frame and shape their individual experiences. When mothers talk about their experiences with the systems that frame family life, the complex relationship between agency and structure emerges. In this chapter we focus on three features of this relationship as these are revealed by mothers' occupational activism work.

The first feature is the active nature of the individual's engagement with societal structures. As the stories demonstrate, this is not simply a case of mothers reacting to the demands of social systems. Mothers also proactively engage with these systems to meet desired goals for their children. Thus, in the stories that follow, we see examples of mothers' proactive and reactive occupational work as they encounter social systems. The second feature is the way in which the experiences of individuals as they engage with broader social systems in turn shape and frame their everyday lives. Through the stories, we hear how mothers' experiences shaped and framed their lives and the lives of their families: for example, by making a decision to change schools, to move to a new location, to employ a home tutor, and so on. The third feature is the varying loci of the individual's engagement with broader social relationships. Here we see how mothers' occupational activism work can be focused on their own child, or can include other disabled children or further extend to the interests of disabled people in society more generally.

Bronfenbrenner's ecological systems model provides a conceptual framework within which to examine the location of an individual's engagement with social systems (Bronfenbrenner, 1979; Bronfenbrenner & Morris, 1988). This model posits everwidening and interrelated circles of relationships that make up society. Closest to home is the most intimate circle, the microsystem, which is made up of the systems with which families engage on a daily basis and the relationship between these systems. Taking school as an example, these systems include the family and the classroom. In the next circle out,

the exosystem, we find the school systems, policies, legislative directives, and so on. The outside circle, the macrosystem, speaks to the larger societal influences such as attitudes toward disability and the gendered nature of caring for people with a disability.

Using this conceptual approach, we differentiated mothers into three groups. The first group of mothers is those who are primarily activists at the most intimate (microsystem) level for their own child and family. In the second group are mothers who extend their activism to situations involving other disabled children (exosystem). The final group are mothers who hold a broader world view of a more just society—one in which disabled children (and adults) are valued, cared about as well as cared for, and included as equal citizens. These mothers are more likely to join parent organizations, become leaders and disability advocates, and add social change activism to their repertoire (macrosystem). Figure 14–1 illustrates the application of the ecological systems model to mother activism. The innermost circle is described as "on behalf of my child." The next circle out, the exosystem, is labeled "extending concerns to others." The outermost circle, the macrosystem, is described as "making the world a better place for disabled people."

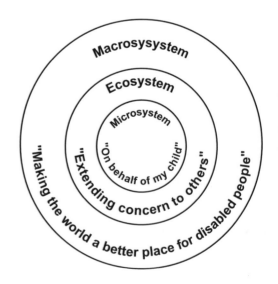

Figure 14–1 *Ever-widening circles of mother activism.*

For ease of presentation we assigned the mothers to one of the conceptual circles illustrated in Figure 14–1 based on where they talked about placing most of their activism efforts. Although the mothers tended to focus their occupational activism primarily in one circle (system), we caution that the circles framework is, of course, artificially imposed on these mothers' lives and that the lines dividing the circles must be considered somewhat fluid. Mothers may engage in one or more types of activism simultaneously, swap from one to another as the situation demands, or engage in all three types, as illustrated in Figure 14–2.

𝕃 Mothers' Stories

To illustrate mother activism, we present vignettes of nine mothers who spontaneously identified in their own words their activism on behalf of their own child, other disabled children, and to seek institutional change. These mothers were chosen from the 81 caregivers in our study because their stories and their language clearly identify the importance they place on their occupational activism work. We trust that, by presenting these examples, we will encourage readers to think about and explore the occupational work of activism in the lives of mothers of disabled children.

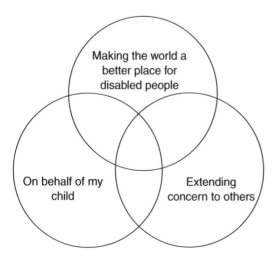

Figure 14–2 *Single and potential multiple loci for mothers' activism.*

We illustrate the three groups of mothers by providing brief accounts from their interview transcripts. Some identifying information has been altered to ensure anonymity and protect their privacy. These vignettes illustrate the actions that mothers take, the catalysts for their actions, and the purposes and goals that mothers pursue in their occupational work.

On Behalf of My Child

This first group of mothers is made up of those whose stories reflect their primary focus on serving the interests of their child and family. In Australia, children with disabilities are now primarily educated in local community schools, with a smaller number still attending special schools for disabled children. Although terms such as "mainstreaming" are frequently used in other parts of the world, "integration" is the term typically used in Australia. Integration means the inclusion of the disabled child with his or her typically developing peers in a regular class or the inclusion of a child in a special (or support) class in a regular school. In the former instance, the disabled child typically receives additional assistance of varying intensity from a teacher's assistant; in the latter, a teacher with special education qualifications and a teacher's assistant staff the classroom. Related services such as occupational therapy, physiotherapy, and speech pathology are typically supplied to both regular classes and special (support) classes as well as to the few remaining special schools.

⌘ Vignette: *Jenny and David*

When Jenny learned that her first child, David, had mild cerebral palsy at around the age of $3 \frac{1}{2}$, she had no idea what that meant. On finding out about services for spastic children, she became involved with therapy for around 15 hours a week in the preschool years. Enrolling David at the local school was her "initiation" into activism.

> The greatest shock was when they said he is not able-bodied, he has to be assessed by the school counsellor, even though it was the

local school about 100 meters down the road. You don't realize, you are so flat out trying to work out this child's abilities and then you have to confront these things. That's why I am involved with integration.

Jenny, with her husband's support, continues to advocate for the therapy and support that David needs to develop his potential. Initially, she focused on getting these in the state-provided system. However, she finally chose a private school known for pastoral care. At home, she developed a plan for each skill that he needed to learn and set out to achieve realistic goals. At school, Jenny consciously decided to be seen as helpful and supportive, for example, regularly making sandwiches for the canteen "to build up brownie points" rather than, in her own words, "being the mother from hell."

By her own admission, she is constantly seeking information and having to translate it into terms that are useful to her son's teachers. She feels that she often becomes obsessed with a particular issue, and then she is grateful for having a really supportive husband who brings her back to reality. He helps her look at longer-term goals, not only immediate results. She is also aware of how constant all of this is and that many parents she meets do not continue on as she has because it is so physically and mentally exhausting. On the other hand, she feels particularly strongly that she has been blessed and that as a couple they have become more compassionate people. She feels passionately about giving back for all that she has gained and is now working with children integrated in the state school system to put this into practice.

Jenny's focus is now on her son's self-esteem. Her concern at school is that he gets opportunities to participate along with the other boys and that:

> He can see that he can make a contribution. That's important. So as a parent you are constantly battling someone. Nobody else has that longer-term outlook for them. We know the sort of adult we want—a nice thoughtful human being who doesn't get frustrated because of his disability, but is kind to others.

For Jenny, the unexpected rejection of her son by the school system was the catalyst that propelled her into action. Out of this grew her constant and ongoing battle to seek the opportunities that her son, as a young child, deserves. Building on her and her husband's long-term goal for their son as a person has helped her identify the activities she feels are important to his personal growth. She works hard at ensuring that these occur naturally within the school environment. One way she does this is by extending her traditional mother task of preparing and serving food to the school canteen to ensure positive acceptance (DeVault, 1991). She also acts as go-between, interpreting specialist information from therapists employed to work with her son in ways that his teachers can understand and apply in the classroom. ⌘

⌘ *Vignette:* **Jane and Michael**

Jane is in a different situation. She has three young children. Her middle child, Michael, who is 8, has a rare syndrome that includes intellectual disability, slow growth, and general slowness of development. As Jane describes this syndrome, the most difficult part is that these children have great difficulty in learning to talk or do not talk at all. Michael needs one-to-one assistance and a specific method of instruction. Although he attends a state-provided special school, the amount of speech therapy available is minimal, and private therapy, prohibitively expensive, is out of the question. In response, Jane took action as she explains here:

> Three days a week I bring him home at lunchtime and we have a good solid hour session. Sally (Michael's younger sister) used to sleep at that time but now she joins in. I can't get her to sleep anymore but she's old enough now and I just give her the same things. The main reason for that is that I am working on his sounds. I have been doing most of his sounds, saying them and looking at the written letters as well, which he does at school as well. I am doing that because if he is going to have a chance of speaking at all it is going to be through a different

method than children normally pick it up. I am getting advice from the speech therapist at school who is able to tell me if I am going in the right direction or not. But he needs one to one and as often as possible and there is no way I can afford three hours of speech therapy a week. He needs motivating activities to go with it. So the only way to do that is to do it myself. School is co-operating in that. They have been good about that. Their afternoons are short anyway so he is not missing out on much.

Jane's activism began when she was confronted with a practical challenge, her son's inability to talk. Faced with a school system unable to provide a solution, Jane took action and initiated part-time home schooling. As Read (2000) has noted, mothers of disabled children frequently act as "their children's allies on the ground." Her proposed solution proved to be acceptable to the school because "not much goes on after lunch anyway." Their approval of this unusual situation is publicly confirmed in two ways: first, by allowing Jane to remove her child for the afternoon period from legally required school attendance; second, by approval for the speech pathologist to design a speech and language program to be carried out at home by his mother rather than in the classroom.

After recently watching Michael's teacher trying to manage her class of seven severely disabled but active boys, Jane offered to help at school. She recalled that many other mothers also help out if they are not working full time. One of the mothers, for example, helped when the children go to "integrated swimming" at a mainstream school. Each child can only go swimming if they have an adult with them. Confronted by the low adult-child class ratio Jane now works with the class, as do other mothers, to give more children an opportunity for one-to-one assistance. ⌘

⌘ *Vignette:* **Peg and Warwick**

There are four young children in Peg's family and all, including the youngest, Warwick, who has cerebral palsy, attend the same mainstream

school. Peg and her husband searched for a school for around 18 months to find the one that they felt would be able to accommodate their son's needs. Peg drives her children to school, spends most of the day there, and brings them home in the afternoon. Although she sometimes leaves the school for a short time to do some errands, she is never away more than an hour or so.

She helps Warwick with toileting and classroom activities because he does not have a daily teacher's aide. If he had to walk to the toilet by himself, it would take around 20 minutes, which Peg feels is much too long to be out of the classroom. Although he has an allocation of aide funding, this works out to be around 1 hour every 2 weeks and clearly not adequate for toileting assistance! Instead, the school channels this funding into a special needs teacher, who then spends the hour a week working with Warwick. Peg is determined that school will work out and that he will be expected to perform along with his peers. She is very aware that if she were not prepared—or able—to be at school every day, the school would not continue to accept his enrollment.

Her experience is that families need to be proactive and seek out schools that will enroll their children. Families also have to be proactive in getting information because there is no central resource available or easy way to access information. For Peg, this is particularly pertinent now that there are so few special schools. In special schools there was a concentration of expertise, information, and other parents "in the same boat." She reminisces that special schools provided a resource that is no longer available.

> You don't have the older and wiser ones saying this is what it's all about so you are kind of isolated in these pockets of kids with disabilities. Sometimes you can get together and find each other by default but there isn't that kind of co-ordinated thing.

A year later, Peg's isolation from information had become even more frustrating. She was concerned that there was no clear school plan for Warwick's future, and she is unsure what to expect of his development over the next few years. For instance, recently the teacher asked her what they should do with her son in the play-ground. Peg felt that it should be the teacher's job to find out. However, she took on this task, believing it is her responsibility to reduce the teacher's burden. She called a specific specialist center and was passed on from therapist to therapist. Finally, someone told her to call the special education teacher at another school. She did this and subsequently referred her son's teacher as well.

For Peg, her desire for her disabled son to attend school with his brothers and sister led to her activism. Her commitment to being "at school" all day every day, she believes, is main-taining his enrollment. Peg's deeply felt regret is at the loss of expertise and both personal and professional support from the closure of specialized centers. From her perspective, this forces mothers to be even more active because "you get pretty selfish and you want benefit for your child and if other people benefit after your child has got it then that is fine but your reality is your child and you have to fight for their needs first."

Vignette: *Clara and James*

At the first interview with Clara, her older daughter attended the school where James, her young son with severe cerebral palsy, was in a support unit. The family moved to be near to this school so that their daughter (and later their youngest son) could spend time with other disabled children and realize that they were not the only ones with a disabled brother.

Clara comes from a health-care background, which she feels has given her "insider" knowl-edge. This also propelled her into action early on—when James was 9 months old—to get an al-ternative therapy for her son in addition to early intervention services. She has been active in ad-vocating for this alternative therapy to be pro-vided in school, as is currently the case in two other Australian states. Clara has needed to be quite assertive to ensure that the therapists pro-vided by the school accommodate to the pro-gram provided by the alternative therapist, whom they see privately, and she is especially

pleased that the occupational therapist is pre-pared to do that. If money were no object, Clara would also pay for this therapist to work daily with James at school so "he wasn't just sitting in his chair for the school day."

Clara is very conscious of building therapy ac-tivities into the everyday routine, and takes every opportunity to do standing or walking with James without any aids (although this takes much longer) when her other children are otherwise occupied.

Looking toward the future, the family has gone into debt and purchased the house next door with an eye to modifying this for James when he is old enough to live in supported ac-commodation. Clara feels very strongly that James should be included in all family activities, no matter how difficult (such as bushwalking, a favorite family outing), and they do not go to places where he is not welcome.

By the time of the second interview, around a year later, Clara was in the throes of organizing for James to be moved from the support unit into his local mainstream school. This happened because the integration he was experiencing in the support unit was "nothing more than token." The planned move was against the advice of the school and departmental officers. Finally, an agreement was reached among all parties. The school to which James was moving has been modified, and a part-time aide will be pro-vided when he enrolls. Clara enlisted the help of a family advocacy organization and attended a workshop to prime herself with the informa-tion and energy needed to request this change, and stood her ground until it happened. The new school was very resistant at first, and as she says, "tried to put us off." They seemed not to realize that parents just want their disabled children to be treated like any other child and not "kept in cotton wool," as is the case in a support unit. His sister will also change schools to attend with him, and in the new year his younger brother will also be enrolled in this new school.

Clara traces her activism in part to her health-care background and being aware of additional help available outside the school system. However, she identifies that she really became active when seeking the best schooling avail-able. She remains constantly alert to maintain

close collaboration between the school therapists and the alternative therapy she has chosen
for her son. Here Clara is mediating as described by Read (2000) to achieve a desired outcome for her son. Clara identifies a change in
herself and a desire to help others in a similar
situation, although this rarely happens, given
her lack of time and opportunity:

> Certainly James has opened my eyes to
> what's really important. And the people we
> have met just through having James I would
> say have straightened me up, got my priori-
> ties right. While it has been difficult for
> James it certainly has been a blessing (for
> me)... time to help others sort of sharing
> things around rather than keeping everything
> to yourself. There's a lot of help you can give
> rather than taking it all .... Whereas I get up-
> set when I see little kids who have so much
> potential and are not (reaching this), you sort
> of try and give as much to them as you can
> when you are able.   ⌘

Extending Concerns to Others

The second group of mothers is also deeply
committed to seeking opportunities for their
disabled children. Added to this, these mothers also talked about their activism on behalf
of other disabled children. They talked in
terms of holding individuals and the systems
they represent to account when any disabled
child is denied an opportunity available to
other children. This could be described as getting a "fair deal" for disabled children.

⌘ *Vignette:* **Elizabeth and Jessica**

Elizabeth describes her daily family life with
Jessica, an only child of 8 years who has cerebral palsy, as very organized, working to a
timetable, but harmonious and happy. Elizabeth
traces her activism on Jessica's behalf in part to
ensuring that she gets the best possible start in
life, and in part, to the tremendous courage and
strength of her daughter. She begins by describing her:

> I am enormously proud of her; she is a per-
> son I admire so much. She has such courage
> and such strength. I look at her and I think

of her struggle on a daily basis and she
doesn't complain, she gets on with it and
she's happy. I am so proud of her and I am
so proud to be her parent. I always tell people that yes, I have a daughter and yes, and
she has cerebral palsy. Perhaps I would get
as much pleasure if she didn't have a disability, but she has such courage and tenacity and we are privileged to share our lives
with her. She has given me enormous
pleasure.

After shopping around to find a suitable
school (many were actively resistant or not
interested in enrolling a disabled child),
Elizabeth and her husband Peter chose one with
an appropriate physical setting and no boys who
they felt could be too rough. The people at the
school expressed their delight at having a disabled child, saying that they felt this would be
good for the Christian values espoused by the
school community.

Elizabeth felt that Jessica is well accepted
generally because she is blessed with a lovely,
sociable personality. However, she recounts stories of prejudice and discrimination, which she
actively works to discount. Recently, for example, Jessica was excluded from the vacation
care program organized by her school. To respond, Elizabeth put in writing her concern that
this action was contrary to antidiscrimination
legislation. She and Peter sought the assistance
of other parents to raise awareness that, once it
is integrated, the institution is responsible for
accommodating to the needs of each disabled
person.

Peter goes to school every morning to see
that his daughter is settled. Through his frequent presence, he aims to provide opportunities to facilitate open communication and
accountability in relation to their daughter's
education. This regular and ongoing contact,
Elizabeth and Peter believe, keeps the school
on their "best behavior" and prevents any further incidents from happening. Following the
previous incident with vacation care, they felt
they needed to work hard to mend the relationship with the school. They do not have a sense
that they have to do extra work because their
child has a disability or to feel grateful (they pay
fees!), but being there provides an opportunity

to monitor what is going on and to set a good role model for Jessica in working for the common good.

Elizabeth's activism, with support from her husband Peter, was initially directed solely at finding the best schooling opportunity for her daughter. An unexpected refusal to allow Jessica to participate in vacation care by the school catapulted Elizabeth, again supported by Peter, to take action irrespective of the possible "fallout" for their daughter. Their ongoing concern to ensure that the school fulfills its obligations in enrolling children with disabilities suggests that Elizabeth and Peter will need to continue their activism well into the future.   ⌘

Vignette: *Gina, Joe, and Roberto*

Gina describes her family life as fluctuating between relative calm and high tension and drama. Gina has two sons, both of whom have Fragile X syndrome. Joe, who is 12, is the eldest, and he is fully integrated in a mainstream school. The younger son, Roberto, is 9, and he is currently in a support class at his local school after several very difficult years. Even now this is not a happy experience because Gina believes that his teacher seems to have very little idea of how to teach children with special needs or how to relate to their parents. Gina is so dissatisfied with his schooling that she has made an official complaint to the state department of education."to be a trail blazer all the way ... our son is the first one to integrate; others have left and gone elsewhere but we stuck it out." Gina refused to capitulate. She has been very active in agitating for inclusion of children with special needs in mainstream classes through into junior and senior high school. Recently she was asked to participate in a departmental film about children with special needs. Joe was chosen as a successful example of inclusion. However, when she was asked whether she believed that the department would support his continuing successful inclusion into high school, she truthfully answered "No," given her previous experiences of having

to fight hard for every achievement. Here she describes this recent experience:

> This school business, we wrote a letter the other day to the head of the region about discrimination in respect for Joe because he has been integrated he is the last on the list to get classroom support. Everybody before us has done it but we have to keep doing it so the people behind us will benefit. It's consuming me but we are determined that they will get what they deserve and we need to drum into people that they need to think a bit more about what these kids need. We have just taken part in this film as well. It's the department's film, going out to the schools, about how kids operate in support classes, as an integrated child, and in special school. Joe has been chosen as the integrated child because he has been so "successful." I was interviewed which was a dreadful experience. One of the things they said to me was do you have faith in the department doing the right thing by Joe in high school and I said no and he asked me again and I said no. It won't go in the video though. I just wish they would realize just what's involved for the parents and they can't keep stuffing us around and giving us second best. None of it will get in to the film but hopefully some people will see the uncut version.

Gina firmly believes it is her responsibility to keep fighting for her sons, but also for other families too so that all children with disabilities will get a fair deal. She vows to continue to do this, whether it involves letter writing, taking issues to the department and demanding solutions, or joining committees in advocacy groups and speaking out publicly to raise awareness of the difficulties faced by parents of children with disabilities in the educational system.

Gina's story illustrates the commitment many mothers of disabled children have to share what they have learned with others (e.g., Solomon, Pistrang & Barker, 2001; Wickham-Searl, 1992b). For many mothers, particularly those new to powerful institutional systems such as education departments, there is concern that if they speak out, their child will be disadvantaged even further. As we saw in Jenny's story, some mothers respond to this fear by taking on acceptable mother roles to enhance their image in the eyes of the school. Other mothers, such as Jane and Peg, when confronted by a serious deficit in their children's schooling, negotiate solutions that are acceptable to the school but that involve extraordinary demands on mothers' time and resources. Gina has no hesitation about taking on the system on behalf of her sons. She gains support for this from the family advocacy group to which she and her husband belong.

To Make the World a Better Place

Mothers in the third group frame their stories in a social justice perspective. For these mothers, the injustices done to their child and their family have galvanized their action to speak out on behalf of all people disabled by societal structures and relationships.

Vignette: *Beth, Jodie, and Josephine*

In this family there are twin girls who are nearly 12 years old. Both girls have cerebral palsy. Beth talks about Jodie being the sicker of the two in her early years and requiring a lot of therapy. She is now doing very well, and is clever and social. Josephine is very severely handicapped and totally dependent.

All of the help Beth now receives has been hard won. This help includes home care for one hour, four mornings a week to shower and dress Josephine. As she says:

It sounds easy and organized. It makes me cringe almost to say I have this because it was never a smooth process and it was never easy or given to me and at every stage I had to find out without anyone telling me and argue. We have had a lot of problems with home care over the years.

Beth is quite clear on what it takes for home care to be of help. The person needs to be regular, needs to know basic safety and handling procedures, and be prepared to do whatever

tasks need to be done in a manner that fits in with the family routine. Beth's experience has been exactly the opposite: irregular staff, with few safety and handling skills, determined to do the tasks that they perceive need doing in their own way. Beth has fought hard to change this system. Right now, she feels that the help available, although by no means meeting these standards, is better than nothing and allows the rest of the family to achieve their morning routines.

For her, the biggest difficulty is that services assume that families ought to be grateful for whatever help they are given and not cause trouble by refusing to have particular staff members in their home or complaining. Angry at being denied access to vacation care, she lodged a complaint with the antidiscrimination board. Each holiday she has to argue to get her daughter into vacation care because there are complaints that it takes too long to feed and change her—"one hour for the staff, and 43 seconds (timed) for me ... they should be ashamed of themselves."

Like Gina, Beth does not help out in the classroom at her daughter's school. However, she is willing to represent the school in public arenas. She sees her contribution as being able to voice a strong point of view, as she did when the state minister for education recently visited her daughter's school. Beth has a clear view of what to fight for and what to let go. In her words:

You have to choose your fights. If you are going to argue with every person that makes a stupid comment in the supermarket ... I would really like to stop fighting with vacation care but I can't see that in the foreseeable future. Home care is getting better. Respite care is sort of all right—that's the four hours of the irregular supposedly regular woman who comes in on Saturday morning.

However, knowing which fights to fight and persevering do not necessarily mean this is easy. She goes on to say:

It is very wearying. You get so tired having to fight everyone. I went to a lecture once by a guy who had no legs and he was talking about his life and his challenges. I asked him about always taking on the next fight and he said for him when he takes on some fight that each time it gives him a charge—knocking over the flag—and I thought that's how he gets his motivation but that's not how I am. Every one of my battles wearies me. I think I probably win more than I lose but each one is incredibly wearying.

Beth's activism was born out of frustration and denial of basic help at home. Beth identifies her strengths and their usefulness to others in forcing system change. She willingly makes herself available to do this in public situations. She is certain that the best help she has received has come from others in similar situations. Their help has been empowering through sharing experiences and hard-won knowledge. Mothers of disabled children worldwide report similar experiences of learning most by sharing the load and exchanging information about how to be effective in responding to the challenges of day to day care (Cant, 1994; Clear, 1999).

Beth also recognizes changes in herself that have come about as part of the struggle to get what she and her family need. She is ambivalent about these changes. On the one hand, she acknowledges the empowering aspects of activism and the ways in which one's individual contributions have personal meaning. On the other, she speaks of her weariness in continuing the ongoing fights to achieve the opportunities that she desires for her daughter and for others:

I think I am a very different person now than I would have been if I didn't have children with disabilities. I was extremely stressed by my circumstances and I think I have changed as a result. I am certainly pushier and prepared to fight for what I think is right because it's not for me it's my child. Whereas I am not prepared to make a fuss on my behalf I am prepared to make a fuss on her behalf. Certainly my life has worked out in ways I never imagined. It's not necessarily a disaster, not necessarily terrible but different from what I planned. I worry about her future about when she is older. I worry about adolescence when her sister is going out all the times and she is not. I worry about what

happens after school and what that will mean for my working ... I am certainly different. There are a lot of compromises I would not have made. Life goes on. People say you are so wonderful. I think well I do it because they are my kids. And when people say that it's almost as if they are saying the child is not worth it. I find it vaguely insulting. Like I was sitting in a café with my husband and Josephine having lunch and a man in the shop said "you are so wonderful how do you cope?" and I thought leave me alone I am having my lunch. Some of the stupid comments.

The last part of Beth's story also illustrates how not all fights are necessarily with the systems that frame the lives of mothers of disabled children. Some fights are quite personal as mothers fight community attitudes that, on the one hand, devalue mother care and, on the other, regard mothers of disabled children as heroes.

⌘ Vignette: *Philippa and Joshua*

Philippa has a young son, Joshua, who has autism. He attends a special school for autistic children some distance away from home. Public transportation is almost non-existent and Philippa does not drive. She is rarely able to visit the classroom, although she talks about how the school is really helpful in designing programs for her to use at home to manage her son's particularly difficult and antisocial behaviors.

For Philippa, there is no defining moment that propelled her into action. Rather, there is ongoing anger coupled with anxiety about the ambiguous nature of the services and systems for disabled children. She tells the story of the school bus to illustrate her point. The state department of education provides a bus to transport her son from home to school. Although she acknowledges that this is a welcome service, particularly because she does not drive, the shortcomings are also great. For example, the bus driver does not always let her know he has arrived. She may be upstairs and not hear the bus, yet Joshua will run out and get on the bus, particularly if she is busy with the baby. Anxious for his safety, she then has to call the driver on his mobile (cell phone) to check that he has picked up her son. One afternoon recently, the bus broke down for the third time on leaving the school grounds, with smoke billowing from the exhaust. The teachers, concerned for the children's safety, refused to allow the driver to transport the children home. Immediately the mothers had to arrange alternative transport for that afternoon, a difficult task at the last moment, and only made possible for Philippa because her mother was visiting and able to pick up her son.

In the past Philippa was a member of the respite service committee. She was concerned, as were other families, about leaving their children at the respite cottage with staff members they did not know. This came about when a new staff member was employed unbeknown to the families using the service. Philippa suggested that information about each new staff member and their photograph should be included in the weekly newsletter to prepare parents and their children before going to the respite cottage. Despite the service initially going along with this idea, it was not very long before the practice was curtailed. The reason given was the time and cost involved. A similar situation occurred when she suggested that a brief description be sent home with each child of the activities they had done at respite, because this would be helpful for the child and family. This practice was instituted for a brief period and then discontinued on the grounds of unreasonable cost.

Philippa's experience in providing practical solutions to issues of concern to families as service users has fanned her involvement in a local advocacy group. This group is now planning strategies to support a "disability-friendly" political candidate at the next state election. An issue of immediate concern that she is pursuing, with an eye to her son's future, is the lack of reasonable employment opportunities for people with a disability. She is currently taking up the case of a young visually impaired woman who is unable to get a job because of serious epilepsy and is forced to work in a sheltered workshop for only $ 50 per week—way below the level of her abilities.

In contrast to the earlier stories, Philippa's activism at this stage is not directly focused on achieving change for her own child. Rather, she translates the concerns experienced in using services into issues to be solved on behalf of children and their families who are similarly placed. She is focusing her attention on system change. She continues to suggest practical solutions to alleviate parental anxiety as well as working at the political level to bring about institutional change.   ⌘

Vignette: *Joy and Angus*

Joy has three sons. The eldest is 16, the middle child is 13, and the youngest, Angus, who has Down syndrome, is 8 years old. Angus attends the local public school at the end of the street, although this was not Joy's first preference. The other boys had attended the local Catholic school. However, this school rejected Angus at school entry age, arguing that the diocese did not have the funds to support his needs.

Joy was very disappointed that the diocesan school would not accommodate Angus. She was left with her faith but little allegiance to the church. Joy then found a local school that would accept Angus. He is now in a mainstream class with support from a teacher's aide for 12 hours per week, and this is now working well. Initially the school, particularly the deputy principal, "tried very hard to get rid of me" and found all sorts of "silly reasons" to complain about Angus, saying he was not always lining up properly when the bell rang. Joy "stood her ground" despite a difficult 2-hour meeting to sort out issues. After this meeting, she felt confirmed in her actions by the department's integration officer, who was similarly horrified at the way in which the school staff were "bullying" the parents. With a new teacher the next year and then a new principal, the situation changed dramatically for the better. Now if problems arise, the teacher asks, "How can we work on this? What can we do?"

Joy helps out at the school about once weekly as a reading mother. She does this, she says, out of gratitude for Angus being accepted there. Although she acknowledges that mothers of children with disabilities should not feel the need to be grateful, this feeling of "ought to be grateful" pervades her willingness to help out. At the time of the first interview, she was planning on giving up her daytime help at the school because of growing pressure at work. She was considering joining the parents and friends association because the meetings are held in the evenings.

Joy, who is a registered nurse, was involved in clinical teaching at a university when she became pregnant with Angus. Because of the time needed to carry out Angus's early intervention activities at home, she was not able to continue lecturing. Instead, with a colleague, she set up a practice providing training to assistant and enrolled nurses in nursing homes. This provided a great deal of flexibility with teaching hours planned ahead of time and her administrative tasks organized around this schedule and the family's needs.

Joy identifies that her activism began at Angus's early intervention program. Her experience of being shown activities, whether PT, OT, or educational, and these activities being written down with the expectation that she carry them out at home has meant that, in her own words, "I have learned a lot." She now remains on the lookout for behaviors that may be troublesome and makes sure that they include activities within their daily routine to teach Angus the correct behavior.

Joy seeks out others to assist her as needed to advocate for her son. For example, when the school was initially trying to "get rid of" Angus, she called on her departmental case manager to gather support for continuing his integration. She also seeks out information from organizations, for example, the Down Syndrome Association. Joy explains her activism on Angus's behalf quite simply as:

> Not having much choice. You want what is best for him and to do that you want to go and access everything you can. When he was born, someone said to me, but you're so lucky, the kids grow up but he'll be with you forever. They probably meant well but I don't want this child forever I want to make this child independent!

In the early years Joy was involved in support activities, including coffee mornings with other mothers through the Down Syndrome Association. Once Angus began school, life resumed more normality, and she felt less need for these types of support. Joy talks about having a disabled child as a challenge, and one that has made her a much stronger person, more assertive. She is really proud that she stood up to the teachers at Angus's school in the early days. She also feels it is unlikely that she would have started her own business without her experience mothering Angus. So, she said, " it has changed me, it's been rewarding." Everyone in her life (business people from the nursing homes, her students) all know about Angus, which, she feels, adds a more human side to life. They will ask questions such as "Did you think of terminating your pregnancy?" This provides an opportunity to talk quite openly and to help others become aware of disability and associated issues.

By the time of the second interview, 18 months later, there was another new teacher in Angus's life. He was developing some difficult behavior, and it had been suggested that he move to a special unit. With the help of the integration officer and the principal, who likes Angus's personality, Joy held out to continue his placement in the mainstream class, and this now seems to be working better. This incident influenced Joy to begin seeking out a high school for Angus, even though this is a few years away.

Joy's story illustrates the continuing nature of activism in the lives of mothers of disabled children. Although initially bitterly disappointed by the local parochial school rejecting her child, this experience empowered Joy, building on her earlier experiences in the early intervention program. From that time, she has actively worked to ensure that Angus's schooling gives him the best chance in life. Joy's experience amounts to "there is no choice for mothers but to become active." This statement echoes the underlying currents in the other mothers'accounts. As a group, these mothers feel strongly that unless they become active in seeking out what is needed to support their child's needs and ensuring that this is delivered, their children will continue to suffer the social restrictions and discrimination levelled against people with a disability more generally in the community.

Joy's brief account also illustrates, as do Clara and Beth's accounts, how mothers' identities can change through the experience of "fighting" for entitlements for their children. Although Joy considers herself to be a strong person she credits her experiences with Angus and particularly the school system with bringing about a change in her identity. She now describes herself as an assertive person. She values this deeply and sees her work situation as the ideal opportunity to "spread the word— far and wide" about disability and the contribution made by disabled children to the community.   ⌘

⤷ Agency and Structure

Mothers of disabled children are subject to intense scrutiny. Their lives inevitably spill over from the personal to the public arena. Once impairment is identified, either at birth or in the early years, the private life of the family becomes exposed to the public gaze. This is particularly so if the child's impairment is immediately obvious to others. In the richer technological societies, families with a disabled child typically become involved with early intervention, medical, and health services and receive support from the state. In the poorer societies, which house the majority of the world population, impairment and disability almost exclusively result in disadvantage and, in many instances, poverty for the child and the family (e.g., Stone, 2001).

Typically, mothers bear the brunt of discrimination or disadvantage irrespective of society or culture (e.g., Iarskia-Smirnova, 1999). In response, activism weaves its way through the occupations of mothers of disabled children. The complex interrelationships between agency and structure in the mothers' accounts raise four issues to which we now turn. These are: *being alike, but different, experience as a catalyst for activism, change in identity*, and *mother care*. All but the last address mothers' agency in relation to the systems they encounter. The last addresses the broader

societal influences with respect to disability and gender.

Alike but Different

The vignettes presented in this chapter demonstrate the marked influence of childhood impairment on families and particularly mothers. The mothers presented here share many things in common. Each has a school-aged disabled child. They all come from a particular geographical location in a highly urbanized capital city. They are all exposed to the institutional structures and broader social relationships inherent within this society.

Typically, the mothers in this study come from middle-class, Anglo-Australian backgrounds in which the division of labor in the home (when two parents are present) follows a traditional pattern. The fathers are responsible for activities outside the home, providing financially, and doing the yard work. The mothers care for the children and do the inside domestic tasks. Not all these mothers are full-time housewives. Jenny and Joy are in paid part-time employment; Elizabeth and Beth hold down full-time paid positions. All are engaged, however, as are other mothers of young children, in the organization and management of everyday family routines to accommodate their families' needs.

Coordinating the services, benefits, programs, and people involved with their disabled children is an additional demand on the time of these mothers. These demands can be intensive and ongoing and significantly intrude into the everyday activities of family life. The following account from Traustadottir (1991) illustrates the occupational work done by mothers in managing services for their disabled children. This mother, who has a daughter with severe physical disabilities, explained:

> My daughter is seen by 17 professionals, or at least it was the last time I counted. I'm sure it is way up by now because there are all these computer specialists now. Seventeen professionals! Now who is going to take responsibility for making sure that all these professionals are seen? That whatever they say is followed up on? That they coordinate and talk to each other, that they are paid ... If

you are going to survive as a mother ... you become an expert manager" (Traustadottir, 1991, p. 222).

Echoes of this account are heard throughout the interview transcripts in our study. Our analysis, however, suggests that the need for organization of services on the part of mothers of disabled children goes well beyond the administrative and managerial, as suggested here. Indeed, the activism undertaken by the mothers presented here suggests that constant vigilance of services is fundamental to ensuring that their disabled child is not disadvantaged or denied opportunities. The vignettes in this chapter demonstrate that activism is another occupation added to the existing occupational repertoire of mothers of disabled children.

We must be cautious, however, about generalizing that all mothers of disabled children will carry out their mothering occupations in the same way, driven by the same goals, or for the same purposes. Families have already critiqued the well established research tradition of conceptualizing childhood disability unidimensionally as a burden inevitably resulting in family tragedy (Stainton & Besser, 1998; Turnbull et al., 1993). It is imperative that the mothering occupations of mothers of disabled children are not similarly seen in a uniform light. As the vignettes clearly demonstrate and as ecocultural theory predicts, mothers' occupational actions vary considerably and derive in part from their values, goals, and beliefs (ecological) and in part from the ways in which they regard the resources and constraints in the environment in which they live (cultural) (Kellegrew, 2002 & Segal, 2000).

For example, Clara and Joy both regard their health-care backgrounds as resources for their activism. The influence of their respective professional backgrounds, however, plays out quite differently in their ongoing activism. Clara identifies her knowledge of the therapies available and alternative schooling options as instrumental to the actions she has taken for her son James. Joy regards her nursing training and education consultancy as an excellent opportunity to promote acceptance

and inclusion of people with disabilities more widely in the community.

Experience as a Catalyst for Activism

As the vignettes demonstrate, negative or unsatisfactory experiences with professionals and service systems are typical catalysts for mothers' activism. Wickham-Searl (1992b) found similar triggers in the stories of mothers engaged in public disability-related work. Dishearteningly, families' negative experiences continue despite over three decades of an extensive research and practitioner literature promoting collaborative partnerships between professionals and parents of disabled children (e.g., Porter & McKenzie, 2000). It is evident from the mothers' stories that the unequal structures of parent/professional relations continue to exclude parents from full participation in determining the care they desire for their child (Clear, 1999).

It is not surprising, given the children's ages, that the majority of the mothers' frustrations were directed at the school system. Some mothers, such as Elizabeth and Peg, had proactively sought out the "best" schooling they could find for their children. They then went on to work hard, in different ways, to ensure that their children's experiences lived up to their expectations. Peg, in effect, has taken on the role of special aide in her son's classroom. She is available throughout the school day to assist her son so that he does not miss out on class experiences. Elizabeth maintains a constant alert to disadvantage and takes action as needed to overturn any discrimination experienced by disabled children in her daughter's school.

For other mothers, unanticipated and problematic events with their children's schooling propelled them into quite different forms of activism. Jane has taken over part of the school system's responsibility and brought a part of her son's education into the family home as his part-time teacher. Jenny, on the other hand, has taken her domestic tasks, specifically food preparation and serving, into the school environment in her role as canteen assistant. In these examples, the flexibility of occupational context for mothering and the adaptability of occupational tasks is made plain.

The importance of education for disabled children cannot be denied. As the mothers here intuitively know, it is a critical factor in how their children will be accepted into the life of the community. Yet, as at least several of the mothers' accounts demonstrate, disabled children continue to be denied the opportunities open to others. As Priestley (2001) noted this is true irrespective of country or culture:

As global markets and technologies develop in new ways, access to education becomes ever more important, particularly for children and young people. Yet many disabled people have been denied educational opportunities to develop the knowledge and skills required for survival in a changing world (Priestley, 2001, p. 9).

Once a disabled child is in school, his or her placement is not necessarily stable. A large part of the mothers' occupational work reported here focused on monitoring their children's educational experiences and being prepared to act—and to do so quickly—if an undesirable situation arose. One way to describe this is as mothers working hard to make their child's schooling the best it can be, and making sure this continues. Given the 13 or so years of compulsory schooling in countries in the minority world, this suggests that mothers' activism in relation to school systems is likely to be extended over a considerable period of time. For those mothers concerned to have their children included in mainstream classes, recent work on the outcomes of inclusion confirms this view. Hanson et al. (2001) conducted a follow up study of children with disabilities, all of whom were in some level of inclusion in the preschool years. By the second grade, this figure had dropped to 60 percent. Of all the factors responsible, professional opinions and not parents' wishes were the most powerful.

The mothers' stories add support to the dominance of professional influence on disabled children's schooling choices. There is a limited and a priori menu of service delivery

options presented to families that is quite inconsistent with the breadth of opportunities available to nondisabled children. As Jenny found when her son was rejected from his local school, and the other mothers' stories confirm, the philosophy held by the school community is paramount in determining access to educational opportunities.

There is substantial evidence from many countries that organizational structures at the local or state level either facilitate inclusion or raise barriers preventing the full range of educational opportunities being available to disabled children despite legislation or policy directives (e.g., Llewellyn, Thompson & Fante, 2000, 2002; Peck, Furman & Helmsetter, 1993). Mothers' activism in the face of these limitations takes various forms. Mothers' efforts in working actively to at best overcome and otherwise minimize the disadvantage of the limited options speaks to their creativity and commitment: Jane as special aide, Jenny as canteen assistant, Clara as go-between (teacher and therapist), and the list goes on; limited options, philosophical commitment, and organizational structures all become grist for the mill of mothers' activism.

Change In Identity

Identity change is frequently discussed as a consequence of social change activism, and is likely to be particularly profound for those new to activism (Della Porta & Diani, 1999; Herda-Rapp, 2000). Mothers who had undertaken public disability-related work in studies by Wickham-Searl (1992) and Traustadottir (1991) reported coming to recognize and acclaim their expertise, growth in self-confidence and assertiveness, and development of a deeper understanding of the interrelationships between their lives and service systems.

Similar benefits have been reported for the parents, who are mostly mothers, involved in mutual self-help groups. Solomon, Pistrang, & Barker (2001) note three domains of change: the sociopolitical, interpersonal and the intra-individual. Derived from and superordinate to these domains, they propose that identity change occurs in the following way. At the sociopolitical level, members of self-help groups report becoming empowered and developing a sense of control and agency in the world, In the interpersonal domain, changes occur in social identity as parents came to feel part of, and belong to a community of, similarly placed individuals; and finally, in the intra-individual domain, self-change occurs in the form of increased confidence and self-esteem.

Rather than assume generalized benefits to mothers' identity from engaging in activism, we argue that it is critical to understand mothers' identity development within their ongoing relationships. Following Gergen (1994) and social constructionist theory (Blumer, 1969), mothers' narrative accounts offer the ideal opportunity to understand how they portray themselves. Identity is multidimensional and subject to redefinition through experience. As Giddens (1991) suggested, we propose that the mothers' identities, as represented in these brief accounts, can be viewed as constructed and reconstructed in the context of their interactions.

We illustrated this point with the accounts from Clara, Beth, and Joy. Each acknowledged personal changes brought about by taking on activism as a mothering occupation. Each engaged in new tasks and added responsibilities when faced with having a disabled child. Each experienced identity change differently. For Clara, the key to identity change is her recognition of reordering priorities in her life, becoming more open and willing to share with others. Identity change for Joy is recognized in her newfound assertiveness and a steadily developing commitment to changing community attitudes toward disabled children. Beth also reported identity change. However, these changes seem hard won and accepted reluctantly. She expressed regret at "the lot of compromises I would not have made (in the absence of a disabled child)."

Beth's experience added weight to our caution about making too much of or romanticizing positive identity changes. We must not assume that all mothers will be similarly empowered or derive benefits from activism on behalf of their children. Although all the mothers here maintained their activism, often in the face of considerable resistance, they do not necessarily view this as a solely positive influence in their lives. Beth reported weariness at the constant battles with systems and community attitudes. In contrast, Joy talks with obvious delight about her opportunities to spread the word about disability far and wide. These contrasting accounts are a timely reminder of how the relationship between agency and structure is experienced differently. As Traustadottir (2000) also reminds us, "Too much celebration of the personal fulfillment women derive from caring ... can easily turn into celebration of differences that serve as a rationale to keep women in an inferior position" (p. 254).

Mother Care

Mothers still largely do the caring work done by parents of disabled children (Read, 2000). Women continue to bear the largest load of caring work more generally (Bittman, 1998). Do we typically think of mothers of disabled children as caregivers? Generally not, because we assume that mothers will care for their children as a matter of course, without recourse to a title such as carer. How then do we regard mothers of school-age disabled children when their children require much more care than typically developing children? Many mothers of disabled children, especially those with children with high support needs, face a lifetime of care. Studies of older mothers of adult disabled children demonstrate that many women find themselves locked into a lifetime career of caring when they have a disabled child (e.g., Hayden & Heller, 1997; Llewellyn et al., 2002a).

The care work that women do and the meaning that this work has in their lives has been examined in British, North American, and Nordic feminist scholarship (Dalley, 1988; Meyer, 2000; Traustadottir, 1991, 2000; Twigg & Atkin, 1994; Wickham-Searl, 1992a). Of relevance here is the often-blurred distinction between caring for and caring about. Caring for is to do with the tasks of tending another person. Caring about explains the feelings held for another person. This distinction between caring for and caring about someone is rarely made in relation to mothering. Dalley (1988) argued that this is "Because it is considered so perfectly natural that in motherhood, caring for and about are so completely integrated, that it is unnecessary to disentangle them" (p. 8).

Women, particularly mothers, are disadvantaged by the lack of differentiation between caring about and caring for. In family and community care policies in many countries, this has led to the unexamined assumption that those who care about will always care for and vice versa (Schofield et al., 1998; Twigg & Atkin, 1994). This means that women, especially mothers, are regarded as the natural carers of their relatives, and any disagreement with this is seen as unwomanly and deviant. The expectation that this pattern of caring belongs "naturally" to women has placed a substantial and frequently unrecognized burden on women, especially mothers, of all ages (e.g., Traustadottir, 2000; Ungerson, 1987). The understanding that it is women who do the caring ignores and alienates male carers to the extent that they are almost totally neglected in research, policy, and practice.

For mothers of disabled children, there are societal demands in addition to the gendered expectation of women as carers (Llewellyn et al., 1999; Traustadottir, 1991). The first of these comes from the assumption that people with impairments are *ipso facto* dependent for the duration of their lifetime. Stereotyped images of disabled people worldwide conjure up eternal children dependent on others, typically their families, for support, and indeed, in many countries, for survival. Consequently, mothers of disabled children are burdened with an expectation of caring (because they are women) and an expectation of lifelong caring (because they have a dependent child).

Feminist analysis has demonstrated that the social identity of care work is derived from the so-called "feminine" nature of mothers' work (DeVault, 1991). Thus care work is seen as being women's work and particularly that of mothers for the reasons noted (Francis-Connolly, 2000). This is confirmed by census data, which demonstrate that disabled people worldwide are predominantly cared for at home by their mothers or sisters (Priestley, 2001). Additional research on disability workers demonstrates that the majority are women,

and in one study at least, these women were also usually mothers (Traustadottir & Taylor, 1998).

The "feminine" nature of caring work, coupled with women carrying society's major caring responsibilities in their families, further denigrates caregiving work. This is because, as Dalley (1988) noted, all women's work is devalued in society. Others, including the feminist Carol Smart (1996) and philosopher Sara Ruddick (1989), suggested that mothers' work is additionally devalued but may, in certain circumstances, be idealized. Beth's encounter with a man in a café while she was lunching with her husband and daughter illustrates this hero effect. Both devaluation and idealization produce similar results. What mothers do in caring for (and about) their disabled children is rarely regarded as "real" work.

Wickham-Searl (1992b) suggested that mothers of disabled children experience an additional devaluation because of the transfer of the stigma attached to their child. If this is the case, it is not surprising that mother care of disabled children is not considered real. Work not considered real is rendered invisible. The fact that most mothers care of disabled children occurs in the relative isolation of the home compounds its invisibility. In sum, when mothers care for a disabled child, their occupational work is seen as women's work, automatically feminized, stigmatized by association with impairment, and typically carried out behind closed doors.

Mothers in our study extended their mother care beyond the boundaries of the family home. These mothers are engaged in activism, in one sense, in a "public" place. They are no longer invisible in their homes; they are visibly present in classrooms, in school canteens, on committees, in political organizations, and in public arenas. Is their mother care as represented in their activism more likely to be acknowledged as real work? Two examples from the literature suggest this could be the case. The first is the recognition given to mutual self-help groups and the second is disability-related work by mothers in service or advocacy agencies.

Mutual self-help groups for parents of disabled children have long been recognized as providing their members with a sense of belonging to a community and a sense of empowerment, control, and agency in the outside world (for example, Linder, 1970 and more recently, Solomon, Pistrang, & Barker, 2001). Of interest here is the structural and societal approval given to these groups in the form of financial, practical, and psychological support from professionals and service agencies. This is true even for those models that rely on direct parent-to-parent support, for example, when a "veteran" parent who is experienced in caring for disabled child is matched in a one-to-one relationship with a "referred" parent who is new to the role (Llewellyn, Griffin, & Sacco, 1992; Singer et al., 1999). This social condoning of self-help groups suggests recognition of the contribution of mother care in a group setting. Yet, when mothers individually undertake similar supportive actions, these may be undermined. Philippa's story illustrates this point. On two occasions, she presented practical suggestions to the respite care service designed to enhance parents and children's experiences in this form of substitute care. Although both suggestions were initially supported, neither received ongoing support.

Traustadottir (1991) provided one explanation as to why mothers' activism may attract social respect when it is carried out in a public arena in contrast to relatively private and individual activities such as Philippa's. She suggested that, when mothers extend their caring work beyond their own child into a disability-related field, the resultant activities come to be regarded more like a "professional" career. Mothers may join "parents' movement" groups, lobby legislators, argue with school officials, and so on. She goes on to argue that, although these are not normally regarded as female activities, when performed by mothers of disabled children, "they are seen as an extension of the mother's caring role and an expression of the mother's devotion to her child" (Traustadottir, 1991, p. 218), and are thus socially condoned.

The findings from Wickham-Searl's (1992a, 1992b, 1994) interview study with mothers of disabled children suggested an alternative explanation. Each of the mothers had taken on a disability-related career in the public arena. Of the 12 mothers in this study, 4 held volunteer positions, 4 held paid positions in not-for-profit organizations, 3 held paid positions within the disability advocacy field, and 1 was a special needs teacher's assistant. These mothers reported their work in these areas began in small ways, seeking advice from other parents of disabled children, and grown into what they regarded as their career. Whether others regarded the work of these mothers work as a career is, however, doubtful. This is made evident by the poor wages attached to this disability-related work. Poor wages are the case more generally for all disability workers in what is a particularly feminized employment field, as noted previously (Traustadottir, 2000). Although they gained satisfaction and a sense of contribution from their work, some of the mothers in Wickham-Searl's study (1992a) expressed resentment that their work was not valued by society because they were unable to earn "respectable" wages. We would argue that, although their public disability-related pursuits may attract more recognition than the individual activism pursuits of mothers, their work remains interpreted as little more than an extension and indeed a "natural" part of their mother caring role.

Conclusion

For the mothers of disabled children who take on activism as a mothering occupation there is a shift in the locus of their care work. They provide ongoing care for their disabled children and families, and they incorporate another mothering occupation into their caring work. Already busy with families and the personal and societal demands of caring for a disabled child, mother activists work on behalf of their own child, extend their concerns to other disabled children, and attempt to make the world a better place for disabled people. As we have seen in the mothers' stories in this chapter, activism as a mothering occupation can develop from a variety of experiences, serve different purposes, and take many forms, all of which speak to the complex interrelationship between agency and structure in individual mother's lives.

Is mother activism accorded its rightful due? Are mothers seeking recognition by adding activism to their mothering occupations? Some mothers identify identity change as a positive and rewarding outcome; others speak of deeply felt motivation to serve their own child and satisfaction in doing so amid the frustrations of ensuring a fair deal for their children. Institutional structures, such as school systems, reap extensive benefits by accepting the work done in the name of mothers' occupational activism. They benefit from the volume of unpaid labor provided by these mothers, for example, in classrooms, in teaching at home, and as "helpers" on school outings. The mothers' accounts, however, suggest that mothers' occupational activism work, although tolerated, remains invisible to these broader social systems. Mothers regard "fighting" for their children as a natural extension of their mother care. Acceptance of invisible mother labor confirms that their activism in the public arena is legitimized as a "natural" extension of their private caring responsibilities.

We come to the conclusion that activism as a mothering occupation is firmly lodged within a continuing expression of care work. This is despite the increasing awareness of the gendered nature of care and feminization in particular of caring work with disabled people. Our mothers' accounts show that, even though mothers may derive personal satisfaction from this occupation, engaging in activism may not always be freely chosen. Mothers and the institutional structures that frame their own and their children's lives, understand activism as a "natural" extension of being a mother. Although activism potentially provides the opportunity for mothers to promote social change, the solid embedding of care work as women's work only serves to reinforce existing gendered expectations and care practices with disabled children.

Discussion Questions 🙠

- In the Introduction section, we posed three questions. The first was: Can we imagine a world where mothers of disabled children need not engage in activism as a mothering

occupation? Choose any one of the mothers' stories under the heading "On Behalf of My Child" and identify what needs to happen so that the mother would not feel compelled to engage in activism on behalf of her child. In doing this task, keep in mind the third of our earlier questions, which was: What responsibility do practitioners bear to join with mothers and work toward making the campaign (for better social conditions for her child and her family) redundant?

- Mothers in the third group framed their stories in a social justice perspective. Read through their stories again and decide whether they achieved their goal to make the world a better place for disabled people. If not, why not? What barriers existed to prevent them from reaching this goal? What role do practitioners have in removing these barriers?

- Given that the mothers' stories speak to the power of social systems and the professionals that are part of these systems, what strategies can practitioners use to defuse professional power and, in turn, empower mothers as they seek desired goals for their disabled son or daughter?

References

Bittman, M. (1998). Changing family responsibilities. The role of social attitudes, markets and the state. *Family Matters, 50*, 31–37.

Blumer, H. (1969). *Symbolic interactionism. Perspective and method*. Englewood Cliffs: Prentice-Hall, Inc.

Bronfenbrenner, U. (1979). *The ecology of human development*. Cambridge, MA: Harvard University Press.

Bronfenbrenner, U., & Morris, P. (1988). Ecological systems theory. In R. Lesner (Ed.). *Handbook of child psychology: Vol 1: Theoretical models of human development* (5th ed., pp. 993–1028). New York: Wiley & Sons.

Cant, R. (1994). Just care-giving: whose work, whose control? In C. Wadell & A. R. Petersen (Eds.). *Just health. Inequality in illness, care and prevention* (Chapter 18). Melbourne: Churchill Livingstone.

Clear, M. (1999). Caring culture and the politics of parent/professional relations. *Australian Journal of Social Issues, 34*(2), 119–130.

Corker, M. & French, S. (Eds.)(1999). *Disability discourse*. Milton Keynes: Open University Press.

Dalley, G. (1988). *Ideologies of caring. Rethinking community and collectivism*. London (UK): Macmillan.

Della Porta, D., & Diani, M. (1999). *Social movements*. Oxford (UK): Blackwell.

De Vault, M. L. (1991). *Feeding the family. The social organization of family as gendered work*. Chicago: University of Chicago Press.

Driedger, D. (1989). *The last civil rights movement: Disabled People's International.* London (UK): Hurst & Co.

Francis-Connolly, E. (2000). Toward an understanding of mothering: A comparison of two motherhood stages. *American Journal of Occupational Therapy, 54*(3), 281–289.

Gallimore, R., Weisner, T. S., Kaufman, S. Z., & Bernheimer, L. P. (1989). The social construction of ecocultural niches: Family accommodation of developmentally delayed children. *American Journal on Mental Retardation, 94*(3), 216–230.

Gallimore, R., Weisner, T. S., Bernheimer, L. P., Guthrie, D., & Nihira, K. (1993). Family responses to young children with developmental delays: Accommodation activity in ecological and cultural context. *American Journal on Mental Retardation, 98*(2), 185–206.

Gergen, K. J. (1994). *Realities and relationships: Soundings in social construction.* Cambridge: Harvard University Press.

Giddens, A. (1991). *Modernity and self-identity.* Stanford, CA: Stanford University Press.

Hanson, M. J., Horn, E., Sandall, S., Beckman, P., Morgan, M., Marquart, J., Barnwell, D., & Chou, H. (2001). After preschool inclusion: Children's educational pathways over the early school years. *Exceptional Children, 69*(1), 65–83.

Hayden, M. F., & Heller, T. (1997). Support, problem-solving/coping ability, and personal burden of younger and older caregivers of adults with mental retardation. *Mental Retardation, 35*(5), 264–372.

Herda-Rapp, A. (2000). The impact of social activism on gender identity and care work. In M. H. Meyer (Ed.), *Care work. Gender, class and the welfare state* (pp. 45–64). New York: Routledge.

Iarskia-Smirnova, E. (1999). "What the future will bring I do not know": mothering children with disabilities in Russia and the politics of exclusion'. *Frontiers: A Journal for Women's Studies, XX* (2), 68–86.

Kasnitz, D. (2001). Life event histories and the US independent living movement. In M. Priestley (Ed). *Disability and the life course. Global perspectives* (pp. 67–78). Cambridge: Cambridge University Press.

Kellegrew, D. H. (2000). Constructing daily routines: A qualitative examination of mothers with young children with disabilities. *American Journal of Occupational Therapy, 54*(3), 252–259.

Linder, R. (1970). Mothers of disabled children: The value of weekly group meetings. *Developmental Medicine and Child Neurology, 12,* 202–206.

Llewellyn, G., Bratel, J., Thompson, K., Whybrow, S., Coles, D., Wearing, C., & McConnell, D. (2002). *Supporting families. Family well being in families of children with disabilities and high support needs.* Final report, ARC-SPIRT Project Grant, 1998–2000.

Llewellyn, G., Dunn, P., Fante, M., Turnbull, L., & Grace, R. (1999). Family factors influencing out-of-home placement decisions. *Journal of Intellectual Disability Research, 43*(3), 219–241.

Llewellyn, G., Gething, L., Cant, R., & Kendig, H. (2002). Progress report, NHMRC Project Grant 107305, *Service pathways for ageing caregivers of adults with intellectual disability.*

Llewellyn, G., Griffin, S., & Sacco, M. (1992). The Parent-to-Parent model in Australia, *Australian Disability Review, 3,* 42–50.

Llewellyn, G., Thompson, K., & Fante, M. (2002). Inclusion in early childhood services: ongoing challenges. *Australian Journal of Early Childhood,* 27(3), 18–23.

Llewellyn, G., Thompson, K., & Fante, M. (2000). Young children with disabilities in NSW Children's Services. In NSW Department of Community Services, *Insights into research. Four studies on early childhood issues and children's services.* Sydney: Author.

Meyer, M. H. (Ed.) (2000). *Care work. Gender, class and the welfare state* (pp. 45–64). New York: Routledge.

Nihira, K., Weisner, T. S, & Bernheimer, L. P. (1994). Ecocultural assessment in families of children with developmental delays: Construct and concurrent validities, *American Journal of Mental Retardation, 98*(5), 551–556.

Peck, C. A., Furman, G. C., & Helmsetter, E. (1993). Integrated early childhood programs: Research on the implementation of change in organizational contexts. In C. A. Peck, S. L. Odom, & D. D. Bricker (Eds.). *Integrating young children with disabilities into community programs: Ecological perspectives on research and implementation* (pp. 187–205). Baltimore: Paul H Brookes.

Porter, L., & McKenzie, S. (2000). *Professional collaboration with parents of children with disabilities.* Sydney: Maclennan and Petty.

Priestley, M. (2001). Introduction: the global context of disability. In M. Priestley (Ed.). *Disability and the life course. Global perspectives* (pp. 3–14). Cambridge: Cambridge University Press.

Read, J. (2000). *Disability, the family and society. Listening to mothers.* Buckingham: Open University Press.

Ruddick, S. (1989). *Maternal thinking. Toward a politics of peace.* New York: Ballantine Books.

Schofield, H., Bloch, S., Herman, H., Murphy, B., Nankervis, J., & Singh, B. (1998). *Family caregivers. Disability, illness and ageing.* Melbourne: Allen and Unwin, Victorian Health Promotion Foundation.

Segal, R. (2000). Adaptive strategies of mothers of children with attention deficit hyperactivity disorder: enfolding and unfolding occupations. *American Journal of Occupational Therapy, 54*(3), 300–306.

Singer, G. H. S., Marquis, J., Powers, K. L., Blanchard, L., Divenere, N., Santelli, B., Ainbinder, J. G., & Sharp, M. (1999). A multi-site evaluation of parent-to-parent programs for parents of children with disabilities. *Journal of Early Intervention, 22,* 217–229.

Smart, C. (1996). Deconstructing motherhood. In E.B. Silva (Ed.). *Good enough mothering* (pp. 37-57), London (UK): Routledge.

Smith, D. (1987). *The everyday world as problematic: A feminist sociology.* Boston: Northeastern University Press.

Solomon, M. N., Pistrang, N., & Barker, C. (2001). The benefits of mutual support groups for parents of children with disabilities. *American Journal of Community Psychology, 29*(1), 113–120.

Stainton, T., & Besser, H. (1998). The positive impact of children with an intellectual disability on the family. *Journal of Intellectual and Developmental Disability, 23*(1), 57–70.

Stone, E. (2001). A complicated struggle: disability, survival and social change in the majority world. In M. Priestley (Ed), *Disability and the life course. Global perspectives* (pp. 50–66). Cambridge: Cambridge University Press.

Traustadottir, R. (2000). Disability reform and women's caring work. In M. H. Meyer (Ed.). *Care work. Gender, class and the welfare state* (pp. 249–269). New York: Routledge.

Traustadottir, R. (1991). Mothers who care. Gender, disability and family life. *Journal of Family Issues, 12*(2), 211–228.

Traustadottir, R., & Taylor, S. J. (1998). Invisible women, invisible work: Women's caring work in developmental disability services. In S. J. Taylor and R. Bogdan (Eds.). *Introduction to qualitative research methods: A guidebook*

and resource (3rd ed.) (pp. 205–220). New York: John Wiley and Sons.

Turnbull, A. P., Patterson, J. M., Behr, S., Murphy, S. K., Murphy, D. L., Marquis, J. G., & Blue-Banning, M. J. (Eds.) (1993). *Cognitive coping, families & disability.* Baltimore, MA: Paul Brookes Publishing Co.

Twigg, J., & Atkin, K. (1994). *Carers perceived. Policy and practice in informal care.* Buckingham: Open University Press.

Ungerson, C. (1987). *Policy is personal: Sex, gender, and informal care.* London (UK): Tavistock.

Wickham-Searl, P. (1994). Mothers of children with disabilities and the construction of expertise. *Research in Sociology of Health Care,* 11, *175–187.*

Wickham-Searl, P. (1992a). Careers in caring: Mothers of children with disabilities. *Disability, Handicap & Society,* 7(1), 5–17.

Wickham-Searl, P. (1992b). Mothers with a mission. In P. Ferguson, D. Ferguson, and S. J. Taylor (Eds.). *Interpreting disability. A qualitative reader* (pp. 251–274). New York: Teachers College Press.

CHAPTER 15

Mothering Work: Negotiating Health Care, Illness and Disability, and Development

Mary C. Lawlor, ScD, OTR, FAOTA

 Anticipated Outcomes

We anticipate that, after reading this chapter, readers will:

- Describe characteristics of partnering up in health-care encounters

- Identify several characteristics of mothering experiences related to health-care encounters

- Analyze ways in which meanings of illness and disability and beliefs about development influence health-care encounters

- Discuss the complexity of mothering work and the implications for clinical practices

Introduction

I remember quite vividly the very first home visit I made as a novice occupational therapist. I had seen this mother and her toddler daughter several times in the interdisciplinary community clinic where I worked. This young mother always presented herself as calm, poised, and proficient in managing her daughter's many medical and developmental needs. The purpose of the home visit was to evaluate needs for such equipment as bathing and positioning devices as this child grew larger, but continued to show little developmental progress. As best as I can remember,

this child was 2, but had shown very limited abilities to move, to interact, or to respond to happenings in her environment. I had packed my new Toyota with various pieces of equipment to try out if needed. I entered the house with my clipboard and tape measure and a few other clinical artifacts. When I came into the kitchen, this mother, whom I will call Abby, asked me if I wanted to have some tea. In fact, I remember it more clearly as a kind of directive to take a seat and have some tea.

Although parts of this scene are still quite clear, other parts require a degree of reconstruction. I do remember the time sitting at the kitchen table and my anxiety over feeling that I should be doing something other than sitting and talking with Abby. I also recall furtive glances at my watch as the time ticked by while we sat and drank tea. Perhaps what I remember most clearly is my sense of deep ambivalence about how I should be spending my time. I remember worrying about whether I could get everything done if I continued to sit and talk. I also remember being conscious of my sense that something important was happening as we sat at the kitchen table. Abby talked quite openly about her daily struggles and her worries about the future. She was conveying to me more of who she was and how she saw her life. I remember being touched by her willingness to share her stories. I also wanted to listen. I sensed that she was telling me things that she wanted me to know about her life and her family, things that I needed to know if I was going to be more helpful. I was also hearing what she needed and wanted in her own way, on her own terms. I not only learned a lot, I learned how little I knew. I also realized how my attempts to prepare for this visit had been misguided.

How could I have known, or understood, so little about this mother's day-to-day world and her experiences of being a mother with this child, who had so many complex medical and developmental needs? What could it have been like for her to come regularly to therapy appointments and receive suggestions or home instructions? How did the act of sitting at the kitchen table and drinking tea generate such new and different understandings of how we might better work together? Why did I feel so ambivalent about whether this exchange was how I should have been using my time?

This story is one of many recalled encounters that continue to provoke my reflections about practices with children and their families and generate questions about the experiences of mothers of children who have illnesses or disabilities. I have spent much of the last dozen years thinking about and studying family-centered care practices and the ways in which practitioners and family members come to know *enough* about each other to effectively partner up in health-care and educational settings (Lawlor & Mattingly, 1998, 2001; Mattingly & Lawlor, 1998, 2001). While on this trajectory, I have increasingly been fo-

cusing on ways of trying to understand the experiences of mothers as they care for their children in both home and institutional worlds. Drawing upon ethnographic data, I will share some insights about the experiences of mothers engaged in "partnering up" with practitioners. The purposes of this chapter are to:

- Describe characteristics of partnering up in health-care encounters
- Present several characteristics of mothering experiences related to health-care encounters
- Provide an overview of a research project to study experiences of African American families
- Analyze ways in which meanings of illness and disability and beliefs about development influence health-care encounters
- Discuss implications for enhancing understanding of mothering experiences

Recent trends in services for children with special health-care needs have emphasized models of family-centered care (e.g., Hanft, 1989; Lawlor, & Mattingly, 1998; Rosenbaum, King, Law, King, & Evans, 1998). Descriptions of proposed partnership models are often framed in terms of empowerment of family members (e.g., Dunst, Trivette, & Deal, 1988; Turnbull, Turbiville, & Turnbull, 2000). These service delivery models require sophisticated forms of collaboration. The partnering-up process creates pressure on both parties to be understanding, skillful, cooperative, respectful of the other's perspective, and a "good enough" partner and collaborator. For both practitioners and parents, it is often difficult to enact this collaborative role, particularly when there are divergent perspectives on the nature of the clinical problem or course of intervention. Challenges to the collaborative process may be heightened in situations in which families and practitioners come from different lived worlds (Mattingly & Lawlor, 1998). Engaging family members as partners in intervention necessitates fundamental shifts in service delivery processes, including a reconceptualization of the nature of the work, expertise, and practitioner-parent relationships (Lawlor & Mattingly, 1998). The work for practitioners is not merely technical, in the sense that a procedure is done or a therapy or other intervention is provided; nor does the work just entail drawing upon clinical expertise. Rather, "partnering up" requires skilled relational work and involves the drawing upon a range of social skills, including intersubjectivity, communication, engagement, and understanding. These forms of collaborative relationships are also built on an appreciation that the involved parties share expertise and that parents and practitioners each bring valuable and complementary expertise to the clinical encounter.

The meanings of illness and disability are shaped by cultural beliefs (e.g., Garro, 2000; Morris, 1998.) Moments that emerge in the course of routine interactions related to health care or in the process of providing interventions over time can reveal cultural influences on illness and disability and health-care services. They can also foreground cultural issues related to family life, parenting, and child development. As Laderman and Roseman (1996) argue, "All medical encounters, no matter how mundane are dramatic events" (p. 1). Health-care encounters often generate narrative accounts or stories that provide rich data related to cultural influences. In the research described in this chapter, we rely heavily on both stories about life and health care and observations of moments that emerge in health-care encounters which reveal that something of significance is happening here to explore meanings of illness and disability, cross cultural communication, and negotiation of health care.

Recently, anthropologists and other social scientists have critiqued conceptualizations of culture that incorporated essentialism, reification or "thingness," and determinism, among other structural features (e.g., Fox & King, 2002; Ortner, 1999). This rethinking of culture allows for conceptualizations that acknowledge that people live in and negotiate multiple cultural worlds and identities. Participation in cultural worlds is enacted through practices, shaped by identities, and marked by social locations framed by cultures and social structures and institutions. Mattingly (2002) has recently argued that the clinic is a cultural border zone where culture is negotiated. Health-care worlds are a kind of meeting place where many cultures, practices, and social worlds intersect. Ortner (1999) also argued for the study of culture at the borders or intersections of cultural worlds, at "zones of friction," "in which the clash of power and meaning and identities is the stuff of change and transformation" (p. 8).

For all the tensions and conflicts at cultural borders, I would argue that health-care encounters also uncover "moments of meeting," to borrow from Tronick (1998), a phrase that is used to describe jointly constructed, complementary actions in which each participant contributes something unique and there is a shared state of consciousness. Moments of meeting occur when partnering up is most successful.

✒ Overview of Ethnographic Research Study

In the arguments that I present in the following paragraphs, I draw upon ethnographic data collected over the past 6 years through *Boundary Crossing: A Longitudinal and Ethnographic Study* (# R01 HD38878, 2000–2004) funded by the National Center for Medical Rehabilitation Research, National Institute of Child Health and Human Development, National Institutes of Health, and *Crossing Cultural Boundaries: An Ethnographic Study* (# MCJ 060745, 1996-1999), funded by the Maternal and Child Health Bureau. The purpose of these collaborative and interdisciplinary studies is to examine how the problems of children with special health-care needs are variously understood or "framed" by family members and health-care practitioners, the influence of different frames or understandings on the intervention process, the processes undertaken by family members and practitioners to negotiate or impose alternate views, and how partnerships with health-care providers alter over time as family structures and resources shift and children's needs change.

We are focusing on the intersections between family changes, changes in the personal lives of key caregivers, changes in health-care services, and child development. This interdisciplinary study is about "lives in motion," a phrase coined by Elder (1998, p. 7). As Elder argues, lives are "linked" and multiple life course trajectories intersect in the everyday lives of people and their social transactions. We recognize that individuals who are ill or have a disability are not the only people to have an experience related to illness or disability. Caregivers, family members, close friends, and other significant people in an individual's social world also have illness- or disability- related life experiences (Mattingly & Lawlor, 1998). We are gathering multiple perspectives on events such as health-care encounters, as well as perceptions about the children, their families, and their illness and development experiences.

The conceptual framework for the study draws heavily on narrative, interpretive, and phenomenological approaches to understanding human experience. Several related assumptions are relevant to the data shared in the following paragraphs. We are studying not only how people live their lives, but also how illness and disability, family life, health care, development, and culture are interrelated. In this study, special health-care needs are not defined in purely diagnostic terms. Rather, in line with a strong tradition in medical anthropology (Good, 1994; Kleinman, 1988; Lawlor & Mattingly, 1998; Mattingly, 1998; Mattingly & Lawlor, 1998), we are examining commonalities of the disability experience that transcend diagnostic categories. In linking commonality to experience rather than biomedically defined disease categories, we follow the important distinction made in anthropology between a "disease" (or diagnostic condition) and an "illness experience" (or the cultural meaning and subjective experience of the condition). An understanding of patterns found in the data is not grounded in the diagnostic condition per se, but rather the "illness experience" or "disability experience" that these diagnostic conditions engender.

This is a longitudinal, urban ethnographic study carried out in many home, community, and institutional settings such as hospitals, outpatient clinics, and schools. As is typical with ethnographic research, prolonged and in-depth participant observations are being conducted. These are supplemented with videotaping, which enables fine-grained microethnographic analysis of interactions and action scenes. Interview methods rely heavily on narrative approaches, which generate insights into how participants are making sense of their experiences, beliefs, motives, hopes and desires, personal theories and explanations, emotional world, and selfhood and identity (e.g., Bruner, 1990a, 1990b; Freeman, 1993; Ochs & Capps, 2001; Polkinghorne, 1988). In addition, narrative approaches foster exploration of perspectives on the multiple identities revealed across cultural worlds and people's perceptions of their social locations (Mattingly, 1998; Mattingly & Lawlor, 2000; Mattingly, Lawlor, & Jacobs-Huey, 2002, Riesman, 2000). Narratives are not just about how stories are told; they also reflect how experiences are enacted (Mattingly, 1998, 2000).

The study cohort is comprised of over 30 African American families, their children who have an illness or disability, their extended family networks, and the practitioners who serve them. In this chapter, I am focusing on the perspectives of African American mothers of children who have special health-care needs and their experiences in navigating the health-care world and negotiating the "partnering-up" process. The mothers in this study represent a wide age range and include some grandmothers as primary caregivers. Although the majority of women and their families in this study have a low household income, there is collectively a wide range of income levels. Educational levels also vary considerably with a number of the women in the study indicating some college course work or completion of a college degree. Our longitudinal and ethnographic work reveals the fluid nature of both household incomes and education and work practices for this urban population who have children with special health- care needs. The caregiving needs and illness trajectories for their children have often directly affected work status and participation in educational programs, with several women reporting loss of job and subsequent decreases in household income due to illness crises or ongoing management of the complex work of managing multiple medical appointments and hospital and clinic visits.

The research described is part of a decade-long effort to examine cultural influences on health, health care, illness and disability, caregiving, family life, and development. Our current work with African American families is designed to generate insights into meanings of health, illness, and disability in family life; family caregiving; health disparities; collaboration among health-care providers and African American families; strengths and resiliency; changes over time; and how changes in family life, child development and illness trajectories influence health care. Historically, African American children and families have been underrepresented in studies of health, health care, disability, and human development.

In this chapter, I will draw upon the experiences and words of several of the African American women in this study. Their experiences highlight the richness and complexity of maternal work in mothering children who have special health-care needs. I am focusing on several aspects that relate closely to the work of practitioners. I hope that my representations of their stories will prompt greater understanding of the scope and nature of mothering work, broaden meanings of illness and disability, and facilitate reflections on how practitioners can promote better partnerships. As is typical with ethnographic data, the richness of the data provides vehicles for interpreting complex dimensions of human experience and interrelated phenomena. New, and often surprising, understandings of phenomena typically emerge.

In a comprehensive rendering of the data, interpretive work would present theoretical arguments of how the findings from individuals or a select group of participants relate to understanding of a broader collective of people, social structures and institutions, and society. I want to be clear that in this brief chapter I am encouraging the reader(s) to "listen to" and appreciate the representations of the experiences of these women and asking that the reader(s) not attempt to generalize to a broader category such as African American mothers or families. Topics such as ethnicity,

race, gender, and social class are only briefly expressed as they emerge in the data below and therefore are not rendered with enough substance here to explore these topics in the manner that is warranted. A more complex discussion of these topics would enhance the reader's ability to more fully understand how the African American women represented here negotiate health care, illness and disability, and development. However, this exploration exceeds the scope of this chapter. As Collins (1998) has persuasively argued, consideration of the influences of race or social class on topics such as health care should incorporate analysis of the intersections of gender, social class, race, and nation rather than attempting to deal with these constructs in isolation or in an overly operationalized manner.

In the following sections, I describe aspects of the mothering experiences of several African American women who have a child or children with special health-care needs and who are negotiating health care and meanings of illness and/or disability. The themes presented are intended to reflect key areas that are surfacing in analyzing and interpreting these longitudinal and complex data. The list is not all-inclusive, and this chapter is not intended as a summative report of findings. Data examples that are presented are intended to be illustrative of key points related to mothering work and to provide the reader with some access to the experiences of the participants in this study at times, conveyed in their own words.[1]

♣ Perspectives on Mothers and Mothering Work

Throughout this chapter, I speak of mothers, mothering, and mothering experiences as if these terms are all self evident. As reflected through many of the chapters in this collection, these terms are socially constructed subject to interpretation, negotiation, redefinition, and contestation (e.g., Francis-Connolly, 2000; Glenn, 1994; Nelson, 1994;

---

[1]Pseudonyms are used and, in a few instances, slight modifications, which do not affect the representation of the experience or the interpretation, were made to the data to protect anonymity.

Ruddick, 1989, 1995). My perspectives on mothering follow social constructivist views prevalent in anthropology and other social sciences that mothering is a practice rather than a biologically determined role. As Ruddick (1994) has argued, mothering as a practice is "gender free." To be a "mother" means to "see" children as demanding protection, nurturance, and training and then commit oneself to the work of trying to meet these demands" (Ruddick, 1994, p. 33). The quotes provided to illustrate mothering experiences in the following paragraphs are primarily drawn from interviews with women who are the primary caregivers and who are also biological parents. Many of the women in the study also talk about mothering in ways that are compatible with social constructivist perspectives. For example, one mother recently left phone messages for me and a Co-Principal Investigator in this research on our answering machines, wishing us a "Happy Mother's Day." This act, and others like this, was couched in comments about the fact that, although neither of us have children, we care for the children in this study.

I would also like to note that I primarily speak of mothers in this chapter as "mothers" rather than "mothers of children with disabilities" or a similar descriptor that would demarcate their experiences in a specific way. I present the mothers' own descriptors of their perceptions of the mothering experience where feasible. In professional worlds, there is a tendency to be specific and objective in ways that can result in a categorization or labeling process that marks difference. In essence, there is a narrowing of the frame or lens through which experience is filtered. Mothers of children who have an illness or disability can be framed as mothers of children with problems, a frame that tends to limit the understanding of the full breadth and range of their life experiences as mothers. The following passages illustrate that nurturing the development of a child is not limited to managing an illness or disability condition. Although mothering children who have an illness or disability may involve experiences that are not shared by all mothers, and some mothers may "aspire to a more typical experi-

ence of mothering" (Larson, 2000a, p. 273), many of the women whose experiences are described below both demonstrate and indicate the centrality of mothering in their lives. Their stories often include aspects of the mothering experience that may or may not be directly related to the ongoing management of an illness or disability. A similar finding was reported by Bower & Hayes (1998) in their study of the experiences of mothers of normally developing children, children with a physical disability, and children with an intellectual impairment. Many of the mothers' descriptions in this study also serve to counter the tendency to view a child with special health-care needs as a special child in ways that also constrain the view of the children. Their children are children, not "a cerebral palsied child" or an autistic or spina bifida patient as commonly expressed in clinical worlds. This need as a mother to convey the full humanity of their children is discussed in more detail below.

In addition, I would also note that the caregiving and mothering aspects of women's lives often extend well beyond the demands of routine care for a child with special health-care needs. Many of the African American women who participate in our research study are simultaneously managing the illness trajectories of several, or at times, many family members. Many of these women also manage their own health problems in such ways that we have come to understand that some of the mothers in our study are "vulnerable caregivers." Although I am concentrating on how mothers negotiate health-care services for their children who have special health-care needs in this chapter, an understanding of how these African American women negotiate health care must involve considerations of intergenerational caregiving, or the distribution of caregiving work across family and kinship networks (Stack & Burton, 1994), and caregiving dyads. Caregiving dyads is a theme of our current research in which mothering tasks may be shared and coordinated in a team often comprised of a grandmother and mother. Even though these important aspects of women's lives will be dealt with only briefly, women's stories about negotiating health care for their children often reflect the caregiving of other family members, and, at times, the deferral of addressing their own health concerns or care contributing to their own health vulnerabilities. Culture brokering, caregiving, and negotiating health care are not only central aspects of the mothering work of many of the women in this study related to a child with special health-care needs. They are complex, often demanding, and highly valued practices that are integral to many dimensions of family life and reflect the pervasiveness of "mothering work" in the daily lives of many of the women in this study.

The following story is illustrative of ways in which many of the women in this study simultaneously care for other family members, such as a parent, while providing the ongoing and special care required for their child who has an illness or disability. This woman, who is in her twenties, is telling a story about the unexpected need to return to the hospital one morning with her daughter. I am using the term *unexpected* because the child developed a problem that needed immediate attention and the necessary trip to the hospital had not been previously scheduled. However, this circumstance was not that unusual because various chronic and acute problems often required that this mother change plans to accommodate the complex care needs of her child. During this time period, this mother was also participating in the care and decision making for her very ill mother, who was dying due to cancer. This mother, whom I will call Sasha, described how, even though her sister and aunt were very much involved in the care of Dora, Sasha's mother, much of the daily work would be done by her. As Sasha explained, on the morning when she needed to take her daughter to the hospital unexpectedly, her sister and aunt were arranging Dora's discharge because she wanted to be home. Sasha shared past experiences and how she wasn't ready. The following excerpt is drawn from narrative interviews conducted with Sasha.

> Because I knew as soon as she came home, everything is on me. I had the little bit of help, but we were in the same apartment complex. I was just right around the corner.

Everything was on me. From day one until she was diagnosed, everything was on me. I just wasn't ready, because I was tired…But I told myself, you know, this is my mother. Would you rather she stay in the hospital or be at home? So you know, we called hospice and set that up and we brought her home. And, she was only in hospice a day and a half before she died.

Sasha credits her experiences with her daughter for preparing her for the intimate, at times technical, demands inherent in caring for her dying mother. As in so many of the stories uncovered in this research, a simple descriptor of mothering experiences is inadequate for capturing these complex and dynamic aspects of experiences that also evoke multiple and sometimes conflicting emotions. Such a brief rendering of this story involving intergenerational caregiving might also obscure the profound relational aspects of this experience, the "love from a mother for a mother."[2]

✦ Bridging Social Worlds

When mothers bring their children for therapy or for other health-care visits such as doctor's appointments, they often become engaged in a complicated communication process. Their role entails serving as the family representative and conveying perspectives on family issues, as well as representing the practitioner's perspective and clinical events to the family. This is a complex role in which the family representative becomes, in effect, a "culture broker" whose difficult task is to bridge the clinic culture with the family world (Brinker, 1992; Lawlor & Mattingly, 1998). Mothers must both represent home life and health concerns to institutionally based practitioners in such a way that effective care can be given and represent clinical encounters back to family members to let them know what happened or what was discussed. This role as culture broker often places the mother or primary caregiver in the position of interpreting for others both the information ex-

---

[2] The quotation marks reflect the insights of a research colleague, Dr. Lanita Jacobs-Huey.

changed and the meanings behind complex sets of experiences. In addition, the mother often acts as messenger in attempting to modify the expectations of either the practitioners or family members to accommodate the needs of the other party. Although family-centered care presumes that practitioners are involved with the entire family system, our experiences indicate that a model is needed that more realistically reflects the central role of one family member and the complexities inherent in that member's role as culture broker (Lawlor & Mattingly, 1998; Mattingly & Lawlor, 1998).

Often there will be more than one perspective within a family and, somewhat similarly, there may often be more than one perspective held by various members of a health-care team (i.e., doctors, therapists, nurses). Previous research confirms that multiple perspectives characterize clinical encounters in which family members and professionals strive to negotiate care for a child (Lawlor & Mattingly, 1998; Mattingly, 1998). But negotiation and conflict among competing perspectives also characterize family life. Thus, understanding the evolution of how a family cares for a child and works with health-care professionals requires attending to the multiple perspectives within a family and how these are negotiated in a family's daily decision making. Such within-family negotiations have their own history, fluctuating in response to modifications in household configuration, household economies and power, as well as influences from larger sociocultural arenas. These within-family world negotiations are an additional form of cultural brokering and a form in which the mother or primary caregiver plays a central role.

Part of the challenge for practitioners who work with children with special health-care needs is the imperative to make health-care encounters meaningful, not only in the moments of actual contact time in the clinical setting, but also in other times in home, school, or community life. The challenges for mothers include connecting happenings in the clinical world with day-to-day life for their children, themselves, and their families. Metaphorically, bridges must be made between the multiple cultural worlds of children and families and clinic life. In the many hours that I have spent in therapy clinics, I have seen many skillful attempts at building bridges between clinic life and home life initiated by practitioners, family members, and children. Practitioners whose success and continued practice is dependent on their ability to partner up with families and engage them in bringing therapeutic principles into the home are trying to design programs to unseen, unknown, and in many ways imaginary worlds. As Mattingly (1998) has argued, therapists are often in positions in which they need to make judgments with little known data, but a wealth of imagined possibilities.

Bridging social worlds, a major component of mothering work as argued here, often involves creating bridges and experiences that will facilitate the integration of social worlds. Mothers are often bridge-makers. They often try directly to bridge home life with clinic life. These metaphorical bridges take many forms and vary in their design, size, and complexity, like real bridges. The creation of bridges may involve facilitating the inclusion of people from one arena to another or the carrying of objects and material representations between different social worlds that foster greater understanding and at times participation. Mothers often must also help their children negotiate the many social worlds that typically comprise childhood life. They must support their child's travel across bridges between clinic, home, and community life.

In the following example, one mother describes her design solution to the problem of bridging home life and clinic life. In her story, she acknowledges her concern that what happens in the clinic must be integrated into family life at home.

> …as the therapy process proceeded on and I had made up in my mind that she sees the therapist once a week. There is no way that she is going to recover if I don't do anything those other six days of the week.

She then proceeded to describe her strategy for bridging home life and clinic life and for maximizing the incorporation of therapy ideas in daily life at home.

> So, what I did is, I became very personal with my therapist. She just wasn't a lady I saw once a

week, she was adopted into my family. And I brought my family to therapy with me. I brought children, I brought my grandma (laughs). So that she could be in on what it is that we would be trying to achieve, what it was that we need my daughter to accomplish. I brought children, aunties, uncles, close neighbors—everybody that was a part of my close daily surroundings, went to therapy. And that's just the way it was. So that the therapy was not just once a week, it was seven days a week. It was from the minute we woke up to the minute we went to bed.

This mother, in essence, brought the entire family into the clinic world. In some ways, this strategy lessened her need to be a culture broker because many family members had direct experience with the therapist and the clinical activities and procedures. The involvement of many family members served to heighten the therapist's awareness of family life and provided her with more direct experience in bridging therapeutic activities in the clinic with life at home. This therapist's direct experience with family members both lessened and expanded her imagining of possibilities for partnering up with this family.

In the following example, one mother, whom I will call Nina, describes her maternal work related to bridging home, school, and an outpatient therapy clinic. Her concern here is, in some ways, the opposite of the story presented above. This mother is trying to understand more about what happens in the school world. Without being there or receiving good communication about what went on at school, she is left to her imagination about what the school world in general, and any one school day in particular, might be like for her daughter. Her mothering work is further complicated by her desire to also bridge school life and clinic life for her daughter. Because her child receives therapy in multiple sites, she is also hopeful that she can facilitate an integration of her therapy experiences and understanding among the practitioners who have come to know her child in one or more social worlds, but not others.

You know, and I wish I could get them to communicate better. We have a little blue notebook.

And my team, the behavior team, writes in there everyday. … every movement she is making, anything unusual with her day. And I take it (the blue notebook) to therapy and Margo will read about her day and they will try and fix it, that kind of thing. But if I could get the speech therapist (the school-based speech therapist) to write what she's doing… and get Margo (the clinic-based therapist) to write what she's working on, you know some kind of way they can be on the same page… You know and even the activities, because Sandy, the occupational therapist, when she reads it…. . how it was that Deanna was disconnected here and how they dealt with it… says where they are helping or not. …she's able to look at the notes and take it from there.

Charting the Developmental Pathways

Mothering work related to bridging worlds is multifaceted. One of the most complex and compelling aspects of this work relates to how mothers chart desired developmental pathways and manage the multiple contingencies that could potentially interfere with the hoped-for achievements. In bridging social worlds, mothers must nurture the pursuit of the desired pathways by negotiating perspectives about their children and presenting views of their children, and at times family, that will facilitate the recruitment of practitioners to participate in co-creating and enacting the desired developmental pathway. For mothers of children with disabilities, pathway work also entails managing sociocultural constructions of disability.

Mothers guide the development of their children, a process that entails crafting, negotiating, and at times contesting, possible futures, possible selves. There are many models and metaphors in developmental literature that are used to describe this aspect of "maternal work," to borrow a phrase from Ruddick (1994) (Also see Larson, 2000b). For example, Bruner (e.g., 1990a) emphasizes socialization models and is credited with coining the phrase "scaffolding" to describe adult-child learning. Rogoff (1993) speaks of "guided participation" in describing adult and child learning (Rogoff, Radziszewska, & Masiello, 1995).

Terms such as "developmental agenda" and "developmental trajectory" are also found in the literature. I am using the term "pathway"[3] metaphorically here to portray a sense of movement in a desired direction, the improvisational nature of plotting and navigating a developmental course, and perception that there are many twists and turns over unexpected terrain.

As Ruddick (1994) notes, a mother's ability to be responsive to the changing needs of a child or children is a central aspect of maternal work. Kellegrew (2000), who conducted a qualitative study with 6 mothers of children with disabilities, also noted the finely calibrated attunement of mothers to the changing needs of their children as they orchestrated routine caregiving tasks. In this longitudinal study of children and families, I am struck with the complexity of the work of mothers to envision possible futures for their children, create experiences that will propel the desired developmental trajectory, and manage the contingencies that threaten to alter or derail a desired developmental pathway. The following examples illustrate aspects of maternal work related to charting developmental pathways for their children. As these mothers indicate, creating a pathway for their child is not enough. Ensuring that a desired outcome will be realized often involves intense negotiation, contesting particular perceptions of their children, and clearing obstacles. Co-creating, navigating, protecting, and where necessary, redesigning pathways is central to mothering work related to nurturing a child with a disability and a major aspect of negotiating health care and developmental services. It is also a critical dimension of bridging social worlds.

The following brief example illustrates the intricacies involved in bridging worlds and navigating pathways. This excerpt is taken from an interview with a mother whom I will call Shareen and her daughter Chandra. Like many skilled storytellers, Shareen provides particulars through her presentation of dialogue in a "she said," "I said" kind of manner. Although all of the next passage is verbatim, quotes are used to highlight the statements made by Chandra as told by Shareen.

> "My legs, I can't walk." And I was like, "Do you wanna walk?" She is like, "Yeah!" And I was like, "You wanna run and play with people, huh?" She is like "Yeah." And I'm like, "what happened to your feet?" And she'll say, "I had surgery. I had blisters." And I was like, "How did the blisters get there?" And she'll sometimes go "I don't know." And I'm just like, "do you want your feet rubbed?" And she is like, "Yeah." And so I have a little tub and I'll sit her in her little chair and put her feet in her chair, put her feet in the little tub and just give her a little pedicure. She'll be like "My toes are polished. I look pretty."

In this brief story, Shareen is conveying both the complexity and richness of her maternal work. Although in one way she is simply recreating a brief exchange she had with her 4-year-old daughter for the interviewer, she is also presenting key aspects of her mothering. She is tenacious in her efforts to understand what her child, who has spina bifida, might be experiencing. She both elicits her child's sense making by asking her about what she knows or understands (e.g., "What happened to your feet?") and seeks ways of experiencing life through her daughter's eyes and, in many ways, her body. The following excerpt is drawn from field notes in which Shareen tells how she tried to feel what her daughter Chandra feels when she must wear long leg casts on both her legs.

> I went to the hardware store and bought two pieces of wood and strapped them to my legs for several hours. I wanted to feel what Chandra feels. It was hard and painful. I don't know how she does it.

Shareen's brief story also sheds light on her maternal work related to co-creating developmental pathways, including her efforts to create desired possible futures. When Shareen is asking Chandra if she wants to walk, she is trying to find out the extent to which walking is important to Chandra. This is both a question about possible futures and a question about

---

[3]Weisner (2002) uses the term "developmental pathway" in his conceptualization of cultural pathways comprised of the routines of everyday life, cultural activities and practices, and development.

mothering as Shareen ponders the impact of medical procedures, therapy, and equipment alternatives on Chandra's experiences of childhood and day-to-day life, such as disruptions in the school day required by the application and removal of braces. The simple act of applying nail polish and Chandra's response (i.e., "I look pretty.") are both routine and compelling. This is both fairly typical of the ways in which this mother and child interact, play, and "be" with each other, and indicative of the work of this mother to mediate the effects of Chandra's disability on her childhood and future development. Her feet are not only the site of medical interventions and blisters, they are a part of the body to be adorned and appreciated.

In the following passage, a mother describes her work to chart a developmental pathway grounded in confidence and directed toward success. Her daughter Bella had a brachial plexus injury, which prior to surgery and therapy significantly affected her ability to use her shoulder, arm, and hand. Her bridging work here is also complex, involving a kind of negotiation about how she would like her child to be seen by the world and anticipating that sociocultural conceptions of disability could constrain her daughter's achievements and impede travel on the desired developmental pathway.

> Bella is going to be OK. Even if she, what's the word I am looking for, even if she didn't get any more usage than what she has and it is obvious to those in the outside world, she's still going to be able to achieve because she has been taught that you can do it. See, 'cause in our house you can't say "can't." I don't like that word. Or, you can't say "I'll try," because to me "try" leaves room for failure. No, "you can do it," "you can do," "but I can't," "yes you can." I am telling you that you can and the confidence that you don't have in yourself, I have it for you so I know you can do it.

Not only must this mother install confidence in this child; she has the confidence *for* her when the child doesn't yet have it in herself. Her work to mediate the effects of her child's birth injury on her development is multifaceted. The passage quoted above reflects her determination that her child achieve. It also alludes to another theme that permeates this mother's stories about her parenting and hopes for her daughter, her hopes that society won't see her daughter as disabled and constrain her development. Her determination to protect her child from any limitations imposed by societal views about disability is fierce and is often tested. Over the years that I have known this mother, child, and family, I have heard many stories and witnessed events in which concerns about how her child is perceived and misperceived are conveyed. The following quote is an example of this aspect of her mothering work.

> First of all I've never looked at her as being disabled because I don't like that term. Disabled means you are not able to do something…She's not disabled and I wasn't accepting it from anybody. To tell you the truth, I have a very strong faith in God and *God* couldn't even tell me my child was disabled and that she was not going to be 100%. He couldn't come down and tell me that. No, I was not going to accept it and [I was] willing to suffer any consequences of living in Hell forever to stand up for what I thought, and what I believed, and what I know to be true.

Carole, the mother who is quoted above, expresses the depth of her determination by asserting that even God is not allowed to call her child disabled.

For many of the mothers in this study, their maternal work involves recruiting practitioners and others to see their child in ways that will foreground their child's strengths. I have referred to these themes as the *likeability of the child*, which involves the presentation of positive attributes, and *giving voice* to the child, which involves saying things that the child might say if he or she were able to express himself or herself clearly (Lawlor & Mattingly, 1998). The following example illustrates features of both of these themes as a mother tells a story about a frustrating exchange with a therapist. As Linda tells this story, she reveals her belief in the need to be vigilant about the perceptions practitioners have of her young daughter, who has many complex medical and developmental needs.

They don't even know Malena so I was like, I had to like watch them clear and carefully and stuff you know. That's why I have to go.

She continues with an explanation.

…'cause people don't understand, [Here she turns to Malena] "people don't understand huh, they just tell you anything." You know, they are just rude. And she's going to therapy. You know, Malena puts her head down if she doesn't like what's going on. Then the therapist is going to say, "Well maybe her head is too heavy and that's why she can't hold it." And I was like, "What?!" You know, how rude! I said "She's got her head down because she doesn't like what you are doing. Whatever it is that you're doing." 'Cause they weren't talking to her, trying to keep her interested in the therapy.

This mother has a view of her child that she wants the therapist to share. Malena is not able to speak, but her mother is able to give voice to her child by indicating that Malena concurs that the therapist doesn't understand her and that she is bored. Linda also enacts her beliefs about the capabilities of her child by seamlessly including her in the interview process by addressing her and saying "huh" indexing her child's understanding and concurrence. As told in this story, this mother is contesting the view that she believes the therapist holds that her daughter is not capable of holding her head up and engaging with this therapist in purposeful activities. Her concerns have consequences, both in the moments of therapy sessions and over time. Linda wants her child to be engaged and learning from therapy. She wants therapy to be effective. She is also conveying her deep concern that the therapist see her child as capable of engaging and learning more. She wants the therapist to be participating in promoting the child's development in a manner that is consistent with her desired developmental pathway. She contests what she perceives as the therapist's assessment that her child doesn't have the head control to sit up and engage in the therapy by positing that the problem with the therapy session is that her child hasn't been captivated by what is going on and is bored. This reframing portrays her child as having many untapped capabilities.

Mothers in this study have also shared many stories about practitioners who seemed to "get" their children and really like their children. "You can tell" is a phrase that is repeated throughout much of the data. For example, one mother of a child who had multiple hospitalizations related to her cancer treatment shared the following story related to doctors who stopped by her child's bedside:

… And say hello, and everything. And then she'd give them a hug maybe, you know. And I mean that made them feel good too, the closeness that they had. You know, they just liked to show, like she was not just a patient. You know. They showed that she was somebody, too, you know? And then um, I mean it's just a feeling that the parents get, to know that they … the parents already know that their children are special to them… But when they see that, you know, someone else thinks the same, then it just makes the parents feel extra good too.

Implicit in this statement, as well as many others, is the belief that the achievement of developmental outcomes, progress on a developmental pathway, is enhanced when professionals like and connect with their children.

Many of these shared examples deal with how mothers work to mediate perceptions about disability and negative or contested perceptions about their children. When mothers work to foster their children's growth on developmental pathways, they manage many other contingencies beyond illness or disability. In the research study described previously, many families live in urban neighborhoods where navigation on developmental pathways may involve protection against violence or other possible dangers. In the following example, a mother whose infant daughter had recently died due to many health problems, described her efforts to protect her other children.

She began by talking about her reluctance to let her children spend the night at someone else's house. She made an exception by occasionally letting her children spend one night at her sister's house. She said, "I don't want them without me. I'm just not that kind of person. I'd rather for my kids to be with me whatever I'm doing. You know?" She continued to talk about wanting her children ("my people") to be near and in the following excerpt further elaborated:

> So my people...they...they stay in my yard, and all the kids come to my house. Because I don't like my kids at other people's houses. I don't want my kids to be saying somebody touched me. So they come into my house and I can watch them. And I know I ain't gonna touch them. You know? I just talk to them. I just don't like all that, "Can I go spend the night over (____)?" "No way. Tell (____) to come over here."

As she continued to explain her parenting she told a story of an exchange with her children. The quotations reflect statements made by one of her children.

> "Mom, you...you stick around too much." But I play basketball with them. I play whatever they want to play. "Let's play Nintendo." I play that. Ain't none of them I can't take.

In another part of her story, she described how her children tell her what other children, like their friends are allowed to do. The word "they" in this passage has two references; her children as in the first "they" and their friends as in the second "they."

> They be like, "Mama, they want to do this." "Oh, okay, let them go do that, and when they get back, they'll tell you how it was." I take them, you know, to parks. But this year, I didn't take them to the beach, because I was scared, you know, the water, and the sharks were biting. And they kept saying, "Mama..."

As she continued to describe how she navigates their developmental pathways and negotiates solutions, she shared another illustrative story.

> I go to the movies with them. My oldest son is 13. He's like, "Mama, I don't want you going with me." It's what I want. "I'm going to be happy that you're at the movies with me. Once you go with somebody else, you aren't going to enjoy it because I'll probably be in the back."

This mother, who is a skillful storyteller, somewhat humorously recounted conversations with her children in which she asserted her need to have her children where she can watch them and protect them. The humor in this passage covers over the deep fears that she may not be able to protect her children from all potential dangers. Many of the women in this study have shared stories about their concerns related to violence, playground bullying, vulnerabilities for abuse, racial discrimination, discrimination or stigmatization related to disability, or peer pressure. Maternal work does not only involve mediating societal attitudes and developmental factors related to illness and disability. Protection against a host of possible harms is a central dimension of maternal work (Ruddick, 1989, 1995).

✒ Managing Perceptions of Parenting

I observed a mother of a 3-year-old child early on in what is now an almost 6-year period fretting over her child's hair and inspecting her appearance carefully while waiting for a medical appointment. I have made many similar observations with this dyad over time. Her anxiety about her child's appearance seemed related to her perception that how her child looked mattered with a capital M, and that how her mothering would be judged related to her child's appearance. This example is plucked from a wealth of data in which this mother and this child, and their health-care practitioners have enacted and acted in ways designed to persuade the other to adopt particular views about themselves and to alter courses of action. Part of the maternal work of mothers who have children with illnesses or disabilities is managing the perceptions of others about them and about their parenting.

Women who have participated in this research often work to construct positive identities with the professionals with whom they interact. These presentations of self involve not only portraying positive attributes, but also demonstrating what one is *not*, a critical aspect of many health-care encounters in which judgments about the beliefs, competencies, and motives of parents become central factors in decision-making processes that significantly affect the illness and developmental trajectories of infants and young children. This crafting of how to act in the clinic is complicated when the need to advocate or present alternative views to the "expert's" perspective arises. The parent must try to advocate and negotiate in ways that maintain the "good parent" persona and risk being perceived by self or the practitioner as a "bad parent" (Lawlor & Mattingly, 1998). The terms "good parent" and "bad parent" are bounded by quotation marks to indicate how these terms emerge in both mothers' and practitioners' descriptions of the partnering-up process. They often are used when people are conveying the intersubjective nature of collaboration and conveying perceptions about the perceptions of others about their parenting, collaboration, and sometimes compliance or cooperation.

Mothers and other family members often work hard to avoid being labeled by professionals in negative ways, to promote a positive view of themselves as caregivers, and work to construct a positive identity with the professionals with whom they interact (Lawlor & Mattingly, 1998). At the same time, they often face a double bind because, if they feel their child is not receiving proper care, they may find their advocacy framed as "noncompliance" by professional staff. There is also a danger in presenting an overly compliant, cooperative attitude to professionals. Being the "good parent" may result in poor care for their child.

The following excerpts capture one mother's assessment of this particularly complicated and consequential aspect of mothering work.

> And by that time, I'm all stressed out, anxious, I feel bad now because I've yelled at the nurse. Now they think, "oh my God she's just a really loud parent," and now I go in there I wonder what these people think of me. I wonder, and this is a constant thing, it's just this juggling thing, well you be nice to the nurses so they'll take care of your daughter. But when you assert yourself and say, "Look I want this and I want this now." What damage have you caused between the relationship that you have with the nurses, the doctors and everything else, and how are you gonna fix that?

This mother, whom I will call Marla, has spent many days and often weeks in several different hospital settings related to the medical care of her young daughter, who requires both chronic and acute care, sometimes of a critical and life-threatening nature. She often articulates the extent of her work to manage her relationships with health-care practitioners and to ensure that her daughter is receiving desired and necessary care. Her knowledge of biomedical cultural worlds and institutional cultures is vast, and she will draw on this expertise in her maternal and relational work. Even with all of this expertise and experience, the work is challenging. Even one's own deep sense of mothering may be called into question.

> But, I know, this is what I have to deal with and it's very very hard. I don't know how any other parents do it. I am sure they think "oh she's a bitch, she's a, a know everything (know-it-all)," but I know I take that in and it hurts. But I still think I have to do this, I can't not do it, I can't stop being who I am, I can't stop fighting for Cara. I can't, because if I stop doing that, then I feel like I'm failing as a parent. I haven't done my job and part of it, too, I think I've said this before, there's this guilt that goes on, too. You feel guilty because your kid has to go through all this.

The above passage was taken from a transcript in which this mother is describing her careful calibration of how much to challenge nurses. Her maternal work is more than advocating for her daughter; it is a complex, intersubjective task that requires a kind of mind reading about what the nurses might be thinking. Her challenge is to decide how much to push for and when to push. Miscalculations could result in negative judgments about the kind of mother that she is that could be highly consequential for both her and Cara. But, as Marla also conveys, mistakes in how and when to be aggressive or challenging could result in harm to her daughter. Several of the parents in this study anguish over regrets that they did not challenge professionals or care decisions sooner or harder.

Managing the perceptions of others about their parenting, for some women in this study, involves countering perceptions about being young or not being smart or competent at required medical procedures. As one mother explains:

> And yes I'm young, but I'm not dumb, and that's what I hate. When they look at me, I'll come in and tell them, tell them first thing, they don't want to admit to certain things. I'm like, I know what I'm talking about, I know what I'm talking about, so don't even, I know I'm right. They don't want to give me the benefit of the doubt. "She's young, she's dumb," "she don't know," "we're professional, she's not." "We're the staff, we do it all, you're just the parent."

In this brief quote, this mother is describing the need to challenge the perceptions that she believes some practitioners hold based on her experiences with them. The quotations reflect her statements about what she thinks practitioners think of her. Throughout many of her stories, her work to manage and redirect these erroneous and harmful perceptions is evident. Her desire to change perceptions is not just because she wishes that everyone would perceive her more positively and more accurately. She knows that perceptions of her abilities and parenting might affect the care her daughter receives. The following story illustrates both her work to manage practitioners' perceptions of her child and her work to manage their perceptions of her mothering competence.

She begins recalling an incident during one hospital visit in which she was concerned that her child had an orthopedic problem. She worried that this could be serious and really wanted to make sure that her child received an x ray to rule out the possibility of a bone deformity or other type of problem. She persisted in trying to have her concerns addressed.

> So, he still tried to shoo me off. And I was like, "You know what, I'm not leaving this hospital until you talk to me." He would diagnose something or say something and then walk away, go to the next patient. I followed that man… I followed him all over that hospital until he sat

there and talked to me and listened to me. I was like, "I know what I'm talking about. I live with this child."

As is true with many stories collected as part of this research, the plot line is complicated. This mother not only needs to have the immediate problem addressed; she desires to ensure that this physician sees her daughter in a way that reflects all of her humanity, not just her clinical problems or diagnostic category. She wants him to see her daughter as the loved child of this mother.

> I'm taking care of her. I know who she is. She's not just a cerebral palsy patient. She knows. You know, she's a child. And he… at first, he was kind of thrown off. After I talked to him, he really finally started, you know, paying attention. He still, you know, calls her by her last name, and he'll do the quick run-in, but she's not just Smith the cerebral palsy patient. She's Monica. She was born with cerebral palsy, but she's my child.

Tenacity is a desired, and sometimes necessary, attribute of many of the mothers in this study. In this research project, we conduct collective narrative groups, a method we have developed that is a form of group narrative interviewing (Mattingly, Lawlor, & Jacobs-Huey, 2002). Their stories about health-care encounters often involve vivid examples of how they had to act in order to acquire the desired services for their children. For example, one mother contributed to the group discussion by sharing the following:

> …Well, if I could give you the names and addresses of all the health-care professionals that I have dealt with, they would tell you—"Not her!"… Because, I will follow them into the office. I will follow them while they are trying to see another patient. I will call them. I will page them. I will do anything I have to to understand what is going on with my child. And I'm not just going to accept those big medical words, which mean nothing to me. You're going to put it to where I understand. Like I said, if you have to draw me a picture, I'm cool with that. If you think I'm stupid, I'm cool with that. But I am not going to leave your face until you help me understand what is going on right here, right now.

In this story, the intersections of managing possible perceptions of practitioners and negotiating what is needed for a child are evident. In this brief example, this mother also indicates what she is willing to tolerate to ensure she gets what she needs, information, and her child gets the necessary care. Being a "not her!" person or withstanding views that she might be "stupid" are perceived to be possible costs of pursuing answers and explanations in a determined and assertive manner.

Conclusion

In this chapter I have emphasized several ways in which mothers bridge social and cultural worlds, create and navigate developmental pathways, and manage perceptions and contest misperceptions related to them or their mothering. Health-care encounters reveal ways in which cultural beliefs are negotiated as a central dimension of collaboration and partnering up. The themes that I have highlighted are representative of the multifaceted maternal work inherent in nurturing and raising children with special health-care needs.

One hopefully self evident conclusion is that mothering work is complex and multifaceted. The negotiation of health-care, illness, and disability and the navigation of desired developmental pathways are demanding aspects of mothering practices for women who have a child with an illness, disability, and/or special health-care need. The stories of these mothers reveal aspects of their experiences that warrant more attention both from practitioners and from researchers.

Although I have focused on the stories of African American mothers related to the care and nurturance of their children, I have tried to convey that mothering work is intertwined with family culture and family life, including intergenerational caregiving processes and distribution of family work and resources. The collapsing of the lens of analysis to the mothers and their maternal work employed for this chapter potentially obscures the profound influence of broader family networks and the specific contributions of fathers, grandparents, siblings, and extended kin on negotia-

tions of health care, illness and disability, and development. These limitations parallel problems encountered in the clinical world where practitioners often meet or come to know a mother and child and try to develop an understanding of family life and culture.

The brief rendering of issues related to race, gender, racial identity, class, and culture and their interrelatedness also constrain the representations of the experiences of these African American women in this chapter. Such a constraint may unfortunately limit the reader's appreciation of the richness and complexity of their maternal work and experiences.

Finally, many of the mothers in this study often eloquently describe how their experiences in negotiating health care for their children have been identity shaping and have transformed their lives. A full discussion of the ways in which mothering experiences have altered their lives also goes beyond the scope of this chapter. However, to completely ignore this powerful dimension of their experiences would be a kind of misrepresentation of the mothering experience and an inadequate representation of the extent to which lives are linked and multiple developmental trajectories intersect.

Discussion Questions

- What are identified aspects of mothering work that warrant more attention in clinical practices?
- How might practitioners come to know enough about mothers and children to more effectively partner up?
- Are there aspects of these mothers' experiences or stories that remind you of clinical encounters within your own practice? If so, how might you reflect on these experiences in a new or different way?
- How might practitioners actively support the co-creation and enactment of desired developmental pathways?

References
Bower, A. M., & Hayes, A. (1998). Mothering in families with and without a child with a disability. *International*

Journal of Disability, Development and Education, 45(3), 313–322.

Brinker, R. P. (1992). Family involvement in early intervention: Accepting the unchangeable, changing the changeable, and knowing the difference. *Topics in Early Childhood Special Education, 12,* 307–332.

Bruner, J. (1990a). Culture and human development: A new look. *Human Development, 33,* 344–355.

Bruner, J. (1990b). A narrative model of self-construction. *Annals of the New York Academy of Sciences, 818,* 145–161.

Collins, P.H. (1998). Intersections of race, class, gender, and nation: Some implications for Black family studies. *Journal of Comparative Family Studies, XXIX*(1), 27–36.

Dunst, C., Trivette, C., & Deal, A. (1988). *Enabling and empowering families: Principles and guidelines for practice.* Cambridge, MA: Brookline.

Elder, G. H. (1998). The life course as developmental theory. *Child Development, 69*(1), 1–12.

Fox, R.G., & King, B.J. (Eds.) (2002). *Anthropology beyond culture.* New York: Berg.

Francis-Connolly, E. (2000). Toward an understanding of mothering: A comparison of two motherhood stages. *American Journal of Occupational Therapy, 54*(3), 281–289.

Freeman, M. (1993). *Rewriting the self: History, memory, narrative.* London (UK) Routledge.

Garro, L.C. (2000). Cultural knowledge as resource in illness narratives: Remembering through accounts of illness. In C. Mattingly & L. Garro (Eds.). *Narrative and the cultural construction of illness and healing* (pp. 70–87). Berkeley, CA: University of California.

Glenn, E.N. (1994). Social constructions of mothering: A thematic overview. In E. Glenn, C. Chang, & L. Forcey (Eds.). Mothering: Ideology, experience, and agency (pp. 1–29). New York, NY: Routledge.

Good, B. J. (1994). *Medicine, rationality, and experience: An anthropological perspective.* Cambridge (UK): Cambridge University.

Hanft B. (1989). *Family-centered care: An early intervention resource manual.* Rockville, MD: American Occupational Therapy Association.

Kellegrew, D. H. (2000). Constructing daily routines: A qualitative examination of mothers with young children with disabilities. *American Journal of Occupational Therapy, 54*(3), 252–259.

Kleinman, A. (1988). *The illness narratives: Suffering, healing, and the human condition.* New York: Basic Books.

Laderman, C. & Roseman, M. (1996). Introduction. In C. Laderman & M. Roseman (Eds.). *The performance of healing* (pp. 1–16). New York: Routledge.

Larson, E. A. (2000a). The orchestration of occupation: The dance of mothers. *American Journal of Occupational Therapy, 54*(3), 269–280.

Larson, E. A. (2000b). Mothering: Letting go of the past ideal and valuing the real. *American Journal of Occupational Therapy, 54*(3), 249–251.

Lawlor, M. C., & Mattingly, C. F. (1998). The complexities embedded in family-centered care. *American Journal of Occupational Therapy, 52*(4), 259–267.

Lawlor, M.C., & Mattingly, C.F. (2001). Beyond the unobtrusive observer: Reflections on researcher-informant relationships in urban ethnography. *American Journal of Occupational Therapy, 55,* 147–154.

Mattingly, C. (1998). *Healing dramas and clinical plots: The narrative structure of experience.* Cambridge (UK): Cambridge University Press.

Mattingly, C. (2000). Emergent narratives. In C. Mattingly & L. Garro (Eds.). *Narrative and the cultural construction of illness and healing* (pp. 181–211). Berkeley, CA: University of California.

Mattingly, C. F. (2002). Pocahontas goes to the clinic. *2002 Abstracts of the American Anthropological Association.* Arlington, VA: American Anthropological Association.

Mattingly, C. F., & Lawlor, M. C. (1998). Disability experience from a family perspective. In M. Neistadt & E. Crepeau (Eds.). *Willard & Spackman's occupational therapy* (9th ed.) (pp. 43–55). Philadelphia: Lippincott.

Mattingly, C., & Lawlor, M. (2000). Learning from stories: Narrative interviewing in cross-cultural research. *The Scandinavian Journal of Occupational Therapy, 7,* 4–14.

Mattingly, C., & Lawlor, M. (2001). The fragility of healing. *Ethos, 29*(1), 30–57.

Mattingly, C., Lawlor, M., & Jacobs-Huey, L. (2002). Narrating September 11: Race, gender, and the play of cultural identities. *American Anthropologist, 104*(3), 743–753.

Morris, D. B. (1998). *Illness and culture in the postmodern age.* Berkeley, CA: University of California.

Nelson, M.K. (1994). Family day care providers: Dilemmas of daily practice. In E. Glenn, C. Chang, & L. Forcey (Eds.). *Mothering: Ideology, experience, and agency* (pp.181–209). New York: Routledge.

Ochs, E., & Capps, L. (2001). *Living narrative: Creating lives in everyday storytelling.* Cambridge, MA: Harvard.

Ortner, S. B. (1999). Introduction. In S. Ortner (Ed.). *The fate of culture: Geertz and beyond* (pp. 1–13). Berkeley, CA: University of California.

Polkinghorne, D. E. (1988). *Narrative knowing and the human sciences.* Albany: State University of New York.

Riesman, C. K. (2000). "Even if we don't have children [we] can live." In C. Mattingly & L. Garro (Eds.). *Narrative and the cultural construction of illness and healing* (pp. 128–152). Berkeley, CA: University of California.

Rogoff, B. (1993). Children's guided participation and participatory appropriation in sociocultural activity. In R. Wozniak & K. Fischer (Eds.). *Development in context: Acting and thinking in specific environments* (pp. 121–153). Hillsdale, NJ: Lawrence Erlbaum.

Rogoff, B., Radziszewska, B., & Masiello, T. (1995). Analysis of developmental processes in sociocultural activity. In L. Martin, K. Nelson, & E. Tobach (Eds.). *Sociocultural psychology: Theory and practice of doing and knowing* (pp. 125–149). Cambridge (UK): Cambridge University.

Rosenbaum, P., King, S., Law, M., King, G., & Evans, J. (1998). Family-centred service: A conceptual framework and research review. *Physical & Occupational Therapy in Pediatrics, 18*(1), 1–20.

Ruddick, S. (1989, 1995). *Maternal thinking: Toward a politics of peace.* Boston, MA; Beacon.

Ruddick, S. (1994). Thinking mothers/conceiving birth. In D. Bassin, M. Honey, & M. Kaplan, (Eds.). *Representations of motherhood* (pp. 29–45). New Haven, CT: Yale University.

Stack, C.B. & Burton, L. M. (1994). Kinscripts: Reflections on family, generation, and culture. In E. Glenn, C. Chang, & L. Forcey (Eds.). *Mothering: Ideology, experience, and agency* (pp. 33–44). New York: Routledge.

Turnbull, A. P., Turbiville, V. & Turnbull, H.R. (2000). Evolution of family-professional partnerships: Collective empowerment as the model for the early twenty-first century. In J. Shonkoff & S. Meisels (Eds.). *Handbook of early childhood intervention* (pp. 630–650). Cambridge (UK): Cambridge University.

Tronick, E.Z. (1998). Interventions that effect change in psychotherapy: A model based on infant research. *Infant Mental Health Journal, 19*(3), 277–279.

Weisner, T.S. (2002). Ecocultural understanding of children's developmental pathways. *Human Development, 45,* 275–281.

Acknowledgments

Data presented were collected through a NIH supported research project entitled: Boundary Crossing: An Ethnographic and Longitudinal Study National Center for Medical Rehabilitation Research, National Institute of Child Health and Human Development, National Institutes of Health (# R01 HD 38878) and a Maternal and Child Health Bureau funded research project conducted with Dr. Cheryl Mattingly entitled: Crossing Cultural Boundaries; An Ethnographic Study (MCJ # 060745). Dr. Lawlor would like to express appreciation to the many children, families, therapists, and practitioners who have participated in this research effort and who have willingly shared their experiences, perspectives, and expertise. In addition, she would like to express gratitude to Dr. Cheryl Mattingly, Dr. Lanita Jacobs-Huey, Dr. Ann Neville-Jan, Erica Angert, Nancy Bagatell, Jeanne Gaines, Jeanine Blanchard, Kim Wilkinson, Melissa Park, Susan Stouffer, and Amy Buffington for their assistance.

CHAPTER 16

Mother Time: The Art and Skill of Scheduling in Families of Children with Attention Deficit Hyperactivity Disorder

Ruth Segal, PhD, OTR

 Anticipated Outcomes

I anticipate that, after reading this chapter, readers will:

🖝 Understand the cultural and social nature of family schedules

🖝 Understand the dynamic and responsive nature of family schedules

🖝 Have an understanding of *mother time*, the mothering occupation of facilitating the family's daily round of activities through time use

🛰 Introduction

In this chapter a conceptual framework of the function of time use in families of children with attention deficit hyperactivity disorder (ADHD) is presented. In order to use time, we organize activities and occupations into schedules that represent our daily round of activities. The focus of this research is on women, who are usually the primary caregivers and organizers of families with children in the home. The conceptual framework consists of maternal construction and adaptation of anchored and responsive schedules, and the maternal strategies of time use of enfolding (engaging in several occupations simultaneously) and unfolding (putting aside all occupations to focus on a single task). This mothering occupation of facilitating the family time use is called *Mother Time* and discussed in the final section.

Mothering is an occupational role that consists of many occupations and activities. Direct care giving is the most commonly discussed aspect of mothering; however, it reflects only an observable aspect of this occupational role. In this chapter, I present and discuss an indirect and unobservable mothering occupation that I call *Mother Time*, which refers to the mothering occupation of facilitating the occupations and activities of the family and its members. This work is similar to the work of the chief executive officer in a business. The chief executive officer is responsible for developing and implementing strategic plans and policies to achieve future goals and for managing the day-to-day operation of the business. Mothers, typically, carry similar responsibilities at home with their families. In families, day-to-day operation consists of family members' survival and successful participation in daily life. Future goals, when raising children, include the successful socialization of the children into society (Gallimore et al., 1989; Ruddick, 1995).

The chief executive officer of a family is different from the chief executive officer of a business. Mothers, unlike chief executive officers of a business, are not paid for their work and they cannot change jobs. Additionally, their work has emotional and psychological aspects of love and care that make it qualitatively different from that of a business manager.

To highlight this qualitative difference, I decided to name this aspect of mothering occupations *Mother Time*, a paraphrase of *Father Time*, the cultural symbol that reminds us to use our time on earth wisely because we do not know what will happen in the hereafter (Macey, 1987). Mother time, on the other hand, is about mothers managing their children's time use to enhance the future opportunities.

Nothing in my professional education prepared me for the lifestyle changes resulting from being a parent. Not only there was there another person in our lives, there were many new activities and occupations that we needed to add to our daily lives and many activities we stopped doing completely or stopped doing as frequently. Our daily lives changed as a matter of fact with no discussions, crises, or questions. It just happened. Or did it?

At the time of the birth of my first child, I already planned to return to the University of Southern California to pursue doctoral studies in occupational science. After the birth of my first child, I knew that my dissertation would be about families. In the course of my studies, I interviewed mothers of children with ADHD for a class project in a seminar on temporal adaptation. At that time, I did not have an interest in children with ADHD. I selected mothers of children with ADHD because access to this population was easy for me and I had to finish the project within one term. This convenience consideration, however, was the decisive experience for the evolution of my dissertation. My dissertation examined the temporal adaptations of families of children with ADHD (a more detailed description of my research journey appears in Segal, 2001).

Mothers' time use in families with children with special needs has been studied using quantitative methods (Breslau, 1983; Crowe, 1993; Eriksen & Upshur, 1989) These studies compared the time use of mothers of children with different disabilities with the time use of mothers of typically developing children. In general, the findings suggest that mothers' time use depends on the children's age and disability. Additionally, it can be surmised that raising children with special needs does not necessarily mean that the mothers allocate more time to childcare than mothers of typically developing children. The existence of these variations in the time allocated to childcare and its relationship to children's age and disability indicates that mothers use time strategically to ensure that the children's needs are met. Therefore, knowing that raising children with special needs takes more time is not enough. I wanted to learn more about the *processes* that guide mothers' decisions on how they allot that extra time to the care of their children and what they give up and why. In more general terms, what are the processes and values that guide families in constructing their daily schedules? In this chapter I describe what I learned about these processes from mothers of children with ADHD.

Social and Cultural Perspectives

In this introduction I present the social, cultural, and familial functions of time. I begin by reviewing the literature on time from the social and cultural perspectives, and then I review the literature on the functions of time in the context of families. Although time and space are important research topics in the natural sciences, philosophy, and sociology, there are remarkably few studies that investigate the functions and use of time in the context of families and in relation to their health and well-being.

There are many discussions on the changes in patterns of time use that occurred in the last decade with the increased use of technologies to replace the way many activities and occupations are performed (e.g., Eriksen, 2001; Kreitzman, 1999). These changes, however, only amplify the importance of cultural and social practices to the way we use time.

The social rhythms of time use appear in the calendars we use. The calendar itself is a linear representation of the annual cycle of time (Fraser, 1987; Young, 1988). The annual cycle of time is based on the movement of the stars and the seasons or nature (Young, 1988). This cycle has been integrated into cultural practices that seem removed from nature (e.g., summer vacation of school). Regardless of the origin and historical development of calendars, they represent various social practices that regulate the behavior of individuals in society. These social practices may have religious, national, or natural origins. For example, in the typical calendar in Western society, Christmas is a day in which government offices, schools, and businesses are closed. The rules that require such closures are civic rather than religious laws. That is, the cultural practices of the majority of the people in these countries influence the social practices of society. National events such as national independence days are often marked with annual celebrations that shape social and individual behavior.

Calendars are further particularized as individuals join a variety of social groups and institutions. For example, the dates of religious holidays may be marked on regular calendars, but when an individual joins a specific church, the time of the day of services is specified. Additionally, each church may offer social activities and functions beyond these religious activities. These events offer individuals opportunities to participate in social activities and occupations at given times and locations. Another example for the particularization of calendars is children's school. Once parents choose a school for their children, they and their children have to follow the school calendar. That is, there are set times and dates in which the children must be in school. Teacher conferences, holidays, and school vacations are also set and advertised in the academic calendar. There are additional events such as parent-teacher association meetings, school plays, and team sports that occur outside these hours.

Another important aspect of the calendar is regulated by work schedules. Different jobs offer different work schedules. Some jobs are from 9 to 5, some persons work in shifts, and others have flexible time. Regardless of the type of work schedule, work commitment comes with a work schedule—a time commitment that is given to individuals once they accept the job. Zerubavel (1981) suggests that this function of calendars separates public time from private time. Once public time is portioned off the calendar, families and individuals are left with their private time to use as they see fit.

The Functions of Time in the Family

The function of time use in families was presented and discussed in 1975 by Kantor and Lehr in their book, *Inside the family: Toward a theory of family process.* Since then, this issue was not the focus of family studies until 1996 when Daly published his study, *Families and time: Keeping pace in a hurried culture.* Daly discussed many aspects of time and families. However, his discussion of organizing time use presents Kantor and Lehr's treatment of the issue.

Clocking and synchronization are the functions of time use in families (Kantor & Lehr, 1975). *Clocking* determines the sequencing, frequency, duration, and pacing of activities as represented by schedules or the daily rounds of activities. Each one of these aspects is embedded in values and knowledge. Participating in the daily rounds of activities reveals and reinforces these values and knowledge to family members, and in particular, to children. For example, brushing one's teeth before going to sleep is a sequencing of activities that is based on current medical knowledge of oral hygiene. If children's participation in this sequence of activities is reinforced with an explanation, they learn and participate in a culturally and socially appropriate sequence of activities.

Frequency and duration determine how often activities occur and for how long, respectively (Kantor & Lehr, 1975). Continuing with the example of brushing teeth, this activity should occur at least twice a day (frequency), once after breakfast and once before going to sleep (sequencing), and it should last at least two minutes (duration). Thus, the sequencing, frequency, and duration of brushing teeth guide the scheduling of the activities of daily oral hygiene.

Pacing is the overall rhythm of life in families (Kantor & Lehr, 1975). Some families are fast and some are slow. Pacing also relates to age. Typically, older people are slower than young children. Pacing is most evident when family members move from one activity to another at a different pace. For example, this may occur when a family is ready to go out to a movie and one family member is not ready. Everyone is waiting and some members may

become angry, leading to an argument. In this case, the family member's different pace evoked a tension in the family. This may have a very different effect on family dynamics if it is a one-time or regularly occurring event.

Lastly, scheduling is the designed organization of time use or the designed slotting of occupations and activities. Schedules are the reference mechanism of clocking (Kantor & Lehr, 1975). They establish deadlines for the completion of occupations and activities and thus create an order (i.e., sequence, frequency, duration, and pace) in the life of the family.

Synchronizing, the second function of time in the family, is the mechanism of regulating the family's total use of time (Kantor & Lehr, 1975). Priority setting, planning, and coordinating are three aspects of synchronizing. In priority setting, the family decides on the relative importance of occupations and activities and uses it as a guide to choose among them. In planning, the family decides on how to change its lifestyle by making long-term changes in their occupational engagement. Lastly, coordinating is the work of ensuring that the individual family members' streams of activities adhere to family's plan.

An example for the importance of synchronization in the family can be seen in DeVault's book, *Feeding the family: The social organization of caring as gendered work* (1991). One of the aspects of feeding the family that DeVault describes is coordinating the schedules of family members so that family meals can occur. Family meals afford the opportunity for the family members to meet and interact. As DeVault writes, these family meals provide "the time and space" for the individual family members to cohere into a family. Kantor and Lehr (1975) indicate that without finding the time to meet regularly, family members cannot cohere into a family or even fight with each other.

✒ Constructing Daily Life in Families of Children with Attention Deficit Hyperactivity Disorder

The above discussion of the functions of time in families highlights the importance of studying how families construct their time use. Occupations and activities occur in the stream of time (Clark et al., 1991). Their organization in time is the way we use time. The following discussion, therefore, will focus on the selection and organization of activities and occupations. The definition of activities and occupations is currently debated in the occupational therapy literature (e.g., Canadian Association of Occupational Therapy, 1997; Pierce, 2001). Because the focus of my chapter is on the organization of activities and occupations into schedules and daily routines, I believe that both terms apply, and that the exact definition of each term is unimportant in the context of my perspective.

Families are part of their social and cultural environment and the construction of their schedules is a cultural activity. That is, family schedules have rhythms that are embedded in their cultural and social environments. The construction of family schedules is a continual purposeful process. In addition to maintaining the social and cultural rhythms, schedules are used to improve the quality of life of the family and its members and to enhance the members' future opportunities (Frank, 1996; Gallimore et al., 1989; Segal, 1995; Segal & Frank, 1998; Zerubavel, 1979).

Families of children with ADHD are "ordinary families with special children" as Seligman and Darling (1997) titled their book. That is, families with children with special needs behave and function just like other families in their social and cultural environment (Gallimore et al., 1989; Seligman & Darling, 1997). In this chapter, "ordinary families" means that families of children with ADHD strive to construct and maintain a family schedule that will be embedded in cultural and familial values, will allow participation of society, and will support the construction of family identity and the future opportunities for the children (Segal, 1995; 1999; Segal & Frank, 1998).

ᡠᢥ The Study

The purpose of this qualitative study was to describe and understand the constructions of

daily schedules and routines in families of children with ADHD. Seventeen families from Southern California participated in the study. Five families were single-parent families consisting of mothers and children. Two of these mothers were divorced; one was separated; and the other two were widowed. In both cases, the husbands' cause of death was medical complications caused by alcoholism. One of the husbands was in his early 40s and the other was in his early 30s.

Mothers participated in all the interviews. In four cases, the fathers participated as well, at least part of the time, and in one case the father was interviewed separately. Fifteen families were interviewed twice and two families were interviewed four times. In the first interview, the participants were asked to tell the interviewer "the story of their family." In the semi-structured second interview, the participants were asked to describe a typical day and a particular day, usually the day before the interview. During the interview, the participants were also asked to describe how their occupations were performed. Most of the interviews lasted between 1 and 1 $\frac{1}{2}$ hours. The interviews were audiotaped and transcribed verbatim by a professional transcriptionist. The researcher listened to the audiotapes while reviewing the transcript for accuracy (Table 16–1).

The analysis followed the constant comparative method (Glaser & Strauss, 1967; Strauss & Corbin, 1998). An audit trail was kept and the research supervisor did the verification of analysis. All names used in this chapter are pseudonyms.

Attention Deficit Hyperactivity Disorder as a Challenge to Family Schedules

The two most common avenues of treating children with ADHD are medications and behavioral interventions. According to Hinshaw (1994), the most prevalent type of behavioral program for intervention with children with ADHD is "individual and group consultation in pertinent strategies to the key adults—parents and teachers—who interact with the child on a daily basis" (p. 115). The purpose of this intervention is to change the children's envi-

Table 16–1 Demographic data on the study participants

	Marital status (years married)	Age	Religion	Education (highest degree achieved)	Number of children	Age of children with ADHD	Gender of children with ADHD	Diagnosis	Medications	Type of school	Interventions
Berg	Married (8.5)	M: 42 F: 43	Jewish	M: Bachelor's F: Master's	2	7 5	Female Male	ADHD ADHD, OB	Ritalin® —	Public Private	
Casey	Widowed	M: 38	Protestant	M: High school	1	10	Male	ADHD, Anxiety, OCD	Ritalin®	Private	Counselor at school
Huberman	Married (18)	M: 41 F: 41	Mormon	M: Bachelor's F: Doctorate (DDS)	4	10	Male	ADD	—	Private	Tutor
Harriot	Divorced	M: 29	Christian	M: High school	1	7	Male	ADD	Ritalin®	Public	
Jameson	Married (2.5)	M: 32 F: 35	Interfaith	M: High school F: High school	2	8	Male	ADHD	Ritalin®	Public	Psychiatrist
Laury	Married (8)	M: 39 F: 46	Baptist	M: High school F: High school	2	7	Male	ADD	—	Public	
Marshall	Married (12)	M: 33 F: 39	Methodist	M: High school F: High school	2	9	Male	ADHD, TS	—	Private	
Mayfair	Separated	M: 32	—	M: College	2	6	Female	ADHD, Aphasia	Ritalin®	Public	Aphasia program
McCowen	Married (18)	M: 47 M: 47	Catholic	M: Bachelor's F: High school	2	7	Male	ADHD	Ritalin®	Private	OT, EC, psychologist
Merriott	Married (11)	M: 40 F: 45	M: Catholic F: Methodist	M: Master's F: Master's	2	9	Female	ADHD	Ritalin®, Asthma medications	Private	Speech therapy
Nether	Married (15)	M: 30 F: 40	Christian	M: Master's F: High school	2	7	Female	ADD	—	Private	Educational therapy

(Continued)

Table 16–1 Demographic data on the study participants *(Continued)*

	Marital status (years married)	Age	Religion	Education (highest degree achieved)	Number of children	Age of children with ADHD	Gender of children with ADHD	Diagnosis	Medications	Type of school	Interventions
Samuel	Married (7)	M: 48 F: 47	Jewish	M: Master's F: High school	1	9	Male	ADD	Ritalin® Haldon	Public	Group
Sandor	Widowed	M: 31	Mormon	M: High school	2	10 8	Male Female	ADHD, TS ADHD	Ritalin® Clonidine	Public Public	Family counselor
Singer	Divorced	M: 36	Catholic	M: Master's	2	6 4	Male Female	ADHD ADHD	Ritalin® Ritalin®	Private Private	BT BT
Walter	Married (16)	M: 43 F: 48	Catholic	M: High school F: High school	2	9	Male	ADHD	Ritalin®	Private	Family therapy
Wendell	Married (14)	M: 36 F: 39	Catholic	M: High school F: Master's	3	7	Male	ADHD	—	Private	Speech therapy, tutor
Wilbor	Married (24)	M: 48 F: 52	Catholic	M: High school F: High school	2	7	Male	ADHD	Ritalin®	Private	OT, Family therapy

ADD = attention deficit disorder; ADHD = attention deficit hyperactivity disorder; BT = behavioral therapy; EC = educational consultant; F = father, M = mother; OB = oppositional behavior; OCD = obsessive-compulsive disorder; OT = occupational therapy; TS = Tourette's syndrome ronment to promote the desired behavioral changes. The shortcomings of this approach are that the gains in behavioral changes are very small, they do not produce an overall behavioral change, and they are "not an easy treatment to implement, given its demands on parent and teacher time" (Hinshaw, 1994, p. 116). The two contradicting points that Hinshaw (1994) mentions are that this is the most difficult intervention for parents and teachers to assume, yet it is the most commonly used. This contradiction can be understood from stories of the families in this study. Almost all the families had reservations about the use of stimulant medications, the most effective treatment for the symptoms of ADHD. Most families explored alternatives to medications such as biofeedback, behavioral optometrists, or diets. These explorations did not reflect parental denial of the children's diagnosis, but rather their reluctance to use the medications. An example for this is Peggy's description of her family's attitude toward giving medication to her daughter who has ADHD:

> Well, her Dad is 100% against it [medication]. I did a lot of reading on it and there are side effects. I know they say in most cases there is no problem, but ... I, myself, don't take medicine unless I absolutely have to. I'd rather just deal with vitamins and exercise and eating right. The reason we tried the biofeedback is I had hoped that she could conquer this through biofeedback. That's more working inwardly than having to depend on drugs as an answer to her problems. So we wanted to take that route if we could and avoid medication. My feeling was if she really was just falling apart at school, then I would go for it. But I know I would have had a real battle with my husband on that—and grandmother too.

In this case, Peggy presents her family's value of using medication only after all alternative avenues have been tried. This value is applied to all family members, including the child with ADHD. Most of the families in the study reported here went through similar routes of exploring other avenues for helping their children before giving them stimulant medication. Eventually, most of the parents

gave their children the medication and reported that it was effective.

The children in this study who received medication took methylphenidate, which is better known in its brand name, Ritalin®. Methylphenidate is the most commonly used medication (Barkley, 1998; Hinshaw, 1994) because it has been shown to be the most effective in many studies over the years (e.g., McMaster University Evidence-Based Practice Center, 1998; MTA Cooperative Group, 1999; Schachar & Tannock, 1993). It is a short-acting stimulant medication (half-life of 2 to 3 hours), and its most common side effects are lack of appetite and insomnia (Barkley, 1998; Hinshaw, 1994). Therefore, the typical medication regimen for most of the children in this study consisted of two dosages, one taken in the morning before school and the other at lunchtime during school. Such medication regimens ensured that the children's symptoms were controlled during school hours, with the effects wearing off around 4 or 5 in the afternoon. That is, to ensure that the children are able to eat at least one meal and sleep, the children could not be medicated while they were at home. An additional influence on the time at home is known as the "rebound effect" (Barkley, 1998). That is, as the medication is wearing off, the symptoms of ADHD are more severe than the children's typical symptoms.

Parents, therefore, have to be with, attend to, and care for their children with ADHD during the hours when their symptoms are not controlled by the medications—in the mornings and in the afternoons and evenings. This raises the question of how they do it, and what the effects are on the quality of life of the family. In the study reported here, only one family took courses on how to deal with children with special needs. The other 16 families worked with their children during these hours with varying degrees of perceived success.

All the mothers in this study said that when the children with ADHD needed their attention that attention had to be *undivided*. When they described difficult experiences at home, the mothers explained that they occurred because they did not give their children their undivided attention. It seemed to me that giving undivided attention was a challenge in the context of maternal practices. I could not find current studies about the allocation of maternal attention in the home. There are three brief descriptions of how mothers use their time. Bateson (1996) indicates that in various societies, mothers typically engage in several occupations simultaneously. She named this phenomenon *enfolding occupations*. Before her, both Hall (1983) and Zerubavel (1981) mentioned that this phenomenon of time use exists in households in Western societies.

Linear schedules, in which activities follow each another successively, are the time use typical of business in Western cultures. Therefore, the need of children with ADHD for maternal undivided attention may not easily fit within the way time is used in the household. To attend to that need, mothers had to construct family schedules that would give them time to give their children the needed undivided attention.

Anchoring the Family Schedule

As described previously, public time consists of those parts of the day in which family members work and attend school. I call these sections of the family schedule the *anchored schedule*. Like a ship, the family schedule is anchored to the schedules of social and cultural institutions. The social and cultural schedules engulf the family's schedule, setting the general guidelines of time use like the port that engulfs the anchored ship. If the general social and cultural schedules interfere with family values and needs, families may change their anchoring. Similar to a ship sailing to another port, the family needs to decide on its goals and plan the route of change, as described by Kantor and Lehr (1975).

Time use in families is taken for granted until a challenge arises (Daly, 1996). Therefore the anchoring of family schedules occurs as a result of search for jobs and schools without much attention to how it affects the use of family time outside work and school hours. Schools in particular have a significant effect on how time is used and experienced during nonschool hours. For example, it might be difficult to leave children at a school they do not like, as Irene said:

It was really devastating because ... I mean I was going through ... I was extremely stressed; I couldn't eat, I couldn't sleep. I couldn't face leaving my child at school ... he would start crying and telling me, "Mom, don't leave." ...
I mean this kid ran off [after] the car so fast – he would run all the way down the sidewalk across the street, almost without looking. He could have [been] hit by a car ... I said, this was not worth it.

Irene describes her emotional anguish because of her son's unhappiness and her fear for his life because of his impulsive behavior. Irene and her husband searched for another school and decided to move their son from the public school to a private school that was affiliated with a church. Similarly, another mother reported that her son did not get out of bed for months in his first grade because of depression, and she eventually moved her son to a private school as well. In both cases, changing school was a process that took about a year to implement.

In this study of 17 families, 4 mothers reported on changing the children's school because the environment did not meet the needs of the children with ADHD. In all four cases, the mothers reported extreme distress on the part of the children because the school failed to respond to their emotional needs or caused emotional distress because of the way the teachers responded to the children's hyperactivity and impulsiveness.

Such difficulties occurred even when mothers searched for a school that would be best for their children and their special needs. The search for schools among families who send their children to private schools began with visiting private schools, observing classes, and interviewing teachers and principals to find out about their attitudes and approaches to children with special needs. Families who did not send their children to private school began the process of testing their children in the public school district to ensure that the children would be placed in appropriate classes with the needed support. Those who were informed also got information about the various special needs programs and visited those classrooms. They used their knowledge in the meetings to ensure that their children were placed appropriately.

The decision of what is appropriate is often based on the mothers' knowledge of their children and what they believe would be best for them. The decisions, therefore, are subjective and varied. Some mothers wanted their children to be in a regular class, with additional services given in the class. Other mothers wanted their children to get services in special rooms during school hours. And others preferred that their children attend regular classes and that the additional services not be provided in the school. In some cases, the children with ADHD had severe co-morbid disorders and needs that necessitated their enrollment in special schools. When mothers concluded that there was a need to change school, the search process was repeated, but with additional knowledge and experience.

In summary, the most common change in the anchored schedules was moving the children to a different school. These changes in the anchored schedule required mothers to invest an extensive amount of time in searching for an alternative school. Once such a change was made, there might be a period of getting into the new routine and schedule, but once the new routine was established, the anchored schedule was taken for granted and not dealt with. There was one family in this study that changed its work schedule as a result of the distress of raising a child with ADHD. In a later discussion, the experience of this family is discussed in detail.

Constructing the Responsive Schedules

Once the family schedule has been anchored within a social and cultural rhythm, the rest of the available time is allocated between wakeful and sleep time. Sleep is an activity that is essential for life, and as diurnal creatures, most humans sleep at night (Fraser, 1987).

The rest of the time is spent in other necessary life-sustaining activities (e.g., eating) and discretionary activities and occupations. Mothers construct and continually adapt the responsive schedule. The responsive schedule consists of all the nonanchored time in the family schedule, that is, the parts of their

schedule in which families have control of the types, lengths, physical location, and sequencing of their occupations. The responsive schedule is tailored to family needs and values. Further, it can respond to immediate needs. For example, the decision to allow a child to take a break while doing homework can be done in response to the child's frustration while doing the homework, and there is no need for advance planning.

The construction and changes in the responsive schedule occur in the three dimensions of adaptation: selection, organization, and performance of occupations (Frank, 1996; Segal, 1995). The selection and organization of occupations relate to Kantor and Lehr's (1975) concepts of clocking and synchronization. When discussing and describing their family's daily schedules and routines, the mothers in this study embedded their choices in their values and priorities. For example, one mother said that "at 6:30 everything stops and we have dinner together. We eat dinner as a family." It is clear from this statement that dinner is an important family occupation because "everything stops" when dinnertime comes and the family sits together. In the following section, I focus on the organization of occupations into the responsive schedules.

The performance of occupations is not related to any of the aspects of time use identified by Kantor and Lehr (1975), and it is embedded in occupational therapy's knowledge. In occupational therapy, activities and occupations are analyzed for the components and skills it takes to perform them. In this study, I looked at the way mothers perform their occupations in terms of time use.

Organizing the Responsive Schedule

Organizing occupations is an adaptive process in which selected occupations are temporally located so that they construct a meaningful and sustainable routine (Gallimore et al., 1989). This process corresponds to Kantor and Lehr's (1975) clocking that was described above.

A common reason for tailoring routines was the physiological needs of children with ADHD. Most of the children in this sample were taking Ritalin®. The side effects of loss of appetite and insomnia disappear when the medication wears off. Therefore, in the afternoons, when the last dosage of Ritalin® is wearing off, the children are hungry. Additionally, homework should be done while the medication is still controlling their symptoms. This leads to a rather common basic afternoon routine: snack or dinner after school, homework, dinner or snack, bath, and bedtime. This basic routine consists of self-care occupations and participation in school. The inclusion of other occupations and their temporal location within the basic routine differs among families. These occupations include free play time, television time, breaks, sports, and music (Segal, 1995; Segal & Frank, 1998).

I have chosen four families to describe the variations in afternoon routines: the Wendell, Merriott, Walter, and McCowen families. The Wendell and Merriott families' afternoon routines include only snack, homework, breaks, dinner, bath, and bedtime. The Walter and McCowen families include other activities in their afternoon routines. The Walter family has sports and music activities for their child, and the McCowen family takes their child to therapy in that part of the day.

Mary and Chris Wendell have three children. The oldest child is 9 years old; the second child, Henry, is 7 years old; and the youngest child is 5 years old. In the previous year, homework was done after dinner. This arrangement worked well for the older child. However, this year Henry started to get homework, and a change was needed. Mary explained:

> This year we have had to implement doing homework right after school, or, "you can take a half an hour break, but then everything goes off and you have to come do your homework." We have to do it that way, because if we wait until after dinner, like last year, Henry just will not lock on to homework, he wants to still play, and you know, I don't know why it was like that, but we just decided it's homework first, and then, "you can play the whole rest of the night just to do what you want." And that makes him feel better. Or if we get stuck on homework, we know we have time instead of saying, "get it

done because you have to get a bath and go to bed."

In this instance, the temporal relocation of homework was a change that improved the family's quality of life. The change resulted from Henry's needs, but it included the routine of his older brother. Thus the family's responsive schedule was changed to address the needs of a child, and at the same time the quality of life of the family has improved. The new organization had another advantage: Mary could allow Henry to take breaks during homework if he needed them because it did not affect his bedtime.

Another feature of Mary's routine is the temporal location of her time alone. Mary scheduled her time alone between 9:00 PM and midnight:

> Because sometimes, Henry wakes up with nightmares. So if I go to bed early, he'll wake and then I'll wake up anyways. So until he is really solidly asleep, you know, I don't go to bed until then.

Mary, who is a full-time homemaker, could have scheduled her time alone at other parts of day. However, this temporal location allows her to attend to Henry's needs if he has nightmares while addressing her own need for uninterrupted sleep. Again, the family schedule responds to the needs of the child with ADHD in a manner that enhances the quality of life of the child, other family members, and the family as a unit.

Donna Merriott tailors many parts of the day around Mirabelle's needs. Mirabelle is 9 years old and has asthma and ADHD. In the afternoons, Donna organizes homework, snack, dinner, and bedtime around Mirabelle's physiological and emotional needs and her ability to concentrate. After she described the daily routine, Donna said: "I can't be rigid, but I try to keep those certain formulas." She also said, about the process of learning not to be rigid, "But you have to learn to be more flexible with them. They are not flexible, so you have to be." When she talked about Mirabelle's inflexibility, she referred to the fits, destruction of homework, and screaming that erupt if Mirabelle loses her self-control. This occurs when she is rushed.

Donna usually picks up Mirabelle from school at about quarter to three, and they arrive home between 3:00 and 3:15.

> She has to eat and it usually takes her about 45 minutes to an hour to decompensate after a day at school because she tries really hard at school. So by 4:00 we have to be starting homework. The only problem is at 4:00, *Reading Rainbow* comes on and that's her favorite show. So if I can get her to eat and start homework by 3:30, ... at 4:00 she gets a break to watch *Reading Rainbow* and then at 4:30 there's another show on but she knows that if she hasn't finished her homework, she has to do the rest of the homework ... By 5:00 she can't do it [homework].

Donna described how she was trying to temporally locate homework and snack so that Mirabelle: (1) will not be hungry, (2) will be able to do her homework, (3) will have a break before beginning homework, and (4) will have a break during homework to watch a favorite television show.

Donna and Mary include breaks in the afternoon routines as a response to the needs of the child with ADHD. However, their style of including these breaks differs. Donna schedules the breaks to certain hours, and she uses this schedule to direct and focus her work with Mirabelle. Mary does not schedule the breaks, but she allows them if they are needed. Both styles achieve the same goal: the children's levels of stress and frustration with homework are manageable, and this increases the family's quality of life. The Walter family includes many more activities in their son's afternoon schedule than do either Donna Merriott or Mary Wendell. Nine-year-old Andrew Walter has some activity scheduled every day of the week during baseball season. Shirley Walter, his mother, describes:

> At 3:00 I pick him up usually every day. If he has an activity, he goes to the activity. Like today [Friday] he has piano at 3:00. He has baseball—he just started this week on Mondays, Thursdays, and Saturdays—he has practice.
> Wednesday night is Awanah and that is from right after dinner he leaves here—he has to be there at 6:20 and it gets out at 8:15. Then the next morning he gets up for choir at school.

This very busy schedule has advantages and disadvantages as Shirley says in the same paragraph:

> Andrew has a pretty tough schedule when baseball season starts because he has—actually he does better in school and does better at doing what we want him to do and everything because he knows he's—he likes it and he's not going to be playing if he doesn't do it. Plus he physically gets out all that aggression ... The thing that I worry most is about him not getting enough rest and I think part of that is why he's so cranky.

Shirley Walter does not schedule or allow for breaks in the afternoons. At another point in the interview, she said that Andrew's extracurricular activities enhance the family's quality of life. That is, they have the same function as the breaks in the schedules that Donna Merriott and Mary Wendell developed.

The inclusion of breaks in a very busy schedule is possible, as the afternoon routine of the McCowen family shows. Seven-year-old Simon goes to occupational therapy on Mondays and Fridays. On Wednesdays, he sees an educational specialist, and on Saturdays he sees a developmental psychologist. Rhoda described the afternoon routine on the days that they go to the occupational therapy clinic:

> We come home from school at 2:30. By the time I get actually to the house [after] dropping off the car-pool it's about ten to three. He watches television for a half hour and calms down. It's fun for him because he likes to do that. And then for the [OT] clinic we have to leave the house at 3:30; the appointment is at 4:00. So we leave the clinic at about 5:00, get home by 5:30 and have dinner. Sometimes he'll have a snack after school. He doesn't eat much mid-day because of the Ritalin®. After dinner any homework that he has gets done.

Simon gets a break after school and before he goes to any of the therapies he has during the week. There are two temporal locations for food in Simon's afternoon: after school and after therapy when the family has dinner. He does his homework after dinner. Simon gets Ritalin® in the afternoons which makes it possible for him to do homework later. Rhoda, like the other three mothers discussed above, includes some kind of break or enjoyable activities to help the child with ADHD perform demanding or difficult occupations.

The four examples show how the responsive schedule is used to address needs of children with ADHD while enhancing the quality of life of the child, the family, and the other family members. In addition to organizing the responsive schedule with these concerns in mind, the mothers needed to find a way to give the children with ADHD the undivided attention they needed. This required the mothers to address the way they use their time.

❧ Managing the Responsive Schedule and Unfolding: An Adaptive Strategy for the Reorganization of Routines

In this section, I explore how families reorganized their routine to address the needs of their children with ADHD (Segal, R., 2000). The guiding concept used is *enfolded occupations* (Bateson, 1996). The use of this concept to understand routine reorganization emerged from family stories of how difficult it is for their children when they do not get undivided attention.

Unfolding is an adaptive strategy of removing chunks of action out of previously established routines. The chunks of the routines that are removed may be temporally relocated to another part of the day, or they may be done by another person.

Temporal Unfolding

Temporal unfolding is the removal of occupations out of a routine to be performed at another time. This adaptive strategy is used either for particular parts of the day or as a rule of household organization. When temporal unfolding is used for a specific part of the day, it often has been devised for an

usually difficult or potentially difficult part of the day.

For example, Donna Merriott does her morning hygiene, grooming, and dressing after she takes Mirabelle to school. This unfolding allows Donna to give Mirabelle her undivided attention. Statements such as "we are going to be late for school" only upset Mirabelle because it is very important for her to be early to school. Therefore, Donna uses her focus and attention for distracting and humoring Mirabelle through the morning routine. Donna described the mornings:

> She [Mirabelle] does not do well if you wake her up. She also does not do well if you try to hurry her. So I try to always make sure there's time in the mornings. My needs go last. I'll go to the bathroom when I can and brush my teeth and wash my face after I've already said hello to her. Then typically I'll not get dressed; I'll put a coat on or I'll put on sweats and take her to school. I don't worry about how I look. Because to me it is more important for her to have as much time as possible in the morning.[1]

Other mothers used temporal unfolding to accomplish things like shopping, errands, housecleaning, baking, reading the mail, paying the bills, and talking on the phone with friends. These occupations fall into two categories. The first category includes occupations that foster the continued functioning of the household and family (e.g., food shopping, housecleaning, and paying bills). The second category includes occupations that are fun and satisfying for the mother (e.g., talking on the phone with friends).

Temporal unfolding is the single most important adaptive strategy used by Rita Singer. This strategy was used to organize the routines so that Rita can accomplish everything by herself. She is the divorced mother of Robert and Louisa. Robert is 6 years old and Louisa is 4 years old. Both children have been diagnosed with ADHD and are treated with medications. Rita is a professional military officer and works full time.

Rita temporally unfolds the daily routine at home so that she can focus on the children while they are awake:

My weekdays start about 4:45 in the morning. I get up, take my shower, get everything ready for the day. Pull their snack packs, put their ice packs in there, put them by the door—just get it organized. Around 6:30–6:45 in the morning I wake them up. I usually dress them—at least once because they will take something off and throw it around and around the house. Both of the children —I do this individually to each of the children. I come downstairs and we normally eat breakfast. We are out of the house somewhere around 7:30, if I'm lucky, and they remember to leave everything at the door …

[We] get home around 6:45–7:00 in the evening. Right away … normally on the weekend I cook enough so I just pull out a portion; defrost it in the microwave and heat it up. That's their first meal of the night.

I put them down initially for bedtime around 8:30 but they have difficulty going to sleep at night so between 8:30 and about 11:00 they are constantly up, walking down(stairs); I put them back to bed—they'll come down, put them back to bed; they'll come down, I'll put them back to bed. There's usually another snack in there. Up, down, back to bed. Around 11:00 at night that's when I get a chance to finish my ironing—finishing their snack packs for the next day and their lunches. That's all set up in the fridge. I just line it all up in there and it's ready to go. Put all the clothes out for the next day before I get to bed. I normally don't get more than about five hours of sleep a night. If I'm lucky, five.[1]

Rita's adaptive strategy of accomplishing the daily routine was based on temporal unfolding. She prepared as much as possible the night before, after the children were asleep. In the mornings she had her shower and got everything ready to go by the door before she woke up the children. Further, she cooked on the weekends only and froze the food in portions. This allowed her to avoid cooking and to give her undivided attention to the children when they arrived home.

Besides the daily routine, Rita did other things using the same adaptive strategy. To do her shopping, Rita planned for one long lunch break (1 $1/2$ hours) every other week. During this lunch break she did all her shopping for the next 2 weeks. That meant that she had to plan for 2 weeks at a time and prepare ice packs to keep for the frozen food frozen in the picnic box. The children went to their father every other weekend. During these weekends, Rita did the housecleaning and the home and car maintenance work.

Temporal unfolding was the dominant adaptive strategy that Rita used. However, it did not eliminate enfolded occupations or the need to use other strategies. For example, while they are driving from home to school and back, Robert had to practice his reading: Rita supervised Robert while driving. She also had a point system at school and home for the children. They had a list of things that they have to do at home, and they got a cent for every item that they have accomplished.

Rita chose temporal unfolding as the main adaptive strategy because this strategy made it possible for her to accomplish everything by herself. There are two explanations for this choice. One is that Rita's divorce required her to pay off the bills of that divorce.

Therefore, she could not afford to pay someone to help her around the house or with shopping. Another reason was that Rita's lifelong style of adaptation was self-sufficiency. She said that her parents were disabled: "I did a lot of physical labor growing up along with sacrificing to get through my schooling. All I'm doing is starting again. And I know I can make it. So that's not a problem." Although Rita was certain that she could make it by herself, her adaptive style was not without a price. The price is lack of sleep, lack of time for herself, and a lot of stress. Rita described it: "my boss has been telling me I need a vacation away from the kids."

Temporal unfolding is the removal of occupations out of a routine to be performed at another time. This strategy can be used to accomplish parts of the daily routine or the complete household routine. The findings show that when temporal unfolding occurs, it helps the family accomplish the daily routine and reduce family stress. However, it displaces the stress from the interaction between a mother and the children to the mother only.

Unfolding by Inclusion

Unfolding by inclusion occurs when there is more than one adult responsible for the daily routines. In this strategy, one adult gives undivided attention to the child with ADHD and the other does the activities that need to be done simultaneously. The mother is always one of the adults responsible for the daily routine, and the individual who shares the responsibility may be the child's father, an older child, a paid housekeeper, a friend, a tutor, or a teacher.

Similar to temporal unfolding, the adaptive strategy of unfolding by inclusion may be used to accomplish particular sections of the daily routine or to organize the household as a whole. The most typical example of unfolding by inclusion is that the husband does homework with the child while the mother is preparing dinner. In another family, a 15-year-old boy picks up his stepsister and stepbrother from the after-school program at 4:00 PM. He gives the 7-year-old stepsister her medicine and helps her with homework. If everything works well, the homework is done by the time the mother comes home from work. That is, homework and dinner preparations are typically unfolded by the inclusion of the older child as helper to the mother.

Another solution for homework is to disengage from it. The mothers leave the homework to be an issue between the children and their teachers or tutors. Disengaging from the homework means that mothers may remind the children that they need to do the homework and give them a choice of when and where to do it. However, they do not sit with the children and help them through with the homework or even check if they are done. If the children do not hand in the homework on time or if they have made mistakes, the teachers and the children resolve that issue. That is, the mothers unfold their afternoons by symbolically including the teachers in homework. This inclusion does not involve the physical appearance of teachers at home during the afternoon. The consequences of doing or not doing homework are carried over to school hours. For the mothers, this unfolding means that the children are not engaged in activity that demands parental undivided attention. All the children in this study could engage in play with only periodic attention; therefore, enfolding cooking and supervision of children's play was not a stressful situation.

A second way in which mothers disengage from homework is hiring somebody to help the children with homework. Some families hire tutors and others get the child involved with education specialists that are expected to work with the children all the way through high school. In this form of unfolding by inclusion, another person is included in the afternoon routine. This individual gives the children undivided attention while they are doing their homework.

Two families organized the household using unfolding by inclusion. One family has a live-in housekeeper, and in the other family, the mothers share the household routine. At the McCowen household, a month before Rhoda had to return to work after her maternity leave, she hired a full-time, live-in helper at home. This occurred before anyone suspected that Simon had any problems.

Rhoda was 40 years old when Simon was born, and she describes her happiness: "To say I embraced motherhood is an understatement." This embracing of motherhood meant that Rhoda planned on becoming very involved with Simon. Roger, the father, says about Rhoda's mothering style: "If there wasn't anything wrong with him [Simon], instead of going to the [therapy] he'd be training to be an Olympic something. God knows what."

This mothering style required the unfolding of homemaking and childcare activities. The adaptive strategy that Rhoda chose was unfolding by the inclusion of a housekeeper. The housekeeper does all the home-making activities and some child supervision. This complete unfolding is manifested in the difficulties that Rhoda had to find chores around the house for 7-year-old Simon. The psychologist suggested that Rhoda would give Simon chores to empower him and give him a sense of responsibility. Rhoda says about the process of finding chores for Simon: "It's a challenge to think of things when you have full-time help. I don't even make my own bed."

The Wilbor family also uses unfolding by inclusion. Their household organization changed for both parents about a year before the study. The husband, Harry, says:

> We actually have changed our life drastically in the last year. I, from a job that I was putting in 60 hours a week, I'm now doing about 60 hours a month. Sharon went back to work a few days a week. So it gives a break to both of us so that we are not always [under] pressure to deal with him all the time. Because before, Sharon was always doing everything with him and I was at work most of the time.

Sharon and Harry Wilbor have two children. Randy is 20 years old and is not living at home, and David is 7 years old and has been diagnosed with ADHD. In the previous quotation, Harry describes the changes in their lifestyles that occurred after he and Sharon felt the family was falling apart. Sharon, in particular, felt that she was "engulfed" and "devoured" by David. So, when the opportunity for Harry's partial retirement and Sharon's part-time job arose, they seized it.

Now that both Sharon and Harry are involved in the household routine, they unfold the occupations: In the mornings they discuss who is better able to handle David that morning, and the other person will make breakfast and lunch. On the day of the interview, Sharon and Harry said that the last few mornings had been particularly difficult. Therefore, unfolding the morning routine was different: "So it kind of like very early in the morning, Harry and I will determine that this is going to be one of those mornings where we'll have to juggle who's prompting. Either he'll do the whole breakfast thing and I'll do, 'OK, David, it's time to get dressed.'" Harry and Sharon consistently use the adaptive strategy of unfolding by inclusion; however, its application varies with the situation at hand. Sometimes one adult is doing only childcare and the other is doing the homemaking activities. When an entire morning of childcare may be too stressful, the unfolding changes to taking turns with David.

Unfolding by inclusion occurs at the Wilbor's household in the afternoons as well. Sharon picks up David from school and takes him to occupational and physical therapy on Tuesdays and Wednesdays. Harry picks up David from school on Mondays, Thursdays, and Fridays. Monday and Friday afternoons are free and on Thursday afternoons David has soccer. Dinner is prepared by the parent who does not spend the early afternoon with David. David's appetite fluctuates because of the medicine. If he is hungry, David has to eat before he can do his homework. Sharon describes the afternoons when they are all at home:

> A lot of times we don't sit down as a family and eat together because his [David's] requirement after the medication is that he be fed first because he's really usually very hungry. And that distracts him from being able to concentrate. So he has to have his physical needs met with eating. And then we … I'm usually the person that does the homework with him while Harry is either fixing our dinner or cleaning up — depends on how we are running. Our whole goal is to get him to bed by 8:30 which is a major goal we are working on because it could go on — the night ritual could go on until 10 or 11 at night with a child like this.

And the night ritual is:

> Quality time with Daddy first, because he usually wants to wrestle with Daddy and with me he'll do something more quiet, where I'll stroke his back and kind of get him ready to relax. And then we'll read a story as a family and then I'll say his prayers with him and rub his back.

Similar to the mornings, the routine in the afternoons is also unfolded by inclusion. Each parent does something with David while the other is occupied with homemaking. This way, when David is asleep, there is no more work around the house and Sharon and Harry have some time for themselves before they "collapse."

Harry goes to ride his bicycle with friends on Saturday mornings, and Sharon does something "nice and quiet" with David. When Harry comes home, Sharon goes grocery shopping and Harry does something with

David. Sharon works on Sundays, and Harry spends the day with David. The adaptive strategy used most by Sharon and Harry Wilbor is unfolding by inclusion: There is always one parent that gives David undivided attention, while the other parent is busy with the relevant home-making occupations or is at work.

The purpose of unfolding by inclusion for Sharon and Harry is to improve the family's quality of life. Sharon and Harry were so stressed that they were beginning to consider getting a divorce. Their adaptive strategy is the result of parenting classes and family and individual therapy. Sharon says that they go to therapy whenever they feel that there is too much stress. It has improved their quality of life. During the interviews Sharon kept saying that she and her husband work as a team, and both Sharon and Harry agree that the quality of their marriage has never been better.

In the two families in which complete unfolding by inclusion occurs as the main adaptive strategy, the mothers are in their 40s and are economically well established. That is, both complete inclusion of the father and of a live-in housekeeper require economic resources. Further, in the scenario of complete inclusion by the husband, the father agreed to take partial retirement at an early age and to participate in childcare and homemaking activities.

In sum, enfolded occupations are a familiar phenomenon of the daily routines at home. They make it possible for mothers to use time efficiently and have some time left for leisure and sleep. For parents raising a child with ADHD, enfolded occupations may be a source of stress because such children often need undivided attention. This study of families raising children with ADHD shows that mothers use two strategic avenues: making enfolded occupations work and unfolding occupations. Making enfolded occupations work is done with the more traditional measures of consequences, timers, and reminders.

Unfolding is an adaptive strategy in which a part of the routine is moved away to another part of the day or to another person to do. The purpose of unfolding is to accomplish daily occupations while enhancing the quality of life of each family member (Frank, 1996).

Unfolding strategies may be used within a section of the daily routine or as a rule of household organization. Either way, unfolding strategies may help the family accomplish the routines and enhance their quality of life.

Performing Occupations: Adaptive Strategies of Working with Child with Attention Deficit Hyperactivity Disorder

Performing occupations refers to the mothers' work in managing the way in which their children perform occupations. This process is important because productive management leads to children's competence and independence. One set of adaptive strategies is aimed at managing occupational performance of enfolded and single occupations. I will first discuss the performance of enfolded occupations and continue with the performance of single occupations.

A result of being engaged in enfolded occupations is that none of the occupations get undivided attention. One finding of this study is that stressful situations often occur when the child with ADHD cannot get a parent's undivided attention. Therefore, enfolding childcare or supervision with another occupation may cause stress in the family.

Mothers often judge that morning rush and homework are the most difficult parts of the day. The common features of these parts of the day are that there are numerous tasks that need to be accomplished within a given time frame. The inability of children with ADHD to stay on tasks and complete them makes these parts of the day difficult for them. Furthermore, mothers often cannot give the children undivided attention in the mornings or during homework. During these parts of the day, mothers have to engage in other activities such as self-care, assisting other children, or preparing dinner. That is, the need to engage in enfolded occupations in the mornings and during homework increases difficulties during these periods. In the present section, the enfolded morning routines at the Laury and Casey families and the enfolded homework period at the Walter family are described to illustrate how mothers help their children to perform occupations during these typically busy and potentially stressful times.

The Laury family has two children. Tommy is 7 years old and has been diagnosed with attention deficit disorder with some hyperactivity. Tina is 4 years old, has some articulation problems and sees a speech therapist, but otherwise her behavior is unremarkable. In the mornings, the children wake up by themselves around 6, and they turn on the television and keep themselves busy. If Tommy is hungry, he gets himself a bowl of cereal. Jennifer, the mother, wakes up when the children and the television become too noisy. At 7:30 AM, Jennifer sends the children to their room to get dressed. While they are dressing, Jennifer lets them know that she is going to the bathroom to get ready too, and that she doesn't want to have to come out to deal with them. However, she always has to come out to separate the children. When she is dressed up, she has to "nag" Tommy a lot to get dressed. Often she has to separate the children by putting them in different rooms, and it is not uncommon for her to yell at them.

Jennifer's occupations from 7:30 AM are: getting herself ready to take Tommy to school, supervising Tommy, and separating Tommy and Tina so that Tommy will be ready to go to school by 8:15 AM Tina dresses herself in the mornings, and if she is not ready, she may stay at home with her father, who is sleeping during that time. Jennifer reported that this part of the day is consistently stressful. The family's morning routine is composed of enfolded occupations that do not allow Jennifer to give Tommy her undivided attention, and, therefore he continually gets off his task.

In another case, Vera Casey and her son, Ethan, live with his maternal grandmother. Ethan is 10 years old and has been diagnosed with ADHD. Vera says that mornings are the most difficult part of the day. Vera gets up around 5:30 AM to have some breathing room and coffee, read the paper, take a shower, and prepare lunch for her and for Ethan. Ethan gets up around 6:00 AM. He vies for attention, and he is very hyperactive because he has not had his medication yet. Vera tries to get Ethan to eat some breakfast while making her bed and getting ready to leave at 7:30 a.m.

Vera and her mother give him periodic warnings about the time left until the school bus comes.

Although Ethan does not hurt anyone or destroy anything while he is so active, he does move around and try to get attention any way he can. A typical thing that Ethan does in the mornings is to get into Vera's car and lock the automatic locks from inside. Once he lets her in, he refuses to go out. Vera says that mornings are: "Kind of like earthquake, while you're in the midst of an earthquake you just take cover and you just wait for it to end. And that's the way it is with him, while, in time, his medication kicks in, that's it."

Although Ethan needs only periodic reminders to start his morning routine, his behavior is difficult because Vera cannot give him undivided attention in the mornings. Vera gets up early to complete some of her morning occupations before Ethan gets up. However, Ethan wakes up early as well, and Vera does not have enough time to complete all the morning activities that do not involve him. Therefore, Vera must engage in enfolded occupations in the mornings and give Ethan only partial attention.

The morning routines of both families, the Laurys and the Caseys, are typical of the sample. Families describe mornings as very stressful and the need to remind and prompt the children as very irritating. The need to prompt the children to stay on task occurs at other parts of the day as well. These parts are not as difficult. The most typical feature of the most difficult part of the day is that the mothers engage in enfolded occupations.

Another frequent difficult part of the day is homework. Homework is an activity that has to be completed, often before dinner. It is common for mothers to prepare dinner during that time. If there are other children in the family, they are also at home and need some supervision as well. That is, usually the mothers engage in enfolded occupations.

In the Walter family, homework is a particularly difficult part of the day. During that time, one child does homework and the other plays the piano, and then they switch places. The child who does homework is in the kitchen with Shirley while she is preparing dinner.

Often this situation turns out to be very stressful because 9-year-old Andrew misbehaves: He teases his sister and responds to his mother with meaningless syllables. Usually, by the time her husband, James, comes home, Shirley cannot handle Andrew any more, and she asks James to take him away from her. However, James needs about half an hour for himself to make the transition from work to home.

Shirley plans the afternoons so that Andrew will be done with homework by the time James comes home. If this happens, Andrew has play time; Shirley has time to prepare dinner; and James has his quiet time. Shirley focuses her planning on this half hour. She and James agree that this period is "a very crucial time in that that's when probably most of the arguments, most of the upsets and what will, can happen. Because that's when you either make the transition easy or you make it rough." Shirley's plans for a smooth transition rarely work. Shirley suggests that the partial attention she gives Andrew while he is doing his homework is the reason for his misbehavior. That is, Shirley says that her engagement in enfolded occupations is a source of stress.

In all three examples, the mothers identified these periods of necessarily enfolded occupations as the most difficult part of the day. These situations occur regardless of gender or hyperactivity, and all families use adaptive strategies to ease these stressful situations. Adaptive strategies are sequences of action used to achieve adaptation's goal of increasing quality of life and enhancing life opportunities (Frank, 1996). In this study, families use adaptive strategies to accomplish daily routines while reducing stress in the family. These strategies have two broad goals: The first goal is fostering the child's independence and general well-being, and the second goal is reducing the stress in the family or enhancing the family's quality of life. The findings show that there are two major routes that families take: trying to reduce to stress when engaging in enfolded occupations and unfolding the occupations. Unfolding has been discussed in a previous section. In the following subsections, the management of enfolded and single occupations is discussed.

Management of Enfolded Occupations

In trying to make enfolded occupations work, families adopted or developed strategies to make these routines less stressful to avoid shouting, engaging, yelling, and anger. Their adaptive strategies focus on teaching the children to complete tasks without the mothers' continual intervention.

A timer system is used at the Nethers' house. Peggy, the mother, gets up at 6:00 AM and exercises for an hour. She prepares breakfast for 7-year-old Daisy and wakes her up at 7:00 AM Daisy has been diagnosed as having attention deficit disorder without hyperactivity. Peggy has to physically stand Daisy up, put her robe on, guide her to the table, and "plop" her on a chair. Once Daisy is at the table, Peggy sets the timer for 10 minutes, and tells Daisy that she has to finish before the timer rings. Peggy sits with Daisy and talks with her or eats breakfast as well.

Once breakfast is done, Peggy begins to enfold occupations. She begins to get dressed while she supervising Daisy's and her 5-year-old brother's morning routine:

> [I just put] her in this front bathroom and I close the door and I say, "You cannot come out until you are dressed." And [I do] it with her brother too, because he will play around … Her brother, I let him sleep a little longer because he's a little quicker and he doesn't want to eat breakfast. So I do the same thing with him. I tell her, "OK, when the bell rings [you have to be dressed]." If she gets everything done then she earns points. If she doesn't then she doesn't get any of the points for the morning. Then I put it [the timer] on for another 10 minutes and in that time she's got to make her bed, brush her teeth, and do her hair. Ideally if she … they got all this done then they'd have some playtime. But it rarely works out.[1]

Peggy started the timer system to reduce her clashes with Daisy, using the timer as an objective third party that announces the consequences of being late. She was familiar with the timer system from her background in special education. In assessing this timer system,

Peggy said that it works "fairly well." However, she has never stopped reminding the children to stay on tasks. That is, the adaptive strategy at the Nether house includes fostering the children's responsibility (timer and points), limiting distractions to make dressing achievable within the given time frame (dressing in the front bathroom), and taking control when it seems that the children are not achieving the goals within the time limits (reminders).

In another household, the timer system did not work because the child threw the timer against the wall. The family therapist helped the mother establish a chip system. In this system, the two children (both with ADHD) get chips for accomplishing things, and if they don't complete activities, chips get taken away. For example, while I was interviewing the mother, she told the children that they would get two chips if they let her go through the interview without interruptions. The children did not enter the room after the two chips were promised.

Two other adaptive strategies used to foster enfolded routines are going to the car and waiting for the child, and a contest. Some mothers simply leave for the car and let the children know that they are waiting there. One parent reminds the child that school is within walking distance. Therefore, if he is not coming within a couple of minutes, she is going to leave and he can walk. Whatever the mothers say to the child as they leave for the car, when they leave the children are able to finish dressing up within few minutes.

A contest of "who gets dressed the fastest" was established by Clara. She is the widowed mother of two children. Alexander is 10 years old and has ADHD and Tourette's syndrome, and Sophia is 8 years old and has attention deficit disorder without hyperactivity. Clara describes the contest and how she manipulates the situation to keep both children involved in it:

> I've gotten to where I kind of have a contest—who gets dressed first—who can get dressed the fastest and of course, I'm always the last. I have to put on [more clothes than they do]. They are pretty good. Alexander is usually the first, which sometimes bothers Sophia—sometimes if

he's asleep when I wake up, I'll wake her up first so that she gets her chance to be first too. So it's not so one-sided. He doesn't like that at all. He has to be first every single day.[1]

Clara manipulates the contest to have Sophia win because Sophia says that there is no point in trying if she never wins. Clara's adaptive strategy is to keep the children involved and interested in the contest rather than fulfill Alexander's need for being the constant winner fully satisfied. As long as the children are participating in the contest, the morning routine is completed in time for her to get to work on time.

Conclusion

As presented in this chapter, mothers construct the family schedule and adapt the use of their own time so that the family will become a cohesive functioning social unit that is appropriate in its social and cultural environment. The focus in this chapter was on the socialization of children into society through time use. According to Parsons (1989/1991), the family is a social institution whose major role in society is to ensure that children internalize values. In other words, families are the social agency responsible for the socialization of their children into society. This social function of families is used to understand their actions in theories such as the ecocultural theory of family accommodation (Gallimore et al., 1989). Socialization, however, is not a result of direct teaching and recitation of values. It is acquired through participation in occupations (Gallimore et al., 1989; Segal, 1999) and through participation in carefully organized daily rounds of activities or schedules (Daly, 1996; DeVault, 1991; Segal & Frank, 1998).

The organization of the daily rounds of activities is a carefully constructed system of time use that takes into account the survival and socialization needs of children. Identifying and addressing these needs is the dialectical process in mother time. Mothers construct the daily life based on previous experience, knowledge of family members and understanding of the demands of the physical and social internal and external worlds. The work is commonly practiced but rarely discussed.

Discussion Questions 🖐

- How would the nature of mother time differ when children have other disabilities?

- How do the cultural and social environments influence the nature of mother time?

- How do family values and beliefs influence the construction of daily schedules and routines?

References

Barkely, R. (1998). *Attention-deficit hyperactivity disorder: A handbook for diagnosis and treatment* (2nd ed.). New York: Guilford Press.

Bateson, M. C. (1996). Enfolded activity and the concept of occupation. In R. Zemke & Clark, F. (Eds.). *Occupational Science: The evolving discipline.* (pp. 5–12). Philadelphia: F. A. Davis.

Breslau, N. (1983). Care of children with disabilities and women's time use. *Medical Care, 21,* 620–629.

Canadian Association of Occupational Therapists (1997). *Enabling occupation: An* occupational therapy perspective. Ottawa, Canada: Author.

Clark, F., Parham, D., Carlson, M., Frank, G., Jackson, J., Pierce, D., Wolfe, R., & Zemke, R. (1991). Occupational science: Academic innovation in the service of occupational therapy's future. *American Journal of Occupational Therapy, 45,* 300–310.

Crowe, T. K. (1993). Time use of mothers with young children: The impact of a child's disability. *Developmental Medicine and Child Neurology, 35,* 621–630.

Daly, K. (1996). *Families and time: Keeping pace in a hurried culture.* Newberry Park, CA: Sage.

DeVault, M. L. (1991). *Feeding the family: The social organization of caring as gendered work.* Chicago, IL: University of Chicago Press.

Eriksen, T. H. (2001). *Tyranny of the moment: Fast and slow time in the information age.* London (UK): Pluto Press.

Eriksen, M., & Upshur, C. C. (1989). Caretaking burden and social support: Comparison of mothers of infants with and without disabilities. *American Journal of Mental Retardation, 94,* 250–258.

Fraser, J. T. (1987). *Time the familiar stranger.* Amherst, MA: University of Massachusetts Press.

Frank, G. (1996). The concept of adaptation as a foundation for occupational science research. In R. Zemke & F. Clark (Eds.). *Occupational Science: The evolving discipline.* Philadelphia: F. A. Davis (pp. 47–55).

Gallimore, R., Weisner, T., Kauffman, S., & Bernheimer, L. P. (1989). The social construction of ecocultural niches: Family accommodation of developmentally delayed children. *American Journal on Mental Retardation, 94,* 216–230.

Glaser, B. G., & Strauss, A. L. (1967). *The discovery of grounded theory: Strategies for qualitative research.* New York: Aldine De Gruyter.

Hall, E. T. (1983). *The dance of life: The other dimension of time.* New York: Anchor Books.

Hinshaw, S.P. (1994). *Attention deficit and hyperactivity in children.* Thousand Oaks, CA: Sage.

Kantor, D., & Lehr, W. (1975). *Inside the family: Toward a theory of family process.* San Francisco, CA: Jossey-Bass.

Kreitzman, L. (1999). *The 24 hour society.* London (UK): Profile Books.

Macey, S. L. (1987). *Patriarchs of time: Dualism in Saturn-Cronus, Father Time, the Watchmaker God, and Father Christmas.* Athens, GA: The University of Georgia Press.

McMaster University Evidence-Based Practice Center (1998). *The treatment of attention-deficit/hyperactivity disorder: An evidence report (Contract 290-97-0017).* Washington, DC: Agency for Health Care Policy and Research.

The MTA Cooperative Group (1999). A 14-month randomized clinical trial of treatment strategies for attention-deficit/hyperactivity disorder. *Archives of General Psychiatry, 56,* 1073–1086.

Parsons, T. (1989/1991). A tentative outline of American values. In R. Robertson & Turner, B. S. (Eds.). (1989) *Talcott Parsons: Theorist of Modernity* (pp. 37–65). Newbury Park, CA: Sage (Reprinted from *Theory, Culture & Society, 4,* 577–512).

Pierce, D. (2001). Untangling occupation and activity. *American Journal of Occupational Therapy, 55,* 138–146.

Ruddick, S. (1995). *Maternal thinking: Toward a politics of peace.* Boston, MA: Beacon.

Schachar, R., & Tannock, R. (1993). Childhood hyperactivity and psychostimulants: A review of extended treatment studies. *Journal of Child and Adolescent Psychopharmacology, 3,* 81–97.

Segal, R. (1995). *Family adaptation to a child with attention deficit hyperactivity disorder.* Unpublished doctoral dissertation, University of Southern California, Los Angeles.

Segal, R. (1999). Doing for others Occupations within families with children with special needs. *Journal of Occupational Science, 6,* 53–60.

Segal, R. (2000). Adaptive strategies of mothers with children with ADHD: Enfolding and unfolding occupations. *American Journal of Occupational Therapy,(54),* 300–306.

Segal, R. (2001). From a personal interest to a research program. In JV. Cook (Ed.). *Qualitative research in occupational therapy (Chapter 9)* (pp. 122–131). Albany, NY: Delmar.

Segal, R., & Frank, G. (1998). The extraordinary construction of ordinary experience: Scheduling daily life in families with children with attention deficit hyperactivity disorder. *Scandinavian Journal of Occupational Therapy, 5,* 141–147.

Seligman, M., & Darling, R. B. (1997). *Ordinary families, special children: A systems approach to childhood disability* (2nd ed.). NY: Guilford Press.

Strauss, A., & Corbin, J. (1998). *Basics of qualitative research: Techniques and procedures for developing grounded theory.* Thousand Oaks, CA: Sage.

Vuchinich, S. (1987). Starting and stopping spontaneous family conflicts. *Journal of Marriage and the Family, 49,* 591–601.

Young, M. (1988). *The metronomic society.* Cambridge, MA: Harvard University Press.

Zerubavel, E. (1981). *Hidden rhythms: Schedules and calendars in social life.* Los Angeles, CA: University of California Press.

Source Credits

Family-centered Care, Mothers' Occupations of Caregiving and Home Therapy Programs

Gillian Brown, MSc, DipCOT, SROT

Introduction
Background to the Context of Family-centered Care
Compliance and Adherence
Parents and Professionals as Learners Together
Mothering Occupations
A Mother as Her Child's Teacher
Use of Home Space as a Performance Context
Home as a Context for Intervention: Constructing Daily Routines
Understanding Family Functioning
Working with Families from a Different Culture
Home Programs: Home Therapy Programs
Family-centered Care: Implications for Professional Practice and Possible Ways to Move Forward
Continuum of Participation
Conclusion

𝒥 *Anticipated Outcomes*

I anticipate that, after reading this chapter, readers will:

- Appreciate the interwoven threads of meaning involved in the processes of collaborative partnership with a family and their child

- Recognize the impact of intervention and use of home programs on family functioning and family occupational well-being and balance

- Link theory and practice with the principles of individualized, negotiated "home programs"

🪱 Introduction

In my first job working with children as a pediatric occupational therapist in the early years of my career, I can remember specific events that made me feel uncomfortable about what was happening. Members of the multidisciplinary team would see a child and the child's family during a morning visit to a children's center. As the morning ended, the members of the multidisciplinary team joined the family in the pediatrician's room. One by one, we would be asked to give our opinion. Finally, the pediatrician would summarize what had been said and comment on the findings, say something about what could be done, and offer various interventions. I particularly remember watching one mother's reactions to what she was hearing about her child. Her facial expression and body language revealed the pain she clearly felt as each opinion she heard confirmed her own worst fears. Although I might have spent about an hour with the child and the mother, there was little opportunity to get to know more about the family before finding myself in the meeting, responding with much trepidation to the expectation to give an opinion on the child's performance and to make recommendations. This was considered "best practice" because, as a new child development center, we did have a multidisciplinary team to offer. That was very forward looking at the time. I was very fortunate to be working alongside a number of very experienced health professionals who had been working with children and their families for some years. I soon learned how important it was to find out as much as I could about the family and their concerns for their child, and that it was unwise to make sweeping recommendations until I had a deeper understanding of a family's situation.

These experiences certainly made me feel uncomfortable, but at that time I was not fully aware of the reason why this was so. The way I worked as part of that team changed over time, as did the way the team worked. We gained insights into what was unhelpful and worked on improving our skills while thinking through both good and bad experiences.

From that center I moved on to work at a residential home and school run by a world-famous childcare organization. This setting gave me a totally different view on family life. The children that I met rarely had regular contact with their birth mother; for one reason or another, family life had broken down, leading to the child being placed in residential care. Because these children had significant physical disability, often associated with complex health needs together with sensory and learning impairments, they were in residential placements. This kind of resource is scarce, and for many children the placement meant leaving their own towns and moving hundreds of miles away from their families. About the same time, societal beliefs about the need to maintain children in their own family group were changing practice away from placement in distant institutions toward strate-

gies that supported families in being able to take care of their own children. It was envisaged that a family would be supported by resources provided by local agencies in the form of care packages for use in the family home and by providing shared care. For the children whose early years were spent in the residential school, their experience of family life came from their placement within family groups and through adult residential social care staff members taking parental roles. Close and often interdependent relationships were formed between the care staff and the child. These relationships were sustained when it was time for a young person to leave the residential care setting for life with a family through adoption, or for an alternative group home setting. As an occupational therapist I found that my role bridged the home and school aspects of the residential setting. Daily experiences extended my appreciation of the complexities of the child's day as attempts to address care and well-being, family life routines, and learning were juggled. Observing families engaged in doing this made me aware of the number of hours of "work" involved and the number of different roles undertaken by the "housemothers" and "housefathers." They supported the child throughout the day and often through the night. It was important to address the way that my suggestions or recommendations could be integrated into the child's life and the house group routines. Feedback from my working colleagues at the time certainly shaped later practice within a community children's service setting.

Other events have shaped my practice. These might be considered "critical incidents" and, if the process of identifying and analyzing such incidents had been available earlier in my career, it is clear that I may have learned more from these events. As it is, the events that arose through my contact with families that had children who had identified childhood conditions still remind me that even "best practice" at any given time will not meet the needs of each and every family.

After some years working in the community setting, I elected to enroll in a post-professional master's program in occupational therapy at a local university. The program offered many opportunities to explore aspects of clinical practice within the community setting. My master's thesis went some way to help me consider the parent as a learner and to hear mothers' perspectives about what they had found useful or unhelpful. This work has enabled me to share these insights with early career stage therapists joining the local service and with other professionals working in the local service and more widely among pediatric occupational therapists. Building on this work and keeping in touch with other research findings and published work have confirmed my belief that family-centered care is a highly complex phenomenon. Reflecting on my own experiences and my own learning, I now view current service and national-level policy developments that seek to ensure that practice and service delivery are family-centered with some caution. Although aspirations for family-centered care are central to initiatives to "modernize" childcare services, I believe that too little attention is being paid to the true nature of family-centered care and to how these aspirations will be achieved. The opportunity to contribute this chapter in this textbook provides a forum in which to share further insights into family-centered care and to attempt to pull together some pointers as to the essence of family-centered care as a context for practice. The future realities for best practice *family-centered care* are threatened by services leaping on a *common needs approach* bandwagon that will overlook the fundamental issues (Dale, 1996).

❧ Background to the Context of Family-centered Care

The expansion of practice toward family-centered care since the second half of the 1980s has been prompted by strong parent lobbying and driven by legislation in the United States (American Occupational Therapy Association 1999; Education of the Handicapped Act Amendments of 1990); the United Kingdom (Department of Health, 2000, 2001) and other countries such as Australia and Canada. Family-centered care is

an approach to health and social care that offers new ways of thinking about the relationships between families and service providers. Thinking about working with families who have a child who has an exceptionality or a special need will be the focus of the themes in this chapter.

Research has highlighted that working collaboratively with parents within a family-centered framework can be challenging because this requires a significant shift in thinking from the previously widely accepted and traditional child-focused approaches (Bailey, McWilliam, & Winton, 1992). Lawlor and Mattingly (1998) also contended that these dramatic changes pose considerable challenges to professionals trained in client-centered models of delivery in that professional understanding of family-centered care lags behind attempts to deliver effective services.

Practice that aspires to be *family centered* "is ahead of theory" (Lawlor & Mattingly, 1998, p. 266). For a family engaging with services, the interwoven occupational roles of a child's mother are now attracting attention (Esdaile, 1994; Francis-Connolly, 2000).

While developing this chapter, it was easy to identify with the complexities of becoming family centered (Lawlor & Mattingly, 1998). When one looks at the literature from the academic arena and from government policy papers, a potentially confusing array of names or terms appear. So it seems important to explore exactly what is meant by the term *family-centered care*. Being aware of the local and international context of professional practice and local health, welfare, disability, and legal systems (Hocking & Ness, 2002) may help to rationalize the terms and relate them to personal situations. Readers may be familiar with any of the following terms: family-centered care, family-centered practice, family focused care, family-friendly services, or parent empowerment. I have chosen to use the term *family-centered care* because it seems to be the one most commonly used in the United States.

The term *family-centered care* seems to be applied to a range of theoretical frameworks used in practice and research. This is problematic when trying to tease out theory-and-practice or practice-and-theory links. It is not clear what, in essence, the term means in daily practice with a family, for that particular family and for their unique child, or what the term means for the professional working with the family. The wide spectrum of meanings for the term *family-centered care* offers professionals a variety of ways in which they can consider themselves as family centered. If the term is considered a philosophy, then it becomes an overriding aspect of professional practice and is accepted as "a theory." On the other hand, if it is seen as a model of service delivery, then it has implications for everyday practice. Used as a mission/vision statement, it may provide an overall vision of how a service might be or the term may be used to imply an anticipated outcome.

In this chapter it is suggested that *family-centered care is* perceived as *a context* that professionals and a family create and evolve together. An interaction paradigm (Hanna & Rodger, 2002) may exist between a professional and parent, but the broader context of family-centered care will shape this interaction. Where a family has contact with a multidisciplinary or interdisciplinary team there can sometimes be 5, 10, 15, or even 20 people offering intervention and support. An individual professional may have evolved a collaborative working relationship with a child's mother, but this can be compromised if a cohesive approach to provide intervention and support from a team of professionals is not achieved. Even when considering family-centered care as a context, we have to acknowledge the influences of legislative frameworks that a professional is obliged to respect. Commonly held rules and laws about the centrality of a child's welfare are paramount. They define but also challenge our thinking about safe practice and family-centered care.

Lawlor and Mattingly's (1998) critique of current family-centered models highlights fundamental issues about the complexity of this construct. If these complexities are not acknowledged, family-centered care may be seen as only a supplement or an "add-on" to traditional health or social care models. These authors argue that family-centered care can-

not be achieved without fundamental changes in the practice of those who work in services for children and their families. They give the example of shifting decision-making power to the consumer (i.e., the family). This shift requires that professionals devote time to negotiating decisions with a family and therefore shift time and attention from direct "hands-on" treatment. This is a significant challenge for agencies and organizations delivering services that focus on a child's specific physical needs at the expense of other aspects of child development or the concerns of the child's family or primary caregivers.

The impact of organizational and operational structures on individual professionals' capacity to implement creative strategies to work in collaboration cannot be underestimated (Lawlor & Mattingly (1998). Challenges to these structures may be perceived as stepping outside "best practice." Traditional structures set up the profession as the authoritarian expert assuming a hierarchical position over the parent (Cunningham & Davis, 1985). This constrains negotiation around the focus and process of their contact, interaction, and intervention.

Family-centered care can be characterized by a collection of interrelated attributes required for supportive partnerships (Hanna & Rodger, 2002). These are:

- The unit of support and intervention is considered to be the family rather than the individual child.
- Parent and child diversity is celebrated and recognized.
- Services are provided in ways that are flexible and responsive to family needs, concerns, and priorities.
- Decision making occurs in a collaborative partnership between parents and professionals, reflecting family rather than professional goals.
- Services are expected to incorporate practices that strengthen family systems and encourage use of wider community resources.

Therefore, as we see a shift in emphasis from the child to the family with a child, the demands placed on a child's parent(s) are extended. Most importantly, the level of demands on the child's mother increase because she has to extend caregiving roles. Support for the parental role(s) among other occupational roles, especially mothering, enhances family-centered care. The discussion about family-centered care also extends to the arena of care of older adults (Hasselkus 1991). For particular families, there may be family members at all life cycle stages when their care has an impact on family occupations and the occupations of individual family members as they incorporate extended roles into their lives.

For many families, a child's mother holds the role of primary caregiver for her child and the responsibility for day-to-day care. It is the child's mother who feeds, washes, clothes, and ensures the physical and emotional well-being of her child. Family structures and care arrangements for a child will be individual to a family's situation at any given time. For example, a biological mother may not always hold the maternal parenting role, and a close family member such as a grandmother may be a child's primary carer. Given that best practice within child and family services holds the ideal of individualizing intervention, the term mother, parent, child, and family will be used in the singular form where appropriate in preference to referring to mothers, parents, families, and children. Practice changes toward family-centered care have been guided by the development of family-centered care models, which support collaboration between professionals and parents. The work of Schaaf and Mulrooney (1989) is an example. Using an integrated, family-oriented model, they demonstrated effects that enhance a child's ability to interact competently in his or her environment. Models such as Schaaf and Mulrooney's are in contrast to the earlier practice that focused on compliance with medical expertise.

Compliance and Adherence

These concepts are associated with the medical model of practice that perceived the parent as a passive receiver of advice. These terms are out of place in the context of family-centered care and within professionals' growing appreciation of the impact of parental rights and well as the impact of evolving Human Rights Legislation (e.g., Her Majesty's Stationary Office, 1998). Collaborative partnership and negotiation do not sit comfortably with compliance. Professionals will be expected to justify their recommendations and balance ethical and moral reasoning to provide a child's family with every opportunity to learn about their child and to learn about how to help their child. Developments in favor of family-centered care will need to establish new ways of identifying when it appears that a parent is seen as not carrying out recommendations made about the care of a child. Family-centered care demands that new understandings are sought about the nature and consequences of apparent breakdown in collaboration or where there are specific concerns about a parent's care of a child.

Changing Appreciation of the Role of the Parent

The importance of including a child's mother and father in intervention for a child is not new in occupational therapy or other fields of practice. Over 30 years ago, Bobath and Finnie (1970), both physiotherapists working in the United Kingdom, stated, "the cooperation of parents plays an important part in the treatment and management of children with cerebral palsy"(p. 629). Aiming to improve "co-operation," they investigated problems of communication between parents and staff. Although it is recognized that they were working at a time when the medical expert model was widely adopted, their findings confirmed the need for clear communication, taking care when making choices about treatment use, giving of information, and treatment recommendations in order to ensure that these aspects of treatment are linked to the everyday activities of the family. Approaches related to how a child's mother and/or father are "included" in intervention have changed over time. Different terms have been used to describe the level of collaboration perceived and terms such as "included," "involved," and "working with" are in use. This is another area of confusion. Opinions differ regarding what is meant by "a parent is in-

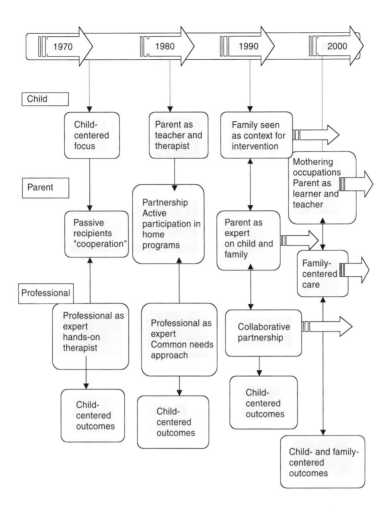

Figure 17–1 *Historical perspectives—influences on parent professional relationship.*

cluded" or "a parent is involved" or what we mean by "working with a family" in considering partnership, participation, and collaboration. The changes in the role of the parent and that of the professional are illustrated in Figure 17–1. Professionals' own perceptions of their roles in helping a mother help her child have also changed over time. Rethinking therapy and shifting to new roles (Snow, 2001) has provided opportunities to evolve collaborative partnerships.

Bazyk (1989) explored the changing attitudes and beliefs regarding parental participation in home programs. She identified three key shifts in attitudes and beliefs, beginning with the medical model, moving on to parents as teachers and therapists, and ultimately to family-centered parent participation. The growth in the use of home therapy programs signifies the time when professionals perceived parents as teachers and therapists. Home therapy programs were prescribed and designed to be carried out by a parent, usually a mother, within the family home. Since the early 1990s, the idea of parent participation has extended toward partnership, collaboration, and collaborative partnership. The more recent focus on mothering as an ongoing occupation (Francis-Connolly, 1998) further challenges our appreciation of the role of a child's mother, in relation to family-centered intervention strategies, that involve additional caregiving tasks such as home therapy programs.

Parent-therapist collaboration has been viewed as one key aspect of family-centered care (Hanna & Rodger, 2002). Humphry and Case-Smith (1996) defined collaboration as "working together towards a common goal" (p. 86). Case-Smith (1998) raised two key points about promoting partnerships and collaboration. First, partnerships are developed and grow over time. This confirms that partnership does not simply happen as soon as the first contact between a mother and a professional takes place. The early stages of contact with a family will involve the incorporation of different approaches at different stages and the negotiation and exchange of information to allow this working partnership to evolve. Case-Smith illustrated this by highlighting the shift in role for a professional from providing advice and recommendation to that of facilitating the mother's own problem solving. Second, a number of factors can influence a partnership. These factors can include past experiences of contacts with professionals, cultural values, and personalities. Case-Smith stated that "collaboration is a skill" (p. 16), and went on to discuss the developmental process of "finding a professional balance between promoting competence and independence in families and providing expertise and emotional support" (p. 16). She acknowledged the link between developing a partnership with a family and achieving a balance between being a source of technical expertise and a source of emotional support. If we accept the complexity of this process, we also need to acknowledge the complex mix of skills and knowledge required to practice in this way. This also prompts a question about how far this "working together" or "collaboration" can extend. If the professional and the parent are working together, it would seem that there is a level of cooperation and partnership. Hanna and Rodger (2002) commented on the lack of clarity from the literature as to whether parents and therapists enter such a relationship on an equal basis. Perhaps this is because the nature of the collaborative relationship is unique to the people involved and to the family's circumstances, and it is therefore inappropriate to draw similarities or to make comparisons. It is the quality of the relationships between professionals and a family that is pivotal in delivering effective family-centered services (McWilliam, Tocci, & Harbin, 1998). From a mother's point of view, "the goal of a relationship with a professional is to help her child" (Snow, 2001, p. 268).

The attitudes and values of parents and professionals working in partnership have been explored by several authors (Humphry & Thigpen-Beck, 1998; Hinojosa, Sproat, Mankhetwit, & Anderson, 2002). Values and attitudes about parenting differ between parents and professionals. Bailey (1987) postulated the factors that may account for the differences in parent and professional priorities and how these factors can affect parental motivation when parents do not see the relevance of recommended activities. These factors include lack of time, resources, energy, or skill to follow through programs or recommendations for a family, but also extend to the professional having limited insight into family needs and priorities, together with limited ability to motivate and challenge parents. Bailey went on to report that differences and most conflicts involve multiple components, especially in these two aspects: goals of intervention and the methods by which these goals are to be achieved. These differences may be fueled by disagreement over either priorities for intervention or values related to intervention. The most difficult types of conflict to resolve arise from value conflicts, and if these are not resolved, the efficacy of intervention will be affected.

Values in the context of family therapy include "the social standards by which therapists define problems, establish criteria for evaluation, fix parameters for technical interventions, and select therapeutic goals" (Aponte, 1985, p. 323). Whether moral, cultural, or political, these standards affect the evolving value systems of the therapist and the family.

The factors that contribute to these differences include the following:

- Personal experiences of parenting
- The extent of experience working with families and young children
- The priority placed on independence and self-respect or developmental outcomes
- Beliefs about conformity and potential for a child's success

Family-related factors can inform practice where strategies to bring about changes in a child's behavior might be negotiated. A mother's expectations for her child to cooperate and participate in activities might be unrealistic. But professionals' expectations may also be unrealistic. These findings are supported by those of Mattingly and Fleming (1994) that a professional socialization process occurs over time rather than a priority developed before entering practice. Less experienced "therapists" focus on developmental outcomes over independence and self-respect. This finding was also supported by reports of the participants in a study that examined how therapists make a difference in parent-child relationships (Mayer, White, Ward, & Barnaby, 2002). However, it was suggested that this change over time arose from a willingness to be open to change and to learn from their experiences.

New insights were gained about the difficulties faced by professionals when working with families in a recent study that replicated earlier work (Hinojosa, Sproat, Mankhetwit, & Anderson, 2002). Professionals now recognized that there are multiple stressors present in a family, not directly related to the intervention for the child, but having significant impacts on the child. Providing help for parents regarding resources, knowledge, and support was seen as an extended role for the professional and served to empower the parents in meeting their child's and family's needs. Family-centered care had recognized the family's needs, in contrast to focusing on the child's needs alone. These factors are pertinent when a therapist and a parent of a child with a disability are trying to establish a working relationship. Misunderstandings may prevent sharing of beliefs about parenting and may lead to conflict situations about how best to help a child. It is the understanding of these values and that conflicts will always exist that supports collaborative goal setting through recognizing and respecting what is seen as strength, a need, or a problem.

The stage of problem setting has received little attention because the recognition that collaboration between professionals and parents has to be established over time is recent. It begins with agreeing what the concerns

about a child are and whether these concerns require attention (Lawlor & Mattingly, 1998). Establishing collaborative practice remains a challenge for professionals, who also need to consider the consequences of not achieving collaborative goal setting. Parents report feeling pressured to engage in activities even when they do not believe these to be important. Extracts from the mother's stories present some of these issues (Brown 1996; Brown, 1997). Lucy and Clare both have sons who have cerebral palsy.

Vignette: *Lucy and Clare*

Lucy recalled how she had struggled to understand why she had been told that her son needed therapy input. It took her a long time to understand fully what cerebral palsy involved and what the implications and outcome might entail. Only when she was able to accept this was she really able to accept the need for the therapist's input.

Clare gave an example of being advised that her daughter should never sit between her knees in a particular way (i.e., sitting with her buttocks on the floor, her hips internally rotated and legs externally rotated at the knees, like a W shape), but she felt that she never really understood why she was told this. It was an achievement in her own yoga class to be able to sit like that. Clare needed to know the reason why her daughter should not sit in a particular way and what the significance and consequences of this might be.

Shared decision making in program planning, service delivery, and evaluation is believed to result in more relevant and meaningful outcomes to both the child and the family (Bazyk, 1989; Wallen and Doyle, 1996). This might be extended not only to include the involvement of families as stakeholders in program design and delivery, but also to ensure that the parents of a child are also an intrinsic part of discovering and establishing the nature, the extent, and the possible consequences of what it is that is different about their child. Gaining a diagnosis is tradionally seen as the domain or role of the medical expert pediatricians, or specialists in childhood illnesses or medical conditions. Giving a professional assessment of a specific area of concern (e.g. speech delay, sensory processing, motor skill acquisition) has often followed. For parents, this is only part of their need for information. There is also a need for a shared understanding of what this means in the first weeks and months for their child and their family and then also what this will mean for the future. So this shared understanding will most effectively be evolved if parents are supported and enabled to see their own knowledge and experiences about the child as an essential part of this process of discovery. Parents will expect respect and constructive use of contributions of knowledge and understanding of the child that they bring to the professionals.

Schön's work from the field of adult learning gives us the term "problem setting" as a precursor to problem solving (1983). Goal-setting stages adopted in the field of education and early intervention can be said to follow from the problem setting stages when the parent and professional have reached a shared understanding through naming and framing the "problems."

> The use of language around these stages of problem setting and problem solving deserves some thought as we consider the impact on a parent and on a child. Thinking from the perspective of the social disability model a child does not have problem. It is society and the environment that disables a child. There are issues about the nature of problems that encompass identifying where the problem is sited and the exclusive impact activated from a single individual's perspective. (Snow, 2001)

Parents and Professionals as Learners Together

Partnerships are based on a premise that two heads are better than one. However, sharing the knowledge that each person has is not an easy thing to do. McConkey (1985, p. 42) cites Newson (1976):

> We should start from the basic assumption that parents in fact have information to impart; that parents are experts on

their own children. This is not to say that they know of their own children in any systematic or integrated form; one cannot ask a parent to bring along an ordered case history... Nonetheless, they know more about the child, on a very intimate level, than anyone else does; the fact that their knowledge may be diffuse and unstructured does not matter, so long as it is available. It is the professional's job to make it available; structuring can come later (p. 105).

Hanna and Rodger's (2002) exploration of the literature on how to incorporate the parent's perspectives into practice revealed the emergent use of a narrative approach or parent story telling. This approach has been used as an ongoing process of parent-therapist collaboration (Burke & Schaaf, 1997). It echoes Newson's (1976) premise cited previously. Further evaluation to determine how professionals can provide narrative frameworks to support a child's family in giving information seems indicated. Ryan and McKay (1999) discussed ways in which this approach can be implemented in practice.

The issue of a parent and a professional learning together is a contentious one (Lyons, 1994: Humphry and Case-Smith, 1996). The debate is complicated by the question, who is the client within "children's services?" Is the child the client? Is the parent the client? Authors have explored how the sense of "patient" and also "client" has evolved (Sumsion, 1999; Schultz-Krohn & Cara, 2000). When we consider family-centered care, this debate has to be extended to include who is being referred and hence who is the patient or client. Professionals respecting the legal context of their work will seek parental permission to have contact and to engage in a "therapeutic relationship" with a child. When one is working in a family-centered way, the nature of the relationship with the child may be direct engagement, or it may be indirect by enabling, for example, a mother to help and teach her child. It may be family focused, when the parent and child are the clients and intervention is not restricted to child-related outcomes (Schultz-Krohn & Cara, 2000).

The factors that motivate the professional

on entering the parent-professional relationship are also important. Traditionally, therapists have adopted a position of child advocacy and commitment to the child's needs (Anderson & Hinojosa, 1984). However, this viewpoint can restrict a therapist's capacity to acknowledge a parent as an expert about her child. There are risks associated with trying to achieve partnership in learning about a child and demonstrating professional knowledge and professional expertise. Although intended to be helpful, the importance of consulting with parents and recognizing their expertise can be overlooked (Peterson & Cooper, 1989).

Professionals working in multidisciplinary or interdisciplinary teams have to be aware of how the different professional background of their colleagues will affect the type of family-centered roles that they can play. It is wise to acknowledge where confusion about these differences can generate real difficulties for a child's family. Parents and professionals need each other's skills and knowledge (Lyons 1994) if an equal collaborative working partnership is to evolve. Featherstone (1980) asked that professionals recognize their own needs. This may include the amount of time available to talk about a child with a mother before another commitment or the impact of personal reactions on discovering some information about a child's health or perhaps the child's future having consequences for the way that they share the information with a child's family. These are challenges for family-centered professionals.

Many of the ideals of family-centered care focus on the development of parental understanding of the child's needs and supporting a parent in meeting those needs. Having acknowledged that a child's mother is the person who cares for her child requires that professionals understand how to support a mother in the parental roles of learner and teacher along with the other roles a mother fulfills.

Mothers' experience of learning about their child was the subject of my research (Brown, 1996; Brown, 1997), in which I used a phenomenological methodology to explore the experiences of five mothers who had a child with cerebral palsy. The key findings of

this study that inform practice highlighted the need to:

- Consider the effects of all events associated with a mother learning about her child because both the mother and her child may perceive these experiences as intrusive, frightening, or painful
- Consider the issue of timing of professional contact and information giving
- Be aware of how a professional's attitude and approach can block or enhance a parent's learning
- Make information and explanations available and meaningful for a mother
- Find ways to enable a mother to learn more about the future for her child and about herself
- Consider a mother's learning needs in relation to enabling her to be competent in her mothering

The fact that timing of information giving was one of the key findings is important because this adds to our understanding of the need to allow flexibility in service provision and for professionals to be aware of a mother's readiness to raise, discuss, or address issues. The study also highlighted that further research into the impact of individual reactions of a mother to her learning about her child's special problems and needs was indicated.

Mothering Occupations

Mothering of a young child is an intense occupation, an enfolded activity with multiple tasks requiring attention simultaneously (Bateson, 1996). A mother of a young child enfolds nurturing, teaching, and daily care tasks in her mothering of her child. The activities involved in mothering change as the child matures, but the mother remains invested in her child's life (Francis-Connolly, 1998). The occupations of mothering contribute to maternal health and are essential to child development (Olson & Esdaile, 2000). Teaching is central to mothering and is enmeshed in the daily routines and the enfolded tasks of feeding; changing diapers, bathing, skin care, and dressing. When there is a child with a disability within the family, mothering will also involve the tasks of learning how to meet that child's exceptional needs. Significantly, mothering will be about preserving or maintaining the life of the child (Ruddick, 1989) and all that this involves. Ruddick's concept of maternal practice includes the preservation of the child, fostering the child's growth and teaching, and molding the child within cultural, societal, and fashion norms. Recognizing and respecting these aspects of maternal practice frames the intervention process. Working toward achieving a truly collaborative partnership with a mother requires a strong foundation of knowledge and sensitivity about a mother's unique perspectives about her child and her family. This is especially so when these perspectives differ from those of other family members and those of professionals.

As an occupation, parenting is simultaneously an "intensely personal and a commonly shared experience" (Llewellyn, 1994, p. 173). Hanna and Roger (2002) held the view that "too often occupational therapists have only considered the *common experience* of parenting and have ignored the personal and individual dimensions" (p. 16). Societal changes have shifted research focus to parenthood and to mothering (e.g. Francis-Connolly, 2000; Lawlor & Mattingly, 1998; Larson, 2000). Through gaining an understanding of mothering occupations, parental perspectives about parenting, the impact of intervention on the parenting process (Hinojosa 1990, Hinojosa & Anderson 1991; Hinojosa et al., 2002; Llewellyn 1994), and about mothers' experience of learning about their child (Brown 1996; Brown, 1997), new understandings have emerged.

Mothering occupations embrace the orchestration of family activities and participation in household chores and in the play of their children. This might include work and play occupations such as preparing meals, housecleaning, car washing, mowing the lawn, reading with the children, watching television, or being a "taxi driver" to access out-of-school activities such as piano lessons. Understanding the impact of interventions such as therapy on the occupations associated with family life has received more attention from researchers recently. The findings suggest that therapists have not always considered this is-

sue (Kellegrew, 2000; Olson & Esdaile, 2000).

Concepts such as mothering occupations, the orchestration of family activity, and the parenting role as an occupation are derived from the field of occupational science (Primeau, Clark, & Pierce, 1989). Occupational science involves the study of a person as an occupational being and addresses the nature of occupation, which encompasses work, play, leisure, self maintenance, and sleep, together with the processes involved in orchestrating daily activities, in order to remain healthy, achieve the necessities of life, and obtain satisfaction (Yerxa, Clarke, Jackson, Pierce, & Zemke, 1990). Mothers' use of time is another example of recent research predicated on occupational science theory. When a mother needs to manage many different activities during the day, the time use strategies of mothers include three adaptive approaches (Segal, 2000). These are enfolding occupations (performing more than one task at a time); unfolding occupations by changing the time sequence; and unfolding occupations by having some one else perform certain occupations.

Expectations placed on mothers to implement a home program add demands within the mothering role, requiring the mothers to make changes in the way they orchestrate family life and to balance the variety of competing demands in their daily lives (Llewellyn, 1994). Thompson (1998) supports the need to recognize that parents make considerable adjustments to accommodate services and that mothers in her study also felt that therapists failed to consider other demands or roles that were not directly related to the provision of direct therapy. This would include considering the impact on a mother herself, the siblings, and other family members. *Occupational scaffolding* was the subject of another study investigating orchestration of work and play within families. The study identified the process of occupational scaffolding, through which mothers may foster their preschool child's competence as adults (Primeau, 1998).

A Mother as Her Child's Teacher

As parents are present in their child's life at the most teachable moments (McConkey, 1985), parents, especially mothers, who are known to spend more time with their young children than fathers, are pivotal in a child's everyday learning of everyday skills. The child's mother is the key person who determines the opportunities available, what stimulation and nurturance the child receives, and also the physical, emotional, social, and nutritional care received. The fact that some mothers are not able to do this supports the need to recognize each individual family's need for help and support.

As a teacher, each mother will have her own teaching style, and therefore mothers should not be expected to teach in the same way as the professional (McConkey, 1985). Professional intervention that focuses on helping a mother extend her ability to help her child learn may enhance her mothering roles. McConkey offered four areas in which a mother can be helped to extend her skills to fulfill her mothering roles. These include selecting precise learning objectives, suggestions for possible teaching contexts, acquiring more techniques to aid a child's learning, and adapting a mother's teaching in the light of a child's learning. Further information about this is given in the section on implications for practice.

🐾 Use of Home Space as a Performance Context

Living in a home creates its unique occupations. Availability of space and beliefs and choices about space use vary between individuals and between families. A glance at a row of houses or a block of apartment houses will demonstrate how each separate dwelling has been transformed into a home. There will be the material, tangible items like blinds or curtains, but there will also be psychological or sociological indicators about the nature and meaning of the home for the occupants. Steward (2000) stated that "the home is not a neutral space" (p. 105), and she proposed that that therapists include a sociological perspective in their work. This perspective can contribute to a deepening understanding of this aspect of family life as the incorporation of new roles and daily activities into the home is negotiated or the therapist is involved in work-

ing on or in the home. Steward highlighted that evidence drawn from the literature about the experiences of "teleworkers" gives useful insights into the meaning of home space. Teleworkers carry out their occupations from their home, using the telephone, and have their office within their home. Steward's findings suggest that households wish to retain the conventional look, feel, and function of the home even when occupants are required to establish new roles and occupations. Professionals may be involved in helping a family look at how they use their home as they orchestrate family activity to incorporate additional roles and activities associated with the care of a child with special needs. Whether negotiating goals, introducing an item of equipment for therapy or management, or helping a family redesign their home to support the day-to-day care of a child, there are many sensitive factors to be considered. The home is the context in which the child and family create and orchestrate their occupations.

Home as a Context for Intervention: Constructing Daily Routines

Adding to Hinojosa and Anderson's (1991) findings about the need to look at the impact of therapist intervention on home life, Larson (2000) indicated that serious consideration needs to be given to how mothers construct a family's daily life if there are to be negotiations about revising these daily routines to accommodate intervention strategies. Appreciating the meanings associated with family routines will assist the professional in seeing the relevant importance of such routines. Occupational therapists have also explored the impact of a child's disability on childcare activity (Crowe, 1993; Crowe, Van Leit, Berghmans, & Mann 1997) and the role demands of caring for a young child with a disability (Crowe, Van Leit, & Bermans, 2000). For some families, these additional demands and the necessity of juggling roles can continue for many years if the child continues to need extensive help and support.

Though the construction of daily routines, a mother provides her child with many opportunities to practice daily routines that promote development. For a child with disabilities, the daily reinforcement of occupations provides a practice component that can be crucial for skill acquisition. Based on the results of a qualitative study Kellegrew (2000) advocated an ecocultural view of the family. She explored the factors that influence the ways in which mothers construct daily routines for their young children with disabilities through exploring the adaptations and adjustments made in family routines. Kellegrew stated that gaining an understanding of the ways in which families construct routines provides useful information that contributes to increased efficacy in designing and integrating intervention into the daily life of the family. Much of the literature about ecocultural theory relied on parental retrospective reports of established routines, and questions were raised as to how this approach might be used to support professionals negotiating changes to family routines. This was particularly important when the opportunities for parents to channel their child's development are sought. Adaptations to family routines might be reviewed to accommodate changes in a child's skills, for example, as a new skill emerges and as the skill develops.

The findings of this study point to the need to individualize interventions and devote time to understanding the specific ways in which a family makes and accommodates adjustments in daily routines. It will be especially important to understand the individual characteristics and cultural context of a family because these affect the activities and routines carried out in the home. For example, the routines and meanings of mealtimes, with or separate from adults, the place where they eat, the range of foods, and the tasks associated with eating them. Another daily routine that can be seen to be unique to an individual family involves self-care, including personal toilet, washing, or bathing. Misunderstandings about the processes and meanings associated with these activities are common and offer the potential mismatch of recommendations pertaining to skill development for the child. For example, before intervening with suggestions about a child's bath time, it is important to discover what is involved in the task of bathing for this child's family. Occupational therapy's

focus on these domains of activity often points to individual professionals developing sensitive and culturally appropriate ways of engaging families in exploring the practical challenges they have in their daily lives.

Kellegrew (2000) identified two processes through which mothers designed and orchestrated daily routines. These are the processes of *accommodation* and *anticipation*. Accommodation is set in the present and implies that mothers adjust and adapt to everyday challenges, most likely to changes in a child's skill level. Participants in the study were seen to use the companion process of anticipation. This process is set in future time in that mothers anticipate the future needs of their child and orchestrate a daily routine that would reinforce and develop the skills perceived by the mother as beneficial to the child's future. These processes may be connected with the maternal role of teacher discussed previously.

Occupations associated with orchestrating daily routines for a child that are interwoven and enfolded with other roles and occupations are hidden by the "merry-go-round" of family life (Widdows, 1997, p. 36) for the family who has a child who has a disability. The following vignette about a mother and her daughter illustrates the weekly merry-go-round in one family.

⌘ *Vignette:* **Mary and Aysha**

Mary and her daughter Aysha, who has special needs, have recently moved into their new home. They chose to move from a third-floor apartment with an unreliable elevator to a house on a new development. Each week brings new challenges. Aysha, now 12 years old, has attended a local mainstream school for the last 4 months. Mary has invested a great deal of time and effort in helping develop Aysha's mobility and independence skills since she was a very small baby. Now Aysha is striving for greater independence, but feels that she is still reliant on her mother's help and care. Mary wants Aysha to continue to develop her skills, but is trying to restructure their home life to allow more time for Aysha to keep up with her studies and homework. With Aysha at school for more of the day, she is trying to help her son and his family and finds that she still has little time for herself. Mary carries out most of the household tasks during the week, aiming to free up time to help Aysha do as much as possible independently by problem solving and planning ahead. She also ensures that Aysha has the time and energy to be able to do her homework as independently as possible. During most days, morning activities have to run like clockwork to ensure that Aysha is ready for school when the school bus arrives. This means that Mary has to get up and be ready to help Aysha by 6:30 AM. Some days Aysha is very stiff and it takes longer for her to carry out personal care and dressing tasks. She often needs direct assistance. After school, Aysha likes to have some time to herself to read or watch television before she is ready to join in with supper and then do her homework. At least two evenings a week and one day on the weekend, Aysha joins in with a local drama group. So mealtimes, homework, and exercises have to be juggled along with time spent with friends and family. ⌘

This vignette is one example of the impact that seemingly simple changes can have on family life. This family was asked to accommodate the arrival of the school bus 20 minutes earlier. It seemed that the students were needed in school earlier. There was no negotiation and no notice. Initially this mother elected to provide the transport herself and take her daughter to school because she felt that it was not practical to extend the day to accommodate this change. She felt that it was often necessary to accommodate the extra demands herself, so that the change did not affect her daughter. Eventually, there was some negotiation, and alternative strategies were implemented. In the end, the school decided that the students were not expected to arrive earlier on the school site after all. In reflecting about this vignette, readers may consider a similar situation within their experience.

Understanding Family Functioning

Family-centered care has its foundations in a professional's understanding of a particular family. A family systems conceptual frame-work, as presented by Turnbull and Turnbull (1990), may be a useful guide in gathering comprehensive and relevant insights into the strengths and needs of a family. It guides by focusing attention to the specific issues for a particular family. The conceptual framework comprises family characteristics, interactions, functions, and family life cycle.

Family-centered care can be most effective when productive interaction takes place between the resources of professionals and the resources of families. This framework is extensively explored and applied in practice by Turnbull and Turnbull (1990). Health-care professionals may consider the inclusion of these components of knowledge about a family to be outside the usual parameter of their practice. Social care professionals may be more comfortable with their inclusion. Family-centered care requires that professionals work together to gather this information. In the United States, the Education of the Handicapped Act Amendments of 1990 have required that the planning of early intervention include the family in the decision-making process. In the United Kingdom, there has been a move to develop a "single-assessment framework" (Department of Health, 2000), that goes some way to address the need for all professionals to understand a family's situation. Further work is under way at government level and locally in the United Kingdom to extend the use of this framework so that it is sensitive to the needs of families who have a member with a disability. It is hoped that this approach will also help agencies work together to support a family and avoid the need for a family to repeat and to share the same information several times over with different agencies or services.

Working with Families from a Different Culture

Working with a family from a culture different from that of the professional requires additional knowledge and skills. Achieving collaboration between the professional and the family may mean recognizing the importance of being sensitive to addressing cultural context (Parker, Tewfik, & Burkhardt, 2002). Paying attention to an individual family's characteristics will highlight specific differences in the meanings attached to tasks and differences in family routines. Various frameworks have been developed that can guide culturally appropriate intervention (Berlin & Fowkes, 1983; Kleineman, 1980). Family routines that may be influenced by a family's culture exist around tasks such as mealtime and personal care. Family beliefs about childrearing, health care, and disability may be shaped by cultural influences. Beliefs about play and other childhood occupations will influence a family's way of orchestrating a child's day and management of a child's behavior. Developing cross-cultural competence and understanding cultural norms and influences within a family may assist in developing shared understandings about a child. Recognizing mismatches between a professional's personal cultural context and beliefs and a child and its family's cultural contexts (Parker, Tewfik, & Burkhardt, 2002) supports individualized problem setting and problem solving, goal setting, and the choice of intervention media. Knowledge of a family's customs and practices leads to adaptation of the intervention process so that the family can understand and implement recommendations and suggestions (Turnbull & Turnbull 1990; Case-Smith, 1998). Communication between a family and a professional when the family home language differs from that of the service provider or immediate community offers many challenges. Effective cross-cultural communication may require careful consideration of the sensitive and appropriate use of strategies such as interpreters, elders, or local advocates. Thinking about the way information is passed on when using, for example, an interpreter is important, particularly when direct translation is used (Cheung, Shah, & Muncer, 2002). The aim of negotiating the use of such strategies would be to ensure that explanations given and information shared does help a family rather than adding confusion.

I have found it helpful to use a sentence that I developed as a memory jogger to recognize and remember the interrelated aspects of family functioning that include the cultural context, and the fact that things can and do change: *"Family-centered care is about this child, in this family; in this home, in this street, in this neighborhood, in this town, in this region, in this country TODAY."*

Home Programs: Home Therapy Programs

A home program is not readily reduced to a definition. There appear to be many misconceptions about the nature and the outcome of home programs. Perhaps this is because there are implicit complexities in the purpose, use, and delivery of home programs. Have home programs been seen as "a sole intervention or adjunct to regular therapy"? (Hamill, 1987, p.51). Do home programs reflect sophisticated appreciation of all that comprises home-situated family-centered care? Do they contain recommendations, strategies, and selected techniques that are geared to the hopes, wishes, or aspirations of an individual family? How have recommendations for activities been developed? Perhaps the important issues arise from the way that knowledge and expertise are shared, as discussed when considering mothers and professionals learning together. What can be helpful? When it is unhelpful? How can a mother be helped to learn how to help her child?

Case-Smith (1998) gave an extensive list of characteristics of successful home programs (p. 88), together with an overview of the typical problems and potential solutions across the areas of performance components (sensory modulation and motor delays) and performance areas (play, feeding, sleeping, dressing, and bathing). This gives useful information about considering the focus, the process involved, and the impact on the family. This work informs the later section on implications for professional practice.

Hamill (1987) recognized the link between mother-child interaction and the effectiveness of traditional home programs. Earlier, Bromwich (1981) used a hierarchical five-stage model of a mother's responsiveness to her child to develop mothers' capacities to carry out home programs. The model explores whether the mother notices what her child does and what the child responds to, and where and when the mother intervenes and modifies her own behavior to bring about changes in her child. Other, more recent parent-child interaction scales examine similar mother-child related factors (e.g., Case-Smith, 1998), although observer reliability is variable. Understanding parent-child interaction, especially mother-child interaction and a mother's capacity to teach her child and to orchestrate activities to help him or her develop skills seems supportive of working in a family-centered way. Mothers "are able to interpret and understand their child's cues and behavioral responses in order to conduct an effective and therapeutic home program activity and to give appropriate feedback on the effectiveness of these activities to the therapist"(Hamill, 1987, pp. 49-50). Importantly, we may now recognize this as actively supporting effective mothering.

Various studies have explored treatment outcomes and roles of professionals working with families (Peterson & Cooper, 1989), the relationships between parents and occupational therapists (Hinojosa, Anderson, & Ranum, 1988; MacClean & Chesson, 1991; Hinojosa, Sproat, Mankhetwit, & Anderson, 2002; Mayer, White, Ward, & Barnaby, 2002); outcomes of intervention (e.g., Mayo, 1981), and parental perceptions of intervention (Hinojosa, 1990; Hinojosa, et al., 2002; Case-Smith & Nastro, 1993, Thompson, 1998). Much of the literature exploring home programs comes from the practice arena of early intervention because many of these programs used a "home program" mode of service delivery. There are methodological concerns around the impact of the implementation of family-centered care over time. Comparative analyses of studies pre-implementation with more recent studies may be unreliable. However, it is helpful to gather insights from the literature in order to prompt questions about current practice.

Early intervention programs were originally designed to take constructive action before a child's problems reached a point where development and learning were seriously compromised (Peterson & Cooper, 1989). The aim was to provide early help in anticipation of the support parents would need and the training their young child would require when a condition is present that is known to interfere with normal development. Early intervention was founded on the recognition that "a primary place for learning is in the home and that parents are responsible for teaching their children many skills that are important for normal development" (Hamill, 1987). The mother has been seen as the primary caregiver, the main constant in the child's life when there are disabilities or special health needs (Leff &Walizer, 1992).

A series of qualitative studies explored how mothers of preschool children with cerebral palsy perceived occupational and physical therapists and their influence on family life and family members (Hinojosa, 1990; Hinojosa & Anderson, 1991). Mothers reported that because of the nature of the daily-care required by their children with cerebral palsy, they did not have the time, energy, or confidence to implement a therapist-directed home program. They did, however, incorporate previously learned treatment strategies into daily interactions with their children. Mother-directed rather than therapist-directed programs were advocated. When these authors replicated their study recently (Hinojosa et al., 2002), they found that professionals are now more aware of the multiple stressors present in a family, not directly related to the direct intervention for the child, but having significant impacts on the child.

Others, for example Case-Smith and Nastro (1993), looked at the effect of occupational therapy on five mothers of children with cerebral palsy. One theme of the findings illustrated the mothers' attitudes toward home programs in which they described their own intensive work with their children when they were infants. As their children reached preschool age, they discontinued their home program routines. None of the participant mothers reported that they felt that therapists had insisted that they carry over the therapeutic regime in their home. They reported that their desire to do so arose from their own need to help their child. The mothers reported that they did not feel that the therapist disapproved of their change in attitude as their child grew older.

Although there seem to be many reasons why professionals seek parental participation, little evidence supports the intuitive acceptance that parental involvement is critically important for successful child-focused outcomes (Parette & Hourcade, 1985; Shonkoff & Hauser-Cram, 1987; White & Castro, 1985). The impact on family interaction patterns of the additional demands on parents arising from their participation in early intervention programs has been questioned (Parette & Hourcade, 1985).

Recollections of five adults with cerebral palsy in a qualitative study (Kibele, 1989) referred to the impact of home therapy programs on mother-child relationships, highlighting the fact that home exercise programs, along with school homework, affected the time available for other activities such as leisure. The life experiences of many families tell a disturbing story about therapy (Featherstone, 1980; Turnbull & Turbull, 1985; Snow, 2001; Britton & Moore, 2002). Recognizing the role strain or burden that may result from requests to mothers to take on additional caregiving tasks such as home therapy programs (Crowe, Van Leit, & Berghmans, 2000) may create support for family-centered working.

This is especially important when many different professionals are making recommendations and giving advice. A family will struggle to make sense of multiple and overlapping interventions, particularly when family routines and occupations are disrupted by the amount of time required to follow recommendations. Contradictory or confusing messages and information will add to the load on a family. Mothers have been considered to be "culture brokers" (Lawlor & Mattingly, 1998, p. 265), in which the role involves bridging the world of the professionals and that of the family. Unfortunately, this often involves sharing both good and bad news arising from the contact of professionals with the family. Effective interdisciplinary working may offer negotiated solutions and avoid overloading a family with unrealistic expectations.

In a review of the literature, the following themes about the professional's role in early intervention home programs emerge:

- Ongoing assistance and education for parents
- Supporting a parent in providing optimal care and stimulation for the child
- Discussing attitudes and feelings with the professional to help the mother achieve positive mother/child interaction
- Enabling parents to learn skills they need for teaching and managing their child
- Helping a mother learn how to set appropriate expectations for her child in the home setting
- Helping parents to nurture and deal constructively with the child as he or she grows and moves into each new developmental stage
- Providing opportunities to share ideas and to learn how and when to intervene through observing their child's reactions to help develop a better understanding of the child
- Offering more than a diagnosis or a label for explaining disorders in young children
- Focusing on helping the child to progress in preparation for the stage of preschool or kindergarten by addressing delays in acquiring critical skills
- Preparing parents to take on new roles and responsibilities as caregivers and teachers in addition to the usual roles
- Creating a home environment where the child feels secure, content, and able to organize himself or herself to develop his or her own role in the family and participate in family life
- Helping the family become and remain a stable, happy, and functional unit
- Supporting the family in integrating the child into the family systems while addressing the child's needs as constructively as possible within family routines

Much of the focus of these professional roles is related to supporting mothering occupations, which include a mother learning about her child and also about a mother teaching her child. Expectations about a mother's capacity to participate in any aspect of her child's intervention are shaped by the mother's readiness to do so and the child's needs (Hamill, 1987).

❧ Family-centered Care: Implications for Professional Practice and Possible Ways to Move Forward

Creating the context of family-centered care requires attention to all elements of professional contact to ensure that all aspects of care are truly family centered. Being responsive to the needs of an individual family requires attention to their hopes, needs, wishes, and aspirations.

Continuum of Participation

At some events in a child's life, at some life cycle stages, or at some family events or life stages, family members may need the freedom to elect to change the way that they manage their lives and the ways in which they care for their child. There may be risks that "best practice" becomes complacent and is constrained by a common-needs approach, thus missing the intent to "individualize" intervention. Authors such as Hamill (1987) and Case-Smith (2001) have alluded to the parents' readiness to participate in their child's care. Recognizing that this readiness may be associated with parental capacity to participate may ensure that parental skills and knowledge, as well as the timing of intervention, are attended to appropriately. Of equal importance is the professional's understanding of parents' reaction(s) to learning about their child (Brown, 1996; Brown, 1997) and caring for their child. Concepts of denial, adjustment, coping, and chronic sorrow have all received attention in the literature. As further exploration of these issues is outside the scope of this chapter, links to relevant material are given in the section on additional reading. All these factors prompt professionals to be aware of a family's need for choice and flexibility in how they can best operate at any one time. For the professional and for service managers, there is also the need to be clear about the approach and the skills and knowledge required to offer appropriate support at appropriate times through integrated and flexible packages of care that can be realistically delivered.

Brown, Humphry, and Taylor (1997) recog-

nized a continuum of involvement and presented a seven-level hierarchy of family therapist involvement. This hierarchy was developed to support educators in preparing entry-level professionals to be prepared for family-centered intervention in recognition that the family plays an important role in rehabilitation of persons with chronic disabilities. Although not originally developed for practice with families and children, it is fundamentally appropriate and gives information about the differences in attitudes and beliefs and skills and knowledge required by the therapist to support a family at each level of family role. When working with a child and his or her family, family-centered care is seen as encompassing all levels of family functioning.

The continuum of involvement has contributed a succinct description of the focus of interaction, the attitude and beliefs supporting this way of thinking, and the knowledge and skills required.

It seems helpful to see *family-centered care* as a "continuum of participation" with mother - professional collaboration being pivotal. This continuum of participation encompasses the following: a child is "looked after" or "in care"; responsibility for the care of a child rests with a statutory agency or their representative; a child's mother may or may not have contact as as informant, assistant, coworker, partner, collaborative partner, or director of services.

Table 17–1 describes a continuum of participation based on the work of Brown, Humphry, and Taylor (1997). This has been evolved to attempt to incorporate insights from the literature and reflects experiences from practice from the author. Each level is not seen as exclusive, and levels are offered only as a guide to prompt professionals' thinking when developing a working relationship with a family. It is anticipated that levels will merge. It is also envisaged that a family would be seen to adopt a point on the continuum that would reflect their overall sense of well-being. As life cycle events occur, and as reactions to events, new understandings or realities are realized, a family may be seen to change the way in which they operate. For example, a mother struggling to juggle the many occupational roles that she performs will, at different times, operate at different points along the continuum. When parents are seen as passive receivers and observers, they are likely to become dependent and to release responsibilities. This may lead to feelings of frustration, incompetence, isolation, and failure.

Table 17–1 Continuum of participation				
	Family role in care of the child	Working toward collaboration	Practitioner's attitudes and beliefs	Skills and knowledge areas desirable to support family-centered care
Continuum of Participation	Child is "looked after" or "in care" Parental responsibility released to agency Fostering arrangements may be in place	Interdisciplinary decisions made about the current and future roles of the birth mother and the extent of her participation	Child's welfare is paramount Effective interagency working arrangements are essential Foster parents are pivotal	Child care and protection legislation Working with foster parents, prospective adoptive parents, and professional carers
	Family as informant	Family contributes information and practitioner leads Practitioner may lead on direct hands-on intervention or seek to arrange resources to support this	Practitioner recognizes family has useful information Works to identify parents' readiness and parenting skills	Readiness Parenting including parent-child interaction Listening and interview skills Family functioning Knowledge of local services
	Family as assistant	Practitioner learns about the family and the child Provides information Makes recommendations about key interventions so that family can carry this through at home	Practitioner takes lead role about what to do and how to do it, through negotiation Family circumstances do not support greater participation	About learning Teaching skills Recognize learning styles of others Communication skills Family functioning Knowledge of local services
	Family as co-worker	Practitioner learns more about the resources available to the family Supports family role in intervention but works to ensure family stability Intervention strategies adjusted to respond to family members needs Monitors impact on family Empathic understanding	Family need support to balance and orchestrate their lives if they are to incorporate interventions into their daily routines	Mothering occupations Family occupations Empathic interpersonal skills Family functioning Knowledge of local services

Table 17–1 Continuum of participation

	Family role in care of the child	Working toward collaboration	Practitioner's attitudes and beliefs	Skills and knowledge areas desirable to support family-centered care
Continuum of Participation	Family as partner	Goal setting and selection of intervention strategies negotiated Goal setting may be supported by problem setting stage over time	Recognizes interaction between family members as it affects the child Family has information about what might work and what will most interest the child	Negotiating skills Family functioning Knowledge of local services
	Family as collaborative partner in team	Problem setting, goal setting, and intervention strategies developed and reviewed collaboratively Supports development of autonomy versus dependence	Recognizes and optimizes parental role from early stages of contact	Negotiating skills Collaboration skills Family functioning Knowledge of local services
	Family as director of service	Consultation and indirect and direct intervention will be negotiated by the family Focus of intervention may not be the child May be in selected contexts that vary over time	Flexible and open to requests for support as appropriate	Negotiating skills Family functioning Knowledge of local services

The most challenging aspect of family-centered care is the development of a collaborative partnership with a parent. Key issues explored and possible answers, listed below, were developed from my practice (Brown, 1996; 1997) with reference to the work of Lawlor and Mattingly (1998) and also Hanna and Rodger (2002).

Strategies for Involving Family Members in the Care of a Child

- Recognizing and actively supporting parental responsibility for care of child
- Recognizing the impact of intervention strategies- dependency—interdependency of parent and professional
- Recognizing the need to adjust expectations to reflect changes in the family situation
- Providing information about resources and options to parents

Key Features of Collaboration with Family Members

- Professionals having a positive attitude towards parents
- Understanding the barriers to partnership
- Understanding "friendship" viewed as an outcome of collaboration

Negotiating Collaboration with Families

- Negotiated models (e.g., Dale, 1996) versus professional as expert model
- Recognizing the appropriate time for the child to be actively involved (e.g., in goal setting) while being sympathetic to conflicts between a parent and a maturing child or young person
- Recognizing that collaboration develops over time

Possible Consequences for the Role of the Professional if Family Members are More Directly Involved

■ Knowledge base and skills—different applications

■ Recognizing parents as learners, teachers, co-learners in shared learning

■ Modes of service delivery—direct/indirect/consultation/education

When Professionals Perceive that Family Members Do Not Want More Involvement

■ Being sensitive and responsive to parents' values, beliefs, and concerns

■ Recognizing continuum of participation

■ Reframing previously accepted notions of compliance and adherence within parameters of "child's welfare is paramount" and "parental responsibility"

■ Being sensitive to parents' reactions to learning about their child

The Effect of Family Inclusion on the Work of the Interdisciplinary Pediatric Team

■ Negotiation about interventions at every stage based on established common goals

■ Services expected to incorporate practices that strengthen family systems and encourage use of wider community resources

■ Recognizing family-centered care as a practice context

The inclusion of "friendship" may be seen to be the most controversial for professionals (McWilliam, Tocci, & Harbin, 1998). Some caution would seem relevant when, placed alongside debates about professionals' growing understanding of the real-life issues associated with client-centered and family-centered practice, comes the issue of professional-client boundaries. Perhaps "treating parents as friends" need not risk professional objectivity. Indeed, the use of the word "treat" (or "deal with" or "care for") is an interesting challenge because it may represent an imbalance in the development of the relationship between parent and professional. Perhaps sensitivity for the care of the parent as a friend is a more acceptable stance when the professional is aware of the impact of his or her actions on the parent/family. From a family's viewpoint, "friend" may also suggest that, for example, a professional may become a companion, a confidant; someone who is not hostile, who is loyal, trustworthy, and sympathetic rather than a foe, with a shared interest in working together for the best interests of the child.

An overview of the literature has suggested that there will be many situations in which there will be potential disagreements between a parent and a professional that will affect the way in which a collaborative working partnership develops or falters. Figure 17–2 provides examples of the daily dilemmas of practice that might arise (e.g., Brown, 1996, 1997; Lawlor & Mattingly, 1998).

For the professional, being aware of these issues may support intervention that is family centered. For the parent, perhaps it signifies the challenges that professionals have to face. For service providers and commissioners, this may enhance their understanding of the complexities of the context of family-centered care.

Dilemmas that do arise will rarely be attributable to one factor alone. Professionals may be able to reflect on their personal practice and use their professional supervision strategies to help unravel complex issues and decide on an appropriate course of action to help resolve the issues involved.

Molding the Intervention Process in Support of Mothering Occupations and Family-centered Care

When we acknowledge that mothers and professionals will "learn together" in order to share understandings about the nature of the concerns about a child, this prompts the need to think about the ways in which services are accessed and delivered. Interactions between mothers or other family members and professionals begin even before a first contact or an initial interview. The process involved in a first contact and afterward will vary and will be influenced by local arrangements for service provision. Revisiting the intervention process allows us to consider the impact of each part of the process on a family and to incorporate specific strategies to support collaborative working. The stages comprising the

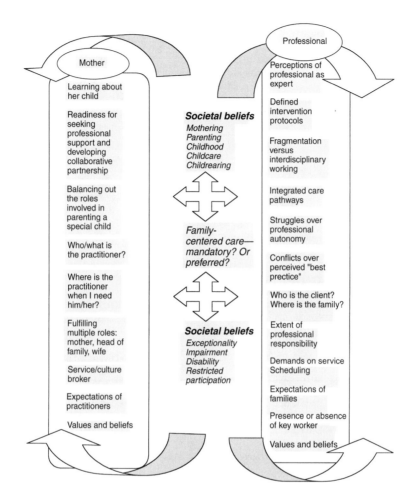

Figure 17–2 *Recognizing the potential for dissonance in collaborative partnerships.*

contact with a family include those that are not directly with the family in all circumstances. For example, the information provided about a service will ideally support the way in which the professionals will wish to work, and therefore careful attention will be paid to the language used to describe how a service might help.

Readers may like to review components of the intervention process that guides practice in their practice setting to consider the extent to which family-centered care is achieved.

As can be seen, the time for negotiating goals and methods of intervention follows problem setting based on a shared understanding of the key issues for a mother and the family. Table 17–2 provides examples of typical strategies for molding these stages in the intervention process in support of family-centered

care; it also incorporates strategies suggested by McConkey (1985) and Case-Smith (1998), together with strategies from my research and practice (Brown, 1996, 1997).

It is relevant to note here that professional literature originating from different countries suggests inconsistent use of terms like objectives, goals, and targets. This has relevance for the way in which words are used to describe intervention when working with families from other countries.

ℐ Conclusion

In conclusion, the importance of honoring families as the experts in the care of their children is essential to the theory and practice of family-centered care. Finding new ways of

Table 17–2 Revisiting the intervention process: Examples of strategies

Stage in intervention process	Working	Collaboratively
Sharing information through the process of problem setting	• Responsive to parents' concerns • Provides opportunities to exchange both a parent's and a practitioner's perspective • Provides opportunity to understand parents priorities	• Consider language used • Consider parent's readiness, timing, and continuum of participation • Consider preferred learning style and preference about presentation of materials
Selecting precise learning objectives (goals)	• Joint decision making about which objectives are selected and rationale made explicit and shared • Short-term achievable goals will lead to sense of achievement for parent and confidence in skills • Decisions about how and when to address other concerns • Focusing teaching to allow goals to be incorporated in everyday routines • Progress easy to monitor, reducing need to include special tests/procedures • Objectives can be shared with other family members	• Consider parent's readiness and continuum of participation • Based on a parent's perspective on concerns that need to be addressed now and those that will affect child's future capacities/abilities • Select a small number (two to three) of activity-based goals at any one time • Consider using ecocultural framework to support parent in constructing routines and activities • Expected outcomes clearly indicated. Attention paid to specific child behaviors • Recommendations do not create more "work" for parent • Responsibility does not fall on one family member
Suggestions for possible teaching contexts	• Identifying a variety of contexts to try to engage the child but also to help generalize the child's learning • During everyday household activities when possible • Selection of readily available materials, equipment, and activities • Being responsive to child's interests (likes and avoiding dislikes if appropriate) • Introducing novel tasks to extend learning opportunities • Adopting a routine except when child/parent is tired or unwell • Consider impact on other family systems	• Consider continuum of participation • Use ecocultural approach to identify appropriate contexts • Recommendations address how a parent holds, feeds, dresses, or plays with a child. • Linked to family's priorities • Activity is enjoyable for both parent and child • Extending child's interests and occupations • Choices address neglected family functions like leisure so activities are not solely child focused
Acquiring more techniques to aid the child's learning	• Task and skill analysis • Identifying child's interests and dislikes	• Provide choices of technique when something does not work as expected
Adapting parent's teaching in the light of the child's learning	• Monitor effectiveness and build on parents' natural style of interacting with their child • Link teaching contexts to teaching style • Provide opportunities for parents to see others teaching. Offer cues and explanations • Focusing on child's point of view can help explain rationale • Offer opportunities to practice with help and supervision • Link changes in teaching style to helping child achieve learning objective • Self-modeling	• Consider use of Parent Behavior Progression, for example, to identify parents' skills • Encourage use of natural conversations and dialogues

utilizing practice knowledge and skills to support a mother in successful mothering occupations, including a mother learning about her child, presents many challenges. Developing collaboration as a skill (Case-Smith, 2001) is fundamental for professionals in being able to work in the context of family-centered care. The realities of delivering family-centered care are daunting when the complexities of the context of family-centered care are appreciated. There is still much to learn. There may be a healthy future for family-centered care if this is so because it will provide opportunities for parents and professionals to pursue collaborative partnerships in family-centered care.

Further research into the realities of the implementation of services that can support such a continuum of participation from both a family and a professional perspective must be a priority.

Discussion Questions 🪶

- What drives the use of the term *family-centered care* in your work place? Is the intent to be child focused, parent and family focused, or service provider led?

- What strategies can professionals in senior and management positions use to support less experienced staff in working with a family in the context of family-centered care?

- How can services ensure that existing staff members can demonstrate the required competencies?

- How can we avoid adopting a common-needs approach in family-centered care?

- What are the resource implications of aspiring to offer *family-centered care* ?

References

American Occupational Therapy Association (1999). *Occupational therapy services for children and youth under the Individuals with Disabilities Education Act* (2nd Ed.). Bethesda, MD: The American Occupational Therapy Association Inc.

Anderson, J., & Hinojosa, J. (1984). Parents and therapists in a professional partnership *American Journal of Occupational Therapy, 38,* 453–461.

Aponte, H. J. (1985). The negotiation of values in therapy. *Family process, 24,* 323–338.

Bailey, D. (1987). Collaborative goal-setting with families: Resolving differences in values and priorities for services. *Topics in Early Childhood Special Education, 7*(2), 59–71. Austin, TX: Pro-Ed, Inc.

Bailey, D. B., McWilliam, P. J., & Winton, P. J. (1992). Building family- centered practices in early intervention: A team-based model for change. *Infants and Young Children, 5,* 73–82.

Bateson, M.C. (1996). Enfolded occupation and the concept of occupation. In R. Zemke & F. Clark (Eds.). *Occupational Science: The evolving discipline* (pp. 5–12). Philadelphia: F. A. Davis.

Bazyk, S. (1989). Changes in attitudes and beliefs regarding parent participation and home programmes: An update. *American Journal of Occupational Therapy, 43,* 723–728.

Berlin, E. A., & Fowkes, W. C. (1983). A teaching framework for cross-cultural health care—Application in family practice. *Western Journal of Medicine, 12*(1930), 93–98.

Bobath, B., & Finnie, N. (1970). Problems of communication between parents and staff in the treatment and management of children with cerebral palsy. *Developmental Medicine and Child Neurology, 12*(5), 629–635.

Britton, C., & Moore, A. (2002). Views from the inside, part 1: Routes to diagnosis—Families' experience of living with a child with arthritis. *British Journal of Occupational Therapy, 65*(8), 374–380.

Britton, C., & Moore, A. (2002). Views from the inside, part 2: What the children with arthritis said, and the experiences of siblings, mothers, fathers and grandparents. *British Journal of Occupational Therapy, 65*(9), 413–419.

Britton, C., & Moore, A. (2002). Views from the inside, part 3: How and why families undertake prescribed exercise and splinting programmes and a new model of the families' experience of living with juvenile arthritis. *British Journal of Occupational Therapy, 65*(10), *453–460.*

Bromwich, R.M. (1981). *Working with parents and infants: An interactional approach.* Baltimore: University Park Press.

Brown, G. (1996). The parent's experience of learning about their child. Master of Science in Pediatric Occupational Therapy. London (UK): University Of East London. Unpublished Dissertation.

Brown, G. (1997). *The parent's experience of learning about their child.* Paper presented at Australian Occupational Therapy Conference, 1997, Perth, Western Australia.

Brown, S. M, Humphry, R., & Taylor, E. (1997). A model of the nature of family-therapist relationships: Implications for education. *American Journal of Occupational Therapy, 51*(7), 597–603.

Burke, J. P., & Schaaf, R. (1997). Family narratives and play assessments. In L. D. Parham & L. S. Fazio (Eds.). *Play in occupational therapy* (pp. 67–84). St. Louis: Mosby.

Case-Smith, J. (Ed).(2001). *Occupational therapy for children* (4th ed.). St Louis: Mosby.

Case-Smith, J. (1998). Pediatric occupational therapy and early intervention. (2nd ed.). Boston: Butterworth Heinemann.

Case-Smith, J., & Nastro, M. A. (1993). The effect of

occupational therapy intervention on mothers of children with cerebral palsy. *American Journal of Occupational Therapy, 47*(9), 811–817.

Cheung, Y., Shah, S., & Muncer, S. (2002). An exploratory investigation of undergraduate students' perceptions of cultural awareness. *British Journal of Occupational Therapy, 65*(12), 543–550.

Crowe,T.K., Van Leit, B., & Berghmans, K.K. (2000). Mothers' perceptions of child care assistance: The impact of a child's disability. *American Journal of Occupational Therapy, 54*(1), 52–58.

Crowe, T. (1993). Time use of mothers with young children: The impact of a child's disability. *Developmental Medicine and Child Neurology, 35,* 621–630

Crowe,T. K., Van Leit, B., Berghmans, K. K, & Mann, P.(1997). Role perceptions of young children: The impact of a child's disability. *American Journal of Occupational Therapy, 51*(8), 651–661.

Cunningham,C., & Davis, H. (1985). Working with parents: Frameworks for collaboration. Open Milton Keynes: University Press.

Dale, N.(1996). Working with families of children with special needs—Partnership and Practice. London (UK): Routledge.

Department of Health (2000). The framework for assessment of children in need and their families. *http://www.doh.gov.uk/scg/cin.htm,* accessed February 7, 2003.

Department of Health (2001). National Service Framework, *http://www.doh.gov.uk/nsf/children.htm,* accessed February 12, 2003.

Esdaile, S. (1994). A focus on mothers, their children with special needs and other caregivers. *Australian Occupational Therapy Journal, 41,* 3–8.

Featherstone, H. (1980). *A difference in the family.* New York: Basic Books Inc.

Francis-Connolly, E. (2000). Towards an understanding of mothering: A comparison of two motherhood stages. *American Journal of Occupational Therapy, 54,* 281–289.

Francis-Connolly, E. (1998). It never ends: Mothering as a lifetime occupation. *Scandinavian Journal of Occupational Therapy, 5,* 149–155.

Hamill, J. S. (1987). Sensory integrative dysfunction: Parental participation in the child's therapy program. *Occupational Therapy in Health Care, 4*(2), 47–59.

Hanna, K., & Rodger, S. (2002). Towards family-centred practice in pediatric occupational therapy: A review of the literature on parent-therapist collaboration. *Australian Occupational Therapy Journal, 49,* 14–24.

Hasselkus, B. R.(1991). Ethical dilemmas in family caregiving for the elderly: Implications for occupational therapy. *American Journal of Occupational Therapy, 45,* 206–212.

Her Majesty's Stationery Office (1998). The Human Rights Act. *hmso.gov.uk/acts1998/19980042.htm,* accessed 7/2/03.

Hinojosa, J. (1990). How mothers of preschool children with cerebral palsy perceive occupational and physical therapists and their influence on family life. *The Occupational Therapy Journal Of Research, 10*(3), 144–162.

Hinojosa, J., & Anderson, J. (1991). Mothers' perceptions of home treatment programs for their preschool children with cerebral palsy. *American Journal of Occupational Therapy. 45,* 273- 279.

Hinojosa, J. Anderson, J., & Ranum, G. W. (1988). Relationships between therapists and parents of preschool children with cerebral palsy: A survey. *Occupational Therapy Journal of Research,* 285–297.

Hinojosa, J., Sproat, C. T., Mankhetwit, S., & Anderson,J. (2002). Shifts in parent-therapist Partnerships : Twelve Years of Change. *American Journal of Occupational Therapy, 56*(5), 556–563.

Hocking,C., & Ness, E. N. (2002). Introduction to the revised minimum standards for the education of occupational therapists (2002). *World Federation of Occupational Therapist Bulletin, November 2002, 46,* 30–33.

Humphry, R., & Case-Smith, J. (1996). Working with families . In J. Case-Smith, A.S. Allen, P. Pratt (Eds.). *Occupational Therapy for Children* (3rd Ed., pp. 67–98). Mosby: St Louis.

Humphry, R, &.Thigpen-Beck, B. (1998). Parenting values and attitudes: Views of therapist and parents. *American Journal of Occupational Therapy, 52*(10), 835–842.

Education of the Handicapped Act Amendments of 1990, Pub. I, 101–476, 20 USC Folio 1400 1400 *et seq.*

Kellegrew, D. (2000). Constructing daily routines: A qualitative examination of mothers with young children with disabilities. *American Journal of Occupational Therapy, 54,* 252–259.

Kibele, A. (1989). Occupational therapy's role in improving the quality of life for persons with cerebral palsy. *American Journal of Occupational Therapy, 43,* 371–377.

Kleineman, A. (1980). Patients and healers in the context of culture. Berkeley,CA: University of California Press.

Lawlor, M. C., & Mattingly, C. F. (1998). The complexities embedded in family centered care. *American Journal Of Occupational Therapy, 52*(4), 259–267.

Larson, E.A. (2000). Mothering: Letting go of the past ideal and valuing the past. *American Journal of Occupational Therapy, 54*(3), 249–251.

Leff, P. T., & Walizer,E. H.(1992). Building the healing partnership: Parents professionals and children with chronic illnesses and disabilities. Cambridge, MA: Brookline.

Llewellyn, G. (1994). Parenting: A neglected human occupation. Parents' voices not yet heard. *Australian Occupational Therapy Journal, 41,* 173–176.

Lyons, M. (1994). Reflections on client-therapist relationships. *Australian Occupational Therapy Journal, 41,* 27–30.

MacClean, M. F., & Chesson, R. (1991) Factors affecting parents' role as co-therapist: A pilot study of parents of children with motor learning difficulties. *British Journal of Occupational Therapy, 54*(7), 262–266.

Mattingly, C., & Fleming, M. H. (1994). *Clinical Reasoning: Forms of inquiry in a therapeutic practice.* Philidelphia: F. A. Davis.

Mayer, M. L., White, B. P., Ward, J. D., & Barnaby, E. M. (2002). Therapist perceptions about making a difference in parent- child relationships in early intervention occupational therapy services. *American Journal Of Occupational Therapy, 56*(4), 411–420.

Mayo, N. E. (1981). The effect of home visits on parental compliance with a home program. *Physical Therapy, 61,* 27–32.

McConkey, R. (1985). *Working with parents—A practical guide for teachers and therapists.* Cambridge MA: Croom Helm, Brookline.

McWilliam, R. A., Tocci, L., & Harbin,.G. L. (1998). Family-centered services: Service providers discourse and behaviour. *Topics in Early Childhood Special Education, 18,* 206–221.

Newson, E. (1976). Parents as a resource in diagnosis and assessment. In T. E.Oppe & F. P Woodford (Eds.) *Early management of handicapping disorders.* (p 105). London (UK): Associated Scientific Publishers.

Olson, J., & Esdaile, S. (2000). Mothering young children with disabilities in a challenging urban environment. *American Journal Of Occupational Therapy, 54,* 307–314.

Parette, H. P., & Hourcade, J. J. (1985). Parental participation in early therapeutic intervention programs for young children with cerebral palsy. *Rehabilitation Literature, 46,* 2–7.

Parker, J. A., Tewfik, D. B., & Burkhardt, A. (2002). Cultural context competency and children(AOTA Continuing Education article). *OT Practice, 7*(22), CE1–CE7.

Peterson, N. L., & Cooper, C. S. (1989). Parent education and involvement in early intervention programs for handicapped children: A different perspective on parent needs and the parent-professional relationship. *The second handbook on parent education.* London (UK): Academic Press, Inc.

Primeau, L. (1998). Orchestration of work and play within families. *American Journal of Occupational Therapy, 52,* 188–195.

Primeau, L. A., Clark, F., & Pierce, D. (1989). Occupational therapy alone has looked upon occupation: Future applications of occupational science to pediatric occupational therapy. *Occupational Therapy in Health Care, 6*(4), 19–32.

Ruddick, S. (1989) *Maternal thinking: Toward a politics of peace.* Boston: Beacon Press.

Ryan, S. E., & McKay, E. A.(Eds.) (1999). *Thinking and reasoning in therapy: Narrative from practice.* Cheltenham (UK): Stanley Thornes Publishers.

Schaaf, C., & Mulrooney, L. L. (1989). Occupational therapy in early intervention: A family-centered approach. *American Journal of Occupational Therapy, 43*(11), 745–753.

Schön, D. (1983). *The reflective practitioner.* New York: Basic Books.

Schultz-Krohn, W., & Cara, E. (2000). Occupational therapy in early intervention: Applying concepts from infant mental health. *American Journal of Occupational Therapy, 54,* 550–554.

Segal, R. (2000). Adaptive strategies of mothers with children with attention deficit hyperactivity disorder. *American Journal of Occupational Therapy, 54,* 300–306.

Shonkoff, J. P., & Hauser-Cram, P.(1987). Early intervention for disabled infants and their families: A quantitative analysis. *Pediatrics, 80,* 650–658.

Snow, K. (2001). *Disability is natural. Revolutionary common sense for raising successful children with disabilities.* Woodland Park, CO: Braveheart Press.

Sumsion, T. (1999). *Client centred practice in occupational therapy. A guide to implementation.* Edinburgh (UK): Churchill Livingstone.

Steward, B. (2000) Living space: The changing meaning of home. *British Journal of Occupational Therapy, 63*(3), 105–111.

Thompson, K. M. (1998). Early intervention services in daily family life: Mother's perceptions of 'ideal' versus 'actual' service provision. *Occupational Therapy International, 5,* 206–221.

Turnbull, A. P., & Turnbull, H. R. (1990). *Families , professionals and exceptionality: A special partnership* (2nd Ed.). Columbus, OH: Merrill Publishing Company.

Turnbull, H. R., & Turnbull, A. P. (1985). *Parents speak out.* New York: Macmillan Publishing Company.

Wallen, M., & Doyle, S.(1996). Performance indicators in pediatrics: The role of standardised assessments and goal setting. *Australian Occupational Therapy Journal, 43,* 172–177.

White, K., & Castro, G. (1985). An integrative review of early intervention efficacy studies with at risk children: Implications for the handicapped. *Analysis and Intervention in Developmental Disabilities, 5,* 7–31.

Widdows, J. (1997). *A special need for inclusion: Children with disabilities, their families and everyday life.* London (UK): The Children's Society.

Yerxa, E., Clarke, F., Jackson, J., Pierce, D., & Zemke, R. (1990). *An introduction to occupational science, a foundation for occupational therapy in the 21st century.* Binghamton, NY: Haworth.

Additional Readings

Dale, N. (1996). *Working with families of children with special needs—Partnership and Practice.* London (UK): Routledge.

Kellegrew, D. H. (1998). Creating opportunities for occupation: An intervention to promote the self -care independence of young children with special needs. *American Journal of Occupational Therapy, 52,* 457–465.

Lynch, E. W., & Hanson, M. J. (1998). *Developing cross-cultural competence. A guide for working with young children and their families* (2nd ed.). Baltimore: Brookes.

Olshansky, S. Chronic sorrow: A response to having a mentally defective child. *Social Casework, 43,* 190–193.

Seligman, M., & Darling, R. B. (1989). *Ordinary families, special children: A systems approach to childhood disability.* New York: The Guildford Press.

CHAPTER *18*

Mothering Children with Disabilities in the Context of Welfare Reform

Barbara W. LeRoy, PhD

 Anticipated Outcomes

I anticipate that, after reading this chapter, readers will:

- Understand the unique characteristics of mothers who receive welfare and who have children with disabilities

- Learn about the impacts and effects of welfare reform on mothers who have children with disabilities

- Learn about the welfare system in the United States, with a particular emphasis on welfare reform since the implementation of the 1996 legislation (Personal Responsibility and Work Opportunity Reconciliation Act [PRWORA])

- Understand the perspectives and issues of serving this unique population from their service providers

- Gain an understanding of policy, service, and familial support strategies to address the needs of these mothers

✦ Introduction

When women are both poor and mothers of a child with disabilities, mothering is a uniquely isolating, stressful, and repetitive occupation. Mothers who have children with disabilities account for more than 12 percent of the United States welfare program. Large-scale research studies have indicated that these women face multiple barriers to self-sufficiency. This chapter presents the results of a Michigan study in which we conducted extensive and longitudinal interviews with 60 mothers who receive welfare and have children with disabilities. We examined their daily realities, their unique mothering situations, and how the requirements of the governmental welfare reform program affected their lives. Mother and child characteristics, their experiences with the welfare system, and findings related to their well-being, self-sufficiency, and employment are presented. Personal stories and concluding reflections complete the chapter.

Although there are numerous studies on the effects of welfare reform on its typical service recipients, few studies have examined the effects on mothers who have children with disabilities. In the research to which we refer in this chapter, we were interested in shining a light on these mothers by presenting a descriptive picture of them and their children and by examining the effects of welfare reform on them and their families. We wanted to know who these women are, what their daily reality is, what is unique about their mothering situations, and how requirements of a governmental program affect their daily lives. We wanted to understand how they cope and what their unique qualities are that make them continue to step up to the plate with a full count of societal strikes against them.

To determine if we could find enough mothers to conduct the study and gain their opinions about essential questions to be included in the interviews, we initially conducted a series of focus groups. We were amazed at how quickly we started to receive telephone calls from mothers who wanted to tell us their stories. They told us that no one had ever asked them about their lives; no one

had seemed to care what they had to say. They were anxious to share their experiences, and they made tremendous sacrifices just to come to our focus groups. The 2-hour focus group sessions could have lasted for 8 hours. Themes of anger, rejection, loneliness, despair, and resilience resonated around the rooms. We heard voices that demanded a larger audience. These mothers have an intuitive sense of the issues with which policy makers and service providers must struggle. They are the welfare system's outliers, the canaries in the gold mine of welfare reform. Our hope is that this chapter illuminates these mothers' stories. For their willingness to take time away from their daily struggles to share their stories, we humbly dedicate our work to them.

✦ Overview

Mothering in Quadruple Jeopardy

Mothering is one of life's supreme occupations, filled with struggles, joys, and rewards. At its basic core, it is no different for mothers who are poor, nor is it different for mothers who have a child with disabilities. However, in its existential reality, mothering is dramatically different for both poor mothers and mothers of children with disabilities. When mothers are poor and have children with disabilities, mothering is a uniquely isolating, stressful, and repetitive occupation. For these mothers, life is like a turntable that keeps spinning the same day over and over, with one day rolling into another with so much repetition and demands that they all start to look the same. Days fall into months and years, and over that time these mothers are lucky if they are able to hold their own in a society that neither recognizes them nor supports them to become economically and emotionally independent citizens.

When welfare reform emerged as a reality in the United States in 1996, there was no mention of disability in the stereotypical images of mothers who use welfare. The media picture of a welfare mother was replete with negative images of lazy, immoral, nonwhite young women who have little education or skills and who have numerous children as their income source at the government's expense. There was no mention of disability in this image. Official reports provided no statistics on the prevalence of these mothers in the welfare population. Perhaps there were none. There was no picture of who these mothers might be and who their children were. The fact that no information existed did not mean these mothers did not exist, but it was indicative of society's blind spot. These mothers are invisible to the system, to their neighbors, and often to their extended families. They live in the margins of society, in quadruple jeopardy. They are marginalized for being poor, nonwhite, and women who cannot even produce healthy babies. Rather, they produce babies who burden society with their care. The daily reality for these mothers is one of depression and social isolation. Yet some of these mothers have amazing resilience and can be buoyed by their ability to see their children as gifts rather than as helpless burdens.

Context of Their Mothering — Policy Reforms

The 1996 Personal Responsibility and Work Opportunity Reconciliation Act (PRWORA) ushered in a new era in welfare reform. PRWORA changed all the rules of eligibility and access, emphasizing work over assistance and education. Under PRWORA states receive block grants of money, known as Temporary Assistance to Needy Families (TANF). TANF differs from its predecessors, Aid to Families with Dependent Children (AFDC) and Job Opportunities and Basic Skills Training Program (JOBS), in that it is a temporary cash assistance program with an emphasis on work as the primary route to self-sufficiency. TANF grants to families are contingent on recipients fulfilling mandatory work requirements (HHS, 1999).

Under the block grants system, states have unprecedented flexibility in designing their cash assistance and welfare-to-work programs. Under PRWORA, states can determine:
- Who is eligible for cash assistance
- Who must participate in welfare-to-work programs and what they are required to do to receive this assistance

- What mix of services they will receive to help them exit welfare

For mothers who have children with disabilities, state decisions about who should be required to participate in welfare-to-work activities and the mix of services are the most important determinants of their future self-sufficiency.

Although PRWORA established state flexibility in work programs, it also made major changes in existing safety net spending (i.e., childcare, food stamps, and Social Security Insurance [SSI]). Specifically, with regard to childcare programs, it eliminated individual childcare assistance for mothers in three categories: former AFDC mothers in work or training programs; mothers making the transition from welfare to work; and low-income mothers. These three programs were consolidated into a single childcare block grant, which each state can allocate as it chooses.

With regard to food subsidies, the law substantially reduced childcare food subsidy for low-income children and reduced eligibility of poor families for food stamps. With regard to SSI, welfare reform legislation changed SSI standards for children. The eligibility standards are more restrictive, attempting to limit the expanded access to SSI that occurred as a result of the 1990 U.S. Supreme Court decision in Zebley vs. Sullivan. Under welfare reform, the definition of childhood disability is disassociated with the definition of disability for adults. The reform legislation also eliminated the eligibility of children with behavioral disorders for SSI. Eligibility for Medicaid was retained.

Finally, with regard to health insurance, PRWORA extended the state's obligation to provide transitional Medicaid (TMA) to TANF participants. Families who exit TANF remain eligible to receive Medicaid for 12 months after exceeding the income ceiling. A second level of the TMA program allows working families to buy into the Medicaid program based on an income scale. The implementation of the federal Children's Health Insurance Program (CHIP) initiative allows children in families that are below 150 percent of the federal poverty level to access health care.

Under the new eligibility rules and require-ments, states began to move recipients off their caseloads at unprecedented rates. For example, in 1992 the welfare caseload in Michigan peaked at 221,884 participants. Since that time, the caseload has continued to decrease to a record low at the end of the year 2000 of less than 50,000 participants, a reduc-tion of more than 70 percent in 8 years.

Mothers of Children with Disabilities on the Caseload

Demographic studies of welfare caseloads indicate that the majority of recipients are women in their 20s who have few job skills and minimal education, are supporting several children, and who experience some form of disability, either personally or within their families. National estimates indicate that up to 60 percent of welfare recipients have disabili-ties and an additional 10 to 20 percent of re-cipients have a dependent family member with a disability (National Council on Disabil-ity, 1997). At the outset of Welfare Reform, caseload statistics in Michigan indicated that 10 to 12 percent of welfare mothers have chil-dren with disabilities (for 1998, n = 12,800 mothers). Less than 2 years later, up to 20 per-cent of the remaining caseload were mothers who have children with disabilities. Although the actual number of welfare mothers who have children with disabilities has not in-creased, they have become disproportionately present in the current caseload. For the large part, these mothers have not been able to exit the system. These percentages and the contin-uation of these mothers in the welfare system is consistent with reports from other states (Urban Institute, 1998; Reischi, 1998).

✍ Literature Review

Few welfare research studies have focused on this specific subpopulation, which again is in-dicative of the fact that these mothers are vir-tually invisible in the system. However, a few studies are starting to highlight what is becom-ing an increasingly larger segment of the wel-fare population, as indicated by recent research by Lee, Sills, and Oh at the Institute

for Women's Policy Research (2002). They found that single mothers receiving TANF are more likely than other low-income mothers to have a child with a disability (20 percent vs. 11 percent, respectively). In addition, they found that TANF mothers themselves were more likely to have a disability than other low-income mothers (38 percent vs. 17 percent, re-spectively). Specifically, they found that nearly half of single-mothers receiving TANF have a disability or a disabled child, but only a small proportion receive government support.

In a longitudinal study of mothers on wel-fare in a largely urban county in Michigan, Danziger and his associates (1998) found that one in five mothers who received TANF had a child with a health, learning, or emotional problem. They also found that many of the mothers in their study had multiple barriers to achieving self-sufficiency (e.g., depression or other mental health problems, a history of abuse, poor job skills, and no transportation). Their results indicated that it was not so much the power of any particular barrier that hin-dered self-sufficiency for these mothers as it was the cumulative effect of multiple barriers. When the family household included a child with a disability, mothers faced multiple and serious obstacles to their potential of moving out of the welfare trap.

Loprest and Zedlewski (1999) and a recent report to Congress from the Department of Health and Human Services (HHS, 1999), both strengthened the finding of multiple bar-riers to self-sufficiency. Loprest and Zedlewski echoed the findings of Danziger and associ-ates by stating that the strongest predictor of not participating in work activity is the pres-ence of multiple obstacles. In reporting to Congress, HHS stated that, although there have been dramatic gains in work for many TANF families, too many families with multi-ple barriers to success are at risk of being left behind.

In a series of studies over the 5 years of wel-fare reform, Eileen Sweeney from the Urban Institute has been tracking the fate of mothers who have children with disabilities (2001, 2002). In her most recent study, Sweeney found that three out of four women in the Institute's urban sample had at least one health barrier to employment and 40 percent had two or more health problems, including the health of a child. With regard to having a child with a disability specifically, she found that one-fourth of welfare mothers had a child with an illness or disability so severe as to limit the mothers' ability to work. She also found that families with multiple barriers were more likely than other recipients to be sanctioned for what the system perceived as noncompliance (e.g., failure to complete work readiness classes; missed appointments with the caseworker; failure to go on job interviews). Mothers who had children with disabilities were among this group of highly sanctioned recipients. As many as one-fourth to one-half of mothers who are no longer receiving TANF because of a sanction for failure to comply with the state's welfare rules indicated that they were unable to comply with the rules because of their own or their child's disability, health condition, or illness. Mothers who have children with disabilities and who had left the welfare system were more likely than others who leave the system to say they had been terminated by the agency rather than having left on their own accord. Sanctioned mothers were less likely to be employed after leaving welfare and, if employed, tended to have lower earnings than nonsanctioned mothers.

In a study of California welfare families, Meyers et al. (1998) found that the presence of chronically ill and disabled children had a significant negative impact on mothers' labor force participation, even after controlling for differences in women's human capital characteristics, household configuration, and other income. The presence of a child with a disability or chronic health problem was associated with a 36 to 90 percent reduction in the odds that the mother worked, depending on the number of children with disabilities in the family. In a follow-up to the 1996 study, Meyers et al. (2000) examined the public and private costs associated with children in Californian families at the intersection of two populations: those served by public welfare programs and those caring for children with disabilities. Similar to other studies, they found that 10 to 12 percent of the welfare population in

California have a child with a disability, and that between 3 and 5 percent of those families have a child with severe limitations. They found that welfare mothers who had children with disabilities were more likely to report experiencing concrete hardships. One-third of the mothers reported that their children had gone hungry in the last year, as compared to 17 percent of welfare mothers with typical children. Additionally, 33 to 73 percent of these mothers reported that they themselves had experienced hunger, as compared to 22 percent of other welfare mothers. Mothers with children who had disabilities were also more likely to report having difficulty paying their housing costs, having experienced eviction or periods of homelessness, and having had phone or utility shutoffs because of an inability to pay their bills. The authors concluded that poor parents who have children with disabilities often face dismaying tradeoffs between meeting the special needs of their children and meeting the basic needs of their families, and between working and caring for their children.

Heymann and Earle (1999) examined the impact of welfare reform on mothers' ability to care for their children's health. Using data from the National Longitudinal Survey of Youth, they examined the availability of benefits that working mothers commonly used to meet the health and developmental needs of their children: paid sick leave, vacation leave, and flexible hours. In comparing mothers who had never received welfare, mothers who had been on AFDC/TANF were more likely to be caring for at least one child with a chronic condition (37 vs. 21 percent, respectively). Yet welfare mothers were more likely to lack sick leave for the entire time they worked (36 vs. 20 percent) and less likely to receive other paid leave or flexibility. They concluded that, under such circumstances, mothers of children with disabilities who are leaving welfare will not find it possible to succeed both at work and in meeting the needs of their children.

The previously cited studies are beginning to paint a picture of the mothers who have children with disabilities and use welfare supports. They have used large, governmental databases to project incidence rates, system uses, and barriers to employment and self-sufficiency. However, these studies fail to paint a picture of the existential reality of a day in the life of these mothers. Who are these mothers who do their mothering against the odds, jeopardized by being poor, needy, and alone in a system that appears to be blind to their existence and their fate?

❧ Michigan Research

Participants

We talked with 60 mothers (45 urban; 15 rural) over the course of 2 years. We recruited them through advertisements posted in community sites in Detroit (urban) and the Upper Peninsula (rural) of Michigan. The advertisement invited mothers to participate in focus groups and/or extended interviews in their homes. The research team completed initial screenings of interested mothers to determine if they met the two criteria of participation (receiving welfare support and having a child with a disability). Subsequently, 21 mothers participated in 3 focus groups to help us refine our interview protocols and the remaining 39 mothers participated in extended interviews in their homes. One year after the initial interviews, 20 of the 39 original urban mothers participated in follow-up interviews.

Interview Questionnaire

The design of the interview questionnaire followed a three-step process. First, a review of the literature was conducted to identify existing research variables and to identify mothering and family disability issues related to self-sufficiency. Second, the focus group participants helped us to refine our questions related to mothering in the context of welfare reform, the implications of welfare program changes, and family needs and supports. Third, the extensive interview questionnaire was developed based on outcomes in the two previous steps. The interview was composed of 9 sections, addressing participant demographics, child demographics, childcare, welfare benefit status and history, work history, self-

sufficiency, future aspirations, perceptions of welfare reform, and personal well-being. The questionnaire was field-tested with three mothers to ensure ease of administration and completeness of design. Approximately 2 hours were required for the administration of each interview.

Findings

The findings are presented for the interview participants only, not the focus group mothers.

Mothers' Characteristics

Table 18–1 presents the characteristics of the 39 mothers who participated in the extended interviews. These mothers were similar to those in the national databases (i.e., majority are minority women, unmarried, have multiple children), except for three characteristics: they were older than the typical mother on welfare, they had more education, and, as a group, they were more ethnically diverse. Only five of these mothers were married at the time of the interviews. The majority were single heads of household, with an average of three children including at least one child who had a disability. As can be seen in the table, just over one-third of these mothers had some college education. Many of the mothers reported that, before the birth of their child with a disability, they had been employed, and some reported that they were on career ladders. The mean yearly household income was similar in both the urban and rural settings, $9,314. Just over half of the mothers rented their homes and one-third owned their homes. Four urban mothers lived with their parents. Equal numbers of urban and rural mothers owned their own cars (n=10).

Although it was not clinically assessed, many of these mothers spoke of being very depressed. They said they felt isolated and spent their days just trying to get through to the next day. One mother said that she had not been out of the house for an extended time since her son with disabilities was born, more than 15 years ago. When we asked how she had heard about our research project, she said that her brother had seen a flyer in the grocery

Table 18–1 Participant characteristics by group

Characteristic	Sample n=39 M	SD	Urban n=24 M	SD	Rural n=15 M	SD
Age (in years)	35.3	7.3	34.3	7.6	37.0	6.7
Gender	n	%	n	%	n	%
Female	39	100.0	24	100.0	15	100.0
Race						
African American	16	41.0	16	66.7	–	–
Caucasian	13	33.3	1	4.2	12	80.0
Latino	6	15.4	6	25.0	–	–
Native American	3	7.7	1	4.2	2	13.3
Other	1	2.6	–	–	1	6.7
Marital Status						
Single	17	43.6	13	54.2	4	26.7
Married	5	12.8	3	12.2	2	13.3
Separated / Divorced	17	43.6	8	33.3	9	60.0
Years of Education						
Less than high school	14	35.9	13	54.2	1	6.7
High school graduate/GED	10	25.6	3	12.5	7	46.7
Some college	12	30.8	7	29.2	5	33.3
College graduate	3	7.7	1	4.2	2	13.3

M = mean; SD = standard deviation

store and he thought she should be talking to someone. Although many of the mothers expressed a strong desire to have other mothers with whom they could share information and support, the majority of them indicated that this concept would be a luxury and that by the time they finished providing the intense care needed by their children, they were too tired to do anything else.

Many of these mothers acknowledged that their lives had taken a totally different turn when their children with disabilities were born. Not unlike other families with disabilities, many of these mothers indicated that their husbands or significant others (the father of the child with disabilities) left shortly after the birth. They were not bitter or angry, simply resigned to their fate in life. Comments such as "He just couldn't take seeing him" or "He just didn't know how to help" were not uncommon. All of these mothers were very clear that they did not blame their fall into welfare on their children with disabilities. In all their comments and actions, their children came

first, even if it meant they were living under the stigma of welfare. All these mothers saw welfare as a stigma and a program they wished they did not have to use. They saw it as their only option when the needs of their children required such full-time commitment. Paid employment was not possible and welfare was perceived as their only safety net.

Mothers' Welfare History and Experiences with the Service System

This group of mothers reported that they had been on welfare for an average of 8 years, which significantly corresponded with the average age of the children with disabilities. In fact, all mothers reported that their reason for using welfare supports was either directly or indirectly related to the birth of their child with disabilities. For the half of the mothers who said there was an indirect connection, 15 percent reported having a disability themselves. They felt that they were not able to cope with the unique needs of their child without the supports. Of the range of possible welfare supports, mothers reported that they received the following types of support, in descending order: health insurance (95 percent); cash assistance (82 percent); food stamps (72 percent); supplemental security income (64 percent); transportation (26 percent); and emergency cash and/or shelter (3 percent each).

A variety of community support services are designed both to benefit the children with disabilities and to provide the mothers with a level of relief from the stress of caring for these children. These services include early intervention (preschool enrichment and therapy), special education, visiting nurses, and respite. Less than one-third of all mothers used any public services that were nominally available to them. The majority of mothers indicated that they were not aware of the availability of these services. Interestingly, 40 percent of the mothers in the rural group used visiting nurses, whereas only 32 percent of urban mothers did. These figures are noteworthy in that the urban mothers had significantly more children with health concerns and the rural mothers had children with mild intellectual concerns. However, caseworker decisions about the need for assistance in the homes of the rural mothers may have been influenced by a self-reported higher incidence of personal disability among those mothers.

Child Characteristics

The 39 mothers who participated in the interviews had a total of 45 children with disabilities. Characteristics of the children for the urban and rural families are presented in Table 18–2. Consistent with other child disability data (US DOE, 2000), two-thirds of the children are male. As a cohort, these children had a lower rate of intellectual disability but a higher rate of behavioral concerns than their typical special education counterparts (Michigan DOE, 2001). Within the two groups, the children were similar on all demographic characteristics, with the exception of age. The children in the rural group were significantly older than the children in the urban group. To determine the level of severity by disability for these children, a severity index was calculated by combining the child's age with his functioning level on eight developmental tasks (e.g., feeding self, dressing, walking, talking, and toileting). The majority of children in the urban families had significant physical and/or mental health disabilities, whereas the majority of children in the rural families had mild intellectual disabilities. However, those rural children also had significant behavioral concerns as reported by their mothers and verified by school records.

Indicators of the severity of the needs among these children abounded in their mothers' stories. One urban mother, who had a child with significant health concerns, reported that she spent 5 to 6 hours a day in taking him through his therapeutic exercises and feeding him. He required a gastric tube for feeding. The mother reported that even when he was in a special class at school, she would be called several days a week to come to school to assist school personnel because of problems with the feeding tube. Another mother worried what would happen to her son, and therefore to her, if he grew much larger. He was 9 years old and already much bigger than she. His anger and tantrums were so severe that the school would often lock him to a desk and then call her to come and take him home. She could always calm him down, but she was afraid of what the future would hold. The school was putting pressure on her to have him institutionalized, but she could not even say the word without tears rolling down her face. A year later, at our second interview, this mother indicated that she had had to institutionalize her son. He had seriously injured her in a struggle, and she was afraid for her own safety. However, she now spent her days going to visit him at the institution. Her need to monitor that program and her depression continued to prevent her from moving ahead with her life. For the majority of these mothers, neither formal childcare arrangements nor school seemed to provide a level of release from their childcaring responsibilities. Many mothers reported that they had very frequent calls for help from these programs and that they felt they were constantly on "pins and needles" waiting for the telephone to ring.

Table 18–2 Child characteristics by group

Characteristic	Sample n=45 M	SD	Urban n=27 M	SD	Rural n=18 M	SD
Age (in years)	8.2	4.3	6.7	3.7	10.6*	4.0
	n	%	n	%	n	%
Gender						
Male	30	66.7	17	63.0	13	72.2
Female	15	33.3	10	37.0	5	27.8
Type of Disability**						
Intellectual	24	48.8	9	33.3	15	83.3
Physical Health	16	35.5	15	55.5	1	5.5
Mental Health	6	13.3	6	22.2	–	–
Sensory	6	13.3	3	11.1	3	16.7
Severity Level						
Mild	23	51.1	9	33.3	14	77.8
Moderate	12	26.7	8	29.6	4	22.2
Severe	10	22.2	10	37.0	–	–
Behavioral Concern	29	64.4	13	48.1	16	88.8

M = mean; SD = standard deviation
*p<.05
**Overlapping categories

❧ Contextual Jeopardy—Mothering in the Face of Welfare Reform's Goal of Self-sufficiency

All of the mothers we interviewed desired, believed in, and supported the goal of self-sufficiency. All of these mothers believed that the welfare system needed serious restructuring. Every one of these mothers wanted a better life for herself and her children. And not one of these mothers felt confident that the system could make self-sufficiency a reality. They could envision how self-sufficiency could be achieved for the *other* mothers on welfare, but for themselves, the mothers of children with disabilities, they did not have a vision or a hope for self-sufficiency. What they hoped for was a system that understood and embraced the concept of interdependence—a hand for their hands.

Mothers identified three systemic barriers to their self-sufficiency: poorly trained welfare caseworkers, limited public transportation, and inadequate childcare. Mothers reported that caseworkers do not have an understanding of the complexities involved in raising a child with a disability. The majority of mothers felt that caseworkers were only focused on the work aspects of welfare and that they were not able to address their unique needs. The caseworkers did not seem to recognize that addressing the support needs of the mothers would help them, in turn, to be able to return to work. The vast majority of mothers indicated that caseworkers did not know what services and supports were available in the community to assist them in meeting the needs of their children. Further, they felt that caseworkers were not motivated to obtain information and to share it with them.

Mothers became quite animated when discussions turned to systemic supports. One mother spoke for the group when she said, "I have to tell them (caseworkers) about the services (e.g., special education, early intervention, respite, home help) that are supposedly available in the community. And I say, supposedly, because where I live (Detroit), these services don't seem to be available to me. I need someone to help me to get them; someone to make the connections. I don't need a class in resume writing or how to dress for success. I dress everyday for the success of my child and that's jeans and a sweatshirt. Until I have a system of support that I can trust, it's jeans and a sweatshirt for me." Another mother said, "They don't have a clue and they don't want to find one, either." These mothers were most frustrated with the perceived unwillingness of their caseworkers to help them to create a plan for their movement toward self-sufficiency: "They want me to work and yet they don't help me find what I need."

Mothers also perceived the lack of transportation as a major barrier in their lives. For rural mothers, public transportation was all but nonexistent. For urban mothers, public transportation was often unreliable, inaccessible, or limited in range. Mothers perceived transportation as a means toward self-sufficiency, but one that remained outside of their daily reality. They indicated that accessible buses would allow them to take their children to a childcare arrangement on their way to work. However, too often the buses did not maintain posted schedules or the handicapped-accessible bus for the route was in repair, causing mothers to wait for extended periods for a bus that never came. Further, many mothers reported that they chose to work during nonstandard hours, between 11:00 PM and 6:00 AM to provide maximum support to their children and therefore to reduce their own anxiety about childcare. Mothers reported that they found little available public transportation at those times. Finally, urban mothers reported that the city buses did not provide services to the suburbs, where the majority of jobs were to be found. One mother, again, captured the sentiment for the group when she said, "I can live with the fact that my bus to work is late or doesn't come, but when I need to get home to my child, it is not a situation I can tolerate. My child needs his therapy or his medication or his feeding and I am the only one who can do that. It's not a choice."

As a group, these mothers found they were very dependent on their extended families, their neighbors, and church friends for transportation to work, doctors' appointments, grocery shopping, and other errands. Often, transportation was not available at the times when the mothers needed it or it was tenuous,

given that their families and friends, themselves, also had economic hardships of their own. Mothers reported that they hated the fact that they always had to be asking for help. They felt they were rarely in the position to return favors, although they tried by offering to take care of their nieces and nephews and their neighbors' children or aging parents. Many times, members of these extended networks told these mothers that they did not like to ask them for help because it seemed their hands were already full. This assumption left these mothers feeling that they were not even on equal footing in terms of giving personal support to others.

More than 70 percent of the mothers we interviewed indicated that childcare was the most significant barrier to their seeking employment. Specifically, they identified availability, costs, quality of care, and knowledge and skills of the providers as barriers to their being comfortable with leaving their children. Although all of the mothers would have qualified for public childcare assistance, less than one-quarter of them received any type of public financial assistance (8 percent received childcare subsidy and 13 percent received respite care). In response to care concerns and the lack of public funding, more than half of the mothers indicated that they rely on relatives and/or neighbors to assist them with their childcare needs. Specifically, in regard to accessing public childcare, mothers indicated that childcare services were not available when needed, not in close proximity to either their homes or work sites, and not accessible for children with disabilities. Because of the unique needs of these children with disabilities and the increased availability of nontraditional jobs, more mothers reported needing childcare at nonstandard hours. Few mothers reported that they were able to find evening or 24-hour childcare in their communities. When mothers did find childcare arrangements, they also found that often the closest childcare program did not have ramp access and the programs were housed in multistory buildings without elevators. Further compounding the availability issue was the fact that childcare options became very limited as the children aged, even though their disabilities required ongoing care and support. While Michigan does fund public childcare for children with disabilities up to age 16, few mothers or care providers were aware of that policy. Ultimately, whether funded or not, few childcare providers wanted to care for older children who had toileting and feeding needs. One mother said, "After age 13, regular childcare is difficult to find. Even after age 6, it is difficult to get childcare, especially if the child is not potty trained. The owners are afraid of bringing liability issues to the center."

Another complication in the system was the issue of who could be funded to provide childcare. The vast majority of mothers said that they preferred to have a family member or close neighbor provide childcare for their children with disabilities. They felt that they could trust them and that they knew how to care for their children. However, licensing restrictions and regulations prohibited childcare subsidy funds from going to family members. One mother said, "I can't leave my kids and not worry about them. It takes more than a book. Some people went to school and have education. While they have book sense, they have no common sense. I need someone I can trust to be around my child."

With regard to costs, mothers reported that they were not able to augment the public childcare subsidy, as required by providers, to support the unique needs of their children. One mother explained the frustration with the system for her: "People think you have so much money when you have a child with a disability, because you receive social security insurance (SSI) and Medicaid. A lady was taking care of my child and wanted money from the Family Independence Agency (FIA) and then $60 extra from me a week to take care of her." In Michigan, the state-allotted subsidy for childcare is $2.95 per hour, which is not differentiated by the needs of the child. However, the average hourly rate for specialized childcare is $4.80 per hour (Michigan League for Human Services, 1998). In fact, the few mothers who found work and who had to augment childcare costs with their earnings actually had less real money to spend per month than those mothers who stayed at home with their children.

Another issue related to cost was reimbursement. For those few mothers who did have the childcare subsidy, they reported it was a "joke." The state was so slow in paying the provider that each mother's story echoed all the other mothers' stories. "One Friday they told me not to come back on Monday. They said they had not received payment and could not continue to carry my child. When I explained it was not my fault and I would lose my job, they said it was not their problem. There were plenty of other children who could pay and who needed child care, and it was too bad."

Even if all the financial issues could be resolved, the majority of mothers expressed their strongest concern and reservation about the quality of care and the knowledge and skills of care providers. All mothers indicated that training was needed to help childcare providers to understand disabilities. Specifically, they indicated that training should address sensitivity, awareness, and how to care for special-needs children. Given that the majority of these children had behavioral concerns, these mothers were particularly worried that providers would not know how to address these needs. One mother reported that she took her child with health-care needs to 15 different childcare settings, and all of them said they were not equipped to handle a child with such needs. They did not have the correct equipment, the skills, or the emotional energy to provide the care. "They told me I would have to provide my own aide and then they would still be concerned about liability issues. I said if I could afford to pay for an aide, I would have someone come to my home." Another mother reported that she tried several childcare programs and in each one, they would call her every afternoon to come and get her child. They did not know how to stop him from hitting and biting other children. She said she was afraid the staff would hit her child. A third mother said, "I called 125 day care centers, looking for childcare which would care for a disabled child, no one would help. Visiting nurses cost $275 per month. I told this to my worker, and she said, I can't help you, so what am I to do?" Her conclusion was that "it was she and her child against the world."

The Impact of Employment on Their Mothering

The basic tenet of welfare reform is that it will promote self-sufficiency for recipients by moving them into employment. Work is the only programmatic goal, and there are severe sanctions for those welfare recipients who do not move in that direction. For welfare recipients who themselves have visible disabilities, the state is allowed to exempt them from employment. For mothers who are caring for children with disabilities, the policy is not so clear. Some of the mothers we interviewed indicated that they had received an exemption from the work policy, others had received sanctions (e.g., cut off from food stamps) for not attending work preparation classes or job interviews, and others had been terminated from the system.

The majority of mothers in our study expressed a desire to work, assuming that they could find safe and reliable supports for their children. At the time of our first interviews, one-third of the mothers were employed to some extent. Half of the mothers were unemployed and the remaining mothers were not seeking employment because of their own disabilities. For the mothers who were employed, the mean length of employment was just over 1 year, working 25 hours per week, at an average hourly wage of $6.77. None of the mothers received benefits through their employers (e.g., health coverage, vacation, medical leave). For the most part, these mothers had jobs that they had found through family members or friends. The jobs were service oriented with no career ladders in sight. Jobs for these mothers included cleaning offices, substitute teaching, factory line assembly, aiding in nursing homes, and making sandwiches at a delicatessen.

At an hourly wage of $6.77, these mothers are remaining in poverty. In a 1998 study by the Michigan League for Human Services economists determined that a single-parent family with two children would need to earn $15.72 per hour in order to be self-sufficient. Most importantly, for these mothers, employment came at a considerable personal price. They struggled with trying to balance family needs with employer requirements, augmenting childcare costs, fretting over the care of their children when they were away, and constantly worrying about potential holes springing through their fragile safety nets. One mother said, "I have been fired so often because my child is in and out of the hospital." With no job leave options, mothers found it difficult to take their children to their numerous doctor and therapy appointments and still hold down their jobs. Another mother commented on the tenuous childcare arrangement she had. "At first, I didn't have any support, because my mother was scared. But she started to feel more comfortable with my child, so I was able to work in the afternoon. My mother passed away in May, so now I don't have anyone who can help me. I want to work and finish school."

For the mothers who were unemployed at the time of our first interviews, most of them had been unemployed for several years. Having to care for their child with a disability was the primary reason these mothers cited for not working. Half of these mothers indicated that they were actively seeking employment. The only characteristic that differentiated employed from unemployed mothers was the age of their child with a disability. Mothers who had older children (10 years vs. 7 years) were more likely to be employed. Other characteristics such as the mothers' age, family size, years receiving welfare supports, education, or number of adults in the household did not predict employment. Presumably, mothers who had older children had more time to establish their support programs, including special education services for the prime work hours. However, many mothers reported that they used the time while their children were in school to catch up on their sleep because they were awake for long hours in the night providing health and/or behavior supports to their children.

❧ One Year Later

One year after the initial interviews, we attempted to conduct a second interview with the urban mothers in our research group (n=24). Indicative of the precarious lives these mothers lead, we were not able to find *any* of the mothers by way of telephone or the mail. All of the telephones had been disconnected and many of the mothers had moved. We were eventually able to connect with 20 of the 24 mothers through neighborhood networks and by contacting the mothers of our interview mothers. In our initial interviews, mothers not only provided their own contact information, but gave us the telephone number for a member of their extended network, which always turned out to be their mother. Several of the mothers told us that they had been evicted from their previous living arrangement, or had had a fire in their apartment, or needed to move in with another adult for more support. However, not all of the stories were ones of sadness and dismay; a few mothers had married during the year and were living in new homes.

Of the 20 mothers in our year 2 interviews, half were employed at the time of the second interview. The average length of employment was 11 months, and they were working 25 hours per week at an average of $8.00 per hour. Three mothers had continued in their same jobs from the previous year. The other mothers had switched jobs for more flexibility in their schedules and increased pay. However, the average pay increase for the group was only 12 cents per hour. Compared to the employment benefits of first-year working mothers, of the 10 employed mothers in year 2, half had vacation time and life insurance; two mothers had health insurance benefits; and three mothers had tuition assistance. Half of the mothers said they did not see any opportunities for advancement in their current jobs. More than half of the mothers believed that they would be able to keep their jobs only if they had family and/or friend support for their child (helping with keeping him or her ready for school; after school care). The major threat to sustained employment for all the mothers was the precarious nature of their children's health. Of the 10 mothers who were not employed at the time of the second interview, 9 of them said they had been exempted from employment by their caseworkers because of their child's needs or their own disability. Nevertheless, six of the exempted mothers said they were actively seeking employment.

Regardless of their employment status, a recurring theme among all mothers was their feeling of vulnerability within an unpredictable system. Many added that often their caseworkers contributed to their feelings of shame about needing government assistance. One mother said, "The workers talk to you like you are crazy. You are controlled in terms of what you can and can't have, and I feel like...hopeless, like lying in the house and doing nothing. It's a pain...degrading, my caseworker makes me feel like scum of the earth. They sometimes put people in categories of being lazy. Welfare is a stigma; helpful, but demeaning. I went there to get on my feet, and a worker who is there to help can also hurt you. They (the system) is good, the worker is bad."

Whether the mothers were employed or not, the prevalence of poverty for these families remained very high, as illustrated in Figure 18–1. Nonworking mothers fell, on average, 23 percent below the poverty line. All part-time employed mothers fell below the poverty line. Only the full-time employed mothers were minimally above the poverty line, yet well within the range for various government supports. Nineteen out of twenty mothers depended on their monthly income from Supplemental Security (SSI) to make ends meet. Additionally, more than half of the mothers used food stamps and cash assistance. In terms of other governmental supports, all mothers relied on Medicaid to take care of their child's medical expenses. Table 18–3 presents a breakdown of monthly income supports, the average amount of those supports, and the number of mothers who received them.

A year into welfare reform, we were curious how these mothers were progressing toward self-sufficiency. We wondered if the rhetoric about welfare reform's ability to improve self-images and self-determination was true for this population. Therefore, in the second interview, we asked the mothers a series of questions related to their well-being. Not sur-

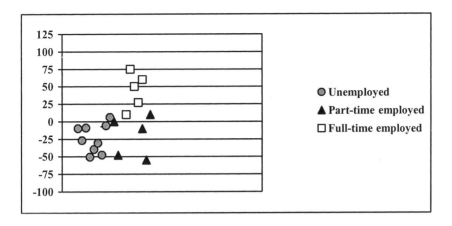

Figure 18–1 *Prevalence of poverty.*

prisingly, mothers who were employed felt better about themselves and their families than those who remained unemployed. Seventy percent of employed mothers said they felt emotionally healthy, as compared to 40 percent of unemployed mothers. Eighty percent also felt that their children had a positive emotional affect, as compared to 60 percent for the unemployed mothers. Mothers,

however, were less optimistic about their own personal health, mostly because of the lack of health-care benefits in their jobs.

Whether employed or not, all mothers felt they were in a tenuous position in their lives and that at any moment their fate could change for the worse. For mothers who were employed and had moved out from welfare supports, 6 of 10 felt reasonably confident in

Table 18–3 Monthly income supports (n=20)					
		Minimum	Maximum	M	SD
Monthly Income From	n	($)	($)	($)	($)
Wages	10	80	2083	800	588
Child Support	4	130	365	216	106
Alimony	1	500	500	500	–
Friends	1	100	100	100	–
Family support subsidy	8	222	222	222	0
Supplemental security income	19	206	1012	508	153
Cash assistance	10	174	580	351	152
Food stamps	10	48	294	180	84
Vendored rent	2	150	385	268	166
Vendored lights	4	10	60	37	27
Vendored gas	3	40	90	37	29
Childcare assistance	1	258	258	258	–
M =mean; SD = standard deviation					

their ability to stay off welfare. One mother's situation spoke for the group. She said, "Right now all the puzzle pieces seem to be in place. I have a job, my child's health is stable, my mother is healthy enough to come over in the morning and help dress and feed Jacob so I can get the other kids ready for school, and the city bus has been running on time for a month. But winter is coming, Jacob usually has lots of infections in the winter, my mother's asthma gets so bad she can't come over, and if we have a snowstorm, I'll be walking to work."

We were particularly curious how those mothers who had left welfare were faring in their day-to-day activities. Although the majority of mothers said they had been able to provide basic necessities (e.g., shelter, food, and clothing) for their families in the past year, some mothers did indicate that there had been months when they had to do without light, heat, school clothes, or their own personal hygiene supplies. Seventy-eight percent of these mothers said they have never been able to afford balanced meals for their families since leaving welfare, and 30 percent of them said they worry that food will run out before the end of the month. One out of nine mothers said that food definitely did not last for the entire month. In terms of the quality and variety of the foods that the mothers prepared, the vast majority indicated that they do not always have the kind of food that they want.

Whether employed or not, whether receiving welfare supports or not, and in spite of life's difficulties, all of the mothers with whom we spoke held on to their dreams. In addition to such universal family themes as child health and home ownership, approximately two-thirds of these mothers maintained a dream of some day being able to work again. Further, nearly half of the mothers cited "personal motivation" as an asset which they possessed to assist them to achieve self-sufficiency. More than half of the urban mothers and 20 percent of the rural mothers reported having job skills, training, certification, or a combination of these with which to market themselves.

Approximately 50 percent of the mothers indicated a desire to obtain additional training in a vocation. Some of the mothers indi-

cated a desire to work at home. One quarter of them indicated a desire to have more education. Specific vocational interests included the computer industry, childcare, or work specifically related to children and disabilities. Mothers felt that their practical education from having to raise their children with disabilities surely must make them attractive to disability employers (e.g., schools, group homes, daycare centers). If they only had the time to apply and such programs had the resources to pay them beyond the government subsidies they were already receiving, they might find employment in such settings. One mother said it best when she said, "Perhaps one day when my child is gone, I will be able to work as an aide in a school for children with disabilities. It will keep him close in my memory. But for now, caring for him is more important than any job. In fact, this is my job and the government is paying me to do it. If the government did not pay me, who would take care of him?"

Snapshots from the Mothers' Perspectives

Mothers who live in poverty and have children with disabilities face multiple struggles and impossible choices every day of their lives. The following snapshots illustrate the existential realities of these mothers. The names of the mothers and their children have been changed to protect their identities.

Julie's and Ruth's stories illustrate how circuitous a mother's life can be when she is living on the edge. Any of life's daily problems has the potential to throw a mother's world into chaos.

Julie's story:

My car was stolen with my child's braces in it, so I was not able to keep a job interview that my caseworker had scheduled for me. And more important than the job interview, my child could not walk and therefore I could not take him to school and had to carry him everywhere. Since my telephone had been cut off the previous month, I had to walk to my mother's house to call my welfare caseworker. I called her as soon as I could to inform her of my situation, and made an appointment to see her. When I arrived for my appointment, I was told I had been cut off from all benefits. I apparently was cut off before I could make the appointment. Without cash assistance, I could not pay for the braces. I didn't have health insurance and the Medicaid office said I was not entitled to a new brace for two years, because my child had just received this one. It's a circle and sometimes I just go round and round, with no relief. Where do you get off this not-so-merry go-round?

Ruth's story:

My lights were about to be shut off and my child needed his breathing machine. I told my caseworker that my lights were about to be turned off and therefore my child would not be able to breathe. My caseworker said the welfare office would take care of it. Things had not been "taken care of" a month later.

Sheila's story illustrates how even an attempt to maintain work is difficult with the challenges posed by her children.

Four months ago my kitchen caught fire, so I had to pack up my three children and move into a hotel. I live in a world of "instants" now, instant oatmeal, instant juice, instant milk, instant everything. There is no place to cook in the hotel. While the kids like to watch the TV in the hotel, the two older boys have ADHD and they fight constantly. The manager told me that if I can't keep them quiet, we will have to move out. Where am I to go? My mother is taking care of my father who has cancer and I can't have noisy boys there. My grandmother helps with my youngest daughter who has physical problems, but she can't keep us all. I go to work when the children are in school, but I get a lot of calls from the school and I end up missing work to go to the school and try to convince them to keep the boys in class. My employer has said if I can't be more consistent, he will have to fill my position. I could be a good worker and he knows this, but I have to take care of my family first. Most days I don't let myself dream of what might be.

Tamar's story illustrates how the system punishes mothers for even the smallest gains.

I have two children with disabilities. Jamie has physical problems. He has had a lot of surgeries and has severe deformities in his limbs. Susan

has ADHD and serious behavior problems. She becomes violent, kicking and biting others, and destroying objects around her. My income consists of a $123 per month stipend that has been decreased from $230 since January. The stipend was reduced because the SSI for my children was increased by $36 a month and I did not inform my welfare caseworker. I was sanctioned for three months, at which time I lost my TANF cash benefit, food stamps, and Medicaid. My church helped me out with food. When I was reinstated, I discovered that my monthly cash assistance was reduced by $50 per month and my food stamps had been cut. Then my stipend was again reduced because I got behind in my utility payments and I was sanctioned for that. My utilities were eventually cut off, and welfare put me on vendored payments. My rent is also vendored and has not been paid in full for three months, so now my landlord wants back rent. Every day I fear an eviction notice is coming.

Becky's story illustrates how the birth of her child with a disability sent her on a downward spiral, without supports.

I was on the same road as all my girlfriends. I went to college for two years. That is where I met my husband. I became pregnant and we decided to marry. I left school to get a job and have my baby. Everything went fine with her and I continued to work part-time after a few months. We were both working and doing ok. In less than a year I became pregnant again. There were lots of complications and I had to quit my job. My husband got laid off shortly after that and then the tensions started. The baby was born and there were lots of problems, physical deformities and surgeries. I also had complications and had to stay in the hospital. The bills kept coming. After the baby came home, he just wasn't the same towards me. Seems like he blamed everyone and he just couldn't get used to looking at the baby with his deformities, so he left. Now, I have two kids, no job, health problems, constant trips to the doctor, no health insurance, bills due. I had to get help and I turned to welfare. Life just seemed to take a downward turn and I'm looking for a sign that things will turn around.

✍ Dreaming of Self-sufficiency

When we asked these mothers about their dreams and what they needed to achieve self-sufficiency, they had ready answers (LeRoy & Johnson, 2000, 2002). They obviously had spent some time thinking about the future and how they might make it brighter for themselves and their families. Clearly, in their minds, welfare was a temporary support system and one they wished to leave behind as soon as possible. However, they were also clear that putting their children in emotional or physical jeopardy was not an option. They were willing to sustain personal hardship and social marginalization to ensure that their children were receiving the best care and treatment that they could provide.

With regard to their personal dreams and hopes, the majority of mothers said that they would like to be working again. Closely related to that wish, they wished that their children with disabilities would be in better health soon. These two wishes are integrally related, in that mothers felt that they could not work without their children being well. One quarter of the mothers wished they had more education because that would lead to better jobs and therefore more options for their families. One-third of the mothers said that a distant dream for them was to own their own homes. They spoke of wanting to be sure that their children would always have a place to live, even if something happened to them. Although only 15 percent of the mothers directly stated that moving off welfare was a dream, they all implied that that would happen if their other wishes fell into place.

In asking mothers what was needed for them to achieve these dreams, nearly half of them said some personal motivation. These mothers are tired and find it difficult to just make it through the day. They are isolated from other mothers and other adults who are working. They do not have an opportunity to hear positive life stories, to receive encouragement to create a life outside of their house and childcare realities. As one mother said, "It is just too hard to take all the steps needed to work. I can't even make a call." More than half of the mothers said that they need to have more training, a certificate, or a college degree. Under welfare reform, education and training are no longer options that caseworkers can authorize, leaving these mothers in a futile trap of unskilled jobs, low pay, no benefits, and no exit.

✍ Conclusion

The national and the State of Michigan research on mothers, their children with disabilities, and welfare reform is beginning to shed a light on the economic and social discrimination that is inherent in their lives. These mothers live in multiple circles of jeopardy, teetering on the edge or falling through their precarious safety nets at any moment. We have documented how state and federal policies and low-wage employment contribute to these mothers' desperate circumstances. They are persistently punished and blamed for simply being the victims of the multitude of their circumstances that are beyond their control: being poor, being minority women, and having given birth to a child with disabilities. If they have "two cents to rub together," the government takes away four cents; if they receive government subsidies, their employers don't provide any benefits.

And yet, faced with these seemingly insurmountable obstacles, these women demonstrate remarkable resilience in support of their children. They find a way to make it through each day and to ensure that their children do not suffer any unnecessary hardships. They piece together their informal networks, relying on their own mothers and neighbors; they work at times when it is least stressful for their families; and they provide the therapies and tutorials that their children need to maintain their health and learning. Most of all, they try to keep a positive outlook, often holding up their children with disabilities as their rays of hope and light in the face of their economic and social plight.

This study was designed to research a day in the life of these women, to open the invisible door to a house to which few policymakers hold a key. Serious attention needs to be paid to the voices and perspectives of these mothers. They have an intuitive sense of the issues with which policy makers must struggle. They are the system's outliers, the canaries in the gold mine of welfare reform. If the system can make a positive change in the lives of poor mothers who have children with disabilities, it can contribute positively to the lives of all its recipients. Several critical questions emerge from this research and are briefly presented below.

- The mothers in this study clearly demonstrate that independence is not a desired or practical reality for them. Rather, they seek a life of interdependence, in which they have a formal and informal network of supports to help them foster a self-actualized family.
- There is no cookie-cutter solution for this population. Rather, each mother needs a family-centered plan that recognizes her unique circumstances and matches her needs with community and personal resources. Making a system that is both dynamic and controlled by the user of the system is a bureaucratic conundrum.
- All of our research has shown that these mothers, like the majority of adults, desire employment. Employment is not just about making money; it is also a social support system and a significant contributor to one's self-esteem. The mothers in our study who worked, regardless of their low pay and lack of benefits, felt good about themselves and their contributions to their family well-being. The challenge for the system is to figure out how employment can be structured to accommodate the unique needs of these families, to financially support them, and to create a viable path out of hardship for them. Clearly, a work policy that keeps families poor creates a perpetual poverty trap for families who have children with disabilities.
- If these mothers are truly the canaries in the gold mine of welfare reform, then the system needs to seriously consider their challenges if it is honestly interested in moving their families toward self-sufficiency. Resilience cannot be a substitute

for government supports or a badge that negates the need for government action on behalf of these mothers.

Discussion Questions ✒

- Is self-sufficiency a feasible goal for the mothers described in this chapter?
- What would a viable and functional service and support system include for mothers who have children with disabilities?
- Is employment a viable option for mothers who have children with challenging needs? How could employment be structured?
- How should the next phase of welfare reform be structured to better support mothers in similar circumstances to those described in this chapter?

References

Danziger, S., Corcoran, M., Danziger, S., Heflin, C., Kalil, A., Levine, J., Rosen, D., Seefeldt, K., Siefert, K., & Tolman, R. (1998). *Barriers to the employment of welfare recipients.* Ann Arbor: Poverty Research and Training Center, the University of Michigan.

Heymann, S. J., & Earle, A. (1999). The impact of welfare reform on parents' ability to care for their children's health. *American Journal of Public Health, 89*(4), 502-505.

Lee, S., Sills, M., & Oh, G. (2002). *Disabilities among children and mothers in low income families.* Syracuse: Institute for Women's Policy Research, Syracuse University.

LeRoy, B., & Johnson, D. (2000). *The perceptions of welfare reform by Michigan families whose children have disabilities and welfare caseworkers.* Detroit: Wayne State University, Developmental Disabilities Institute.

LeRoy, B., & Johnson, D. (2002). Open road or blind alley? Welfare reform, mothers and children with disabilities. *Journal of Family Economics* Issues, *23*(4), 323–337.

Loprest, P. & Zedlewski, S. (1999). *Current and former welfare recipients: How do they differ?* Washington, D. C.: The Urban Institute.

Meyers, M. K., Brady, H. E., & Seto, E. Y. (2000). *Expensive children in poor families: The intersection of childhood disabilities and welfare.* San Francisco: Public Policy Institute of California.

Meyers, M. K., Lukemeyer, A., & Smeeding, T. (1998). The cost of caring: Public and private costs childhood disabilities in poor families. *Social Science Review, 72*(1), 209–233.

Michigan Department of Education (2001). *Michigan special education student database.* Lansing, MI: Office of Special Education.

Michigan League for Human Services (April 1998).

Economic Self-Sufficiency: A Michigan Benchmark. Lansing: Author.

National Council on Disability. (1997). *National disability policy: A progress report.* Washington, DC: Author.

Reischi, T. M. (1998). *Recent studies of AFDC recipients estimate need for specialized childcare.* Durham, NH: Institute on Disability, University of New Hampshire.

Sweeney, E. (2002). *Update on what we know about people with disabilities and TANF.* Washington, DC: The Urban Institute.

Sweeney, E. (2001). *Preserving the safety net: Maintaining services for those with barriers to work.* Washington, DC: The Urban Institute.

Sweeney, E. (2000). *Recent studies indicate that many parents who are current or former welfare recipients have disabilities or other medical conditions.* Washington, D.C.: The Urban Institute.

United States Department of Education (2000). *Twenty-second annual report to Congress on the implementation of Individuals with Disabilities Education Act.* Washington, DC: Author.

United States Department of Health and Human Services. (August 1999). *Temporary Assistance for Needy Families (TANF) Program: Second Annual Report to Congress.* Washington, DC: Author.

Urban Institute (1998). *Welfare policy and research report.* Washington, DC: Author.

Additional Readings

Cancian, M., & Meyer, D. R. (2000). Work after welfare Women work efforts, occupations, and economic well-being. *National Association of Social Workers, Inc., 24*(2), 69–86.

Coll, C. G., Surrey, J. L., & Weingarten, K. (Eds.). (1998). *Mothering Against the Odds.* New York: The Guilford Press.

Danziger, S., & Corcoran, M. (2000). *Barriers to the employment of welfare recipients.* Ann Arbor: Poverty Research and Training Center, the University of Michigan.

Danziger, S., Corcoran, M., Danziger, S., & Heflin, C. M. (1999). *Work, income and material hardship after welfare. For better and for worse state welfare reform and the well-being of low-income families and children.* Ann Arbor: Joint Center for Poverty Research, the University of Michigan.

Kingfisher, C. P. (1996). *Women in the American Welfare Trap.* Philadelphia: University of Pennsylvania Press.

Polakow, V., Kahn, P., & Martin, N. (1998). Struggling to survive: The lives of women and children under the new welfare law. *Journal for a Just and Caring Education, 4*(4), 374–392.

Polakow, V. (1993). *Lives on the Edge: Single Mothers and Their Children in the Other America.* Chicago: University of Chicago Press.

Thompson, T. S., Holcomb, P. A., Loprest, P., & Brennan, K. (1998). *State welfare-to-work policies for people with disabilities: Changes since welfare reform.* Washington, DC: The Urban Institute.

Acknowledgments

In addition to the author, the research team on this study included: Dr. Sharonlyn Harrison, Donna Johnson, and Sandra Meyskens. The research was funded by the Administration on Developmental Disabilities, United States Department of Health and Human Services.

Janice Fialka

"ADVICE TO PROFESSIONALS WHO MUST CONFERENCE CASES"

Before the case conference,
I would look at my almost five-year-old son
And see a golden haired boy
Who giggled at his baby sister's attempts to clap her hands.
Who charmed adults by his spontaneous hugs and hellos,
Who captured his parents with his rapture with music and
His care for white-haired people who walked a walk
a bit slower than younger folks.
Who often became a legend in places visited because of his
exquisite ability to befriend a few special souls,
Who often wanted to play "peace marches,"
And who, at the age of four
went to the Detroit Public library
requesting a book on Martin Luther King.

After the case conference
I looked at my almost five-year-old son.
He seemed to have lost his golden hair.
I saw only words plastered on his face.
Words that drowned us in fear and revolting nausea.

Words like:
Primary expressive speech and language disorder
severe visual, motor delay
sensory integration dysfunction
fine and gross motor delay
developmental dyspraxia and RITALIN now.

I want my son back. That's all.
I want him back now. Then I'll get on with my life.

If you could see the depth of this wrenching pain.
If you could see the depth of our sadness
then you would be moved to return
our almost five-year-old son
who sparkles in the sunlight despite his faulty neurons.
Please give me back my son

Undamaged and untouched by your labels, test results,
descriptions and categories.

If you can't, if you truly cannot give us back our son
Then just be with us quietly,
gently and compassionately as we feel.

Sit patiently and attentively as we grieve and feel powerless.
Sit with us and create a stillness
known only in small, empty chapels at sundown.
Be there with us
As our witness and as our friend.

Please do not give us advice, suggestions, comparisons or
another appointment. (That's for later.)
We want only a quiet shoulder upon which to rest our too-heavy
heads.

If you can't give us back our sweet dream
then comfort us through this darkness
Hold us. Rock us until morning light creeps in.
Then we will rise and begin the work of a new day.

Reprinted with permission from Janice Fialka. Published by J. Fialka: "Advice to Professionals Who Must Conference Cases" from her book *It Matters: Lessons from My Son*, 1997, p. 19.

Epilogue

Within the chapters of our book we have presented many facets of mothering occupations. These range from daily interactions and challenges that include the physical care of young children, as mothers engage in bathing, dressing, feeding, and playing with their children, to more complex activities. When children have special and unique needs, such as a physical disability or attention deficit hyperactivity disorder, everyday occupations require careful time management and design of home space. For some mothers, the occupations of caregiving are extended to include advocacy on behalf of others in similar situations, as well as consideration of the welfare of children more generally.

We have also described how we shared our experiences as clinicians, educators, and researchers with mothers who are themselves challenged by mental health conditions, physical disabilities, chronic health conditions, or intellectual limitations. We have highlighted special situations that challenge participation in mothering occupations such as incarceration, poverty, and conflicting demands, as in the case of teenage mothering. We have also acknowledged the special challenges to mothering involved in partnering with professionals and negotiating health care systems. You, the reader, have been introduced to many mothers as individuals whose voices are distinct as they told their personal stories. These have ranged across the life span of mothering, from pregnancy to mothering young adult children. Repeatedly, these mothers have voiced the ways in which they have worked to claim their agency to overcome obstacles in order to participate fully in their mothering and other chosen occupations and to enable their children to do the same. In editing this book, we have added our voices to the emerging discourse on mothering that centralizes the occupations of mothering. We have spoken out for mothers and mothering occupations. Our primary motivation for doing this has been the importance we place on acting on behalf of the many mothers with whom we collectively have worked, who have shared their lives and stories with us, and have not just allowed but encouraged us to share their stories with our professional communities by writing of their experiences. We believe that our mother-focused work is important and needs to be given priority within our communities at all levels, and that it should result in action on behalf of mothering individuals.

We believe that, as professionals, we have societal as well as individual responsibilities, which include advocating for women whose mothering occupations are compromised because of overwhelming health challenges, their own or their children's, or who are even denied the ability to mother because of intellectual limitations, extreme poverty, or incarceration. Therefore we have a wish list for you, our readers. We wish most fervently that you will be inspired to action on behalf of individuals who are mothering. This action can take many forms:

- Advocacy for services for mothering
- Development of services to all mothering persons
- Support for services to all mothering persons
- A commitment to include mothering persons in a collaborative way in your professional research and practice
- A commitment to research that includes a critical examination of the lived experience of mothering persons and their needs
- A commitment to examine the lives and needs of mothering persons who now operate on the margins of our societies and whose needs are being ignored or are not being met

We urge you to reflect on the issues highlighted in this book and to redesign your future practice to include the consideration of the mothering occupations for all individuals who are mothering.

Susan A. Esdaile
Judith A. Olson

Index

An "f" following a page number indicates a figure; a "t" following a page number indicates a table.